GREENMAN'S PRINCIPLES OF MANUAL MEDICINE

Fourth Edition

GREENMAN'S PRINCIPLES OF MANUAL MEDICINE

Fourth Edition

Lisa A. DeStefano, D.O.

Assistant Professor & Chairperson
Department of Osteopathic Manipulative Medicine
College of Osteopathic Medicine
Michigan State University
East Lansing, Michigan

Wolters Kluwer | Lippincott Williams & Wilkins
Health

Philadelphia • Baltimore • New York • London
Buenos Aires • Hong Kong • Sydney • Tokyo

Acquisitions Editor: Charles W. Mitchell
Product Manager: Jennifer Verbiar
Marketing Manager: Christen Melcher
Designer: Stephen Druding
Compositor: SPi Technologies
Printer: C&C Offset

Fourth Edition

Library of Congress Cataloging-in-Publication Data
DeStefano, Lisa A.
    Greenman's principles of manual medicine. — 4th ed. / Lisa A. DeStefano.
        p. ; cm.
    Rev. ed. of: Principles of manual medicine / Philip E. Greenman. 3rd ed. c2003.
    Includes bibliographical references and index.
    ISBN 978-0-7817-8915-8 (alk. paper)
  1. Manipulation (Therapeutics) 2. Medicine, Physical. I. Greenman, Ph. E., 1928– Principles of manual medicine. II. Title. III. Title: Principles of manual medicine.
    [DNLM: 1. Manipulation, Orthopedic. 2. Physical Medicine. WB 460 D476g 2011]
    RM724.G74   2011
    615.8'2—dc22
                                                                    2009035561

DISCLAIMER
Care has been taken to confirm the accuracy of the information present and to describe generally accepted practices. However, the authors, editors, and publisher are not responsible for errors or omissions or for any consequences from application of the information in this book and make no warranty, expressed or implied, with respect to the currency, completeness, or accuracy of the contents of the publication. Application of this information in a particular situation remains the professional responsibility of the practitioner; the clinical treatments described and recommended may not be considered absolute and universal recommendations.

The authors, editors, and publisher have exerted every effort to ensure that drug selection and dosage set forth in this text are in accordance with the current recommendations and practice at the time of publication. However, in view of ongoing research, changes in government regulations, and the constant flow of information relating to drug therapy and drug reactions, the reader is urged to check the package insert for each drug for any change in indications and dosage and for added warnings and precautions. This is particularly important when the recommended agent is a new or infrequently employed drug.

Some drugs and medical devices presented in this publication have Food and Drug Administration (FDA) clearance for limited use in restricted research settings. It is the responsibility of the health care provider to ascertain the FDA status of each drug or device planned for use in their clinical practice.

This book is dedicated to those passionate about advancing the knowledge of neuromusculoskeletal function.

CONTENTS

The first edition of this book was originally designed to support the Continuing Medical Education's courses offered through Michigan State University and its colleges of osteopathic medicine. Since that time, this publication has been used nationally and internationally in a number of colleges of osteopathic medicine, chiropractic colleges, schools of physical therapy, and schools of massage therapy.

As a second year Family Medicine/Neuromusculoskeletal Medicine Resident, I had the privilege to shadow and treat patients with Dr Greenman in his clinic at Michigan State University. It was during these precious moments in his clinic when I began to recognize my role in facilitating one's process toward improved function; this is the goal of the osteopathic manipulative medicine treatment.

The fourth edition of *Greenman's Principles of Manual Medicine* attempts to help the reader look beyond the general application and pursue the "how" and the "why" technique can improve neuromusculoskeletal system function. The basic principles are maintained and substantially referenced thanks in part to two major scientific contributors to our understanding of manual medicine—the *First International Fascia Conference* and *Movement Stability & Low Back Pain: The Essential Role of the Pelvis,* which originated out of two world congresses on low back and pelvic pain.

Lisa A. DeStefano, D.O.

ACKNOWLEDGMENTS

I am greatly indebted to Philip Greenman, D.O., F.A.A.O., for giving me the opportunity to write the fourth edition of *Greenman's Principles of Manual Medicine*. Thank you, Phil; it's a great honor.

Michigan State University College of Osteopathic Medicine has been my home since matriculating in 1988; I would like to thank the staff and faculty, present and past, for their tenacious pursuit of excellence in osteopathic education. I would especially like to acknowledge my colleagues in the Department of Osteopathic Manipulative Medicine, Jennifer Gilmore, Jacob Rowan, Mark Gugel, Sherman Gorbis, William Golden, Vincent Cipolla, William Pintal, and Timothy Francisco; I am very fortunate to have such a great team. I am particularly grateful to our Dean William Stampel, D.O.; thank you, Bill, for all your support and leadership.

The Continuing Medical Education Program in Michigan State University College of Osteopathic Medicine has been providing the highest quality manual medicine education in the country for more than 30 years. To be given the opportunity to participate as a faculty member in this program is one of greatest joys in my career. Over the years, I have learned from the very best students, faculty, and staff; to you all, I owe a great deal of gratitude.

My greatest teachers in life have been my parents, Jim and Joanne DeStefano. Thank you for providing me with all the tools necessary to excel while allowing me the freedom to use them in a fashion that is uniquely mine; I admire and love you both so very much. I am especially appreciative to my husband Keith; thank you, my love, for your enduring support and encouragement during this adventure.

PRINCIPLES AND CONCEPTS

STRUCTURAL DIAGNOSIS AND MANIPULATIVE MEDICINE HISTORY

HISTORY

Manual medicine is as old as the science and art of medicine itself. There is strong evidence of the use of manual medicine procedures in ancient Thailand, as shown in statuary at least 4,000 years old.[1] The ancient Egyptians practiced the use of the hands in the treatment of injury and disease. Even Hippocrates, the father of modern medicine, was known to use manual medicine procedures, particularly traction and leverage techniques, in the treatment of spinal deformity. The writings of such notable historical figures in medicine as Galen, Celisies, and Oribasius refer to the use of manipulative procedures.[2] There is a void in the reported use of manual medicine procedures corresponding to the approximate time of the split of physicians and barber-surgeons. As physicians became less involved in patient contact and as direct hands-on patient care became the province of the barber-surgeons, the role of manual medicine in the healing art seems to have declined. This period also represents the time of the plagues, and perhaps physicians were reticent to come in close personal contact with their patients.

The 19th century found a renaissance of interest in this field. Early in the 19th century, Dr Edward Harrison, a 1784 graduate of Edinburgh University, developed a sizable reputation in London utilizing manual medicine procedures. Like many other proponents of manual medicine in the 19th century, he became alienated from his colleagues by his continued use of these procedures.[3]

The 19th century was a popular period for "bonesetters" both in England and in the United States. The work of Mr Hutton, a skilled and famous bonesetter, led such eminent physicians as James Paget and Wharton Hood to report in such prestigious medical journals as the *British Medical Journal* and *Lancet* that the medical community should pay attention to the successes of the unorthodox practitioners of bone setting.[4] In the United States, the Sweet family practiced skilled bone setting in the New England region of Rhode Island and Connecticut. It has also been reported that some of the descendants of the Sweet family emigrated west in the mid-19th century.[5] Sir Herbert Barker was a well-known British bonesetter who practiced well into the first quarter of the 20th century and was of such eminence that he was knighted by the crown.

The 19th century was also a time of turmoil and controversy in medical practice. Medical history of the day was replete with many unorthodox systems of healing. Two individuals who would profoundly influence the field of manual medicine were products of this period of medical turmoil. Andrew Taylor Still, M.D., was a medical physician trained in the preceptor fashion of the day, and Daniel David Palmer was a grocer-turned-self-educated manipulative practitioner.

Osteopathic Medicine

Still (1828–1917) first proposed his philosophy and practice of osteopathy in 1874. His disenchantment with the medical practice of the day led to his formulation of a new medical philosophy, which he termed "osteopathic medicine." He appeared to have been a great synthesizer of medical thought and built his new philosophy on both ancient medical truths and current medical successes, while being most vocal in denouncing what he viewed as poor medical practice, primarily the inappropriate use of medications then in use.[6]

Still's strong position against the drug therapy of his day was not well received by his medical colleagues and was certainly not supported by contemporary osteopathic physicians. However, he was not alone in expressing concern about the abuse of drug therapy. In 1861, Oliver Wendell Holmes said, "If all of the MATERIA MEDICA were thrown into the oceans, it will be all the better for mankind, and worse for the fishes."[7] Sir William Osler, one of Still's contemporaries, stated: "One of the first duties of the physician is to educate the masses not to take medicine. Man has an inborn craving for medicine. Heroic dosing for several generations has given his tissues a thirst for drugs. The desire to take medicine is one feature which distinguishes man, the animal, from his fellow creatures."[8]

Still's new philosophy of medicine in essence consisted of the following:

1. The unity of the body.
2. The healing power of nature. He held that the body had within itself all those things necessary for the maintenance of health and recovery from disease. The role of the physician was to enhance this capacity.
3. The somatic component of disease. He felt that the musculoskeletal system was an integral part of the total body and alterations within the musculoskeletal system affected total body health and the ability of the body to recover from injury and disease.
4. Structure–function interrelationship. The interrelationship of structure and function had been espoused by Virchow early in the 19th century,[9] and Still applied this principle within his concept of total body integration. He strongly felt that structure governed function and that function influenced structure.
5. The use of manipulative therapy. This became an integral part of Still's philosophy because he believed that restoration of the body's maximal functional capacity would enhance the level of wellness and assist in recovery from injury and disease.

It is unclear when and how Dr Still added manipulation to his philosophy of osteopathy. It was not until 1879, some 5 years after his announcement of the development of osteopathy, that he became known as the "lightning bonesetter." There is no recorded history that he met or knew the members of the Sweet family as they migrated west. Still never wrote a book on manipulative technique. His writings were extensive, but they focused on the philosophy, principles, and practice of osteopathy.

Still's attempt to interest his medical colleagues in these concepts was rebuffed, particularly when he took them to Baker University in Kansas. As he became more clinically successful, and nationally and internationally well known, many individuals came to study with him and learn the new science of osteopathy. This led to the establishment in 1892 of the first college of osteopathic medicine at Kirksville, Missouri. In 2009, there are 28 osteopathic training sites (including 3 branch campuses) in the United States graduating more than 3,000 students per year.[10] Osteopathy in other parts of the world, particularly in the United Kingdom and in the commonwealth countries of Australia and New Zealand, is a school of practice limited to structural diagnosis and manipulative therapy, although strongly espousing some of the fundamental concepts and principles of Still. Osteopathic medicine in the United States has been from its inception, and continues to be, a total school of medicine and surgery while retaining the basis of osteopathic principles and concepts and continuing the use of structural diagnosis and manipulative therapy in total patient care.

Chiropractic

Palmer (1845–1913) was, like Still, a product of the midwestern portion of the United States in the mid-19th century. Although not schooled in medicine, he was known to practice as a magnetic healer and became a self-educated manipulative therapist. Controversy continues as to whether Palmer was ever a patient or student of Still's at Kirksville, Missouri, but it is known that Palmer and Still met in Clinton, Iowa, early in the 20th century. Palmer moved about the country a great deal and founded his first college in 1896. The early colleges were at Davenport, Iowa, and at Oklahoma City, Oklahoma.

Although Palmer is given credit for the origin of chiropractic, it was his son Bartlett Joshua Palmer (1881–1961) who gave the chiropractic profession its momentum. Palmer's original concepts were that the cause of disease was a variation in the expression of normal neural function. He believed in the "innate intelligence" of the brain and central nervous system and believed that alterations in the spinal column (subluxations) altered neural function, causing disease. Removal of the subluxation by chiropractic adjustment was viewed to be the treatment. Chiropractic has never professed to be a total school of medicine and does not teach surgery or the use of medication beyond vitamins and simple analgesics. There remains a split within the chiropractic profession between the "straights," who continue to espouse and adhere to the original concepts of Palmer, and the "mixers," who believe in a broadened scope of chiropractic that includes other therapeutic interventions such as exercise, physiotherapy, electrotherapy, diet, and vitamins.

In the mid-1970s, the Council on Chiropractic Education (CCE) petitioned the United States Department of Education for recognition as the accrediting agency for chiropractic education. The CCE was strongly influenced by the colleges with a "mixer" orientation, which led to increased educational requirements both before and during chiropractic education. Chiropractic is practiced throughout the world, but the vast majority of chiropractic training continues to be in the United States. The late 1970s found increased recognition of chiropractic in both Australia and New Zealand, and their registries are participants in the health programs in these countries.[11]

MEDICAL MANIPULATORS

The 20th century has found renewed interest in manual medicine in the traditional medical profession. In the first part of the 20th century, James Mennell and Edgar Cyriax brought joint manipulation recognition within the London medical community. John Mennell continued the work of his father and contributed extensively to the manual medicine literature and its teaching worldwide. As one of the founding members of the North American Academy of Manipulative Medicine (NAAMM), he was instrumental in opening the membership in NAAMM to osteopathic physicians in 1977. He strongly advocated the expanded role of appropriately trained physical therapists to work with the medical profession in providing joint manipulation in patient care.

James Cyriax is well known for his textbooks in the field and also fostered the expanded education and scope of physical therapists. He incorporated manual medicine procedures in the practice of "orthopedic medicine" and founded the Society for Orthopedic Medicine. In his later years, Cyriax came to believe that manipulation restored function to derangements of the intervertebral discs and spoke less and less about specific arthrodial joint effects. He had no use for "osteopaths" or other manipulating groups and the influence of his dynamic personality is being felt long after his death in 1985.

John Bourdillon, a British-trained orthopedic surgeon, was first attracted to manual medicine as a student at Oxford University. During his training, he learned to perform manipulation while the patient was under general anesthesia and subsequently used the same techniques without anesthesia. He observed the successful results of non–medically qualified manipulators and began a study of their techniques. A lifelong student and teacher in the field, he published five editions of a text, *Spinal Manipulation*. Subsequent to his death in 1992, a sixth edition of *Spinal Manipulation* was published with Edward Isaacs, M.D., and Mark Bookhout, M.S., P.T., as coauthors.

The NAAMM merged with the American Association of Orthopaedic Medicine in 1992 and continues to represent the United States in the International Federation of Manual Medicine (FIMM).

PRACTICE OF MANUAL MEDICINE

Manual medicine should not be viewed in isolation nor separate from "regular medicine" and clearly is not the panacea for all ills of humans. Manual medicine considers the functional capacity of the human organism, and its practitioners are as interested in the dynamic processes of disease as those who look at the disease process from the static perspective of laboratory data, tissue pathology, and the results of autopsy. Manual medicine focuses on the musculoskeletal system, which comprises more than 60% of the human organism, and through which evaluation of the other organ systems must be made. Structural diagnosis not only evaluates the musculoskeletal system for its particular diseases and dysfunctions, but can also be used to evaluate the somatic manifestations of disease and derangement of the internal viscera. Manipulative procedures are used primarily to increase mobility in restricted areas of musculoskeletal function and to reduce pain. Some practitioners focus on the concept of pain relief, whereas others are more interested in the influence of increased mobility in restricted areas of the musculoskeletal system. When appropriately used, manipulative procedures can be clinically effective in reducing pain within the musculoskeletal system, in increasing the level of wellness of the patient, and in helping patients with a myriad of disease processes.

GOAL OF MANIPULATION

In 1983, in Fischingen, Sweden, a 6-day workshop was held that included approximately 35 experts in manual medicine from throughout the world. They represented many different countries and schools of manual medicine with considerable diversity in clinical experience. The proceedings of this workshop represented the state of the art of manual medicine of the day.[12] That workshop reached a consensus on the goal of manipulation: The goal of manipulation is to restore maximal, painfree movement of the musculoskeletal system in postural balance.

This definition is comprehensive but specific and is well worth consideration by all students in the field.

ROLE OF THE MUSCULOSKELETAL SYSTEM IN HEALTH AND DISEASE

It is indeed unfortunate that much of the medical thinking and teaching look at the musculoskeletal system only as the coat rack on which the other organ systems are held and not as an organ system that is susceptible to its own unique injuries and disease processes. The field of manual medicine looks at the musculoskeletal system in a much broader context, particularly as an integral and interrelated part of the total human organism. Although most physicians would accept the concept of integration of the total body including the musculoskeletal system, specific and usable concepts of how that integration occurs and its relationship in structural diagnosis and manipulative therapy seem to be limited.

There are five basic concepts that this author has found useful. Since the hand is an integral part of the practice of manual medicine and includes five digits, it is easy to recall one concept for each digit in the palpating hand. These concepts are as follows:

1. Holism;
2. Neurologic control;
3. Circulatory function;
4. Energy expenditure; and
5. Self-regulation.

Concept of Holism

The concept of holism has different meanings and usage by different practitioners. In manual medicine, the concept emphasizes that the musculoskeletal system deserves thoughtful and complete evaluation, wherever and whenever the patient is seen, regardless of the nature of the presenting complaint. It is just as inappropriate to avoid evaluating the cardiovascular system in a patient presenting with a primary musculoskeletal complaint as it is to avoid evaluation of the musculoskeletal system in a patient presenting with acute chest pain thought to be cardiac in origin. The concept is one of a sick patient who needs to be evaluated. The musculoskeletal system constitutes most of the human body and alterations within it influence the rest of the human organism; diseases within the internal organs manifest themselves in alterations in the musculoskeletal system, frequently in the form of pain. It is indeed fortunate that holistic concepts have gained increasing popularity in the medical community recently, but the concept expressed here is one that speaks of the integration of the total human organism rather than a summation of parts. We must all remember that our role as health professionals is to treat patients and not to treat disease.

Concept of Neural Control

The concept of neurologic control is based on the fact that humans have the most highly developed and sophisticated nervous system in the animal kingdom. All functions of the body are under some form of control by the nervous system. A patient is constantly responding to stimuli from the internal and external body environments through complex mechanisms within the central and peripheral nervous systems. As freshmen in medical school, we all studied the anatomy and physiology of the nervous system. Let us briefly review a segment of the spinal cord (Fig. 1.1). On the left side are depicted the classic somatosomatic reflex pathways with afferent impulses coming from the skin, muscle, joint, and tendon. Afferent stimuli from the nociceptors, mechanoreceptors, and proprioceptors all feed in through the dorsal root and ultimately synapse, either directly or through a series of interneurons, with an anterior horn cell from which an efferent fiber extends to the skeletal muscle. It is through multiple permutations of the central reflex arc that we respond to external stimuli, including injury, orient our bodies in space, and accomplish many of the physical activities of daily living. The right-hand side of the figure represents the classical viscero-visceral reflex arc wherein the afferents from the visceral sensory system synapse, in the intermediolateral cell column, with the sympathetic lateral chain ganglion or collateral ganglia which then terminate onto a postganglionic motor fiber to the target end organ viscera. Note that the skin viscera also receive efferent stimulation from the lateral chain ganglion.

These sympathetic reflex pathways innervate the pilomotor activity of the skin, the vasomotor tone of the vascular tree, and the secretomotor activity of the sweat glands. Alteration in the sympathetic nervous system activity to the skin viscera results in palpatory changes that are identifiable by the structural diagnostic means.[13] Although this figure separates these two pathways,

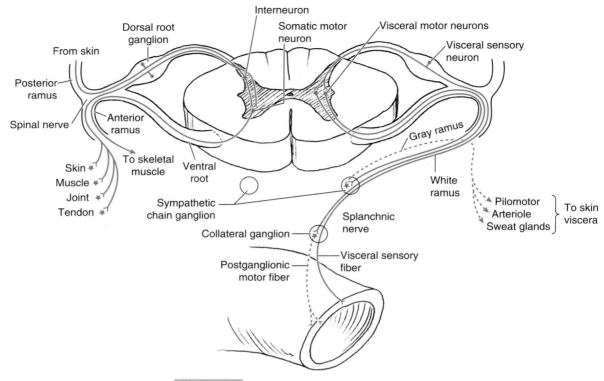

FIGURE 1.1   **Cross section of spinal cord segment.**

they are in fact interrelated so somatic afferents influence visceral efferents and visceral afferents can manifest themselves in somatic efferents. This figure represents the spinal cord in horizontal section and it must be recalled that ascending and descending pathways—from spinal cord segment to spinal cord segment, as well as from the higher centers of the brain—are occurring as well.

Another neurologic concept worth recalling is that of the autonomic nervous system (ANS). The ANS is made up of two divisions, the parasympathetic and sympathetic. The parasympathetic division includes cranial nerves III, VII, VIII, IX, and X and the S2, S3, and S4 levels of the spinal cord. The largest and most extensive nerve of the parasympathetic division is the vagus. The vagus innervates all of the viscera from the root of the neck to the midportion of the descending colon and all glands and smooth muscle of these organs. The vagus nerve (Fig. 1.2) is the primary driving force of the cardiovascular, pulmonary, neuroimmune, endocrine, and gastrointestinal systems[14] and has an extensive distribution. Many pharmaceutical agents alter parasympathetic nervous activity, particularly that of the vagus.

The sympathetic division of the ANS (Fig. 1.3) is represented by preganglionic neurons originating in the spinal cord from T1 to L3 and the lateral chain ganglion including the superior, middle, and inferior cervical ganglia; the thoracolumbar ganglia from T1 to L3; and the collateral ganglia. Sympathetic fibers innervate all of the internal viscera as does the parasympathetic division but are organized differently. The sympathetic division is organized segmentally. It is interesting to note that all of the viscera above the diaphragm receive their sympathetic innervation from preganglionic fibers above T4 and T5, and all of the viscera below the diaphragm receive their sympathetic innervation preganglionic fibers from below T5. It is through this segmental organization that the relationships of certain parts of the musculoskeletal system and certain internal viscera are correlated. Remember that the musculoskeletal system receives only sympathetic division innervation and receives no parasympathetic innervation. Control of all glandular and vascular activity in the musculoskeletal system is mediated through the sympathetic division of the ANS.

Remember that all these reflex mechanisms are constantly under the local and central modifying control of excitation and inhibition. Conscious and subconscious control mechanisms from the brain constantly modify activity throughout the nervous system, responding to stimuli. The nervous system is intimately related to another control system, the endocrine system, and it is useful to think in terms of neuroendocrine control. Recent advances in the knowledge of neurotransmitters, endorphins, enkephalins, and materials such as substance P have enlightened us as to the detail of many of the mechanisms previously not understood and have begun to provide answers for some of the mechanisms through which biomechanical alteration of the musculoskeletal system can alter bodily function.[15]

Emphasis has been placed on the reflex and neural transmission activities of the nervous system, but the nervous system has a powerful trophic function as well. Highly complex protein

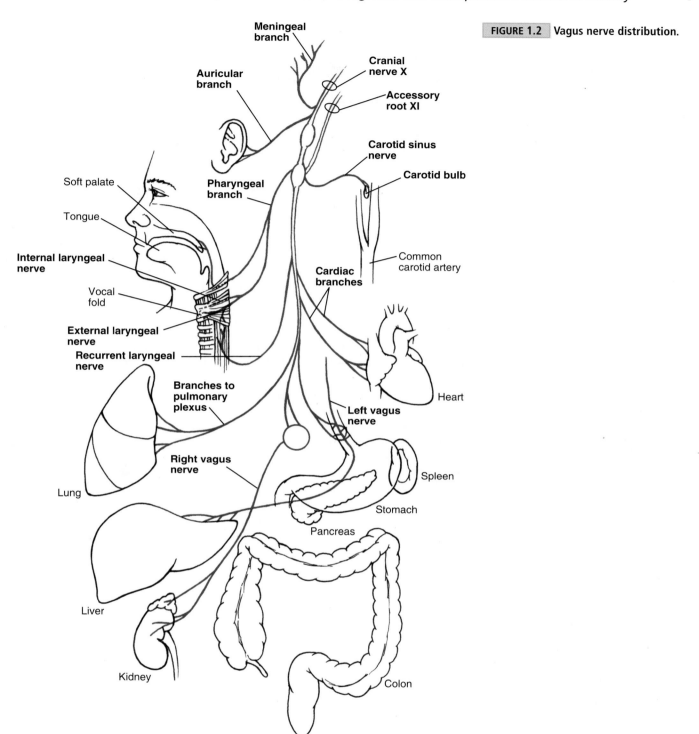

FIGURE 1.2 Vagus nerve distribution.

and lipid substances are transported antegrade and retrograde along neurons and cross over the synapse of the neuron to the target end organ.[16] Alteration in neurotrophin transmission can be detrimental to the health of the target end organ.[17,18]

Circulatory Function

The third concept is that of circulatory function. The concept can be simply described as the maintenance of an appropriate cellular milieu for each cell of the body (Fig. 1.4). Picture a cell, a group of cells making up a tissue, or a group of tissues making up an organ resting in the middle of the "cellular milieu." The cell is dependent for its function, whatever its function is, upon the delivery of oxygen, glucose, and all other substances necessary for its metabolism being supplied by the arterial side of the circulation. The arterial system has a powerful pump, the myocardium of the heart, to propel blood forward. Cardiac pumping

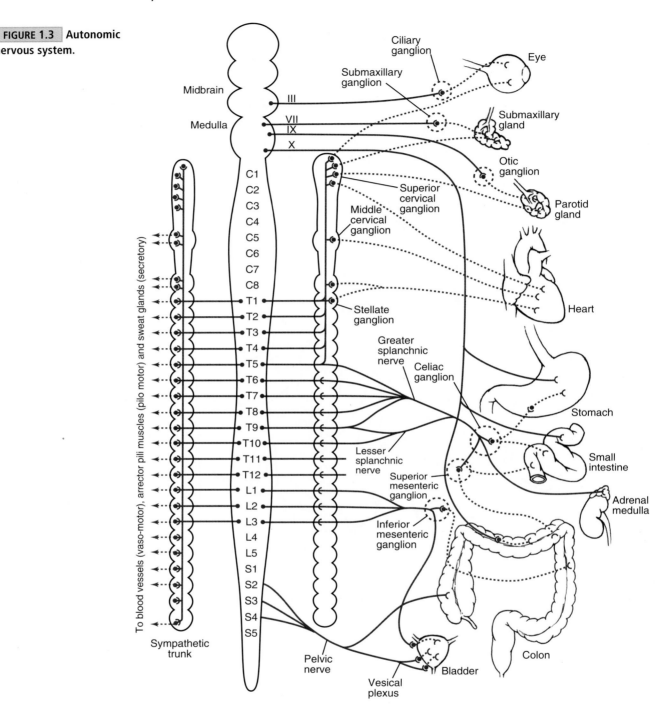

FIGURE 1.3 Autonomic nervous system.

function is intimately controlled by the central nervous system, particularly the ANS, through the cardiac plexus. The vascular tree receives its vasomotor tone control through the sympathetic division of the ANS. Anything that interferes with sympathetic ANS outflow, segmentally mediated, can influence vasomotor tone to a target end organ.[19]

The arteries are also encased in the fascial compartments of the body and are subject to compressive and torsional stress that can interfere with the delivery of arterial blood flow to the target

organ or cell. Once the cell has received its nutrients and proceeded through its normal metabolism, the end products must be removed. The low-pressure circulatory systems, the venous and the lymphatic systems, are responsible for the transport of metabolic waste products. Both the venous and lymphatic systems are much thinner walled than the arteries, and they lack the driving force of the pumping action of the heart, depending instead on the musculoskeletal system for their propelling action.[20] The large muscles of the extremities contribute greatly

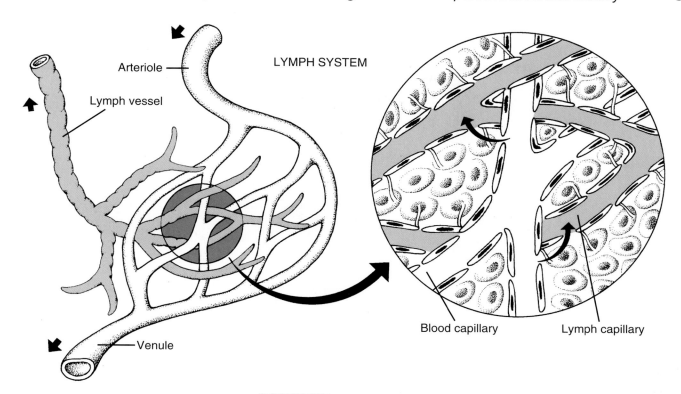

FIGURE 1.4 The cellular milieu.

to this activity, but the major pump of the low-pressure systems is the diaphragm (Fig. 1.5a,b).

The diaphragm has an extensive attachment to the musculoskeletal system, including the upper lumbar vertebra, the lower six ribs, the xiphoid process of the sternum, and, through myofascial connections with the lower extremities, the psoas and quadratus lumborum muscles. The activity of the diaphragm modulates the negative intrathoracic pressure that provides a sucking action on venous and lymphatic return through the vena cava and the cisterna chyli. Because of the extensive attachment of the diaphragm with the musculoskeletal system and its innervation via the phrenic nerve from the cervical spine, alterations in the musculoskeletal system at a number of levels can alter diaphragmatic function and, consequently, venous and lymphatic return. Accumulation of metabolic end products in the cellular milieu interferes with the health of the cell and its recovery from disease or injury. It should be pointed out that the foramen for the inferior vena cava is at the apex of the dome of the diaphragm. There is some evidence that diaphragmatic excursion has a direct squeezing and propelling activity on the inferior vena cava.[21]

Another circulatory concept related to musculoskeletal function concerns the lymphatic system (Fig. 1.6) and the location where it empties into the venous system. The lymph from the right side of the head, right side of the neck, and right upper extremity enters into the right subclavian vein at the thoracic inlet just behind the anterior end of the first rib and the medial end of the clavicle. The lymph from the rest of the body empties into the left subclavian vein at the thoracic inlet behind the anterior extremity of the left first rib and the medial end of the left clavicle. Alteration in the biomechanics of the thoracic inlet, particularly its fascial continuity, can affect the thin-walled lymph vessels as they empty into the venous system. Maximal function of the musculoskeletal system is an important factor in the efficiency of the circulatory system and the maintenance of a normal cellular milieu throughout the body.

Energy Expenditure

The fourth concept is that of energy expenditure primarily through the musculoskeletal system. The musculoskeletal system not only constitutes more than 60% of the human organism but also is the major expender of body energy. Any increase in activity of the musculoskeletal system calls on the internal viscera to develop and deliver energy to sustain that physical activity. The greater the activity of the musculoskeletal system, the greater is the demand. If dysfunction alters the efficiency of the musculoskeletal system, there is an increase in demand for energy, not only for increased activity, but for normal activity as well. If we have a patient with compromised cardiovascular and pulmonary systems who has chronic congestive heart failure, any increase in demand for energy delivery to the musculoskeletal system can be detrimental. For example, a well-compensated chronic congestive heart failure patient who happens to sprain an ankle and attempts to continue normal activity might well have a rapid deterioration of the compensation because of the increased energy demand by the altered gait of the sprained ankle. Obviously, it would make more sense to treat the altered musculoskeletal system by attending to the ankle sprain than to

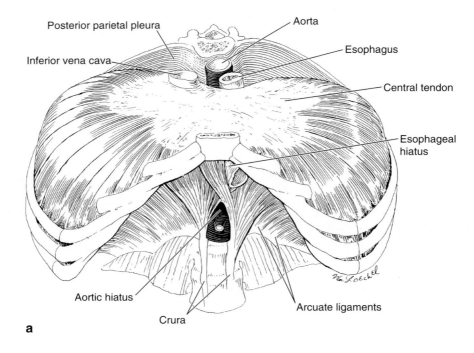

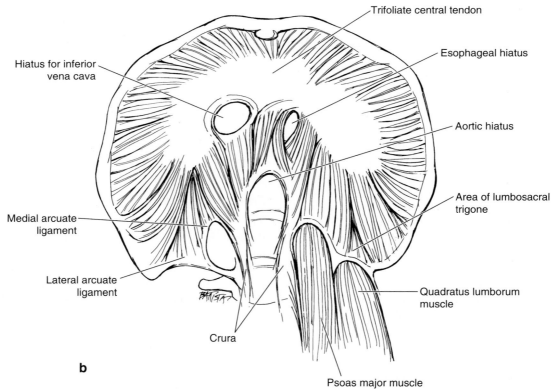

FIGURE 1.5   a,b: Thoracoabdominal diaphragm.

increase the dosage of medications controlling the congestive heart failure. Restriction of one major joint in a lower extremity can increase the energy expenditure of normal walking by as much as 40%[22] and if two major joints are restricted in the same extremity, it can increase by as much as 300%.[23] Multiple minor restrictions of movement of the musculoskeletal system, particularly in the maintenance of normal gait, can also have a detrimental effect on total body function.

Self-Regulation

The fifth concept is that of self-regulation. There are literally thousands of self-regulating mechanisms operative within the

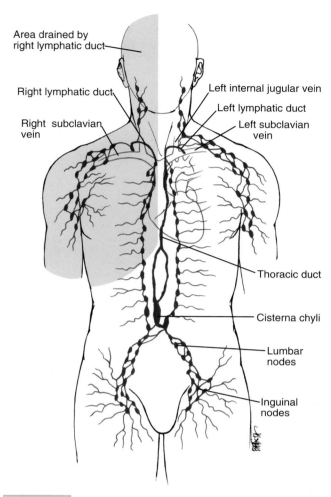

Area drained by
right lymphatic duct

Right lymphatic duct

Right subclavian
vein

Left internal jugular vein

Left lymphatic duct

Left subclavian
vein

Thoracic duct

Cisterna chyli

Lumbar
nodes

Inguinal
nodes

FIGURE 1.6   **Lymphatic system.**

THE MANIPULABLE LESION

Manual medicine deals with the identification of the manipulable lesion and the appropriate use of a manual medicine procedure to resolve the condition. The field of manual medicine has suffered from multiple, divergent, and sometimes confusing definitions of the entity amenable to manipulative intervention. It has been called the "osteopathic lesion," "chiropractic subluxation," "joint blockage," "loss of joint play," "joint dysfunction," and other names. The acceptable term for this entity is somatic dysfunction. It is defined as impaired or altered function of related components of the somatic (body framework) system; skeletal, arthrodial, and myofascial structures; and related vascular, lymphatic, and neural elements.[25] Notice that the emphasis is on altered function of the musculoskeletal system and not on a disease state or pain syndrome. Obviously, if a somatic dysfunction is present that alters vascular, lymphatic, and neural functions, a myriad of symptoms might well be present, including painful conditions and disease entities. The diagnosis of somatic dysfunction can accompany many other diagnoses or can be present as an independent entity. The art of structural diagnosis is to define the presence of somatic dysfunction(s) and determine any significance to the patient's complaint or disease process presenting at the time. If significant, it should be treated by manual medicine intervention just as other diagnostic findings might also need appropriate treatment.

DIAGNOSTIC TRIAD FOR SOMATIC DYSFUNCTION

The mnemonic **ART** can express the diagnostic criteria for identification of somatic dysfunction.

"**A**" stands for asymmetry of related parts of the musculoskeletal system, either structural or functional.

Examples are altered shoulder height, height of the iliac crest, and contour and function of the thoracic cage, usually identified by palpation and observation.

"**R**" stands for range of motion of a joint, several joints, or region of the musculoskeletal system.

The range of motion could be abnormal by being either increased (hypermobility) or restricted (hypomobility). The usual finding in somatic dysfunction is restricted mobility, identified by observation and palpation using both active and passive patient cooperation.

"**T**" stands for tissue texture abnormality of the soft tissues of the musculoskeletal system (skin, fascia, muscle, ligament, etc.).

Tissue texture abnormalities are identified by observation and a number of different palpatory tests.

Some authors add one of two other letters to this mnemonic, "P" or a second "T." "P" stands for pain associated with other findings, and "T" stands for tenderness on palpation of the area.[26] Tenderness is particularly diagnostic if localized to a ligament. A normal ligament is not tender. A tender ligament is always abnormal. However, both pain and tenderness are subjective findings instead of the objective findings of asymmetry, altered range of motion, and tissue texture abnormality. By the use of these criteria, one attempts to identify the presence of

body at all times. These homeostatic mechanisms are essential for the maintenance of health, and if altered by disease or injury, they need to be restored. All physicians are dependent on these self-regulating mechanisms within the patient for successful treatment. The goal of the physician should be to enhance all of the body's self-regulating mechanisms to assist in the recovery from disease. Physicians should not interfere with self-regulating mechanisms more than absolutely necessary during the treatment process. All things that are done to or placed within the human body alter these mechanisms in some fashion. When any foreign substance is given to a patient, the beneficial and detrimental potentials of the substance must be considered. As modern pharmacology grows with evermore-potent pharmacological effects, we must recognize the potential for iatrogenic disease. Many patients are on multiple medications, particularly in the hospital environment, and the actions and interactions of each must be clearly understood to avoid iatrogenic problems. Only physicians cause iatrogenic disease. Reportedly, the incidence of serious adverse drug reactions in hospitalized patients is 6.7% and is considered one of the top ten leading causes of death in the United States.[24]

somatic dysfunctions, their location, whether they are acute or chronic, and particularly whether they are significant for the state of the patient's wellness or illness at that moment in time. In addition to the diagnostic value, changes in these criteria can be of prognostic value in monitoring the response of the patient, not only to manipulative treatment directed toward the somatic dysfunction, but also to other therapeutic interventions.

SUGGESTED READINGS

Buerger AA, Greenman PE, eds. *Empirical Approaches to the Validation of Spinal Manipulation*. Springfield, IL: Charles C. Thomas Publisher, 1985.

Buerger AA, Tobis JS. *Approaches to the Validation of Manipulative Therapy*. Springfield, IL: Charles C. Thomas Publisher, 1977.

Cyriax J. *Textbook of Orthopedic Medicine*. Vol. 1, 7th Ed. East Sussex, England: Bailliere-Tindall, 1978.

Greenman PE. The osteopathic concept in the second century: Is it still germane to specialty practice? *J Am Osteopath Assoc* 1976;75:589–595.

Greenman PE, ed. *Concepts and Mechanisms of Neuromuscular Functions*. Berlin: Springer-Verlag, 1984.

Greenman PE. Models and mechanisms of osteopathic manipulative medicine. *Osteopath Med News* 1987;4(5):1–20.

Grieve GP. *Common Vertebral Joint Problems*. Edinburgh: Churchill Livingstone, 1981.

Hoag JM, Cole WV, Bradford SG. *Osteopathic Medicine*. New York: McGraw-Hill, 1969.

Maigne R. *Orthopedic Medicine*. Springfield, IL: Charles C. Thomas Publisher, 1972.

Maitland GD: *Vertebral Manipulation*. 4th Ed. Stoneham, MA: Butterworths, 1980.

Mennell JM. *Back Pain*. Boston: Little, Brown and Company, 1960.

Mennell JM. *Joint Pain*. Boston: Little, Brown and Company, 1964.

Northup GW, ed. *Osteopathic Research: Growth and Development*. Chicago, IL: American Osteopathic Association, 1987.

Northup GW, Korr IM, Buzzell KA, et al. *The Physiological Basis of Osteopathic Medicine*. New York: Postgraduate Institute of Osteopathic Medicine and Surgery, 1970.

Page LE. *The Principles of Osteopathy*. Kansas City, MO: American Academy of Osteopathy, 1952.

Paris SA. Spinal Manipulative Therapy. *Clin Orthop* 1983;179:55–61.

Schiotz EH, Cyriax J. *Manipulation Past and Present*. London: William Heinemann Medical Books, 1975.

Schneider W, Dvorak J, Dvorak V, et al. *Manual Medicine: Therapy*. New York: Thieme Medical Publishers, 1988.

Stoddard A. *Manual of Osteopathic Technique*. London: Hutchinson Medical Publications, 1959.

Stoddard A. *Manual of Osteopathic Practice*. New York: Harper & Row, 1969.

Ward RC, ed. *Foundations for Osteopathic Medicine*. Baltimore: Williams & Wilkins, 1997.

Zink JG. Respiratory and circulatory care: The conceptual model. *Osteopath Ann* 1977;5:108–124.

REFERENCES

1. Schiotz EH. Manipulation treatment of the spinal column from the medical-historical viewpoint. *Tidsskr Nor Laegeforn* 1958;78:359–372, 429–438, 946–950, 1003 [NIH Library Translation NIH 75–22C, 23C, 24C, 25C].

2. Lomax E. Manipulative therapy: A historical perspective from ancient times to the modern era. In: Goldstein M, ed. *The Research Status of Spinal Manipulative Therapy*. National Institute of Neurological and Communicative Disorders and Stroke, Monograph No. 15. 1975:11–17.

3. Weiner M-F, Silver JR. Edward Harrison and the treatment of spinal deformities in the nineteenth century. *J R Coll Physicians Edinb* 2008;38: 265–271.

4. Hood W. On so-called "bone setting" its nature and results. *Lancet* 1871;Apr 1:336–338, 373–374, 441–443, 499–501.

5. Joy RJT. The natural bonesetters, with special reference to the Sweet family of Rhode Island. *Bull Hist Med* 1965;28:416–441.

6. Hildreth AG. *The Lengthening Shadow of Dr Andrew Taylor Still*. Macon, MO: Hildreth, 1938.

7. Gevitz N. *The D.O.'s: Osteopathic Medicine in America*. 2nd Ed. Baltimore, MD: Johns Hopkins University Press, 2004.

8. Osler W. *Aequanimitas: With Other Addresses to Medical Students, Nurses and Practitioners of Medicine*. 2nd Ed. Philadelphia, PA: The Blakiston Company, 1910.

9. Northup GW. *Osteopathic Medicine: An American Reformation*. 2nd Ed. Chicago, IL: American Osteopathic Association, 1979.

10. The American Association of Colleges of Osteopathic Medicine. 2009 College Information Book for the Entering Class 2009. http://www.aacom.org/resources/bookstore/cib/Pages/default.aspx

11. Haldeman S. *Modern Developments in the Principles and Practice of Chiropractic*. East Norwalk, CT: Appleton-Century-Crofts, 1980.

12. Dvorak J, Dvorak V, Schneider W, eds. *Manual Medicine 1984*. Heidelberg: Springer-Verlag, 1985.

13. Korr IM, ed. *The Neurobiologic Mechanisms in Manipulative Therapy*. New York: Plenum Publishing, 1978.

14. Verberne AJM, Saita M, Sartor DM. Chemical stimulation of vagal afferent neurons and sympathetic vasomotor tone. *Brain Res Rev* 2003;41:288–305.

15. Konttinen Y, Tiainen V-M, Gomez-Barrena E, et al. Innervation of the joint and role of neuropeptides. *Ann N Y Acad Sci* 2006;1069:149–154.

16. Altar CA, DiStefano PS. Neurotrophin trafficking by anterograde transport. *Trends Neurosci* 1998;21(10):433–437.

17. Hagberg H, Mallerd C. Effect of inflammation on central nervous system development and vulnerability. *Curr Opin Neurol* 2005;18(2):117–123.

18. Aller M-A, Arias J-L, Sánchez-Patán F, et al. The inflammatory response: An efficient way of life. *Med Sci Monit* 2006;12(10):RA225–RA234.

19. Tsuru H, Tanimitsu N, Hirai T. Role of perivascular sympathetic nerves and regional differences in the features of sympathetic innervation of the vascular system. *Jpn J Pharmacol* 2002;88:9–13.

20. Gashev AA. Physiologic aspects of lymphatic contractile function: Current perspectives. *Ann N Y Acad Sci* 2002;979:178–187.

21. Takata M, Robotham J. Effects of inspiratory diaphragmatic descent on inferior vena caval venous return. *J Appl Physiol* 1992;72(2):597–607.

22. Waters RL, Perry J, Conaty P, et al. The energy cost of walking with arthritis of the hip and knee. *Clin Orthop Relat Res* 1987;214:278–284.

23. Buzzell KA. The cost of human posture and locomotion. In: Northup GW, Korr IM, Buzzell KA, et al., eds. *The Physiological Basis of Osteopathic Medicine*. New York: Postgraduate Institute of Osteopathic Medicine and Surgery, 1970:63–72.

24. Lazarou J, Pomeranz BH, Corey PN. Adverse drug reactions in hospitalized patients. *JAMA* 1998;279(15):1200–1205.

25. Commission on Professional and Hospital Activities. *Hospital Adaptation of the International Classification of Disease*. 2nd Ed. Ann Arbor, MI, 1973.

26. DiGiovanna EL, Schiowitz S. *An Osteopathic Approach to Diagnosis and Treatment*. Philadelphia, PA: JB Lippincott Co., 1991.

2

PRINCIPLES OF STRUCTURAL DIAGNOSIS

Structural diagnosis in manual medicine is directed toward evaluation of the musculoskeletal system with the goal of identification of the presence and significance of somatic dysfunction(s). It is a component part of the physical examination of the total patient. Most of the evaluation of the internal viscera takes place by evaluation of these structures through the musculoskeletal system. Therefore, it is easy to examine the musculoskeletal system while evaluating the internal viscera of the neck, chest, abdomen, and pelvic regions. Structural diagnosis uses the traditional physical diagnostic methods of observation, palpation, percussion, and auscultation. Of these, observation and palpation are the most useful. Structural diagnosis of the musculoskeletal system should never be done in isolation and should always be done within the context of a total history and physical evaluation of the patient. It has been said that 90% of a physician's decision making is from the history and physical examination.

The diagnostic entity sought by structural diagnosis is somatic dysfunction. It is defined as follows:

Somatic dysfunction: impaired or altered function of related components of the somatic (body framework) system; skeletal, arthrodial, and myofascial structures; and related vascular, lymphatic, and neural elements.

The three classical diagnostic criteria for somatic dysfunction can be identified with the mnemonic **ART** as follows:

"**A**" for asymmetry: asymmetry of related parts of the musculoskeletal system either structural or functional. Examples might be the height of each shoulder by observation, height of iliac crest by palpation, and contour and function of the thoracic cage by observation and palpation. Asymmetry is usually discerned by observation and palpation.

"**R**" for range-of-motion abnormality: Alteration in range of motion of a joint, several joints, or region of the musculoskeletal system is sought. The alteration may be either restricted or increased mobility. Restricted motion is the most common component of somatic dysfunction. Range-of-motion abnormality is determined by observation and palpation, using both active and passive patient cooperation.

"**T**" for tissue texture abnormality (TTA): Alteration in the characteristics of the soft tissues of the musculoskeletal system (skin, fascia, muscle, and ligament) is ascertained by observation and palpation. Percussion is also used in identifying areas of altered tissue texture. A large number of descriptors are used in the literature to express the quality of the abnormal feel of the tissue. There are two primary tissue abnormalities that account for palpable changes, namely muscle hypertonicity, secondary to increased alpha motor neuron stimulation, and altered activity of the "skin viscera," the pilomotor, vasomotor,

and secretomotor functions that are under the control of the sympathetic division of the autonomic nervous system.

HAND–EYE COORDINATION

In structural diagnosis, it is important for the physician to maximize the coordinated use of the palpating hands and the observing eyes. When using vision for observation, it is important to know which eye is dominant so that it can be appropriately placed in relation to the patient for accuracy in visual discrimination. Since most structural diagnosis uses hand–eye coordination with the arms extended, it is best to test for the dominant eye at arm's-length distance (Fig. 2.1). The test is as follows:

1. Extend both arms and form a small circle with the thumb and index finger of each hand.
2. With both eyes open, sight through the circle formed by the thumbs and fingers at an object at the other end of the room. Make the circle as small as possible.
3. Without moving your head, close your left eye only. If the object is still seen through the circle, you are right-eye dominant. If the object is no longer seen through the circle, you are left-eye dominant.
4. Repeat the procedure closing the right eye and note the difference.

When looking for symmetry or asymmetry, it is important that the dominant eye be located midway between the two anatomic parts being observed and/or palpated. For example, when palpating each acromial process to identify the level of the shoulders, the dominant eye should be in the mid-sagittal plane of the patient, equidistant from each palpating hand. In other words, the dominant eye should be on the midline of the two anatomic parts being compared. With a patient supine on the examining table, a right-eye–dominant examiner should stand on the right side of the patient and a left-eye–dominant examiner should stand on the left side of the patient. Remember that the hands and eyes should be on the same reference plane when one is attempting to determine if paired anatomic parts are symmetrically placed. For example, when evaluating the height of the shoulders by palpating the two acromial processes and visualizing a level against the horizontal plane, the eyes should be on the same horizontal plane as the palpating hands. When palpating the two iliac crests to identify if they are level against the horizontal plane, the eyes should be at the level of the iliac crests in the same plane as the palpating hands. Whenever possible, the eyes should be in the plane against which anatomic landmarks are being compared for symmetry or asymmetry.

All physicians use palpation in physical examination of the abdomen for masses, normal organs for size and position, point

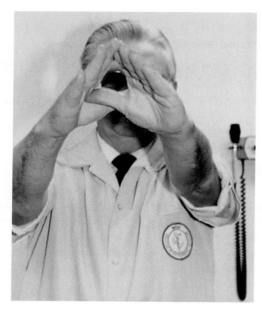

FIGURE 2.1 Test for dominant eye.

of maximum impulse of the heart, tactile fremitus of the lungs, and pulsations of the peripheral vessels. Palpation is also used to identify masses, normal and abnormal lymph nodes, and other changes of the tissues. In structural diagnosis, palpation requires serious consideration and practice to develop high-level diagnostic skills. Palpatory skills affect the following:

1. The ability to detect TTA.
2. The ability to detect asymmetry of position, both visual and tactile.
3. The ability to detect differences of movement in total range, quality of movement during the range, and quality of sensation at the end of the range of movement.
4. The ability to sense position in space of both the patient and examiner.
5. The ability to detect change in palpatory findings, both improvement and worsening, over time.

It is important to develop coordinated and symmetric use of the hands so that they may be linked with the visual sense. In developing palpatory skills, one must be aware that different parts of the hands are valuable for different tests. For example, the palms of the hands are best suited for use in the stereognostic sense of contour; the dorsum of the hands are more sensitive to temperature variations; the finger pads are best for fine discrimination of textural differences, finite skin contour, and so forth; and the tips of the fingers, particularly the thumbs, are useful as pressure probes for the assessment of differences in depth.

Three stages in the development and perception of palpatory sense have been described: reception, transmission, and interpretation. The proprioceptors and mechanoreceptors of the hand receive stimulation from the tissues being palpated. This is the reception phase. These impulses are then transmitted through the peripheral and central nervous systems to the brain where they are analyzed and interpreted. During the palpation process, care must be exercised to ensure efficiency of reception, transmission, and interpretation. Care must be taken of the examiner's hands to protect these sensitive diagnostic instruments. Avoidance of injury abuse is essential, hands should be clean, and nails an appropriate length. During the palpation process, the operator should be relaxed and comfortable to avoid extraneous interference with the transmission of the palpatory impulse. To accurately assess and interpret the palpatory findings, the examiner must concentrate on the act of palpation, the tissue being palpated, and the response of the palpating fingers and hands. Reduce all extraneous sensory stimuli as much as possible. Probably the most common mistake in palpation is the lack of concentration by the examiner.

Tissue palpation can be further divided into light touch and deep touch. In light touch the amount of pressure is very slight and the examiner attempts to assess tissue change both actively and passively. By simply laying hands on the tissue passively, the examiner is able to make tactile observation of the quality of the tissues under the palpating hand. By moving the lightly applied hand in an active fashion, scanning information of multiple areas of the body can be ascertained, both normal and apparently abnormal. Deep touch is the use of additional pressure to palpate deeper into the layers of the tissue of the musculoskeletal system. Compression is palpation through multiple layers of tissue and shear is a movement of tissue between layers. Combinations of active and passive palpation and light and deep touch are used throughout the palpatory diagnostic process.

It is useful to develop appropriate terms to describe the changes in the anatomy being palpated and evaluated. The use of paired descriptors such as superficial–deep, compressible–rigid, moist–dry, warm–cold, painful–nonpainful, circumscribed–diffuse, rough–smooth, among others, are most useful. It is best to define both normal and abnormal palpatory clues in anatomic and physiologic terms. Second, it is useful to define areas of altered palpatory sense by describing the state of the tissue change as acute, subacute, or chronic in nature. Third, it is useful to develop a scale to measure the severity of the altered tissue textures being palpated. Are the tissues normal or are there changes that could be identified as mild, moderate, or severe? A zero, 1+, 2+, and 3+ scale is useful in diagnosing the severity of the problem and in monitoring response to therapeutic intervention over time. Try to use descriptive language that a colleague can comprehend.

LAYER PALPATION

The following describes a practice session that is helpful in learning skill in layer palpation of the tissues of the musculoskeletal system. Two individuals sit across from each other with their arms placed on a narrow table (Fig. 2.2). Each individual's right hand is the examining instrument and the left forearm is the part for the partner to examine. Starting with the left palm on the table, each individual places the right hand (palms and fingers) over the forearm just distal to the elbow.

1. The right hand gently makes contact with the skin. No motion is introduced by the operator's right hand. The

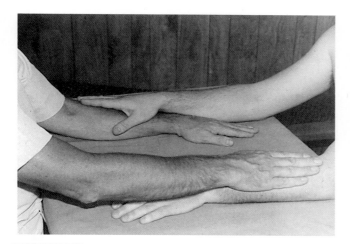

FIGURE 2.2 Layer palpation of dorsal forearm.

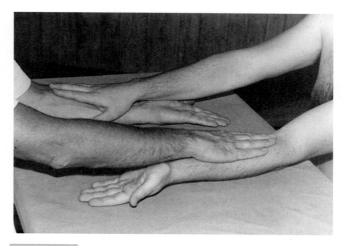

FIGURE 2.3 Layer palpation of volar forearm.

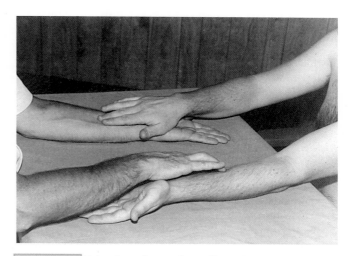

FIGURE 2.4 Palpation of musculotendinous junction.

operator "thinks" skin. How thick or thin is it? How warm or cold is it? How rough or smooth is it? The left forearm is now supinated and the examiner's right hand is placed on the volar surface of the forearm in the same fashion. Again analysis of the skin is made and comparison made between the dorsal and volar aspects (Fig. 2.3). Which is the thickest? Which is the smoothest? Which is the warmest? It is interesting to note the ability to identify significant differences between skin of one area and another by concentration on skin alone.

2. With the right hand firmly in contact with the skin, slight movement of the skin is made, both longitudinally and horizontally, to evaluate the subcutaneous fascia. You now concentrate on the second layer, the subcutaneous fascia. How thick is the layer? How loose is it? Note that with movement in one direction the tissues are more "loose" and in the other direction are more "tight." It is within this layer that many of the TTAs associated with somatic dysfunction are found.

3. Within the subcutaneous fascia layer are found the vessels, arteries, and veins. Palpate these structures for their identification and description.

4. Gently increase the pressure until you sense the deep fascia layer that envelops the underlying structures. Think deep fascia. It can be described as smooth, firm, and continuous. By palpating the deep fascia layer, and moving the hand gently horizontally across the forearm, you can identify areas of thickening that form fascial compartments between bundles of muscle. The ability to define these enveloping layers of deep fascia is helpful, not only in separating one muscle from another, but as a means of getting deeper into underlying structures between muscle.

5. Palpating through the deep fascia, you now concentrate on the underlying muscle and, through concentration, identify individual fibers and the direction in which the fibers run. Move your hands both transversely and longitudinally, sensing for smoothness or roughness. As you palpate across muscle fiber it seems rougher, but as you move in the direction of the muscle fiber it feels smoother. While palpating muscle,

both individuals slowly open and close their left hands, energizing the muscles of the forearm. Your right hand is now palpating contracting and relaxing muscle. Next, squeeze the left hand as hard as possible and palpate muscle during that activity. You are now palpating "hypertonic" muscle. This is the most common TTA feel at the muscle level in areas of somatic dysfunction.

6. While palpating at the muscle level, slowly course down the forearm until you first feel change in the tissue and the loss of ability to the discern muscle fiber. You have now contacted the musculotendinous junction, a point in muscle that is vulnerable to injury (Fig. 2.4).

7. Continue to course down toward the wrist, beyond the musculotendinous junction, and palpate a smooth, round, firm structure called a tendon. Note the transition from muscle through musculotendinous junction to tendon.

8. Follow the tendon distally until you palpate a structure that binds the tendons at the wrist. Palpate that structure (Fig. 2.5). It is the transverse carpal ligament. What are its

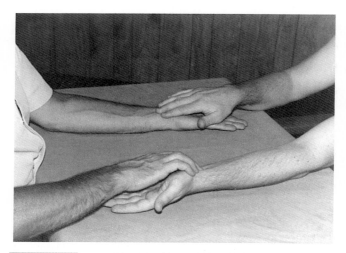

FIGURE 2.5   Palpation of transcarpal ligament.

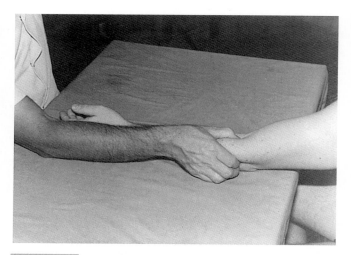

FIGURE 2.6   Palpation of radial head.

characteristics? What direction do its fibers traverse? How thick is it? How firm is it? Ligaments throughout the body feel quite similar.

9. Now return your palpating right hand to the elbow with your middle finger overlying the dimple of the elbow in the dorsal side and your thumb opposite it on the ventral side to palpate the radial head (Fig. 2.6). Stay on bone, and think bone. How hard is it? Is there any "life" in it?

10. Now move just proximal with your palpating thumb and index finger until you fall into the joint space. Underlying your palpating fingers is a structure that you should not be able to feel, namely, the joint capsule. Palpable joint capsules are present in pathologic joints and are not usually found in somatic dysfunction. In fact, some individuals believe that a palpable joint capsule, with the limited exception of the knee joint, is a contraindication to direct-action manipulative treatment.

You have now palpated skin, subcutaneous fascia, blood vessels, deep fascia, muscle, musculotendinous junction, tendon, ligament, bone, and joint space. After using the forearm as the model, these same structures are palpable throughout the body. Practice and experience can enhance your capability as a structural diagnostician.

Vertebral Column Muscles

The muscles overlying the vertebral column are many and layered. They can be described as follows:

Layer 1: the trapezius, latissimus dorsi, and lumbodorsal fascia
Layer 2: the levator scapulae and major and minor rhomboids
Layer 3: the erector spinae mass including the spinalis, semispinalis, longissimus, and iliocostalis
Layer 4: multifidi, rotatores, and intertransversarii

The palpation of these structures is an essential component of structural diagnosis. The following exercise in palpation might

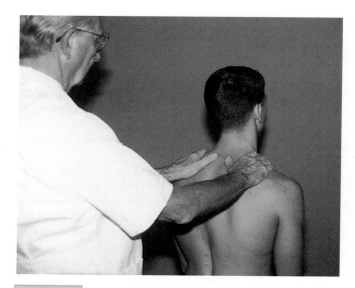

FIGURE 2.7   Layer palpation of shawl area.

be useful in gaining familiarity with some of them for further use both diagnostically and therapeutically.

1. Standing behind a seated patient, place the palms and palmer surfaces of the fingers over the shawl area of the cervicothoracic junction (Fig. 2.7). Palpate the skin for thickness, smoothness, and temperature.

2. Move the skin on the subcutaneous fascia overlying the deep structures in a synchronous and alternating fashion anteroposteriorly and from medial to lateral (Fig. 2.8). Note that in one direction it will be more free and in the other, somewhat tighter. This tight/loose characteristic is a sensation of great significance when using myofascial release technique.

3. Using the thumb and index finger on each hand, pick up the skin and subcutaneous fascia and gently roll the skin over your thumbs by the action of your index fingers coming

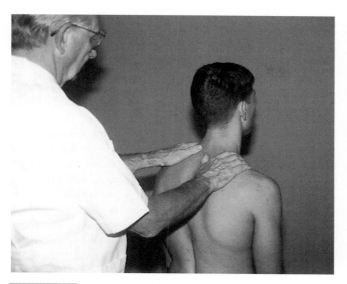

FIGURE 2.8   Skin motion on subcutaneous fascia.

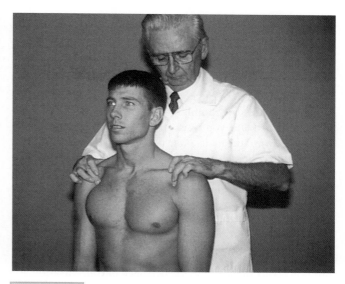

FIGURE 2.10   Palpation of shoulder girdle and coracoid process.

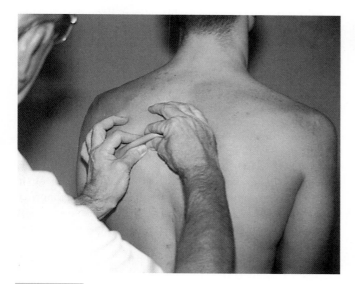

FIGURE 2.9   Skin rolling.

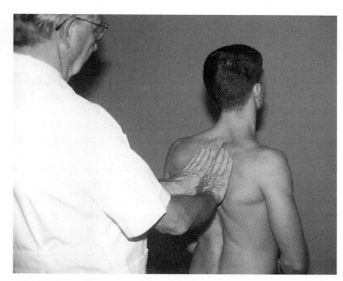

FIGURE 2.11   Layer palpation of trapezius muscle.

from below upward (Fig. 2.9). Repeat starting medially and going laterally. Perform this procedure symmetrically on each side looking for differences in thickness and pliability of the skin and ascertaining if this procedure produces pain for the patient. Skin rolling that identifies tightness and tenderness is a valuable tool in identifying levels of somatic dysfunction.

4. Place the palm of your hand over each acromion process with the long finger extending to the anterior aspect of the shoulder girdle and the finger pad palpating the tip of the coracoid process (Fig. 2.10). Be gentle because this location is quite tender in all subjects. Palpate for the sensation of the resilience of bone. Move your finger pad slightly inferiorly to palpate the rounded, smooth, firm tendon of the

short head of the biceps brachii. Return to the tip of the coracoid process, proceed medially, and palpate the broader, but still smooth and firm tendon of the pectoralis minor muscle.

5. Place the palms of the fingers of both hands overlying the upper thoracic region lateral to the spinous processes and medial to the scapula (Fig. 2.11). Palpate through skin and subcutaneous fascia to palpate the deeper fascia overlying the first layer muscle, the mid portion of the trapezius. Move your fingers from side to side as well as superiorly to inferiorly sensing for muscle fiber direction. This is somewhat easier by having the patient retract the scapulae actively. Note that it appears smoother to move your hands from side to side and more rough when you move your hands from

above to below. That smoothness-versus-roughness characteristic is typical of muscle fiber direction.

6. Place your left hand where your right hand was in the last example and grasp the elbow with your right hand (Fig. 2.12). Palpate through the tissues, including the horizontal portion of the trapezius, and concentrate on the next layer of muscle below, the rhomboids. The rhomboid can be more easily palpable if you resist the patient's effort to push the elbow toward the table. Note that the muscle has a different fiber direction than the trapezius at the same level. It is oblique from medial to lateral and from above downward. The inferior margin is easily palpable to give you the fiber direction.

Development of high-level palpation skill requires considerable practice, which is accumulated over time if a concentrated effort is made. It is also important to avoid the three most common errors in palpation, namely lack of concentration, too much pressure, and too much movement. As stated previously, the most common error is the lack of concentration on the task. The beginner frequently attempts to gain information rapidly and presses much too hard. Remember, the harder you press, the more stimulation you provide to your own mechanoreceptors thus decreasing the amount of sensory impulse being transmitted. To demonstrate, try this simple palpatory exercise; rest the dorsum of your whole hand on the surface of a table. Using the opposite hand gently tap the table top. Notice the location(s) in your palpatory hand where you feel the vibration of tapping the table. Now press your palpatory hand more firmly into the table and notice the diminished sense of feel.

The beginner is also prone to use too much movement in searching for anatomic landmarks and in identifying layers of tissue. This is referred to as the "jiggling hands syndrome." One must remember that the more motion exerted by the

hands, the more stimulation there is in the afferent system to be transmitted and interpreted by the nervous system. Therefore, concentrate, do not push too hard, and do not move too much.

MOTION SENSE

In identifying areas of somatic dysfunction by defining alterations in the diagnostic triad of asymmetry, altered range of motion, and TTA, a combination of observation and palpation is used. In palpation, both static and dynamic dimensions are present. Statically, we look for levels of paired anatomic parts to identify asymmetry. By static and dynamic palpation, we look for alterations in TTA. In palpating tissues without movement, the examiner is interested in such things as skin temperature, smoothness, thickness, and other qualifiers of the state of the tissue. In dynamic palpation, one evaluates, by compression and shear movement within the tissue, the thickness of the tissue, the amount of normal tissue tone, and a sense of which tissues are abnormal. It is within the evaluation of the range of motion that the palpatory sense becomes highly refined. Because restoration of the maximal normal amount of motion possible in the tissue is the desired end point, it is essential that we be able to identify normal and abnormal ranges of motion within both soft tissue and arthrodial structures.

Motion sense is an essential component of the palpatory art in structural diagnosis. The examiner attempts to identify whether there is normal mobility, restricted movement (hypomobility), or too much movement (hypermobility). In motion testing, the examiner may put a region or part of the body through both active and passive movement to ascertain how that part complies with the motion demand placed on it. Information is sought as to whether the mobility is abnormal in a regional sense or confined to one segment. A wide variety of techniques can be used, both actively and passively, to test for motion.

Motion Sense Palpatory Exercise

1. Standing aside a seated patient, palpate the midline of the upper thoracic spine overlying the spinous processes (Fig. 2.13). As you move from above downward, note that the skin is very tightly attached at the midline. As you course from above downward, you will note a bump-and-hollow characteristic. The bumps are the bony spinous processes and the hollow is the interspinous space. Note the tension of the interspinous space reflecting the tension of the supraspinous and intraspinous ligaments.

2. Place three fingers in the interspinous spaces of the upper thoracic spine. Introduce flexion passively through the head, sensing for opening of the interspinous spaces (Fig. 2.14). Reverse the process by taking the head and neck passively into extension and note that the interspinous spaces narrow (Fig. 2.15). Repeat this process several times noting how the interspinous spaces open and close. Attempt to move the head and neck so that you can localize the opening of the

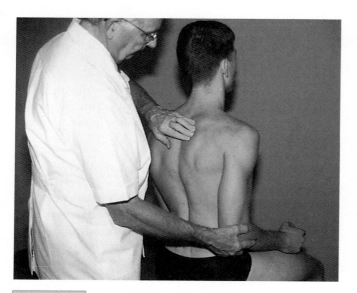

FIGURE 2.12 Layer palpation of rhomboid muscle.

interspinous space beneath the middle finger during flexion, but not the finger below, and repeat the same process in extension so that you can close the interspinous space under the middle finger, but not the one below. This is an important exercise in identifying your capacity to localize to a single vertebral segment.

3. Standing behind a seated patient, place the distal finger pads of your index finger on one side of the spinous process and your middle finger on the other and palpate the fascial groove between the spinous process and the third layer of muscle, the erector spinae mass (Fig. 2.16). Actually, the fascial plane is between the spinalis muscle, which is

intimately attached to the lateral aspect of the spinous processes, and the medial side of the longissimus, the easily palpable "rope" of the erector spinae mass. As you move from cephalad to caudad in this groove, you should feel symmetry and no palpable structure. Should you palpate anything in this medial groove, it is a reflection of hypertonicity of the deeper fourth-layer muscle, primarily at the multifidus layer. Fourth-layer hypertonic muscle is rounded and tense and is about the size of a Tootsie Roll candy. They are usually quite sensitive to the patient and found unilaterally. Occasionally, a bilateral fourth-layer muscle hypertonic area can be palpated in the presence of bilateral flexion or

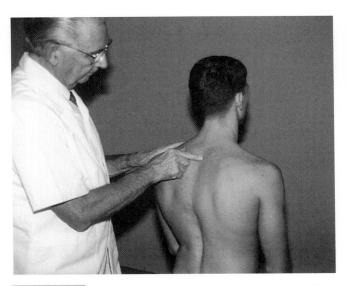

FIGURE 2.13 Layer palpation of the spinous processes.

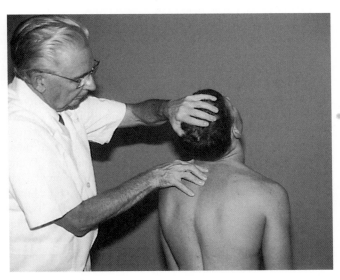

FIGURE 2.15 Palpation of the interspinous spaces during backward bending.

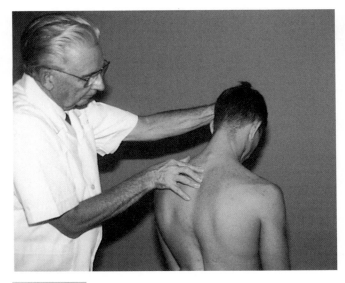

FIGURE 2.14 Palpation of the interspinous spaces during forward bending.

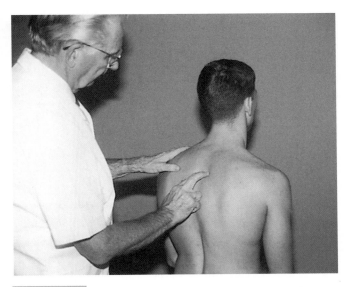

FIGURE 2.16 Palpation of the medial groove erector spinae muscles.

extension restrictions of a vertebral segment. Palpable fourth-layer hypertonic muscle (the "Tootsie Roll" sign) is one of the cardinal diagnostic findings in vertebral segmental somatic dysfunction.[1]

4. Using the same distal finger pad placement as above, (Fig. 2.16) again palpate the medial groove, only this time with a very light and relatively quick motion cephalad to caudad. As you glide your finger pads downward try to perceive any horizontal bands of tissue dampness or tackiness. Autonomic nervous system changes will often be present at the same level as the vertebral segmental somatic dysfunction.[2] In relatively acute situations these areas may be perceived as areas of increase tissue texture such as bogginess, dampness, or tackiness. In more chronic situations these may be perceived as areas of decreased tissue texture such as slickness or smoothness.

5. Move laterally from the medial groove over the rounded mass of the longissimus muscle and note that there is a lateral deep fascial groove separating the lateral aspect of the longissimus from the medial aspect of the iliocostalis muscle. Place your thumbs on the lateral aspect of the longissimus in the lateral groove in a symmetric fashion (Fig. 2.17). Move your thumbs symmetrically in an anteromedial direction until you feel a deep resistance (Fig. 2.18). Note that there has been elevation of the belly of the longissimus. While maintaining your palpation at this deeper level, move your thumbs in a cephalic to caudad direction sensing for a bump and hollow contour similar to that identified over the spinous processes in the midline. At the level you are now palpating, you are overlying the transverse processes of the thoracic vertebrae, which are the bumps. The intertransverse space is the hollow. Try to palpate one pair of transverse processes in a symmetric fashion and ask the patient to actively flex and extend his or her head and neck while you attempt to maintain contact with the transverse processes. Note that it is

easier to feel the transverse process during the extension movement than during flexion. Acquisition of the skill of following transverse processes in three-dimensional space is most valuable in making a diagnosis of vertebral somatic dysfunction.

6. Move your hands more laterally overlying the most posterior aspect of the thoracic cage (Fig. 2.19). You are palpating over the rib angles and the associated attachment of the iliocostalis muscle. Move from cephalad to caudad and note that the rib angles diverge from medial to lateral. Each rib angle should participate in the posterior convexity of the thoracic cage. The finding of one rib angle that is more or less prominent than its fellows above and below is significant in the diagnosis of rib somatic dysfunction. Any palpable hypertonicity of muscle at the rib angle is indicative of hypertonic

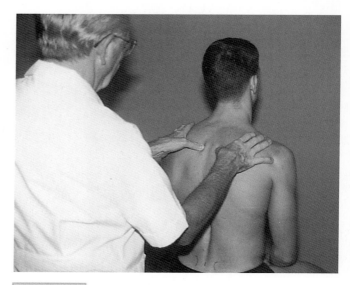

FIGURE 2.18   **Palpation of transverse processes.**

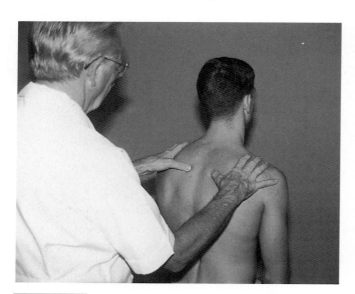

FIGURE 2.17   **Palpation of the lateral groove erector spinae muscles.**

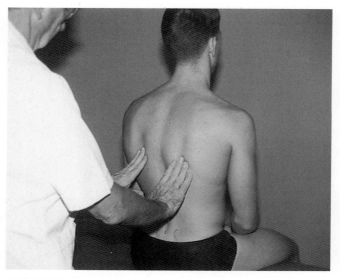

FIGURE 2.19   **Palpation of the rib angles and iliocostalis muscle.**

iliocostalis, which is only found in the presence of rib dysfunction. Again, hypertonic iliocostalis at a rib angle is frequently tender to the patient.

7. Place your thumb overlying the rib angle of the most posterior aspect of the thoracic cage, usually the seventh rib (Fig. 2.20). Move your thumb over the rib shaft at the angle, noting the posterior convexity. Move to the superior and inferior aspect of the rib noting the rib edge. Most commonly, the inferior edge is somewhat more easily palpable than the superior. Of importance is the contour of the rib in comparison to the one above, the one below, and those on the contralateral side. Prominence of the superior or inferior rib edge is significant in the diagnosis of rib somatic dysfunction. Palpate the interspace above and below the rib and compare it with the opposite side. Is one narrower or wider than the other? Palpate the intercostal muscle to see if it is hypertonic and tender. Abnormal width above and below a rib and intercostal hypertonicity are significant findings in certain rib somatic dysfunctions.

8. From the rib angle, continue to monitor rib shaft and move medially with the palm of your thumb on the rib shaft until the tip of your thumb runs into an obstruction (Fig. 2.21). The tip of your thumb has now struck the lateral aspect of the transverse process. The portion of bone from the rib angle to the tip of the transverse process is an important component of the rib that is used in some of the subsequently described techniques for rib somatic dysfunction. Again note that the longissimus muscle becomes more prominent as you have moved from lateral to medial along the rib shaft.

This layer palpation exercise of the back will provide you with the ability to palpate anatomic structures necessary for the accurate diagnosis of vertebral axis and costal cage somatic dysfunction. Particularly important is the ability to follow paired transverse processes through a range of motion and the ability to identify tender, tense hypertonic muscle of the fourth layer. Practice this exercise on a regular basis until it becomes habitual.

The examiner must recognize that there is an inherent tissue motion that is continuous and palpable with practice. Perception of inherent tissue motion is accomplished via the cutaneous and joint mechanoreceptors of the operator's palpatory hand. Cutaneous receptors are very sensitive to stretch or skin displacement. Joint mechanoreceptors are extraordinarily sensitive to joint position sense.[3–7] With this in mind, return to the hand and forearm positions of Figure 2.2 with light consistent whole hand contact such that you cannot determine where your hand ends and their forearm begins. Relax the joints in your palpating hand, close your eyes and concentrate on the behavior of the tissues under your palpating hand. With practice, you will note that the forearm is not static, but is inherently, dynamically moving. This inherent motion is thought to be a compilation of motions from transmission of the arterial pulse, effect of respiration, contraction and relaxation of muscle fibers during normal muscle tone, and the cranial rhythmic impulse.

It is essential that good contact be made with the examiner's hand(s) on the part(s) being palpated; one that appreciates that it is the soft tissues around and within the joint capsules of the examiner's hand that perceive finite motion. As the part is taken through a range of motion, either actively or passively, the examiner is interested in three elements: range of movement, quality of movement during the range, and "end feel." In determining range of movement, one is interested in the quantity of movement. Is it normal, restricted, or increased in range? Second, how does it feel during the movement throughout the range? Is it smooth? Is it "sticky" or "jerky" or "too loose"? There are a number of alterations in movement feel during the range that

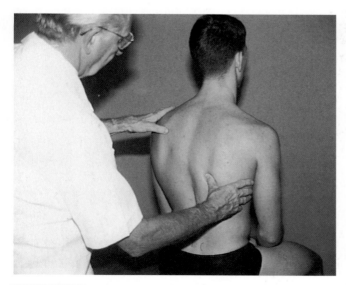

FIGURE 2.20 Palpation of rib angle contour.

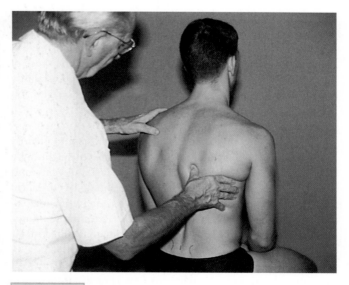

FIGURE 2.21 Palpation of rib shaft to tip of transverse process.

can be of assistance to the examiner in determining what factors might be altering the range of movement. Third, what is the feel at the end point of the range of movement? Is there symmetry to the range and does each extreme of the range of movement feel the same? If there is alteration in the end feel, what are the qualities of the end point? Is it hard? Is it soft? Is it spongy? Is it jerky? There are wide varieties of characteristic end feels that experience will teach the examiner. The quality of the end feel is most helpful in determining the cause of the restrictive movement and the type of manipulative therapy that might be most effective.

Hypermobility

Manual medicine procedures are used to overcome restrictions of movement. Techniques that increase mobility should not be used in the presence of hypermobility. Hypermobility is present when there is an increase in the range of movement, a loose feeling throughout the range of movement, and loss of normal tissue resiliency at the end feel. Hypermobility might be normal in certain highly trained athletes, such as gymnasts and acrobats, but in most individuals, it must be considered abnormal. In the vertebral complex, it is not uncommon to find relative hypermobility of one vertebral motion segment adjacent to a vertebral motion segment that is restricted. This has been described as "compensatory hypermobility" and has been explained as the body's attempt to maintain mobility of the total mechanism in the presence of restricted mobility of a part of the vertebral axis. It is common to find that hypermobile segments are the areas of symptomatology. As such, they gain a great deal of attention from the examiner. Care must be exercised not to provide manual medicine procedures that increase the relative hypermobility of these segments, rather than appropriately applying mobilizing techniques to the segment(s) with restricted mobility. Hypermobility can progress to the stage that can best be described as instability. Instability occurs when the integrity of the tissues supporting the joint structure cannot maintain appropriate functional apposition of the moving parts; thus, the relative stability of the motion unit is lost. The dividing line between hypermobility and instability is not always definite, and good objective measures to quantify instability are not available. Nonetheless, the skilled clinician must develop some sense of normal motion, hypomobility, hypermobility, and instability of anatomic structures within the musculoskeletal system. It is for this reason that the development of a motion sense is worth the effort.

One must also develop the skill of motion sense to identify change in the range of motion, quality of movement during a range, and the end feel after a manual medicine intervention. It is useful in prognosis as well as diagnosis. It should be possible to identify a change in range of motion, and its quality, if a manual medicine intervention has been successful. Retesting the range of motion available is always the last step in any manual medicine therapeutic intervention.

Motion sense is an essential component of the palpatory art in structural diagnosis. As in any art form, practice is the major requirement for mastery.

SCREENING EXAMINATION

The screening examination evaluates the total musculoskeletal system as part of patient examination. It answers the question, "Is there a problem within the musculoskeletal system that deserves additional evaluation?" There are numerous formats for a screening examination. The following 12-step procedure is comprehensive in scope and can be accomplished rapidly.

Step 1. Gait analysis in multiple directions
Step 2. Static posture and palpation of paired anatomic landmarks
Step 3. Dynamic trunk side bending
Step 4. Standing flexion test
Step 5. Stork test
Step 6. Seated flexion test
Step 7. Screening test of upper extremities
Step 8. Trunk rotation
Step 9. Trunk side bending
Step 10. Head and neck mobility
Step 11. Respiration of thoracic cage
Step 12. Lower extremity screening

STEP 1. GAIT ANALYSIS

1. Observe gait with patient walking toward you (Fig. 2.22).
2. Observe patient walking away from you (Fig. 2.23).

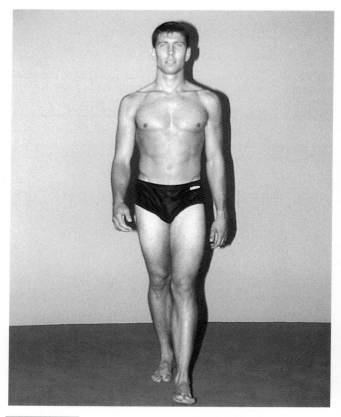

FIGURE 2.22 Observation of gait from the front.

3. Observe patient walking from the side (Figs. 2.24 and 2.25).

4. Observe length of stride, swing of arms, heel strike, toe off, tilting of the pelvis, and adaption of the shoulders.

5. One looks for the functional capacity of the gait, not the usual pathologic conditions. Of particular importance is the cross-patterning of the gait and symmetry of stride.

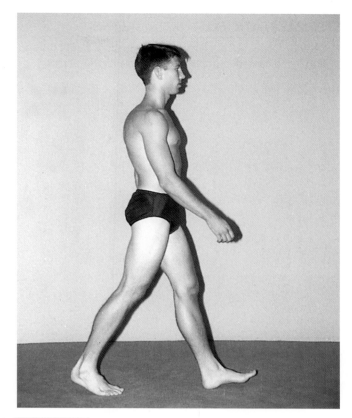

FIGURE 2.24   **Observation of gait from the right side.**

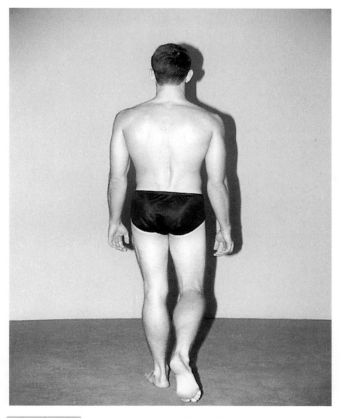

FIGURE 2.23   **Observation of gait from the back.**

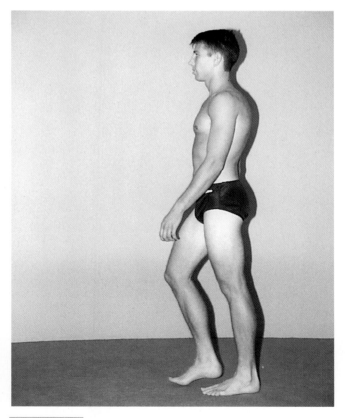

FIGURE 2.25   **Observation of gait from the left side.**

STEP 2A. STATIC POSTURE ANALYSIS

1. Observe from the front (Fig. 2.26), evaluating weight distribution, head carriage, shoulder level, and foot placement.

2. Observe from the back (Fig. 2.27), evaluating head carriage, shoulder height, level of pelvis, and weight distribution of the feet.

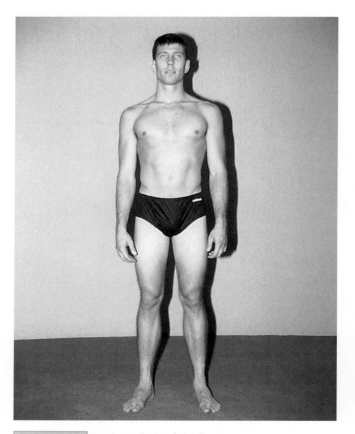

FIGURE 2.26 Static analysis of the front.

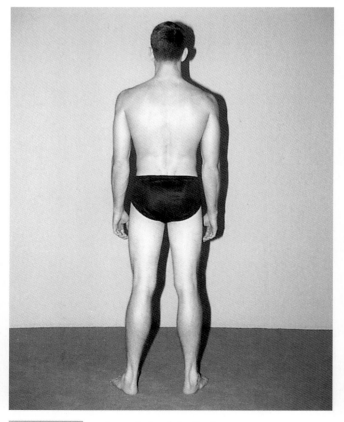

FIGURE 2.27 Static analysis of the back.

3. Observe from the side (Fig. 2.28), evaluating posture against the plumb line that drops from the external auditory meatus to the tip of the acromion through the femoral trochanter to just in front of the medial malleolus.

4. Observe from the opposite side (Fig. 2.29); again assess the plumb line and compare with the opposite side. Note head carriage, anteroposterior spinal curves, and extent of knee extension.

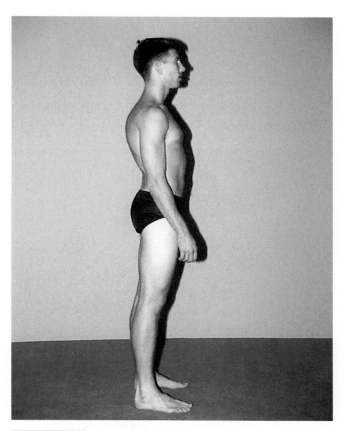

FIGURE 2.28 **Static analysis of the right side.**

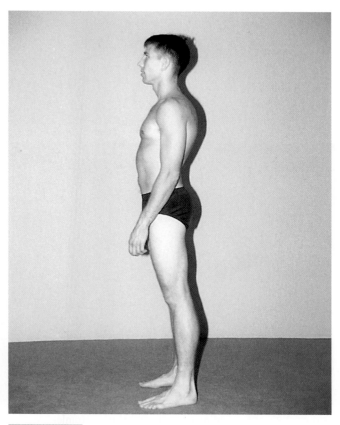

FIGURE 2.29 **Static analysis of the left side.**

STEP 2B. STATIC POSTURE ANATOMIC LEVELS

1. Combined palpation and observation is made of the levels of the acromion process (Fig. 2.30).

2. Palpation of the iliac crest (Fig. 2.31) is performed by pushing soft tissue out of the way from below and placing proximal phalanges of the index fingers on similar portions of the right and left hip bones.

3. Palpation and observation of the top of the greater trochanter require lateral-to-medial compression of the soft tissues of the lateral hip (Fig. 2.32).

4. Unleveling of the iliac crest and greater trochanter in the standing position is the first index of suspicion for a *short-leg–pelvic-tilt syndrome.*

5. Note that the eyes are on the same horizontal plane as the palpating fingers for better hand–eye coordination.

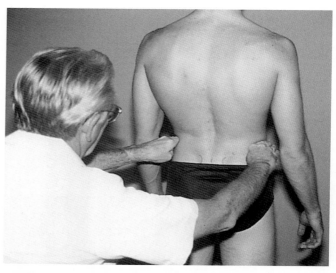

FIGURE 2.31 Palpation and observation of the top of the iliac crests.

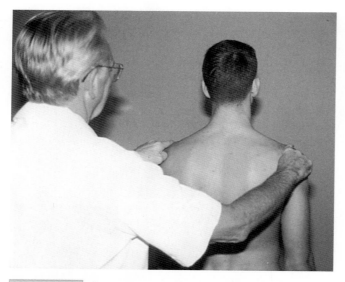

FIGURE 2.30 Observation of the levels of the acromion process.

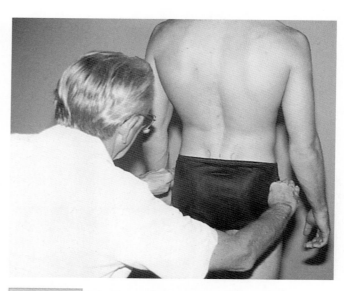

FIGURE 2.32 Palpation and observation of the top of the greater trochanters.

STEP 3. TRUNK SIDE BENDING

1. Observation is made from the back.

2. Patient is asked to side bend to the left (Fig. 2.33) as far as possible without bending forward.

3. The patient repeats the side bending to the right (Fig. 2.34), again without bending forward.

4. Observation is made of the symmetry of range from right to left as a reflection of fingertip distance on the lateral leg.

5. Observation is made of the induced spinal curve, which should be a smooth symmetric C curve with fullness on the side of the induced convexity. Straightening of the segments of the induced curve and fullness on the side of the concavity are highly suggestive of significant vertebral motion segment dysfunction at that level and are an indication that there is a need to scan the area for specific segmental motion loss.

6. Observation is made of the symmetry of the pelvic shift from right to left during the side bending effort and whether the loading of the lower extremities appears symmetric.

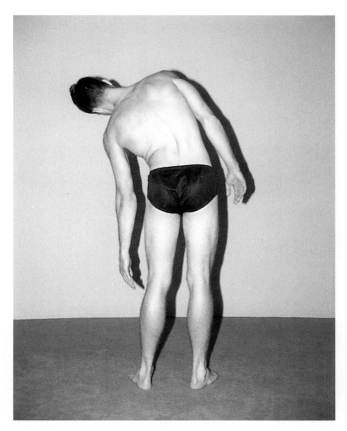

FIGURE 2.33 Observation of left trunk side bending from the back.

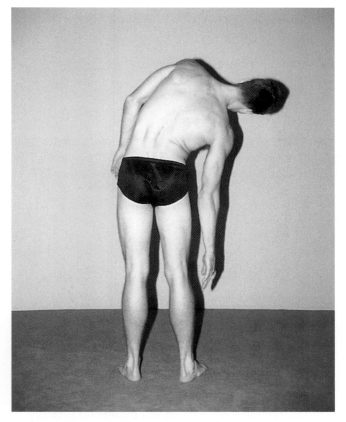

FIGURE 2.34 Observation of right trunk side bending from the back.

STEP 4. STANDING FLEXION TEST

1. Patient stands with feet approximately 4 in. (10 cm) apart with weight under the hip joints (Fig. 2.35).

2. Operator's hands grasp along the posterior aspect of each ilia with the pads of the thumbs placed just under the inferior slope of the posterior superior iliac spine.

3. Patient is instructed to bend forward as smoothly as possible, attempting to touch the floor (Fig. 2.36). Operator's hands follow the motion of the ilia with a visual focus on the thumbs to see whether one appears to move more cephalad than the other.

4. The test is viewed as positive if one posterior superior iliac spine moves further cephalad or ventrally than the other does.

5. Observation is also made of the lower thoracic and lumbar spines for segmental rhythm and for the induction of side bending rotational curves.

6. This test is very sensitive to dysfunctions in the articulations of the bony pelvis. A positive test does not define a specific dysfunction; its value is to lateralize dysfunction from one side to the other of the pelvis.

CLINICAL PEARL

The key to the accuracy of the standing flexion test it to allow the hands to follow motion of the bony pelvis as the patient moves into forward flexion. Monitoring motion of the fascias of the trunk and lower extremity during forward bending is useful in some clinical situations; however, it may give the operator unreliable findings of dysfunction of the bony pelvis. Starting with the thumbs inferior to the posterior superior iliac spines and lifting soft tissue and fascia upward prior to seating the thumbs on the inferior slope of the posterior superior iliac spines limits the potential for the operator's thumbs to be prematurely pulled cephalad by these tissues as the patient bends forward.

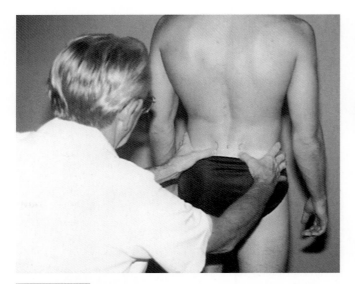

FIGURE 2.35   Palpation of the inferior slope of the posterior superior iliac spines.

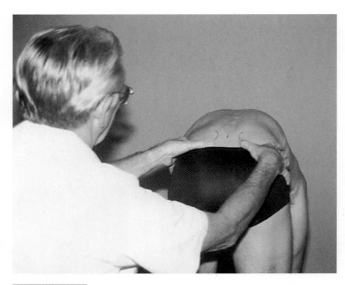

FIGURE 2.36   Standing flexion test.

STEP 5. STORK TEST

1. With the patient standing and the operator sitting behind, the operator's left hand grasps along the posterior aspect of the left ilia with the pads of the thumb placed just under the inferior slope of the posterior superior iliac spine and the right thumb overlying the midline of the sacrum at the same horizontal level (Fig. 2.37).

2. Operator asks the patient to flex the left hip and knee to a minimum of 90 degrees of hip flexion (Fig. 2.38).

3. Motion of the left ilia is followed with a focus on the thumb. A negative test finds the left thumb on the posterior superior iliac spine moving caudad in relation to the right thumb on the sacrum.

4. The thumb placements are reversed, and the patient is asked to raise the right leg in a similar fashion (Fig. 2.39).

5. A positive finding occurs when the thumb on the posterior superior iliac spine fails to move or moves cephalad in relation to the thumb on the sacrum.

6. The findings of this test are correlated with those of the seated flexion test (step 6). The stork test is more specific for upper pole sacroiliac joint restrictions.

7. If the patient has difficulty standing on one foot to perform the test, proprioceptive sensory motor balance deficit should be further evaluated.

CLINICAL PEARL

Although the stork and seated flexion test findings are specific for sacroiliac joint restrictions, the stork test is more specific for upper pole sacroiliac joint dysfunctions such as posterior torsions[8]; whereas the seated flexion test is more specific for lower pole sacroiliac joint dysfunctions, such as anterior torsions or unilateral sacral dysfunctions (see Chapter 17).

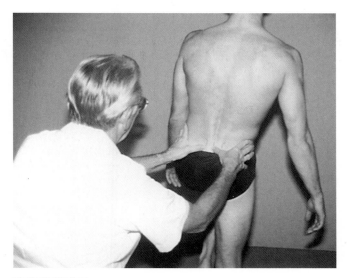

FIGURE 2.38 Left stork test.

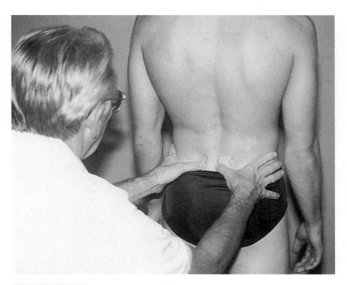

FIGURE 2.37 Preparation for left stork test; left thumb on the inferior slope of the left posterior superior iliac spine, right thumb midline at same level.

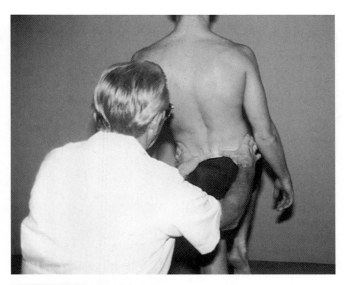

FIGURE 2.39 Right stork test.

STEP 6. SEATED FLEXION TEST

1. Patient sits on the examining stool with knees apart and feet flat on the floor.

2. Operator's hands grasp along the posterior aspect of each ilia with the pads of the thumbs placed just under the inferior slope of the posterior superior iliac spine (Fig. 2.40).

3. Patient is instructed to bend forward with the arms between the knees as far as possible (Fig. 2.41).

4. Operator's hands follow the motion of the ilia with a visual focus on the thumbs to see whether one posterior superior iliac spine appears to move more cephalad than the other (Fig. 2.42). The one that moves the furthest in a cephalad or ventral direction is deemed positive, indicative of restricted mobility of that side of the pelvis.

5. Operator observes the behavior of the lower thoracic and lumbar spines for dysrhythmia and for the introduction of side bending and rotational curves.

6. Comparison of findings with those of a standing flexion test evaluates the behavior of the pelvic girdle and vertebral complex without the influence of the lower extremities as the patient is sitting on the ischial tuberosity.

7. Unleveling of the iliac crest when seated to perform this test is presumptive evidence of inequality in size of the right and left hip bones.

CLINICAL PEARL

This test is very specific for lower pole sacroiliac joint dysfunctions. Its accuracy is highly dependent on prior treatment of any symphysis pubis or innominate shear dysfunctions (see Chapter 17).

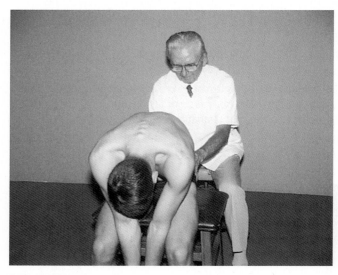

FIGURE 2.41 Seated flexion test, patient's arms dropped between the legs.

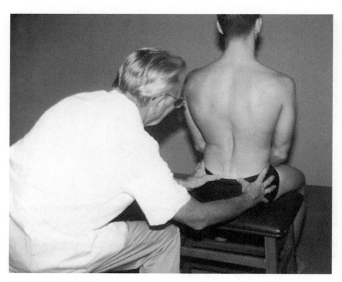

FIGURE 2.40 Preparation for seated flexion test; thumbs placed on the inferior slope of the posterior superior iliac spine.

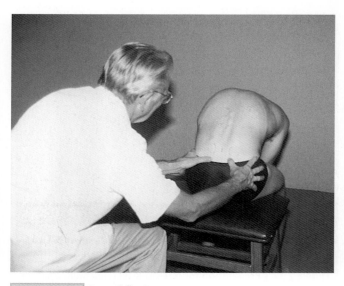

FIGURE 2.42 Seated flexion test.

STEP 7. UPPER EXTREMITY SCREEN

1. Patient is seated on an examining stool or table.

2. Patient is instructed to fully abduct both upper extremities in the coronal plane, reach to the ceiling, and turn the backs of the hands together (Fig. 2.43).

3. Observation is made from the front.

4. Observation is also made from behind (Fig. 2.44).

5. This maneuver requires mobility of the sternoclavicular, acromioclavicular, glenohumeral, elbow, and wrist joints.

6. Any asymmetry indicates the need for additional evaluation.

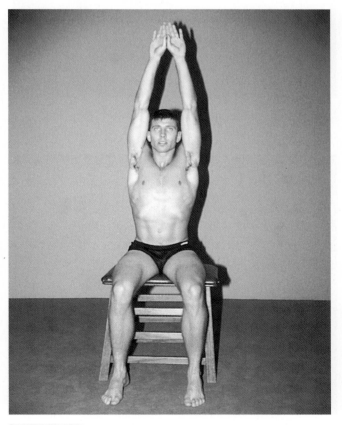

FIGURE 2.43 Observation of the upper extremity screen from the front.

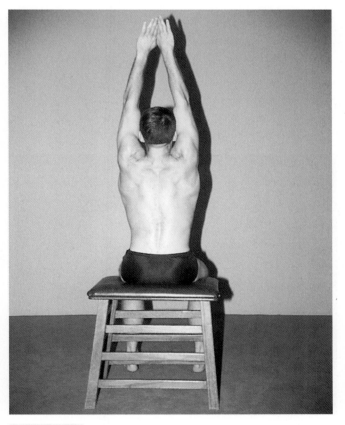

FIGURE 2.44 Observation of the upper extremity screen from the back.

STEP 8. TRUNK ROTATION

1. Patient sits on the table with operator standing behind.

2. Operator grasps each shoulder (Fig. 2.45).

3. Operator introduces trunk rotation through the shoulders (Fig. 2.46), sensing for range, quality of movement, and end feel.

4. Operator rotates trunk to the left (Fig. 2.47), comparing range, quality of movement, and end feel with those of right rotation.

5. Asymmetry of right-to-left rotation indicates additional diagnostic procedures for the vertebral column and rib cage.

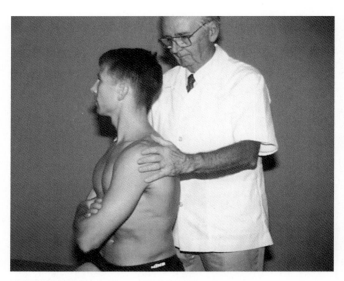

FIGURE 2.46 Trunk rotation right.

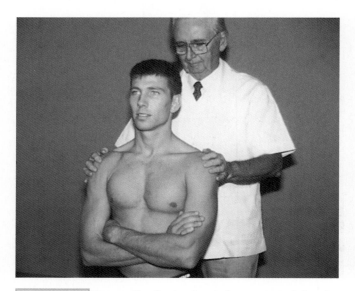

FIGURE 2.45 Preparation for trunk rotation; operator's hands grasp each shoulder.

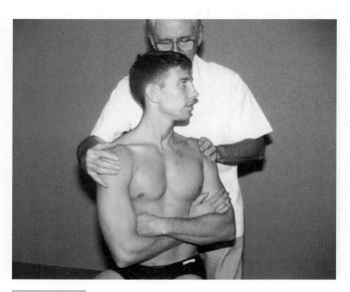

FIGURE 2.47 Trunk rotation left.

STEP 9. TRUNK SIDE BENDING

1. Patient sits with operator behind.

2. Operator grasps each shoulder (Fig. 2.48).

3. Operator presses downward on right shoulder with the right hand, introducing right-side bending (Fig. 2.49), sensing for range, quality of movement, and end feel.

4. Operator pushes left shoulder inferiorly to introduce left-side bending (Fig. 2.50), sensing for range, quality of movement, and end feel.

5. Comparison is made of left- and right-side bending for symmetry or asymmetry. Asymmetry demonstrates a need for additional diagnostic evaluation of the vertebral column and the rib cage.

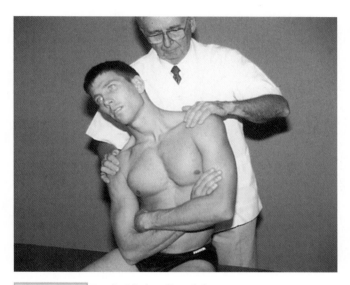

FIGURE 2.49 Trunk side bending right.

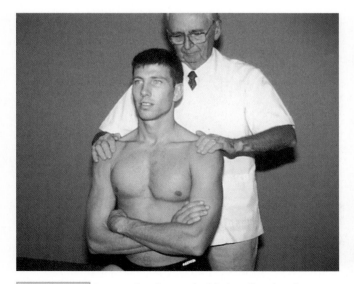

FIGURE 2.48 Preparation for trunk side bending; hands contact the top of each shoulder.

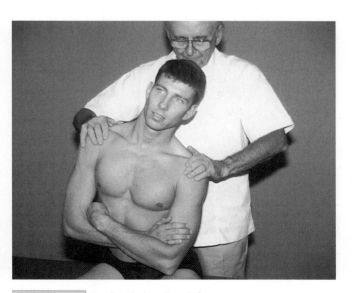

FIGURE 2.50 Trunk side bending left.

STEP 10. MOBILITY OF THE HEAD AND NECK

1. Patient sits on the table with the operator standing behind.
2. Operator grasps head between the two hands (Fig. 2.51).

3. Operator introduces backward bending (Fig. 2.52). Normal extension is 90 degrees.

4. Operator introduces forward bending (Fig. 2.53). Normal range is 45 degrees of flexion.

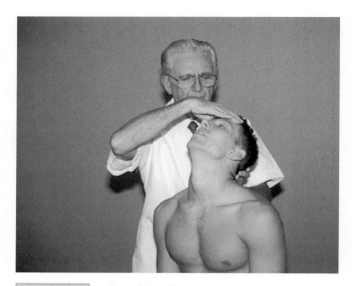

FIGURE 2.52   **Backward bending.**

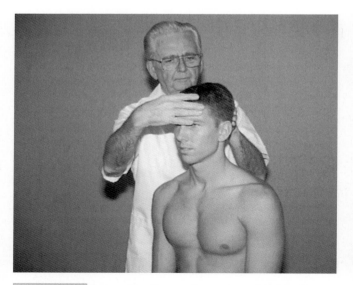

FIGURE 2.51   **Preparation for passive neck motion; hands contact the front and back of the head.**

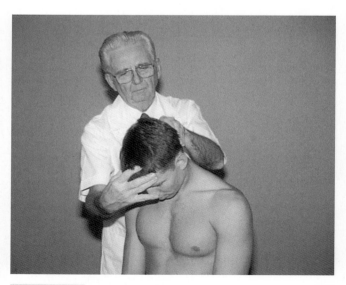

FIGURE 2.53   **Forward bending.**

5. Operator introduces right-side bending (Fig. 2.54) and left-side bending (Fig. 2.55). Normal range is 45 degrees to each side.

6. Operator introduces rotation to the left (Fig. 2.56) and to the right (Fig. 2.57). Normal range is 80 to 90 degrees on each side.

7. Operator evaluates range, quality of movement during the range, and end feel, looking for symmetry or asymmetry. If asymmetric, additional diagnostic evaluations of the cervical spine, upper thoracic spine, and rib cage are necessary.

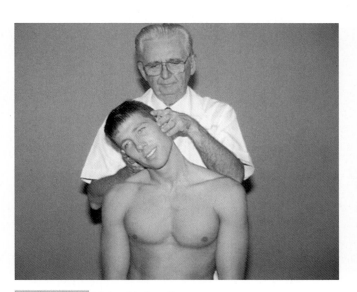

FIGURE 2.54 Right-side bending.

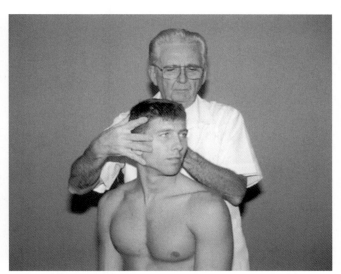

FIGURE 2.56 Left rotation.

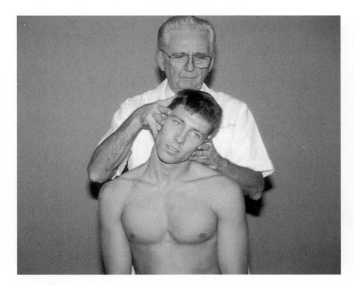

FIGURE 2.55 Left-side bending.

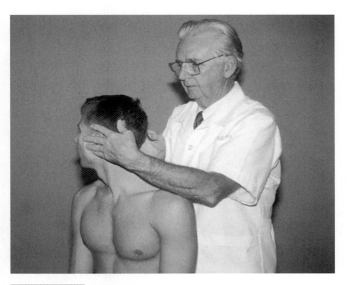

FIGURE 2.57 Right rotation.

STEP 11. RESPIRATORY MOVEMENT OF THORACIC CAGE

1. Patient is supine on the table with operator standing at the side, with dominant eye over the midline of the patient.

2. Operator symmetrically places hands over the anterolateral aspect of the lower rib cage bilaterally (Fig. 2.58).

3. Patient is instructed to deeply inhale and exhale while operator follows lower thoracic cage movement during respiration, looking for symmetry or lack of it.

4. Operator places hands in intercostal spaces of the anterolateral aspect of the upper rib cage (Fig. 2.59) to evaluate bucket-handle movement of the upper ribs during inhalation and exhalation.

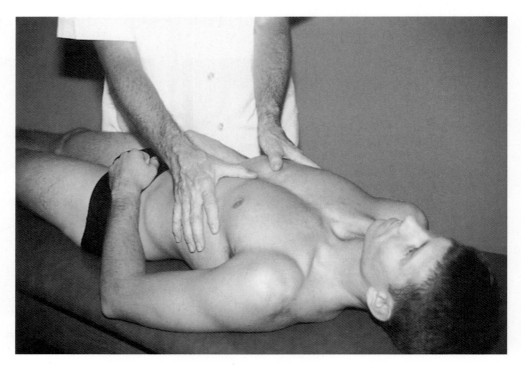

FIGURE 2.58 Observation of lower rib cage motion.

5. Operator's hands are placed vertically over the anterior aspect of the upper rib cage with the longest finger in contact with the cartilage of the first rib under the medial end of the clavicle (Fig. 2.60) and assess pump-handle motion response of the upper ribs to inhalation and exhalation.

6. Asymmetry of movement of inhalation and exhalation efforts calls for more definitive diagnosis of the thoracic spine and rib cage.

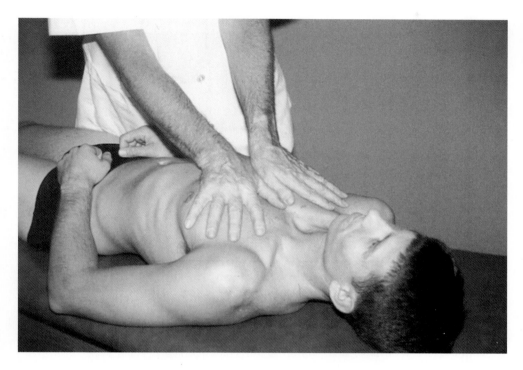

FIGURE 2.59 Observation of bucket-handle motion of the upper rib cage.

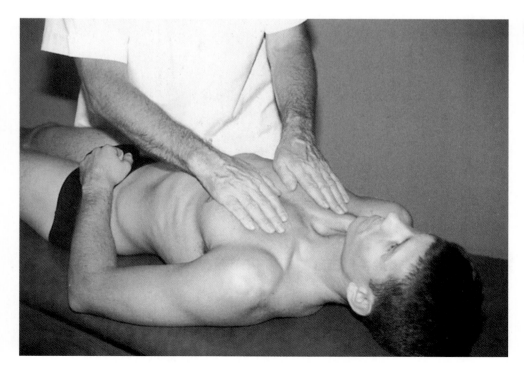

FIGURE 2.60 Observation of pump-handle motion of the upper rib cage.

STEP 12. LOWER EXTREMITY SCREEN

1. Patient is supine on the table with operator standing at the side.

2. Operator grasps left ankle, monitoring the right anterior superior iliac spine (Fig. 2.61).

3. Operator lifts the left leg until the first movement of the right anterior superior iliac spine is felt, indicative of length of the hamstring muscle group (Fig. 2.62).

4. Comparison is made with the opposite side for symmetry or asymmetry.

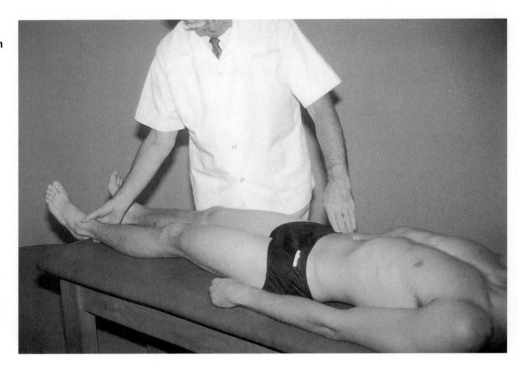

FIGURE 2.61   Monitor the contralateral ASIS in preparation for a straight-leg raise.

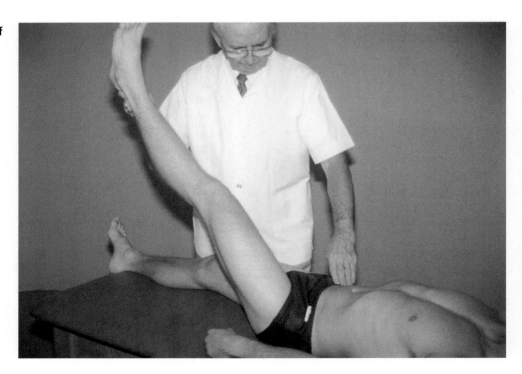

FIGURE 2.62   Monitor for end of range of the hamstrings.

5. Operator flexes, externally rotates, and abducts the patient's right hip (Fig. 2.63). Comparison is made with the opposite side for symmetry or asymmetry. Restricted motion suggests dysfunction and pathology of the right hip joint.

6. Patient is instructed to do a deep knee bend, maintaining the heels on the floor (Fig. 2.64). This squat test requires mobility of the foot, ankle, knee, and hip joints bilaterally. Inability to perform the squat test indicates additional diagnostic evaluation of the lower extremities.

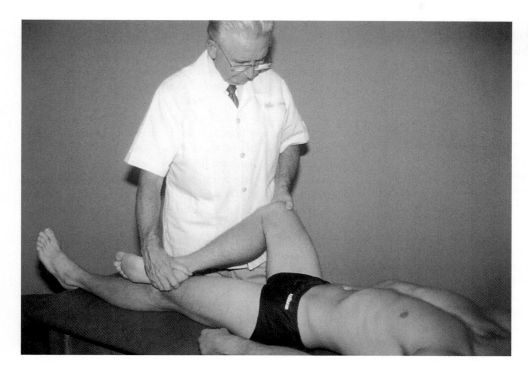

FIGURE 2.63 Flexion, abduction, and external rotation of the right hip.

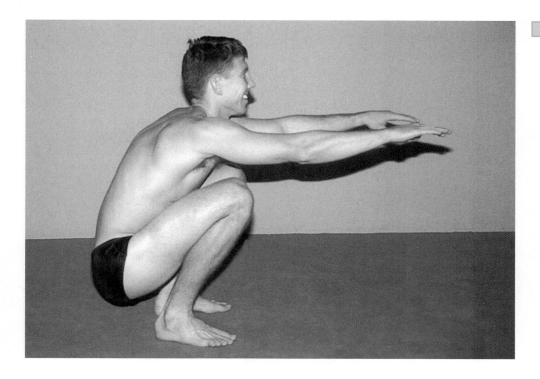

FIGURE 2.64 Squat test.

SCANNING EXAMINATION

Once an area of the musculoskeletal system has been identified during the screening examination as being sufficiently abnormal for further investigation, a scanning procedure of that region is initiated. The scanning examination is designed to answer the following questions: What part of the region, and what tissues within the region, are significantly dysfunctional? The object is to locate the areas that might account for the abnormal finding. By using the analogy of a microscope, we have gone from low power (the screening examination) to high power (scanning examination). More definitive evaluation of soft tissue can be accomplished with active and passive light and deep touch. Thumbs or fingers can be used as a pressure probe searching for areas of tenderness or more specific signs of tissue texture change. Multiple variations of motion scanning can be introduced to look for alterations in symmetry of range, quality of movement, and sensations at end feel. Respiratory effort might be used to evaluate the response of the region to inhalation and exhalation efforts. Responses within the region to demands placed on it from more remote areas of the musculoskeletal system are frequently useful in defining better the area requiring specific attention.

SKIN ROLLING TEST

One valuable diagnostic test for scanning procedures is the skin rolling test. In this examination, a fold of skin is grasped between the thumb and index finger and rolled as if one were rolling a cigarette (Fig. 2.65). Skin rolling can be accomplished symmetrically on each side of the body, testing for normal painfree laxity of the skin and subcutaneous fascia. A positive finding is tenderness and pain provocation in certain dermatomal levels of skin, with tightness and loss of resiliency within the skin and subcutaneous fascia. Frequently, tender nodules will be palpated while accomplishing this test. They are interpreted to represent alteration in dermatomal innervation from dysfunctions within the vertebral axis. In the examination of the thoracic and lumbar

regions of the spine, it is recommended that the skin be rolled in the midline overlying the spinous processes and, more laterally, coursing from below upward, comparing changes on one side to the other. Although defined as a scanning procedure, skin rolling can be quite specific in defining specific segmental dysfunction because of the clinically observable dermatomal relationship to altered vertebral motion segment function.

SEGMENTAL DEFINITION

The third element to the diagnostic process is segmental definition, used to identify the specific vertebral motion segment, or peripheral joint, that is dysfunctional. It is also used to determine the specific motion restriction that is involved. An attempt is made to identify the tissue(s) that is most involved in the dysfunctional segment.

One method of identifying the specific joint that is dysfunctional, and the motion that is lost, is to test for joint-play movements. Mennell has advocated this concept for many years. Joint-play movements are defined as being independent of the action of voluntary muscle and are found within synovial joints. The range of joint play is very small but very precise. Normal joint-play movement allows for easy, painless performance of voluntary movement. The amount of joint play is usually less than one eighth of an inch in any one plane within a synovial joint. Mennell defines joint dysfunction as the loss of joint-play movement that cannot be recovered by the action of voluntary muscles. Once the precise system for identifying joint play is learned, very similar maneuvers can be used therapeutically in restoring anatomic and physiologic function to the joint by reestablishing its normal joint play.

Numerous diagnostic procedures can specifically define, within the vertebral motion segment or the synovial extremity joint, the specific dysfunction that is present. Subsequent chapters will describe the methods most commonly used by this author. The primary goal is to determine which vertebral motion segment is dysfunctional, which joint within that vertebral motion segment is dysfunctional, the direction of altered motion(s), and some estimate of the tissue involved in the restricted motion. Primary emphasis is placed on motion loss and its characteristics. Many diagnostic systems depend upon localization of pain or provocation of pain by certain motion introductions. In the opinion of this author, motion loss and its characteristics are more valuable diagnostic criteria than the presence of pain and the provocation of pain by movement. Pain and its provocation can be of assistance in diagnosis, but they are not diagnostic in and of themselves.

These principles of structural diagnosis need to be studied extensively and mastered by the physician who wishes to be skilled in the field of manual medicine. An accurate and specific diagnosis is essential for successful results from manual medicine therapeutic interventions.

SUGGESTED READINGS

Dvorak J, Dvorak V. *Manual Medicine, Diagnostics*. New York: Thieme-Stratton, 1983.

Dvorak J, Dvorak V, Schneider W, eds. *Manual Medicine 1984*. New York: Springer-Verlag, 1984.

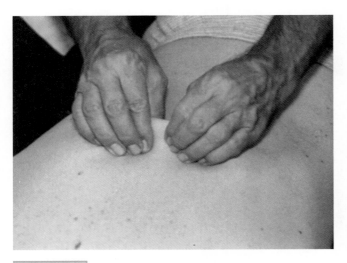

FIGURE 2.65   Skin rolling.

Farfan HF. The scientific basis of manipulative procedures. *Clin Rheum Dis* 1980;6:159–178.

Fisk JW. *The Painful Neck and Back*. Springfield, IL: Charles C Thomas Publisher, 1977.

Greenman PE. Layer palpation. *Mich Osteopath J* 1982;47:936–937.

Mennell J McM. *Joint Pain*. Boston: Little Brown & Co., 1964.

The Glossary Review Committee of the Educational Council on Osteopathic Principles in Allen TW. AOA Yearbook and Directory of Osteopathic Physicians, ed. Chicago, IL: AOA, 1993.

Ward RC, Sprafka S. Glossary of osteopathic terminology. *J Am Osteopath Assoc* 1981;80:552–567.

REFERENCES

1. Avramov AI, Cavanaugh JM, Ozaktay CA, et al. The effects of controlled mechanical loading on group-II, and IV afferent units from the lumbar facet joint and surrounding tissue. *J Bone Joint Surg* 1992;74-A(10):1464–1471.

2. Sato A, Schmidt RF. Somatosympathetic reflexes: Afferent fibers, central pathways, discharge characteristics. *Physiol Rev* 1973;53(4):916–947.

3. Macefield G, Gandevia SC, Burke D. Perceptual responses to microstimulation of single afferents innervating joints, muscles and skin of the human hand. *J Physiol* 1990;429:113–129.

4. Johansson RS, Landstöm U, Lundström R. Responses of mechanoreceptive afferent units in the glabrous skin of the human hand to sinusoidal skin displacements. *Brain Res* 1982;244(1):17–25.

5. Olausson H, Norrsell U. Observations on human tactile directornal sensibility. *J Physiol* 1993;464:545–549.

6. Grill SE, Hallett M. Velocity sensitivity of human muscle spindle afferents and slowly adapting type II cutaneous mechanoreceptors. *J Physiol* 1995;489:593–602.

7. Macefield VG. Physiological characteristics of low-threshold mechanoreceptors in joints, muscle and skin in human subjects. *Clin Exp Pharmacol Physiol* 2005;32:135–144.

8. Isaacs ER, Bookhout MR. *Bourdillion's Spinal Manipulation*. 6th Ed. Woburn, MA: Butterworth Heinemann, 2002.

Within the diagnostic triad of asymmetry, range of motion abnormality, and tissue texture abnormality, perhaps the most significant is the alteration in the range of joint and tissue movement. Loss of normal motion within the tissues of the musculoskeletal system, or one of its component parts, responds most favorably to appropriate manual medicine therapeutic intervention. To achieve the goal of manual medicine intervention and restore maximal, pain-free movement to a musculoskeletal system in postural balance, we must be able to identify both normal and abnormal movements. In the presence of altered movement of the hypomobility type, an appropriate manual medicine intervention might be the treatment of choice. We must strive to improve mobility of all of the tissues of the musculoskeletal system, bone, joint, muscle, ligament, fascia, and fluid, with the anticipated outcome of restoring normal physiologic movement and maximum functional physiology as well.

In the musculoskeletal system, there are inherent movements, voluntary movements, and involuntary movements. The inherent movement has been described by some authors as relating to the recurrent coiling and uncoiling of the brain and longitudinal movement of the spinal cord, together with a fluctuation of the cerebral spinal fluid. Inherent motion is also the movement of the musculoskeletal system in relation to respiration. It has been observed that during inhalation the curves within the vertebral column straighten and with exhalation the curves are increased. With inhalation the extremities rotate externally, and with exhalation, internally. The voluntary movements of the musculoskeletal system are active movements resulting from contraction of muscle from voluntary conscious control. The involuntary movements of the musculoskeletal system are described as passive movements. An external force moving a part of the musculoskeletal system through an arc of motion induces passive movement. The joint-play movements described by Mennell are also involuntary movements. They are not a component of the normal active or passive range of movement but are essential for the accomplishment of normal active and passive movement.

In structural diagnosis, we speak of normal and abnormal barriers to joint and tissue motion. The examiner must be able to identify and characterize normal and abnormal range of movement and normal and abnormal barrier to movement in order to make an accurate diagnosis. Most joints have motion in multiple planes, but for descriptive purposes we describe barriers to movement within one plane of motion for one joint. The total range of motion (Fig. 3.1) from one extreme to the other is limited by the anatomic integrity of the joint and its supporting ligaments, muscles, and fascia. Exceeding the anatomic barrier causes fracture, dislocation, or violation of tissue such as ligamentous tear.

Somewhere within the total range of movement is found a midline neutral point.

Within the total range of motion there is a range of passive movement available that the examiner can extraneously introduce (Fig. 3.2). The limit of this passive range of motion has been described as the "elastic barrier." At this point, all tension has been taken within the joint and its surrounding tissues. There is a small amount of potential space between the elastic barrier and the anatomic barrier described by Sandoz as the paraphysiologic space. It is within this area that the high-velocity, low-amplitude thrust appears to generate the popping sound that results from the maneuver.

The range of active movement (Fig. 3.3) is somewhat less than that available with passive movement, and the end point of the range is called the "physiologic barrier." The normal end feel is due to resilience and tension within the muscle and fascial elements.

Frequently there is reduction in available active motion due primarily to myofascial shortening (Fig. 3.4). This is often seen with aging but it can occur at all ages. It is the stretching of this myofascial shortening that all individuals, particularly athletes, should do as part of physical exercise. Stretching exercise to the muscles and fascia enhances the active motion range available and the efficiency of myofascial function.

When motion is lost within the range it can be described as major (Fig. 3.5) or minimal (Fig. 3.6). The barrier that prevents movement in the direction of motion loss is defined as the "restrictive barrier". The amount of active motion available is limited on one side by the normal physiologic barrier and on the opposite side by the restrictive barrier. The goal of a manual medicine intervention is to move the restrictive barrier as far into the direction of motion loss as possible. Another clinically describable phenomenon associated with motion loss is the shifting of the neutral point from midline to the middle of the available active range. This is described as the "pathologic" neutral and is usually, but not always, in the midrange of active motion available.

Each of the barriers described have palpable findings that can be described as either normal or abnormal end feel. Within a normal range of passive movement, the elastic barrier will have a normal sensation at the end point as a result of the passively induced tension within the joint and its surrounding structures. At the end of the range of active movement, the physiologic barrier likewise has a characteristic feel that results from the voluntary increase in resistance due to the apposition of the joints and the myofascial tension developed during voluntary muscular activity.

Let us return to the layer palpation exercise (see Chapter 2) and begin at the point where one examiner was evaluating the

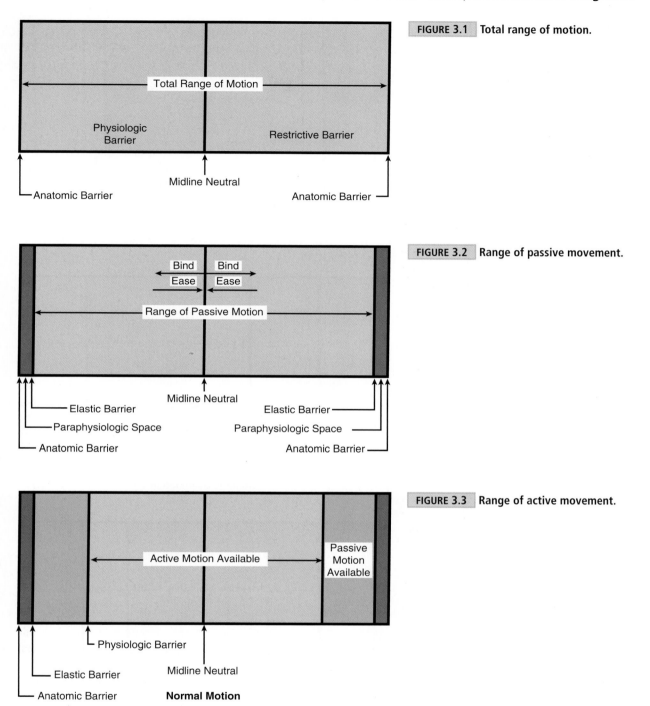

FIGURE 3.1 Total range of motion.

FIGURE 3.2 Range of passive movement.

FIGURE 3.3 Range of active movement.

joint space at the proximal radiohumeral joint (Fig. 3.7). While palpating this joint with the thumb placed anteriorly and the index finger placed posteriorly, have the subject actively introduce pronation and supination (Fig. 3.8). You will note that the range is not symmetric in pronation and supination and that the end feel is not the same at the terminal range of pronation and supination. Which range is greater? Which end feel seems tighter or more abrupt? Now grasp the subject's hand and wrist and passively introduce pronation and supination while monitoring

at the proximal radiohumeral joint (Fig. 3.9). Note that you are now receiving proprioceptive information into your palpating hand as well as into your moving or motor hand as it passively introduces the pronation and supination effort (Fig. 3.10). Again, look for total range of movement, the quality of movement during the range, and the end feel. In supination and pronation, which has the greatest range? Which has the tighter or looser end feel? How does this compare with the active movement? Now let us take it one step further. While passively introducing

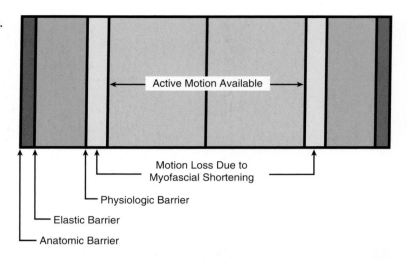

FIGURE 3.4 Reduced range from myofascial shortening.

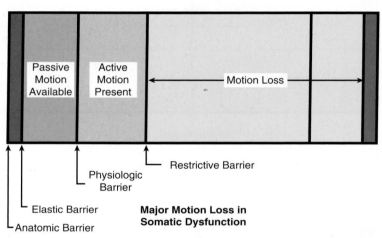

FIGURE 3.5 Major motion loss.

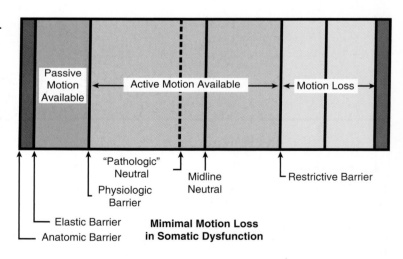

FIGURE 3.6 Minimal motion loss.

pronation and supination you should notice the palpatory sense of tension increase the closer you get to the end points of the range. As you move in the opposite direction, it appears to be easier or freer. See if you can, by decreasing increments of pronation and supination, find the point between the two extremes of movement wherein the joint feel is the freest. Even though pronation and supination are not a symmetric range of movement at this joint, it is possible to find a point within the range that is the freest and could be described as the physiologic neutral point.

We now have another concept of joint motion, the concept of "ease" and "bind" (Fig. 3.11). The more one moves in the direction of the neutral point, whether a midline neutral point in a normal range of motion or a "pathologic" neutral point

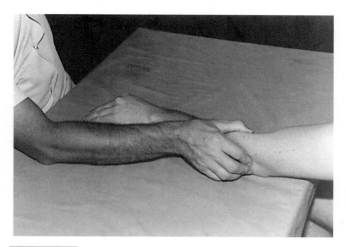

FIGURE 3.7 Palpate radiohumeral joint.

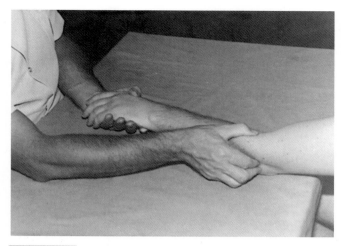

FIGURE 3.9 Passive pronation–supination.

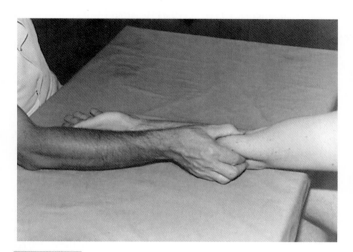

FIGURE 3.8 Active pronation–supination.

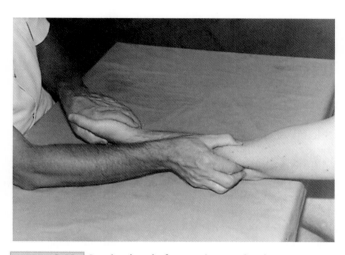

FIGURE 3.10 Sensing hand of pronation–supination.

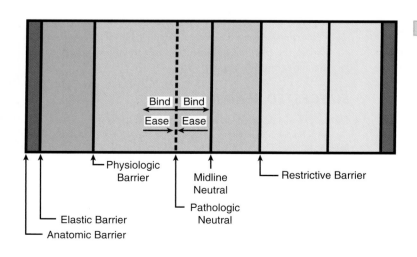

FIGURE 3.11 Neutral ease–bind point.

somewhere within the range of altered motion, it becomes more free, or there is more "ease." Conversely, as one moves away from the neutral "free" point, one begins to sense a certain amount of "bind," or increase in resistance to the induced movement. Understanding this concept of ease and bind, and the ability to sense this phenomenon, is essential to localize to the feather edge of the restrictive barrier before performing a muscle energy technique or in mastering the functional (indirect) techniques (see Chapter 10). In the elbow exercise that you just accomplished, the hand palpating over the proximal radiohumeral joint was the "sensing hand," and your other hand that introduced passive supination and pronation at the subject's hand was the "motor hand."

RESTRICTIVE BARRIERS

The restrictive barriers limit movement within the normal range of motion and have palpatory characteristics different from the normal physiologic, elastic, and anatomic barriers. The restrictive barrier can be within the following tissues:

Skin
Fascia
Muscle, long and short
Ligament
Joint capsule and surfaces

Restrictive barriers can be found within one or more of these tissues and the number and type contribute to the palpable characteristics at the restrictive barrier. Different pathologic changes within these tissues can give quite different end feel sensations. For example, congestion and edema within the tissues will give a diffuse, boggy sensation quite like a sponge filled with water. Chronic fibrosis within these tissues will give a harder, more unyielding, rapidly ascending end feel when compared to the more boggy, edematous sensation. A restrictive barrier due to altered muscle physiology, whether it be spasm, hypertonus, or contracture, will give a more jerky and tightening type of end feel than one due to edema or fibrosis. Do not forget that pain can be a restrictive barrier as well. If a movement is painful, it will result in restriction as the body attempts to compensate for relief of pain by reduction of movement. When examining ranges of movement, and particularly when looking for normal and abnormal barriers to movement, one should constantly keep in mind the potential for hypermobility. The classic feel of a hypermobile range of motion is one of looseness for a greater extent of the range than would be anticipated, and with a rapidly escalating, hard end feel when one approaches the elastic and anatomic barriers.

Restrictive barriers may be long or short. They may involve a single joint or spinal segment, or cross over more than one joint or series of spinal segments. It is important to identify the tissue or tissues involved in the restrictive barrier, their extent, and the functional pathology found within the tissues. Some types of manual medicine intervention are more appropriate for certain restrictive barriers than others.

In structural diagnosis, alteration of range of movement is an essential criterion for a diagnosis of somatic dysfunction. It is necessary to evaluate the total range of movement, the quality of movement available during the range, and the feel at the end point of movement in order to make an accurate diagnosis of the restrictive barrier. Therapeutic intervention by manipulative means can be described as an approach to these pathologic barriers. Multiple methods are available and different activating forces can be used toward the goal of restoring maximal physiologic movement available within the anatomy of the joint(s) and tissue(s).

DEFINITIONS

1. *Active motion*: Movement of an articulation between the physiologic barriers limited to the range produced voluntarily by the patient.
2. *Anatomic barrier*: The bone contour and/or soft tissues, especially ligaments, which serve as the final limit to motion in an articulation beyond which tissue damage occurs.
3. *Barrier*: An obstruction; a factor that tends to restrict free movement.
4. *Elastic barrier*: The resistance felt at the end of passive range of motion when the slack has been taken out.
5. *Motion*: Movement, act, process, or instance of changing places.
6. *Paraphysiologic space*: The sensation of a sudden "give" beyond the elastic barrier of resistance, usually accompanied by a "cracking" sound with a slight amount of movement beyond the usual physiologic limit but within the anatomic barrier.
7. *Passive motion*: Movement induced in an articulation by the operator. This includes the range of active motion as well as the movement between the physiologic and anatomic barriers permitted by soft-tissue resiliency that the patient cannot do voluntarily.
8. *Physiologic barrier*: The soft-tissue tension accumulation that limits the voluntary motion of an articulation. Further motion toward the anatomic barrier can be induced passively.
9. *Restrictive barrier*: An impediment or obstacle to movement within the physiologic limits of an articulation that reduces the active motion range.

SUGGESTED READINGS

Beal MC. Motion sense. *J Am Osteopath Assoc* 1953;53:151–153.
Good AB. Spinal joint blocking. *J Manipulative Physio Ther* 1985;8:1–8.
Sandoz, R. Some physical mechanisms and effects of spinal adjustments. *Ann Swiss Chiro Assoc* 1976;6:91–141.

Chapter 4

THE MANIPULATIVE PRESCRIPTION

In the practice of medicine, it is essential that an accurate diagnosis be made before the institution of either curative or palliative therapy. When a therapeutic intervention is indicated, particularly when using pharmacotherapeutic agents, a specific and accurate prescription must be written. No self-respecting physician would make a diagnosis of throat infection and write a prescription for an antibiotic.

Diagnosis (DX)—Throat infection
Prescription (RX)—Antibiotic

The physician would seek to identify the infectious agent, either bacterial or viral, causing the throat infection. When a specific infectious agent responsive to antibiotic therapy is identified, a specific prescription would be written for the antibiotic agent. The prescription would identify the antibiotic to be used, the strength of each dose, the number of doses per day, and the duration of therapy.

In manual medicine it is common for practitioners to be lax in their specificity for the structural diagnosis and prescription of the manual medicine intervention to be applied. Too often, a diagnosis is made of somatic dysfunction and manual medicine is the prescription, such as

DX—Somatic dysfunction
RX—Manipulative treatment

In manual medicine, it is just as important to know the location, nature, and type of somatic dysfunction before a specific manual medicine therapeutic intervention is prescribed. The same elements are needed for a manual medicine prescription as for a pharmaceutical agent. One wants to be specific about the type of manual medicine, the intensity, the frequency, and the total length of the treatment plan. Therefore, the manipulative prescription requires an accurate diagnosis of the somatic dysfunction to be treated and a specific description of the type of manipulative procedure, the intensity, and the frequency.

Manipulative therapeutic procedures are indicated for the diagnostic entity somatic dysfunction or the manipulable lesion.

SOMATIC DYSFUNCTION

Somatic dysfunction is impaired or altered function of related components of the somatic (body framework) system: skeletal, arthrodial, and myofascial structures, and the related vascular, lymphatic, and neural elements.

MANIPULABLE LESION SYNONYMS

- Joint blockage
- Joint lock
- Chiropractic subluxation
- Osteopathic lesion
- Loss of joint play
- Minor intervertebral derangements

DIAGNOSTIC TRIAD

In defining somatic dysfunction, one uses three elements:

"**A**" for asymmetry of form or function of related parts of the musculoskeletal system.

"**R**" for range of motion, primarily alteration of motion, looking at range, quality of motion during the range, and the "end feel" at the limit of movement.

"**T**" for tissue texture abnormality with alteration in the feel of the soft tissues, mainly muscle hypertonicity, and in skin and connective tissues, described as hot/cold, soft/hard, boggy, doughy, and so forth. Most of the tissue texture abnormalities result from altered nervous system function with increased alpha motor neuron activity maintaining muscle hypertonicity and altered sympathetic autonomic nervous system function to the skin viscera, vasomotor, pseudomotor, and pilomotor activity.

CLINICAL GOALS FOR MANIPULATIVE TREATMENT

As previously stated, the goal of manipulation is the use of the hands in a patient-management process, using instructions and maneuvers to achieve maximal, painless, movement of the musculoskeletal (motor) system in postural balance. In achieving this goal, different types of therapeutic effects upon the patient can be sought. They can be classified as follows:

1. Circulatory effects
   a. Move body fluids
   b. Provide tonic effect
2. Neurologic effect—modify reflexes
   a. Somato-somatic
   b. Somato-visceral
   c. Viscero-somatic
   d. Viscero-visceral
   e. Viscero-somato-visceral
   f. Somato-viscero-somatic
3. Maintenance therapy for irreversible conditions

Depending on the desired outcome, the therapeutic application will use different models of manual medicine.

MODELS AND MECHANISMS OF MANUAL MEDICINE INTERVENTION

Several different conceptual models can be used in determining the manual medicine approach to a patient. Five such models will be described, but it should be evident that when a manual medicine procedure is provided, it has multiple effects and is mediated through a number of different mechanisms.

Postural Structural or Biomechanical Model

The postural structural model is probably the one most familiar to practitioners of manual medicine. In this model, the patient is approached from a biomechanical orientation toward the musculoskeletal system. The osseous skeleton is viewed as a series of building blocks piled one on top of the other, starting with the bones of the foot and ending with the skull. The ligamentous and fascial structures are the tissues that connect the osseous framework, and the muscles are the prime movers of the bones of the skeleton, working across single and multiple joint structures. Alteration of the patient's musculoskeletal system is viewed from the alignment of the bones and joints, the balance of muscles as movers and stabilizers of the skeleton, the symmetry of tone of the ligaments, and the integrity of the continuous bands of fascia throughout. Alteration in joint apposition, alteration in muscle function due to hypertonicity or weakness, tightness or laxity of ligament(s), and shortening or lengthening of fascia are all considered when approaching a patient from this perspective. The manual medicine treatment would be directed toward restoring maximal motion to all joints, symmetry of length and strength to all muscles and ligaments, and symmetry of tension within fascial elements throughout the body. The goal is to restore maximal function of this musculoskeletal system in postural balance. The patient can be approached starting at the feet and ending with the head or vice versa, starting from the top and ending at the feet.

The most important element of the postural structural model in this author's experience has been the restoration of maximum pelvic mechanics in the walking cycle. The pelvis becomes the cornerstone of the postural structural model. Influences from below or above must be considered to achieve symmetric movement of the osseous pelvis during walking.[1]

This model is most useful in approaching patients with pain resulting from either single instances of trauma or microtrauma over time due to postural imbalance from such entities as anatomic shortening of one leg, unilateral fallen arch, and so forth. This conceptual model includes much of the current biomechanical engineering research in the areas of joint mechanics; properties of ligaments, tendons, and fascia; and kinetics and kinematics.[2]

Neurologic Model

The neurologic model concerns influencing neural mechanisms through manual medicine intervention. One mechanism of action is through the autonomic nervous system. There is a large body of basic research regarding the influence of the somatic (motor) system on the function of the autonomic nervous system, primarily the sympathetic division. This basic research is consistent with clinical observations, but additional clinical research is needed into the influence of alteration in function of the musculoskeletal system on total body function

mediated through the sympathetic division of the autonomic nervous system.

Autonomic Nervous System Model

The concept is based on the organization of the sympathetic nervous system. The preganglionic fibers take their origin from the spinal cord from T1 to L3. The lateral chain ganglia are paired and overlie the posterior thoracic and abdominal walls, where synaptic junction occurs with postganglionic fibers. The lateral chain ganglia in the thoracic region are tightly bound by the fascia to the posterior chest wall and overlie the heads of the ribs. Measurable sympathetic nervous system changes have been demonstrated following thoracic manipulation[3]; and it is hypothesized that altered mechanics of the costovertebral articulations could mechanically influence the lateral chain ganglia, or the peripheral ganglia, through which the sympathetic nervous system synapses with postganglionic fibers that are relatively adjacent to the organs being innervated.

The sympathetic nervous system is the sole source of autonomic nervous system activity to the musculoskeletal system. There is no parasympathetic innervation to the somatic tissues. The sympathetic nervous system has wide influence on visceral function, endocrine organs, reticuloendothelial system, circulatory system, peripheral nervous system, central nervous system, and muscle. Korr has worked extensively on the function of the sympathetic nervous system and points out the wide diversity of influence that sympathetic hyperactivity has on target end organs. Many factors can affect sympathetic hypertonia, one of which is afferent impulses from segmentally related areas of soma. It would seem reasonable, therefore, to attempt to reduce aberrant afferent stimulus to hyperirritable sections of the sympathetic nervous system to reduce the hyperactivity on target end organs.[4]

Because the sympathetic nervous system is organized segmentally, it can be used in a maplike fashion to look for both alterations of afferent stimulus and areas that might be influenced through manual medicine intervention. All of the viscera and soma above the diaphragm receive their preganglionic sympathetic nervous system fibers from above cord level T4. All viscera and soma below the diaphragm receive preganglionic sympathetic nervous system fibers from T5 and below. Understanding this anatomy helps in relating the identified somatic dysfunction to the patient's problem and can lead the physician to give appropriate manual medicine treatment to those areas of somatic dysfunction thought to contribute increased somatic afferent stimuli to cord levels with manifestations of increased sympathetic nervous system activity.[5]

The parasympathetic nervous system takes its origin from the brain, brainstem, and sacral segments of the cord. Its organization differs from the segmental aspects of the sympathetic division, but its segmentation relates to the origin of the cranial nerves in the brainstem and the segmentation of the sacral cord. The cranial nerves, including those with parasympathetic activity, exit from the skull through numerous foramina and penetrate the dura. These nerves are at risk for entrapment with alteration of cranial mechanics and dural tension. Often, the clinical goal of craniosacral technique is to improve the function of cranial nerves as they exit the skull and sacrum. The autonomic nervous system neurologic model leads the therapist toward a patient approach based on the anatomy/physiology of the two divisions of the autonomic nervous system and how best to affect them through manual medicine means.

Pain Model A second neurologic model focuses more on the interrelationships of the peripheral and central nervous systems, their reflex patterns, and their multiple pathways. This model is particularly useful in managing patients with pain syndromes, such as back pain. Although controversy remains about the origin of back pain, much is known about the location and type of nociceptors and mechanoreceptors within the musculoskeletal system.[6] The pain stimulus can originate in a number of tissues and be transmitted by peripheral afferent neurons to the spinal cord for integration and organization. Different neurons end in different laminae of the dorsal horn and synapse with interneurons that transmit information up and down the spinal cord, thus affecting other neuronal pools through propriospinal pathways. Transmission up the cord to higher centers can be through the fast or slow pain pathways. Pain is perceived in the brain and stimulatory or inhibitory activities can enhance or reduce the pain perception. These processes are programmed through the brainstem and back down the cord to modulate activity at cord segmental level.

An understanding of the anatomy and physiology of the musculoskeletal system and nervous systems, particularly the spine and paraspinal tissues, is necessary to develop a therapeutic plan to manage the patient's pain syndrome. A clear distinction must be made between acute pain and chronic pain. Acute pain is that which is best known to the clinician. It results from tissue damage, is well localized, has clear objective evidence of injury, and has a sharp pricking quality. There may be some lingering burning and aching. Acute pain responds well to treatment and abates when the tissue damage has resolved. Chronic pain persists despite the lack of ongoing tissue damage. It is poorly localized with no objective evidence present. It has a burning aching quality with a strong associated affective component. Changes have occurred in the central pathways and central endogenous control. It is unclear as to when chronic pain begins, but it is generally accepted that ongoing pain beyond three months results in central pathway changes. Acute and chronic pains respond differently to therapeutic interventions. Manual medicine has a role in the treatment of both acute and chronic musculoskeletal pain syndromes. In the acute condition, manual medicine attempts to reduce the ongoing afferent stimulation of the nociceptive process.[7] If it is determined that muscle contraction and hypertonicity are primary factors, muscle energy procedures might be most beneficial. If it is believed that altered mechanoreceptive behavior in the articular and periarticular structure of the zygapophyseal joint is the primary factor, a mobilizing procedure with or without impulse might be more appropriate. The goal of manual medicine in the patient with chronic pain is to restore the maximum functional capacity of the musculoskeletal system so that exercises and increased activities of daily living can occur. It is difficult for a patient with

chronic pain to undergo exercise therapy and reconditioning rehabilitative processes in the presence of restricted mobility of the musculoskeletal system.

Stability Model The third concept within the neurologic model is that of dynamic stability. Recently, a large focus on trunk control and dynamic joint stabilization has immersed itself on the physical therapy and biomechanical literature.[8] The primary tenet is a respect for the body's utilization of neuromuscular "feedforward" neurologic mechanisms, to prepare it to accomplish a task, and "feedback" neurologic mechanisms, to prevent injury or strain in the case of unexpected perturbation. Dynamic stability of the spine relies on the interdependent relationship of active (muscular), passive (articular/ligamentous), and neuromuscular subsystems defined by Panjabi.[9] The active subsystem component of most importance for dynamic stabilization is the muscles which control "neutral" joint position. These "stabilizer muscles are described as having the characteristics of being monoarticular or segmental, deep, working eccentrically to control movement, and having static holding capacities."[10] The passive subsystem consists of the articular surface, ligaments, and discs which provide structural control, movement checks, and critical afferent kinesthetic information via its mechanoreceptors.[11] The neuromuscular subsystem relies on the central nervous feedforward control as well as feedback neurologic information from the active and passive subsystems. Although joint dysfunction resulting in musculoskeletal pain is often approached from the biomechanical model; there has been a significant amount of research suggesting an association with inhibition of the local stabilizers as well as deficits in feed forward and/or feedback neurologic mechanisms[12] and thus deserves a neurologic consideration.

Neuroendocrine Model

The fourth concept within the neurologic model is that of neuroendocrine control. Since the late 1970s, there has been a rapidly expanding body of knowledge about the role of endorphins, enkephalins, and other neural peptides. These substances are not only active in the nervous system but also profoundly affect the immune system. There appears to be ample evidence that alteration in musculoskeletal activity influences their liberation and activity.[13] It has been hypothesized that some of the beneficial effects of manipulative treatment might result from the release of endorphins and enkephalins with subsequent reduction in the perception of pain. Because of the influence of the substances in areas other than the central nervous system, other systemic effects may result from manual medicine procedures. This neuroendocrine mechanism might explain some of the general body tonic effects of manual medicine interventions.

All of these neurologic mechanisms are highly complex and have been only superficially dealt with here. They can be used, however, as conceptual models to approach a patient with a myriad of problems.

Respiratory Circulatory Model

The respiratory circulatory model looks at a different dimension of musculoskeletal system activity. In this model, the patient is viewed from the perspective of blood and lymph flow. Skeletal muscles and the diaphragm are the pumps of the venous and lymphatic systems. The goal is restoring the functional capacity of the musculoskeletal system to assist return circulation and the work of respiration. The function of the diaphragm to modify the relative negative intrathoracic pressure to assist in inhalation and exhalation requires that the torso, including the thoracic cage and the abdomen, have the capacity to respond to these pressure gradient changes. Thus, the thoracic spine and the rib cage must be functionally flexible, particularly the lower six ribs where the diaphragm attaches. The lumbar spine must be flexible enough to change its anterior curvature for breathing. The abdominal musculature should have symmetric tone and length and the pelvic diaphragm should be balanced and nonrestrictive.

The respiratory circulatory model looks at somatic dysfunction(s) and its influence on fluid movement and ease of respiration, rather than neural entrapment or biomechanical alteration. Thus, some of the techniques applied are less segmentally specific and are more concerned with tissue tension that might impede fluid flow. The guiding principle of this model is the progression from central to distal. The beginning point is usually in the thoracic cage, primarily at the thoracic inlet, so that the tissues of the thoracic cage are able to respond to respiratory effort and the pumping action of the diaphragm to receive the fluids trapped in the peripheral tissues. Attention to the thoracic inlet also aids in the drainage of fluid from the head, neck, and upper extremities. Recall that all of the lymph ultimately drains into the venous system at the thoracic inlet behind the anterior extremity of the first rib and the medial end of the clavicle. When the thoracic cage is functioning at maximal capacity, one progresses to the lumbar spine, pelvis, and lower extremities attempting to remove any potential obstruction to fluid flow that occurs in these tissues. The therapeutic goals of the respiratory–circulatory model are to reduce the work of breathing and to enhance the pumping action of the diaphragm and the extremity muscles to assist lymphatic and venous flow.[14–17]

Bioenergy Model

The bioenergy model is somewhat more ethereal than the preceding and focuses on the inherent energy flow within the body. Some clinicians are skilled at both observing and feeling energy transmission, and the absence of it, from patients. We are all familiar with the phenomena of Kirlian photography that enables us to visualize radiant energy outside the anatomic limits of the body. This may be but one example of perceptible energy that emanates from the human organism. The bioenergy model focuses on the maximization of normal energy flow within the human body and its response to its environment. Many clinicians have reported sensations of release of energy that appear to emanate from the patient during manual medicine procedures.

There is also the element of the transfer of energy from the therapeutic touch of the physician. Many of the ancient, oriental forms of healing have focused on elements of "life force," "energy field," and so forth, and it is within this domain that a manual medicine practitioner can apply this conceptual model.

The craniosacral manual medicine approach is one in which one of the major goals of treatment is to restore the normal inherent force of the central nervous system, including the brain, spinal cord, meninges, and cerebral spinal fluid, to maximize a symmetric, smooth, normal rhythmic CRI (cranial rhythmic impulse).

Psychobehavioral Model

The psychobehavioral model views the patient from the perspective of enhancing the capacity for them to "safely" relate to both the internal and external environments. There are many racial, social, and economic factors that influence the patient's perception of such things as pain, health, illness, disease, disability, and death. The patient's ability or inability to cope with all the stresses of life may manifest itself in a wide variety of symptoms and physical signs. To understand the connection between trauma, stress, and emotion and the somatic system, one would be wise to read Steven Porges' "Polyvagal Theory."[18] His writings help us understand our patients with poor coping skills and chronic pain associated with autonomic nervous system alterations such as bradycardia, hypotension, connective tissue disease, autoimmune dysfunction, and hypoxia. The physician's ability to understand the patient's response to stress and coping skills and the methods to assist the patient with the process are important components of this conceptual model. "Therapeutic touch" is an integral part of the doctor–patient interaction in this model. The influence of manual medicine may be less a biomechanical, neurologic, or circulatory effect than just an important safe and caring function. Awareness of this model is also important in understanding the difficulty in clinical research within manual medicine because of the "placebo" effect of the "laying on of hands."[19]

It is beyond the scope of this volume to do anything but highlight the various models that are available for consideration when using a manual medicine intervention. It should be obvious that more than one model can be operative at the same intervention. It is strongly recommended, however, that the physician use some conceptual model before a manual medicine intervention. I support the contention of F.L. Mitchell, Jr (personal communication, 1974) that manual medicine therapy is more than "a search and destroy mission of somatic dysfunction."

MANUAL MEDICINE ARMAMENTARIUM

Manual medicine procedures are classified and described below.

Soft-Tissue Procedures

The soft-tissue procedures use manual application of force directed toward influencing specific tissue(s) of the musculoskeletal system or, by peripheral stimulation, enhancing some form of reflex mechanism that alters biologic function. The direct procedures include massage, effleurage, kneading, stretching, friction rub, and so forth. These procedures can prepare the tissues for additional specific joint mobilization or can be a therapeutic end in themselves. The therapeutic goals are to overcome congestion, reduce muscle spasm, improve tissue mobility, enhance circulation, and "tonify" the tissue. These procedures are some of the first learned and practiced by manual medicine physicians and can be used effectively in a variety of patient conditions.

A number of reflex mechanisms have been described that stimulate the peripheral tissues of the musculoskeletal system. These include acupuncture, reflex therapy, Chapman reflexes, Travell trigger points, and so forth. In these procedures, a manual, mechanical, or electrical stimulus is applied to certain areas of the body to enhance a therapeutic response. Some of these systems have been postulated for neurologic models, lymphatic models, neuroendocrine models, and in some instances, without any explanation for the observable clinical phenomena. Suffice it to say, many of these peripheral stimulating therapeutic points are consistent across patients, observable by multiple examiners, and provide a predictable response.

Articulatory Procedures

The articulatory procedures (mobilization without impulse) are used extensively in physiotherapy. They consist primarily of putting the elements of the musculoskeletal system, particularly the articulations, through ranges of motion in some graded fashion, with the goal of enhancement of the quantity and quality of motion. These procedures are therapeutic extensions of the diagnostic process of evaluating range of motion. If there appears to be a restriction of motion in one direction, with some alteration in sense of ease of movement in that direction, a series of gentle, rhythmic, operator-directed efforts in the direction of motion restriction can be found to be therapeutically effective. These articulatory procedures are especially useful for their tonic and/or circulatory effect.

Specific Joint Mobilization

The specific joint mobilization procedures all have two common elements: method, that is, the method of approaching the restricted barrier, and activating force, that is, the intrinsic or extrinsic forces(s) exerted.

Methods   The specific joint mobilization methods are as follows.

1. *Direct method*: All direct procedures engage the restrictive barrier and by application of some force attempt to move the restrictive barrier in the direction of motion loss.
2. *Exaggeration method*: This therapeutic effort applies a force against the normal physiologic barrier in the direction opposite that of the motion loss. The force is usually a high-velocity, low-amplitude thrust and has been quite successful. There are systems of manual medicine that only provide therapeutic force in the direction of pain-free movement, and it is within this exaggeration method that such therapy seems to be operative.
3. *Indirect method*: In these procedures, the operator moves the segment away from the restrictive barrier into the range of "freedom" or "ease" of movement to a point of balanced tension ("floating" of the segment(s)). The segment can then be

held in that position for 5 to 90 seconds to relax the tension in the tissues around the articulations so that enhanced mobility occurs. Procedures using this method are termed "functional technique," "balance-and-hold technique," and "release-by-positioning technique."
4. *Combined method*: Sometimes it is useful to use combinations of direct, exaggeration, and indirect methods in sequence to assist in the ultimate therapeutic outcome. Frequently, a combined method series of procedures is more effective than multiple applications of the same method.
5. *Physiologic response method*: These procedures apply patient positioning and movement direction to obtain a therapeutic result. A series of body positions may use nonneutral mechanics to restore neutral mechanics to the spinal complex of the musculoskeletal system. Another example of a physiologic method is the use of respiratory effort to affect mobility of vertebral segments within spinal curvatures. Inhalation effort enhances straightening of the curves and hence backward-bending movement in the thoracic spine and forward bending in the cervical and lumbar spines; exhalation effort causes just the reverse.

Activating Forces   The activating forces can be categorized as extrinsic and intrinsic. The extrinsic forces are those that are applied from outside the patient's body directly to the patient. These can include

1. Operator effort, such as guiding, springing, and thrust;
2. Adjunctive, such as straps, pads, traction, and so on;
3. Gravity, which is the weight of the body part, and the patient position.

The intrinsic group includes those forces that occur from within the patient's body and are used for their therapeutic effectiveness. They are classified as

1. Inherent forces, or nature's tendency toward balance and homeostasis
2. Respiratory force
   a. Inhalation, which straightens curves in vertebral column and externally rotates extremities
   b. Exhalation, which enhances curves in vertebral column and internally rotates extremities
3. Muscle force of the patient
   a. Muscle cooperation
   b. Muscle energy, especially isometrics
4. Reflex activity
   a. Eye movement
   b. Muscle activation

Afferent Reduction Procedures

The afferent reduction procedures appear to work on a model of reducing aberrant afferent activity from the various mechanoreceptors found within the various tissues of the musculoskeletal system. The working hypothesis is that altered behavior of the musculoskeletal system provides aberrant stimulation to the central nervous system that alters the programming of musculoskeletal function. Identifying various positions and maneuvers that reduce the afferent bombardment to the spinal cord and central levels can provide an opportunity to restore more normal behavior. It is thought that many of the indirect approaches, including the dynamic functional techniques, balance-and-hold techniques, and release-by positioning techniques, work through this mechanism.

MANIPULATION UNDER ANESTHESIA

Manipulation under anesthesia has had a long history in manual medicine. It is used for dysfunction within the spinal complex, particularly the lumbosacral and cervical regions, as well as peripheral joints. The procedures performed are mobilization with impulse (high-velocity, low-amplitude thrust technique) with the patient under general, regional, or local anesthesia. Its use requires skilled anesthesia and a high level of competence of the manipulating practitioner. The indications are acute or chronic vertebral dysfunctions that cannot be managed by nonoperative, conservative means. Muscle spasm and irritability may preclude a successful manual medicine procedure without anesthesia. In chronic myofibrositis, manipulation under anesthesia may enhance the response unobtainable by more conservative measures. The indications are not high. Morey reported that only 3% of patients hospitalized with musculoskeletal disorders in a 3-year period required manipulation under anesthesia. Complications are rare, but the procedure is contraindicated in patients who cannot tolerate the anesthetic and those in whom manual medicine is not viewed as appropriate.

It is possible to design multiple variations of method and activating force to achieve the desired clinical goal. All of the procedures in manual medicine can be viewed as having a common goal, which is to reprogram the behavior of the central nervous system. Using the analogy of the computer, manual medicine deals with the "hardware" of the musculoskeletal system and modulates the behavior of the "software" in the central nervous system. The more optimal the behavior of the central nervous system, the better the function of the musculoskeletal system. The anatomy (hardware) may be altered by developmental variant; trauma, both single and repetitive; and surgery. Despite the changes in the anatomy, the goal of manual medicine is to restore the maximum functional capacity that the anatomy will allow. The more skilled one becomes in using different methods and activating forces, the more successful one becomes as a manual medicine therapist.

FACTORS INFLUENCING TYPE OF MANIPULATIVE PROCEDURES

In addition to a wide variety of types and styles of manual medicine procedures available and a number of different clinical goals, other factors influence the type of manual medicine procedure instituted.

1. Age of patient
2. Acuteness or chronicity of problem
3. General physical condition of patient
4. Operator size and ability
5. Location (office, home, hospital, etc.)
6. Effectiveness of previous and/or present therapy

If one were prescribing a pharmaceutical agent, the dosage would be adjusted to the age of the patient. This is also the case in the use of manual medicine. Clearly, one approaches an infant differently from a young adult. In an elderly debilitated patient, one is much more careful and judicious in the use of some of the more forceful direct action types of technique. Osteoporosis in the female is not necessarily a contraindication to manual medicine, but indirect procedures with intrinsic activating forces would be more appropriate.

The type of manual medicine procedure is also modified by the acuteness or chronicity of the problem. In acute conditions, inflammatory swelling and acute muscle spasms are frequently encountered. The physician might use the respiratory–circulatory model to relieve the inflammatory congestion and perhaps some soft-tissue procedure to reduce the amount of acute muscle spasm. In more chronic conditions with long-standing fibrosis in the ligaments, muscles, and fascia, a more direct action myofascial release or direct action mobilization with impulse (high-velocity thrust) procedure might be more appropriate. In the acutely ill patient with reduced capacity to withstand aggressive, intensive therapy, a more conservative approach such as indirect technique might be more appropriate. Remember that manual medicine procedures, particularly those using intrinsic activating forces, result in energy expenditure by the patient. Keep the therapeutic application within the physical capacity of the acutely ill patient. In chronic conditions, do not expect to overcome all of the difficulty with a single manual medicine intervention.

The operator's size, strength, and technical ability will also influence the type of procedure used. Although strength is not necessarily the primary determinant of a successful procedure, the proper application of leverage usually is. Understanding of and ability in a number of manual medicine procedures make a more effective clinician. With only one antibiotic available, the ability to treat an infectious disease is clearly hampered. Likewise, with only one form of manual medicine treatment, one is clearly hampered as an effective manual medicine practitioner.

The physician should have the capacity to provide an effective manual medicine treatment regardless of the location of the patient. Although there are some procedures that are more effective in the office setting with specific therapeutic tables, stools, and other equipment, one should be able to devise an effective procedure anywhere. In a hospital bed or at home on a soft mattress, the capacity to use a high-velocity, low-amplitude thrust is compromised. Muscle energy activating forces and other intrinsic force techniques are more appropriate in such locations.

Past therapy is also highly important in determining the type of procedure to be used. You must know if there has been a previous surgical intervention, manual medicine intervention, or pharmacotherapeutic treatment. If surgery has changed the anatomy, you might wish to modify the therapeutic procedure to meet the altered anatomy. Lack of response to previous manual medicine treatment is not necessarily a reason not to use a different manual medicine treatment. Previous medication, particularly muscle relaxants, tranquilizers, and antiinflammatory agents, might modify the type of procedure to be used. With long-standing steroid therapy, be aware of the potential for laxity of ligaments and softening of cancellous bone.

These are but a few of the factors that affect the choice of a manual medicine procedure. In addition, there are three cardinal rules for any effective manual medicine procedure: control, balance, and localization.

Control includes the physician's control of body position in relationship to the patient, control of the patient in a comfortable position, control of intrinsic or extrinsic forces, and control of the type of therapeutic intervention being applied. Balance of patient and operator ensures adequate patient relaxation and the ability of the operator to engage the restrictive barrier in comfort. Localization refers to adequate engagement of a restrictive barrier in a direct action procedure, localization on the point of maximum ease in a balance-and-hold indirect procedure, and localization of the most painfree position in a release-by-positioning procedure.

CONTRAINDICATION TO MANUAL MEDICINE PROCEDURES

Much has been written about absolute and relative contraindications to manual medicine procedures. This author holds the view that there are none, if—and it is a big if—there is an accurate diagnosis of somatic dysfunction that requires treatment to effect the overall management of the patient, and if the manual medicine procedure is appropriate for that diagnosis and the physical condition of the patient. However, there are a number of conditions that require special precautions. Some of these are as follows:

1. The vertebral artery in the cervical spine.
2. Primary joint disease (e.g., rheumatoid arthritis, infectious arthritis, etc.).
3. Metabolic bone disease (e.g., osteoporosis, etc.).
4. Primary or metastatic malignant bone disease.
5. Genetic disorders (e.g., Down syndrome), particularly in the cervical spine.
6. Hypermobility in the involved segments. This should clearly be avoided. One should look for restricted mobility elsewhere in the presence of hypermobility.

Following these principles, a specific and appropriate manual medicine therapeutic prescription can be written for a diagnosis, much as with traditional therapeutic interventions. Returning to our original example, the thinking physician identifies the infectious agent in a throat infection before deciding on a therapeutic intervention. If, for example, the throat infection was due to a streptococcus, the physician might select ampicillin as the antibiotic of choice. With the specific infectious agent identified and an appropriate antibiotic chosen, then adequate dosage on an appropriate schedule for a sufficient length of time would be ordered.

DX—Throat infection (streptococcal)
RX—Ampicillin 250 mg every 6 hours for 10 days

With an appropriate diagnosis of somatic dysfunction, an accurate manual medicine prescription can be written on the basis of the principles addressed above. One would choose the type of procedure and specify the method, activating force, dosage, length of treatment time, and frequency of treatments.

DX—Somatic dysfunction, T6, extended, rotated, and side bent right (ERS_{right})
RX—Manual medicine, direct action muscle energy type to flexion, left rotation, and left-side bending. Reexamine in 48 hours.

The specific somatic dysfunction has been identified with its position and subsequent motion restriction. A direct procedure and an intrinsic activating force were chosen. It was anticipated that the effectiveness of the procedure would last 48 hours and therefore reexamination at that time was indicated.

COMPLICATIONS

It is difficult to have an accurate estimation of the incidence of complications from manual medicine procedures. Some authors have defined the rate at one to two per million procedures. A well-controlled study by Dvorak and Orelli identified symptom exaggeration as one in 40,000 and a significant complication as one in 400,000. Most of the complications involve vascular and neural structures. Obvious complications occur when a procedure is contraindicated. Many of the complications occur from manipulation in the cervical spine resulting in insult to the vertebrobasilar artery system. Fractures and dislocations as well as spinal cord injury have been identified. Complications of exaggeration of disc herniation with progressive radiculopathy after manipulation are controversial. Some authors view mobilization with impulse as contraindicated in the presence of disc herniation, whereas others believe that it is indicated in certain conditions if appropriately applied. Postmanipulation injury to the vertebral basilar artery system occurs in the 30- to 45-year-old age group with a slight preponderance in the female population. Death rates approach 22% and significant disability occurs in 75% to 80%. Complete recovery is available to only a small number. The avoidance of complications requires the practitioner to be knowledgeable about the patient's diagnosis, have an appreciation of their own level of skill and experience, and have the ability to deal with complications if they occur. Although the incidence is low, they are to be avoided if possible.

As manual medicine practitioners, we should all prescribe our therapy as precisely as we prescribe any other therapeutic agent. It is hoped that these principles will assist in the appropriate use of manual medicine.

SUGGESTED READINGS

Dvorak J, Orelli F. How dangerous is manipulation to the cervical spine? *Man Med* 1985;2:1–4.

Greenman PE. Manipulation with the patient under anesthesia. *J Am Osteopath Assoc* 1992;92:1159–1170.

Kimberly PK. Formulating a prescription for osteopathic manipulative treatment. *J Am Osteopath Assoc* 1976;75:486–499.

Korr IM. *The Segmental Nervous System as a Mediator and Organizer of Disease Processes. The Physiological Basis of Osteopathic Medicine.* New York, NY: Postgraduate Institute of Osteopathic Medicine & Surgery, 1970:73–84.

Mitchell FL Sr. *Motion Discordance*. Carmel, CA: Yearbook of the Academy of Applied Osteopathy, 1967:1–5.

Morey LW Jr. Osteopathic manipulation under general anesthesia. *J Am Osteopath Assoc* 1973;73:84–95.

Morey LW Jr. Manipulation under general anesthesia. *Osteopath Ann* 1976;4: 127–135.

Romney IC. Manipulation of the spine and appendages under anesthesia. *J Am Osteopath Assoc* 1968;68:235–245.

REFERENCES

1. Greenman PE. Syndromes of the lumbar spine, pelvis, and sacrum. *Phys Med Rehabil Clin North Am* 1996;7:773–785.

2. Vleeming A, Mooney V, Snijders CJ, et al. *Movement, Stability and Low Back Pain: The Essential Role of the Pelvis.* Churchill Livingston, 1997.

3. Budgell B, Polus B. The effects of thoracic manipulation on heart rate variability: A controlled crossover trial. *J Manipulative Physiol Ther* 2006;29(8):603–610.

4. Korr IM. The spinal cord as organizer of disease processes: II. The peripheral autonomic nervous system. *J Am Osteopath Assoc* 1979;79(2):82–90.

5. Gwirtz PA, Dickey J, Vick D, et al. Viscerosomatic interaction induced by myocardial ischemia in conscious dogs. *J Appl Physiol* 2007;103:511–517.

6. Riedel W, Neeck G. Nociception, pain, and antinociception: Current concepts. *Z Rheumatol* 2001;60(6):404–415.

7. Shen FH, Samartzis D, Andersson GB. Nonsurgical management of acute and chronic low back pain. *J Am Acad of Orthop Surg* 2006;14(8):477–487.

8. Reeves NP, Narendra KS, Cholewicki J. Spine stability: The six blind men and the elephant. *Clin Biomech* 2007;22(3):266–274.

9. Panjabi MM. The stabilizing system of the spine. part i. function, dysfunction, adaptation, and enhancement. *J Spinal Disord* 1992;5(4):383–389 (discussion 397).

10. Mottram SL, Comerford M. Stability dysfunction and low back pain. *J Orthop Med* 1998;20(2):13–18.

11. Holm S, Indahl A, Solomonow M. Sensorimotor control of the spine. *J Electromyogr Kinesiol* 2002;12(3):219–234.

12. Falla D, Jull G, Hodges PW. Feedforward activity of the cervical flexor muscles during voluntary arm movements is delayed in chronic neck pain. *Exp Brain Res* 2004;157(1):43–48.

13. Khalsa PS. Biomechanics of musculoskeletal pain: Dynamics of the neuromatrix. *J Electromyogr Kinesiol* 2004;14(1):109–120.

14 Knott EM, Tune JD, Stoll ST, et al. Increased lymphatic flow in the thoracic duct during manipulative intervention. *J Am Osteopath Assoc* 2005;105(10): 447–456.

15. Degenhardt BF, Kuchera ML. Update on osteopathic medical concepts and the lymphatic system. *J Am Osteopath Assoc* 1996;96(2):97–100.

16. Takata M, Robotham JL. Effects of inspiratory diaphragmatic descent on inferior vena caval venous return. *J Appl Physiol* 1992;72(2):597–607.

17. Hodges PW, Gandevia SC. Changes in intra-abdominal pressure during postural and respiratory activation of the human diaphragm. *J Appl Physiol* 2000;89(3):967–976.

18. Porges SW. Orienting in a defensive world: Mammalian modifications of our evolutionary heritage. A Polyvagal Theory. *Psychophysiology* 1995;32: 301–318.

19. Robinson J, Biley F, Dolk H. Therapeutic touch for anxiety disorders. *Cochrane Database Syst Rev* (Online) 2007;3:CD006240.

In this chapter, we will focus on the anatomy, kinematics, and biomechanics of the vertebral column. The goal is to give the reader an understanding and appreciation of the role of cardinal plane movement and coupled movement in normal vertebral motion. Comprehension of normal vertebral motion is critical for one to achieve a clinical perspective as to the pathogenesis of vertebral dysfunction.

VERTEBRAL MOTION

Certain conventions are used in describing all vertebral motion. The *vertebral motion segment* consists of the superior and inferior adjacent vertebrae and the intervening disc and ligamentous structures. By convention, motion of the superior vertebra is described in relation to the inferior. Motion is further defined as the movement of the superior or anterior surface of the vertebral body. In describing rotation, the anterior surface is used rather than the elements of the posterior arch. For example, in rotation of T3 to the right in relation to T4, the anterior surface of T3 turns to the right and the spinous process deviates to the left. Therefore, remember that descriptions relate to the anterior or superior surfaces of the vertebral body. In addition to describing characteristics of a vertebral motion segment, we also speak of movement of groups of vertebrae (three or more).

Vertebral motion is also described in relation to the anatomically oriented cardinal planes of the body using the right-handed orthogonal coordinate system (Fig. 5.1a). Most of the clinical literature relates to the anatomically described cardinal planes and axes (Fig. 5.1b), while the biomechanical research literature uses the coordinate system extensively. Motion can be described as rotation around an axis and translation along an axis with the body moving within one of the cardinal planes. By convention the horizontal axis is the x-axis, the vertical axis is the y-axis, and the anteroposterior axis is the z-axis. The coronal plane is the xy plane, the sagittal plane is the yz plane, and the horizontal plane is the xz plane. The ability to rotate around an axis and to translate along an axis results in six degrees of freedom for each vertebra. Vertebral motion can then be described as having an *overturning movement* (rotation around an axis) and/or a *translatory movement* (translation along an axis).

TERMINOLOGY

At the present time, convention in clinical practice describes vertebral motion in the following terms: forward bending, backward bending, side bending right and left, and rotation right and left. These motions are oriented to the cardinal planes of the body. It is imperative that one understands that the context of the following descriptions is kinematical. *Kinematics* is defined as that phase of mechanics concerned with the study of movement of rigid bodies, with no consideration of what has caused the motion.

Forward Bending

In forward bending, the superior vertebra rotates anteriorly around the x-axis and translates somewhat forward along the z-axis. In forward bending (Fig. 5.2), the anterior longitudinal ligament becomes somewhat more lax, anterior pressure is placed upon the intervertebral disk displacing the nucleus posteriorly, and the posterior longitudinal ligament becomes more tense as do the ligamentum flavum and the interspinous and supraspinous ligaments. The transverse processes of the superior segment move more anteriorly. The inferior zygapophysial facet of the superior vertebra moves superiorly in relation to the superior zygapophysial facet of the inferior vertebra. This has been described as "opening" or "flexing" of the facet.

Backward Bending

In backward bending, the vertebra rotates backward around the x-axis and moves posteriorly along the z-axis (Fig. 5.3). The anterior longitudinal ligament becomes more tense. There is less tension on the posterior longitudinal ligament, the ligamentum flavum, and the interspinous and supraspinous ligaments. The transverse processes of the superior segment move more posteriorly. The inferior zygapophysial facet of the superior segment slides inferiorly in relation to the superior zygapophysial facet of the inferior vertebra. The facets are spoken of as having "closed" or "extended." Forward bending and backward bending result in an accordion-type movement of the opening and closing of the zygapophysial joints. If something interferes with the capacity of a facet joint to open or close, restriction of motion of either forward bending or backward bending will result.

Side Bending

In side bending, there is rotation around the anteroposterior z-axis, translation along the horizontal x-axis, and rotation around the vertical y-axis. The z-axis and x-axis directions are dependent on the direction of side bending; however, the y-axis direction (rotation) can vary, as it is dependent on the vertebral segment involved. In side bending to the right, the right zygapophysial joint "closes" and the left zygapophysial joint "opens." Interference with a facet's capacity to open or close can interfere with its segmental side-bending and rotatory movement.

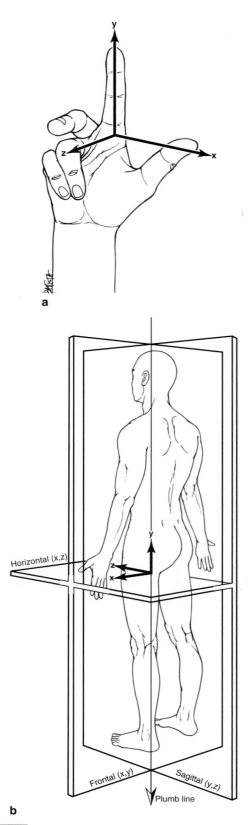

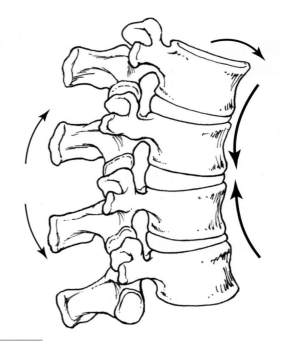

FIGURE 5.2   Vertebral forward bending.

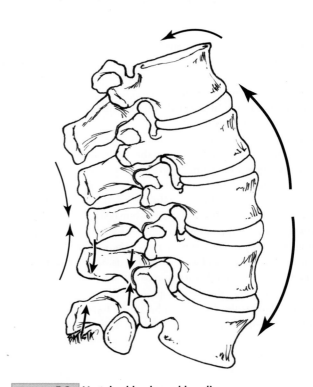

FIGURE 5.3   Vertebral backward bending.

FIGURE 5.1   a. Right-handed orthogonal coordinate system.
b. Anatomically described cardinal planes and axes.
(Taken from White AA III, Panjabi MM. *Clinical Biomechanics of the Spine.* 2nd Ed. Philadelphia, PA: Lippincott Williams & Wilkins, 1990:87.)

Rotation

Rotation of a vertebra is described as rotation around the y-axis with the translatory movement being dependent on the vertebral segment involved. Rotation is always a component of side bending with the exception of the atlantoaxial joint.

COUPLED MOVEMENTS

Coupled motion by definition is the *rotation or translation of a vertebral body about or along one axis that is consistently associated with rotation or translation about a second axis*.[1] Coupling of spinal motion is a phenomenon that is derived from the kinematics of the individual vertebra, the anterior–posterior curvature and the connecting ligaments of the spine. Robert W. Lovett, M.D., in his quest to understand the pathogenesis of scoliosis, dispelled the theory that there are four movements of the spine since neither rotation nor side-bending movements were "pure."[2] Panjabi further discriminated it stating, "When we flex the spine in the sagittal plane, the flexion rotation is the main motion and the accompanying anterior and inferior/superior translatory motions are called the coupled motions."[3] The phenomenon of coupling has been well documented experimentally and clinically in all areas of the vertebral column[4–7]; however, controversy remains regarding the conclusions that Dr Lovett[8,9] and Harrison Fryette[10] made as to the direction of coupled rotation in the various areas of a side-bent spine.

Dr Lovett contributed to our understanding of spinal motion with his observation that two dominant factors controlled spinal motion, one being the articulating facets and the other the bodies of the vertebra. By separating the spine through the pedicles into two columns, he studied the coupling behavior of the anterior part, which consisted of the vertebral bodies and intervertebral disks; and the posterior part which consisted of the laminae and neural arch. When the column of vertebral bodies was side bent under load, they collapsed toward the convexity. When the column of facets were similarly side bent it behaved like a flexible ruler or blade of grass; rotation into the concavity was necessary before it could be side bent. These experiments suggest that in the intact spine, to the degree that the facets are in control they direct and govern rotation.[10] If the facets are not controlling motion, side bending can occur with coupled rotation to the opposite or convex side; if the facets are controlling motion, side bending can occur after the spine rotates into the concavity or into the direction of the side bending. As will be discussed below, the amount of "control" each vertebral segment facet is provided is dependent on the anterior–posterior curvature of the spine and the orientation of the facets to the horizontal plane. An understanding of vertebral anatomy and spine kinematics is crucial in understanding coupling mechanics and vertebral dysfunction.

Neutral Mechanics

Neutral mechanics, or its synonym type I mechanics, results in coupled movement of side bending and rotation to opposite sides. Neutral mechanics occur in the thoracic and lumbar spine; in the absence of dysfunction (or anatomical deviation) when the patient is in the erect position with normal anteroposterior curves, the facets are not controlling motion. For example, in the lumbar spine, with a normal lumbar lordosis present, side bending of the trunk to the left results in rotation of lumbar vertebrae to the right in three-dimensional space (Fig. 5.4).

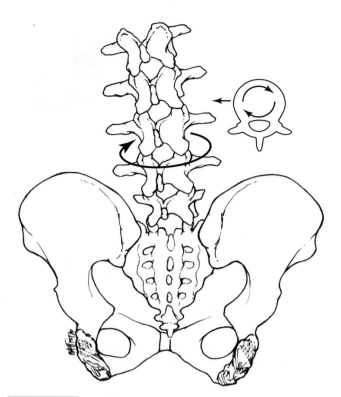

FIGURE 5.4   **Neutral (type I) vertebral motion.**

This motion behavior is derived from bending forces on the vertebral bodies and associated ligaments; the facets do not control motion.

CLINICAL PEARL

You can demonstrate this on yourself by standing erect and placing four fingers of your hand over the posterior aspect of the transverse processes of the lumbar spine. Now side bend to the left and feel the tissues under your right hand become more full. This fullness is interpreted as posterior movement of the right transverse processes of the lumbar vertebrae as they rotate right in response to side bending to the left.

If one looks at the behavior of each of the lumbar vertebra in relation to the segment below, they do not all side bend and rotate to opposite sides. In fact, in this example, the middle segment maximally side bends and rotates to the opposite side. The segments below the apex also side bend and rotate to opposite sides in a gradual fashion. The segments above the apex side bend and rotate to the same side and the curve gradually reduces. However, for descriptive purposes, the neutral mechanical behavior is described as being side bent and rotated to opposite sides in three-dimensional space.

Look at a model of the vertebral column. Now imagine the motion that would occur if the posterior aspect (neural arch) of the vertebra were removed, leaving only the bodies of the vertebra. Because the facets of the thoracic and lumbar spine are oriented at a 60 to 90 degree angle from horizontal, there is a fairly large anteroposterior range in which they have no effect on motion. This is the neutral range. Outside this range the bending forces are placed on the facets allowing them to control motion.

Nonneutral Mechanics

Nonneutral mechanical coupling, or its synonym type II mechanics, results when side bending and rotation of vertebrae occur to the same side. This takes place when there is alteration in the anteroposterior curve into forward or backward bending which places bending forces onto and allows the facets to control motion.

To demonstrate, stand and forward bend at the waist and place both fingers overlying the posterior aspect of the transverse processes of the lumbar spine. Introduce side bending to the right. You will feel fullness occur under the fingers of your right hand, interpreted as resulting from posterior orientation of the right transverse processes during a right rotational response to the right-side bending coupled movement (Fig. 5.5). Return to the midline before returning to the erect posture.

Nonneutral (type II) mechanics include the coupling of all three arcs of vertebral motion and all six degrees of freedom.[11] Nonneutral coupling results in significant reduction in freedom of motion. It is for this reason that the vertebral column appears to be at risk for dysfunction when nonneutral mechanics are operative.

Type III Mechanics

Type III refers to the observation that when motion is introduced in the vertebral column in one direction, motion in all other directions is reduced. To demonstrate the phenomenon, have your patient sit erect on an examining couch and passively introduce rotation of the trunk to the right and left. Ascertain the range and quality of movement. Now have the patient slump on the table with a posterior thoracolumbar convexity and again introduce trunk rotation to the right and left. Note the reduction in range and the restricted quality of movement during the range with the patient in this slumped position. The phenomenon of type III vertebral motion is therapeutically applied during localization to dysfunctional segments. Introduction of motion above and below a dysfunctional vertebral segment can be accurately localized to a single vertebral motion segment that will then be treated by introduction of some activating force.

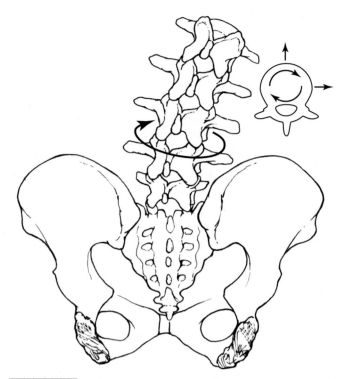

FIGURE 5.5   Nonneutral (type II) vertebral motion.

VERTEBRAL ANATOMY

The vertebral column consists of 33 segments. There are usually 7 cervical segments, 12 thoracic segments, 5 lumbar segments, 5 fused sacral segments, and 4 coccygeal segments. Anomalous development occurs in the spine and is most common in the lumbar region where four or six segments are occasionally found. The lumbar region is also the site of the greatest number of anomalous developmental changes, particularly in the shape of the transverse processes and zygapophysial joints. The *vertebral motion segment* consists of two adjacent vertebrae and the intervening ligamentous structures (Fig. 5.6). The *typical vertebra* consists of two parts, the body and the posterior neural arch. The vertebral body articulates with the intervertebral disk above and below at the vertebral end plate. The posterior arch consists of the two pedicles, two superior and two inferior zygapophysial joints, two laminae, two transverse processes, and a single spinous process. Two adjacent vertebrae are connected, front to back respectively, by the anterior longitudinal ligament, the intervertebral disk with its central nucleus and surrounding annulus, the posterior longitudinal ligament, the articular capsules of the zygapophysial joints, the ligamentum flavum, the interspinous ligament, and the supraspinous ligament.

The anterior–posterior curves of the vertebral column develop over time. The primary curve at birth is convex posteriorly. The first secondary curve to develop is in the cervical region, which becomes convex anteriorly when the infant begins to raise its head. The second curve develops in the lumbar region

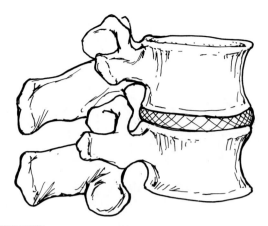

FIGURE 5.6 Vertebral motion segment.

on assuming the biped stance. This curve is convex anteriorly. Appropriate alignment of the three curves of the vertebral axis is an essential component of good posture (Fig. 5.7).

Cervical Region

Atlas

The atlas and axis are structurally and functionally different from the vertebrae in the lower cervical region. The atlas (Fig. 5.8) is considered atypical as it does not have a vertebral body or intervertebral disk and because it consists primarily of a bony ring with two lateral masses. On the posterior aspect of the anterior arch is a small joint structure for articulation with the anterior aspect of the odontoid process of the axis. Each lateral mass consists primarily of the articular processes. The shape of the superior articular process is concave front to back and side to side. The long axis of each superior articulation diverges approximately 30 degrees from anteromedial to posterolateral. This results in an anterior wedging of the long axis of these joints. The superior articular processes articulate with the concave shaped, similarly oriented condyles of the occiput. The inferior articular processes of the atlas are quite flat but when the articular cartilage is attached, they become convex front to back and side to side. These inferior articular processes articulate with the superior articular process of the axis. The transverse processes are quite long and are palpable in the space between the tip of the mastoid process of the temporal bone and the angle of the mandible.

The primary movement of the occipitoatlantal articulation is forward and backward bending. There is a small amount of coupled side bending and rotation to opposite sides. This motion is consistently controlled by the uniquely shaped articulation and its ligamentous attachments. Left rotation of the occiput on the atlas is associated with anterior displacement of the right occipital condyle on the concave and anteriorly convergent right articular process of the atlas, and posterior displacement of the left occipital condyle on the concave and posteriorly divergent left articular process of the atlas. As the occiput turns to the left its articular capsule tightens, displacing the occipital condyles to the left, resulting in side bending to the right[12] (Fig. 5.9).

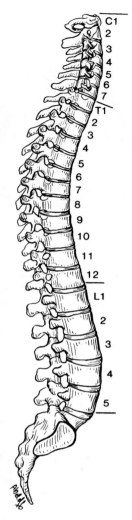

FIGURE 5.7 Normal vertebral curves.

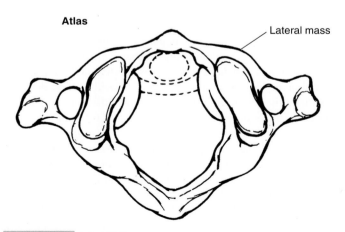

FIGURE 5.8 Atlas (C1).

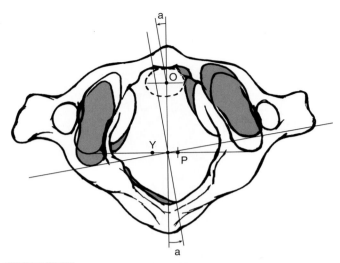

FIGURE 5.9 Left rotation of the occiput over the center of the odontoid O, the base of the occiput is displaced to the left by 2 to 3 mm along the direction indicated by the vector V (right-side bending).

(Taken from Kapandji IA. *The Physiology of the Joints*. Vol. 3. London: Churchill Livingstone, 1974:183.)

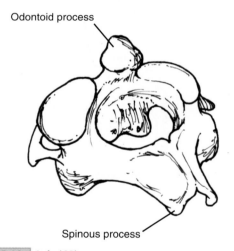

FIGURE 5.10 Axis (C2).

Axis

The axis (C2) (Fig. 5.10) has atypical vertebral characteristics in its superior portion and more typical characteristics in its inferior portion. There is no intervertebral disk between C1 and C2. The vertebral body is surmounted by the odontoid process, developmentally the residuum of the body of the atlas. On the anterior aspect of the odontoid process is an articular facet for the posterior aspect of the anterior arch of the atlas. The posterior aspect of the odontoid process also has an articular facet for the transverse ligament of the atlas which secures the odontoid. The superior articular processes are convex superiorly and slope downward to the front and to the back. They are higher on the medial than lateral aspect and their contour resembles a pair of shoulders. The spinous process of C2 is quite long and is one of the more easily palpable spinous processes in the cervical region.

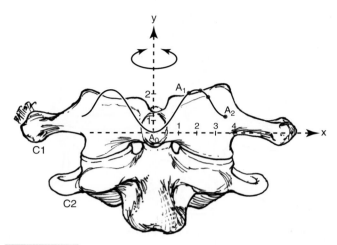

FIGURE 5.11 Upward and downward translatory movements of the anterior aspect of C1 with respect to C2, when the head rotates, around the *y*-axis, to the left and right.

(Taken from White AA III, Panjabi MM. *Clinical Biomechanics of the Spine*. 2nd Ed. Philadelphia, PA: Lippincott Williams & Wilkins, 1990:95.)

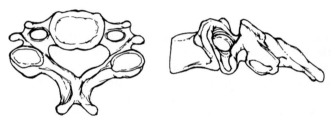

FIGURE 5.12 Typical cervical vertebra.

The geometry and orientation of the C0/C1 and C1/C2 articular processes, as well as the dens/C1 articulation, appear to dictate the type and amount of motion available at the atlanto-axial joint. The primary motion is rotation; however, helical (transverse or *y*-axis) coupling does occur as a result of the convex/convex shape of the superior axial and inferior atlantal articular processes. As the atlas rotates in either direction, its inferior articulation travels downward off the most superior aspect of the convex shaped superior articulation of the axis. This allows for downward helical motion of the inferior articular process of the atlas on the superior articular process of the axis (Fig. 5.11).

Typical Cervical Vertebrae

The typical cervical vertebrae, from the inferior surface of C2 down to the cervical thoracic junction, have the following characteristics (Fig. 5.12). The vertebral body is relatively small in relation to the posterior arch. The superior surface is convex front to back and concave side to side, whereas the inferior surface is concave front to back and convex side to side. When the intervertebral disk joins two typical vertebral bodies, the shape is similar to a universal joint. At the posterolateral corner of each vertebral body is a small synovial joint called the uncovertebral joint of Luschka. These joints are found only in the cervical region and are subject to degenerative changes that

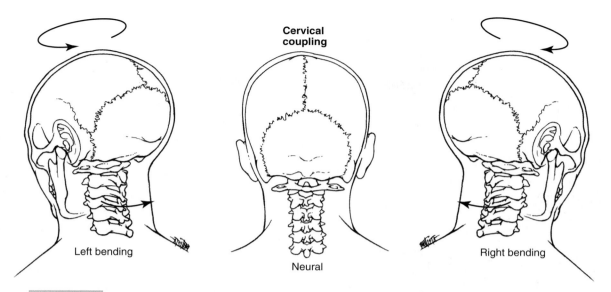

Cervical coupling

Left bending

Neural

Right bending

FIGURE 5.13 Typical cervical coupling pattern; when the head and neck are bent to the right, the spinous processes go to the left. The converse is also shown.
(Taken from White AA III, Panjabi MM. *Clinical Biomechanics of the Spine*. 2nd Ed. Philadelphia, PA: Lippincott Williams & Wilkins, 1990:100.)

occasionally encroach on the intervertebral canal posteriorly. The pedicles are quite short and serve as the roof and floor of the related intervertebral canal. The articular pillars are relatively large and are easily palpable on the posterolateral aspect of the neck. The zygapophysial joints are relatively flat and face backward and upward at approximately a 45-degree angle. The shape and direction of the zygapophysial joints, and the universal joint characteristics between the vertebral bodies, largely determine the type of movement available in the typical cervical spinal segments. The laminae are flat and the spinous processes are usually bifid with the exception of C7. The transverse processes are unique in this region, having on each side the intertransverse foramen for the passage of the vertebral artery. The tips of the transverse processes are bifid and serve as attachments for the deep cervical muscles. They are quite tender to palpation and are not easily used in structural diagnosis of the cervical spine. The intervertebral foramina on each side are ovoid in shape and are limited by the inferior margin of the pedicle above, the posterior aspect of the intervertebral disk and Luschka joints in front, the superior aspect of the pedicle of the vertebral segment or vertebra below, and the anterior aspect of the zygapophysial joints behind. The vertebral canal is relatively large and provides the space necessary for the large area of the spinal cord in the cervical region.

Flexion, extension, side bending, and rotation are all permissible in the typical cervical vertebra; lateral flexion and rotation are always facet controlled regardless of its anteroposterior curvature position.[13] This is due to the relative flatness of the superior articular facets and the limitations of motion allowed by the uncovertebral joints of Luschka. Side bending in one direction will always be coupled with rotation in the opposite direction[12] (Fig. 5.13).

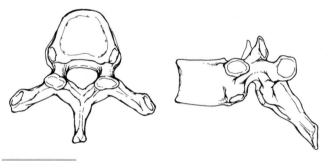

FIGURE 5.14 Thoracic vertebra.

Thoracic Vertebrae

In the thoracic region (Fig. 5.14), the vertebral bodies become somewhat larger as they descend and have unique characteristics for articulation with the heads of the ribs. T1 has a unifacet found posterolaterally for the articulation of the head of the first rib bilaterally. From the inferior surface of T1 down are found demifacets, which together with the intervertebral disk provide an articular fossa for the head of each rib. Asymmetry of facet orientation in the thoracic spine is not uncommon. The zygapophysial joints are vertical (sagittal) in orientation and the superior facets project backward and laterally. The superior articulation has an upward-facing frontal plane orientation (−60 degrees) which is most significant at T1 and T2, then gradually decreases such that T12 faces backward and medially[14] (Fig. 5.15).

The transverse processes have an articular facet on their anterior aspect for articulation with the tubercle of the rib. This forms the costotransverse articulation bilaterally. The transverse processes become progressively narrower in descent, with those at T1 being widest at their tips and those at T12, the narrowest.

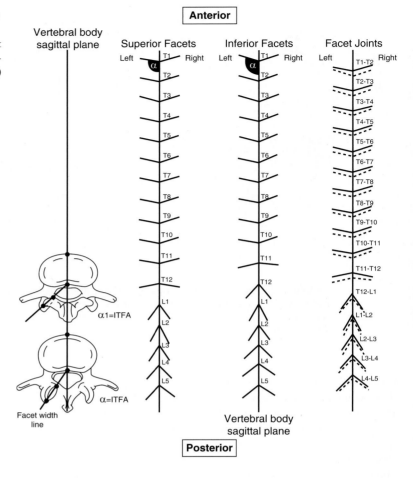

FIGURE 5.15 Facet orientation in the transverse plane along the vertebral column.
(Taken from Masharawi Y, Rothschild, B, Dar, G, et al. Facet orientation in the thoracolumbar spine: Three-dimensional anatomic and biomechanical analysis. *Spine* 2004;29(16):1755–1763.)

The laminae are shingled and continue to the spinous processes, which are also shingled from above downward. The spinous processes are quite long and overlap each other, particularly in the mid to lower region. Conventionally, the relation of the palpable tips of the spinous processes to the thoracic vertebral bodies is referred to as "the rule of 3s" (Fig. 5.16). The purpose of "the rule of 3s" is for one to easily locate the transverse processes. The spinous processes of T1 to T3 are palpable at the same vertebral level as their respective transverse processes. The spinous processes of T4 to T6 project one-half vertebral body below their respective transverse process. The spinous processes of T7 to T9 are located a full vertebral body lower than their respective transverse process. The spinous processes of T10 through T12 return to being palpable at the same vertebral level as their respective transverse processes.[15]

Theoretically, there should be a great deal of freedom of movement in multiple directions in the thoracic spine, but the attachment of the ribs to the thoracic vertebra and sternum markedly restricts the available motion. The coupling behavior of thoracic rotation and side bending has been very controversial. A recent systematic review of studies examining in vivo and in vitro thoracic spine coupled motion showed no consistent coupling patterns when the rotation or side bending was introduced to a neutral (not flexed or extended) spine.[16] Despite this controversy,

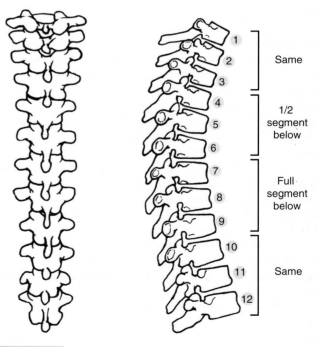

FIGURE 5.16 Thoracic spine rule of 3s. The spinous process segmental relativity to its transverse process.

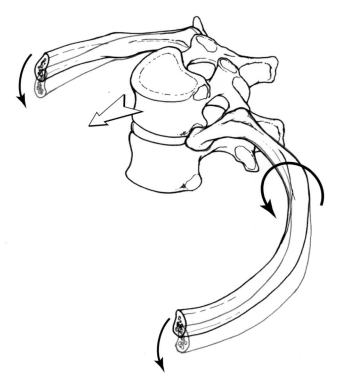

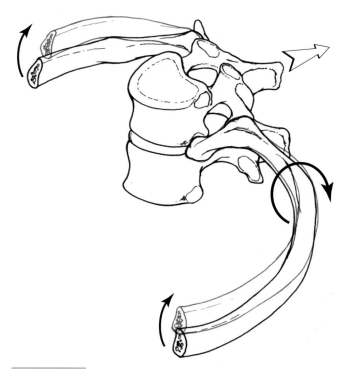

FIGURE 5.17 The osteokinematic and arthrokinematic motion proposed to occur in the thorax during flexion.
(Taken from Lee D. Biomechanics of the thorax: A clinical model of in vivo function. *J Man Manipulative Ther* 1993;1:15.)

FIGURE 5.18 The osteokinematic and arthrokinematic motion proposed to occur in the thorax during extension.
(Taken from Lee D. Biomechanics of the thorax: A clinical model of in vivo function. *J Man Manipulative Ther* 1993;1:15.)

there appears to be some consensus which arises when anatomical, clinical, and experimental data are contributed.[4,17,18]

Coupling mechanics of the thoracic spine motion cannot be complete without elucidation of its effect on the rib cage. During flexion of a vertebral segment the rib attached to the inferior demifacet of the superior segment will follow the superior segment forward. This turns its superior border anteriorly, inducing anterior rotation or internal rotation of the affected rib (i.e., T5 and the sixth rib) (Fig. 5.17). During extension of a vertebral segment the rib attached to the inferior demifacet of the superior segment will follow the superior segment backward. This turns its superior border posteriorly, inducing posterior rotation or external rotation of the affected rib (Fig. 5.18).

Because of the limitations of motion due to the rib cage, flexion and extension of the thoracic spine quickly deliver control of motion to the facets, such that any side bending from a forward or backward bent position will couple ipsilaterally. In the absence of dysfunction and alteration in the anterior posterior curvature, side bending of the thoracic spine will behave similar to a flexible rod and couple with rotation in the opposite direction. This motion is permitted because the facets in the upright posture are not controlling motion and because the ribs on the convex side internally rotate and those on the concave side externally rotate in response to compressive/distractive forces on the respective ribs laterally. This torsioning of the ribs delivers contralateral rotational forces back into the costovertebral joints and vertebral body[18] (Fig. 5.19).

In the absence of dysfunction or alteration in the anterior–posterior curvature, rotation of the thoracic spine quickly delivers control to the facets. In addition; right rotation of T4 on T5 torsions the right fifth rib posteriorly, as it travels posteriorly with the right inferior demifacet of T4, and the left fifth rib anteriorly, as it travels anterior with the left inferior demifacet of T4. The rib influence on rotation becomes significant as it exerts a pulling force onto the right transverse process, via its superior costotransverse ligament, toward the side of rotation, adding to right-side bending[17,18] (Fig. 5.20).

Lumbar Vertebrae

In the lumbar region, the vertebral bodies (Fig. 5.21) become even more massive and support a great deal of weight. The spinous processes project posteriorly in relation to the vertebral body to which they are attached and are broad, rounded, and easily palpable. The transverse processes project laterally, with those attached to L3 being the broadest in range. The lumbar zygapophysial joint superior articular surface is convex and inferior articular surface is concave; the orientation of the superior articular surface is backward and medially limiting the amount of side bending and rotation available. Given the orientation of the facets, flexion delivers control to the facets whereas physiological extension allows the bodies of the vertebra to maintain control.

In the lumbar region, asymmetric facing of the zygapophysial joints or "tropism" is not uncommon. In the absence of tropism, vertebral dysfunction, or alterations in the anteroposterior curvature of the spine, side bending will couple with rotation to

FIGURE 5.19 During right-side bending; the bilateral costal rotation in opposing directions tends to drive the superior vertebra into left rotation.
(Taken from Lee D. Biomechanics of the thorax: A clinical model of in vivo function. *J Man Manipulative Ther* 1993;1:15.)

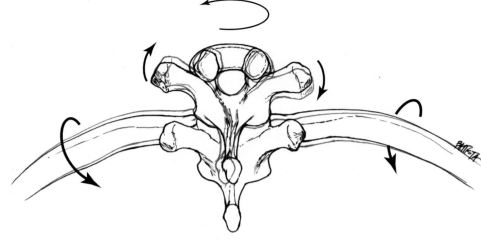

FIGURE 5.20 As the superior thoracic vertebra rotates to the right, it translates to the left. The right rib posteriorly rotates and the left rib anteriorly rotates as a consequence of the vertebral rotation.
(Taken from Lee D. Biomechanics of the thorax: A clinical model of in vivo function. *J Man Manipulative Ther* 1993;1:15.)

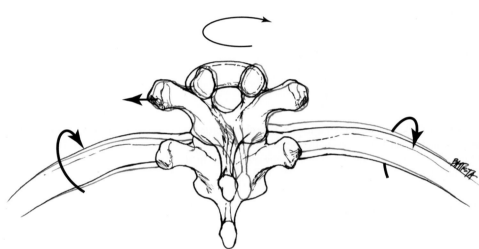

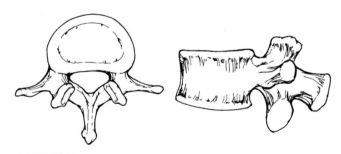

FIGURE 5.21 Lumbar vertebra.

the opposite side.[12] The lumbar vertebral segments have large intervertebral disks and vertically oriented articular facets. The side bending forces are directed into the disc on the side of convexity and onto the lateral vertebral body ligamentous structures of the concavity. Rotation into the concavity reduces the pressure within the disc and minimizes the stretch of the lateral vertebral ligaments.

In the absence of tropism, vertebral dysfunction, or alterations in the anteroposterior curvature of the spine; axial rotation from above to the right will couple with side bending to the left at L1-L3 and side bending to the right at L3-L5.[3,19] The transition at L3-L4 likely resolves the reciprocal left rotation from below, generated from fixation of the lumbar spine at the sacrum.

With the spine in the flexed position, side bending quickly directs control of motion to the facets and couples rotation to the same side.[20] With the spine in the extended position, side bending forces are maintained by the bodies of the vertebra and couple rotation to the opposite side. In the lumbar region, non-neutral coupling results in significant reduction in freedom of motion. With the trunk forward bent, side bent, and rotated to the same side, any additional movement places the lumbar spine at risk for muscle strain, zygapophysial joint dysfunction, annular tear of the intervertebral disk, or posterolateral protrusion of nuclear material in a previously compromised disc annulus.

The Sacrum

The sacrum is formed by the five fused elements of the sacral vertebrae and articulates superiorly with the last lumbar vertebra and caudally with the coccyx. The sacrum should be viewed as a component part of the vertebral axis.

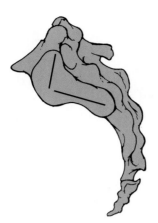

FIGURE 5.22 Sacroiliac joint configuration.
(Adapted from Kapandji IA. *The Physiology of the Joints*. Vol. 3. London: Churchill Livingstone, 1974:67.)

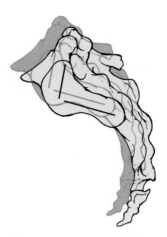

FIGURE 5.23 The sacrum nutates by gliding anteriorly along the short arm of its articulation and inferiorly along the long arm of its articulation.
(Adapted from Kapandji IA. *The Physiology of the Joints*. Vol. 3. London: Churchill Livingstone, 1974:67.)

The sacroiliac joints are true arthrodial joints with a joint space, synovial capsule, and articular cartilage. They are unique in that the cartilage on the sacral side is hyaline cartilage and the cartilage on the ilial side is fibrocartilage. The articular cartilage on the sacral side is much thicker than that on the ilial side. The joints are L-shaped in contour with a shorter upper arm and a longer lower arm (Fig. 5.22). The joint contour usually has a depression on the sacral side at approximately S2 and a corresponding prominence on the ilial side. The sacroiliac joints are relatively flat and like most flat articular surfaces they lack the ability to resist shear forces. Given the location of the sacrum, the lack of resistance to shear forces can be a problem. The shape of the sacrum and its relationship to the ilia protect it from shear, but the sacrum requires sophisticated continuous muscular and ligamentous tensile forces to protect it from vulnerability and yet allow function. The sacrum is wider superiorly than it is inferiorly and wider anteriorly than posteriorly. This "keystone-shape" configuration is necessary for the sacrum to wedge itself anteriorly between the ilia.[21]

Sacroiliac motion is the movement of the sacrum between the two hip bones and requires the participation of both sacroiliac joints. Nutation (nodding) and counternutation are the sacral motion about which the most is known from biomechanical and radiographic research.[22] Nutation (anterior nutation) is anterior movement of the sacrum between the hip bones. This motion of the sacrum occurs with extension of the lumbar spine. The sacrum moves into nutation by gliding anteriorly along the short arm of its articulation and inferiorly along the long arm of its articulation (Fig. 5.23). Nutation allows for sacral stability as it generates medial compression of the ilia between the sacrum; essentially wedging itself between the ilia.

Counternutation (posterior nutation) is a backward movement of the sacrum between the hip bones. This motion of the sacrum occurs with flexion of the lumbar spine. The sacrum moves into counternutation by gliding superiorly along the long

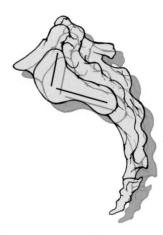

FIGURE 5.24 The sacrum moves into counternutation by gliding superiorly along the long arm of its articulation and posteriorly along the short arm of its articulation.
(Adapted from Kapandji IA. *The Physiology of the Joints*. Vol. 3. London: Churchill Livingstone, 1974:67.)

arm of its articulation and posteriorly along the short arm of its articulation (Fig. 5.24). Counternutation places the sacrum into a vulnerable shearing state by "unlocking" it from its protective ilial compression.

The third motion of the sacrum is axial rotation. Because the sacrum is five fused vertebral segments that have very little motion independent of their ilial attachments, its rotation is always coupled with side bending. This sacral motion has been described as "torsion" to describe the coupling of side bending and rotation to opposite sides. For descriptive purposes, this complex, polyaxial, torsional movement is considered to occur around an oblique axis. The left oblique axis runs from the upper extremity of the left sacroiliac joint to the lower end of

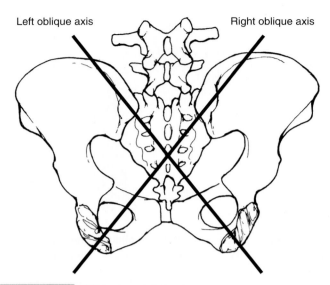

FIGURE 5.25 Oblique axes of the sacrum.

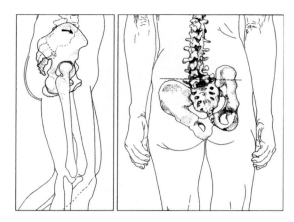

FIGURE 5.26 At right mid-stance (mid-left swing phase), the sacral base on the left begins to move into anterior nutation as it is carried forward by the advancing left ilia. As it begins to rotate to the right it side bends to the left. The oblique hypothetical torsional axis that is produced from this polyaxial movement is right. So during right mid-stance gait, the sacrum begins to move into right rotation about a right oblique axis. The lumbar spine will concurrently rotate to the left and side bend to the right.

(Taken from Greenman PE. Clinical aspects of sacroiliac function in human walking. In: Vleeming A, Mooney V, Snijders CJ, Dorman T, Stoeckart R, eds. *Movement Stability and low Back Pain: The Essential Role of the Pelvis.* Churchill-Livingstone, 1997.)

the right sacroiliac joint, and the right oblique axis runs from the upper end of the right sacroiliac joint to the lower extremity of the left sacroiliac joint. Although the exact biomechanics of the torsional movements of the sacrum are unknown, the hypothetical left and right oblique axes are useful for descriptive purposes (Fig. 5.25).

The sacrum has anterior torsional motions and posterior torsional motions. Anterior torsional motion occurs physiologically with lumbar extension and side bending. It also occurs physiologically with gait[23] (Fig. 5.26).

Posterior torsional movement of the sacrum occurs when the trunk is forward bent and side bent or rotated to one side. This maneuver results in the nonneutral behavior of the lumbar spine with side bending and rotation coupled to the same side. The sacrum between the hip bones participates in this maneuver by backward or posterior torsional movement. For example, as the trunk is forward bent and rotated to the left, coupled with lumbar side bending to the left; the right sacral base will move into posterior nutation and the sacrum will rotate to the right and side bend to the left. The hypothetical torsional axis that is produced is to the left. So flexion, left-side bending and left rotation of the lumbar spine,

takes the sacrum into posterior torsion to the right on a left oblique axis.

TYPES OF MOTION AVAILABLE

The type of coupled movement available in the vertebral column varies from region to region and from posture to posture. In the areas of the vertebral column that have both neutral and nonneutral movement capability, the vertebral segments can become dysfunctional with either type of motion characteristic (Table 5.1). An understanding of the anatomy of the vertebral column, the ability to palpate the tissues therein, and an understanding of the concepts of vertebral motion are essential to understand and diagnose vertebral dysfunctions.

TABLE 5.1	*Summary of Spinal Coupled Mechanics*			
Segment	No AP Curve/Side Bending	Flexion/Side Bending	Extension/Side Bending	Axial Rotation
C2–C7	Nonneutral	Nonneutral	Nonneutral	Nonneutral
T1–T12	Neutral	Nonneutral	Nonneutral	Neutral
L1–L5	Neutral	Nonneutral	Neutral	Neutral above L3 nonneutral below L3
Sacrum	Neutral	Posterior torsion	Anterior torsion	Neutral

REFERENCES

1. White AA III, Panjabi MM. *Clinical Biomechanics of the Spine*. 2nd Ed. Philadelphia, PA: Lippincott Williams & Wilkins, 1990:646.
2. Lovett RW. *Lateral Curvature of the Spine and Shoulders*. 4th Ed. Philadelphia, PA: P. Blakiston's Son & Co.
3. White AA III, Panjabi MM. *Clinical Biomechanics of the Spine*. 2nd Ed. Philadelphia, PA: Lippincott Williams & Wilkins, 1990:53.
4. Panjabi MM, Brand RA, White AA. Mechanical properties of the human thoracic spine: As shown by three-dimensional load–displacement curves. *J Bone Joint Surg* 1976:58A:642–652.
5. Panjabi MM, Summers DJ, Pelker RR, et al. Three dimensional load displacement curves due to forces on the cervical spine. *J Orthop Res* 1986;4:152.
6. Panjabi MM, Krag MH, White AA, et al. Effects of preload on load displacement curves of the lumbar spine. Orthop. *Clin North Am* 1977;88:181.
7. Stevens A. Sidebending and axial rotation of the sacrum inside the pelvic girdle. In: Vleeming A, Mooney V, Snijders CJ, Dorman T, eds. *First Interdisciplinary World Congress on Low Back Pain and Its Relation to the Sacroiliac Joint*. 1992, San Diego, CA, 5–6 November, 209–230.
8. Lovett RW. The study of the mechanics of the spine. *Am J Anat* 1902;2:457–462.
9. Lovett RW. The mechanism of the normal spine and its relation to scoliosis. *Med Surg J* 1905;153:349.
10. Fryette HH. *Principles of Osteopathic Technique*. Carmel, CA: American Academy of Osteopathy, 1954.
11. Harrison DE, Harrison DD, Troyanovich SJ. Three-dimensional spinal coupling mechanics: Part I. A review of the literature. *J Manipulative Physiol Ther* 1999;22(5):350–352.
12. Kapandji IA. *The Physiology of the Joints*. Vol. 3. London: Churchill Livingstone, 1974.
13. Mimura M, Moriya H, Watanabe T, et al. Three-dimensional motion analysis of the cervical spine with special reference to the axial rotation. *Spine* 1989;14(11):1135–1139.
14. Masharawi Y, Rothschild B, Dar G, et al. Facet orientation in the thoracolumbar spine: Three-dimensional anatomic and biomechanical analysis. *Spine* 2004;29(16):1755–1763.
15. Isaacs ER, Bookhout MR. *Bourdillon's Spinal Manipulation*. 6th Ed. Woburn, MA: Butterworth-Heinemann, 2002.
16. Sizer PS Jr, Brismée JM, Cook C. Coupling behavior of the thoracic spine: A systematic review of the literature. *J Manipulative Physiol Ther* 2007;30(5):390–399.
17. Flynn TW. *The Thoracic Spine and Rib Cage: Musculoskeletal Evaluation and Treatment*. Woburn, MA: Butterworth-Heinemann, 1996.
18. Lee D. Biomechanics of the thorax: A clinical model of in vivo function. *J Man Manipulative Ther* 1993;1:13–21.
19. Pearcy M, Tibrewal S. Axial rotation and lumbar sidebending in the normal lumbar spine measured by three-dimensional radiography. *Spine* 1984;9:582–587.
20. Vicenzino G, Twomey L. Sideflexion and induced lumbar spine conjunct rotation and its influencing factors. *Aust Physiother* 1993;39:299–306.
21. Vleeming A. Stoeckaert R, Volkers ACW, et al. Relation between form and function in the sacroiliac joint. Part I: Clinical Anatomic Aspects & Part II: Biomechanical Aspects. *Spine* 1990;15(2):130–136.
22. Sturesson B, Selvick G, Uden A. Movements of the sacroiliac joints. A roentgen stereophotogrammetric analysis. *Spine* 1989;14:162–165.
23. Greenman PE. Clinical aspects of sacroiliac function in human walking. In: Vleeming A, Mooney V, Snijders CJ, Dorman T, Stoeckart R, eds. *Movement Stability and Low Back Pain: The Essential Role of the Pelvis*. New York, NY: Churchill-Livingstone, 1997:235–242.

6

CONCEPTS OF VERTEBRAL MOTION DYSFUNCTION

In the application of manual medicine procedures to the vertebral column, it is essential to make appropriate, accurate diagnosis of vertebral somatic dysfunction.

> Somatic dysfunction is defined as: Impaired or altered function of related components of the somatic (body framework) system; skeletal, arthrodial, and myofascial structures; and related vascular, lymphatic, and neural elements.

This term is codable under current classification systems, International Classification of Diseases, Ninth Revision, Clinical Modification, (ICD-9-CM) codes 739.0 through 739.9.[1] Somatic dysfunction replaces old terms such as "osteopathic lesion," "chiropractic subluxation," "joint blockage," "joint lock," "loss of joint play," or "minor vertebral derangement." Concern for the function of the musculoskeletal system requires a method of evaluating motion within the vertebral complex to determine if it is normal, increased, or decreased. The motion spectrum advances from ankylosis to hypomobility, to normal motion, to hypermobility, to instability. Manual medicine procedures are most appropriate for segments with hypomobility that retain the capacity to move.

THEORIES OF VERTEBRAL MOTION DYSFUNCTION

Many theories have been proposed to explain the clinically observed phenomenon of hypomobility.[2] One theory proposes that there is entrapment of synovial material or a synovial meniscoid between the two opposing joint surfaces. There is some anatomic evidence that meniscoids do occur but whether they actually cause joint restriction has not been demonstrated. The joint meniscoid has innervation by C-fibers that suggest nociception function.

A second theory suggests that there is a lack of congruence in the point-to-point contact of the opposing joint surfaces. This theory postulates alteration in the normal tracking mechanism between the joint surfaces and that the role of manual medicine is to restore the joint to the "right track."

A third theory suggests an alteration in the physical and chemical properties of the synovial fluid and synovial surfaces. In essence, the smooth gliding capacity has been lost because the opposing surfaces have become "sticky." Following a mobilization with impulse (high-velocity, low-amplitude thrust) procedure, in both vertebral and extremity joints in which separation of the joint surfaces has occurred, the "cavitation" phenomenon has been demonstrated. In addition to the audible popping sound, there has been the observation of a negative density within the joint on X-ray. This "vacuum phenomenon" appears

to have the density of nitrogen and this gaseous shadow is present for a variable period before it is no longer observable. This observation suggests a change from liquid to gaseous state as a result of the thrusting procedure.

A fourth theory regards the restriction of motion as a result of altered length and tone of muscle. Some muscles can become hypertonic and shortened in position, whereas others become lengthened and weaker. Of greatest significance is the loss of muscle control. Physiologic control of muscle is highly complex and includes the behavior of mechanoreceptors in joints and related soft tissue, muscle spindle and Golgi tendon apparatus, cord level and propriospinal pathway reflexes, pathways to the motor cortex, corticobulbar and corticospinal pathways modulated by the cerebellum, and the final common pathway of the alpha motor neuron to muscle fiber. Any alteration in afferent stimulus to this complex mechanism or alteration of function within the system can result in dysfunctional muscle activity and ultimately affect joint mechanics and dynamic stability. Any alteration in muscle tone then restricts normal motion and serves as a perpetuating factor in altered joint movement. Whether the abnormal muscle activity is primary or secondary to the vertebral dysfunction is purely conjectural. However, altered muscle component of a vertebral dysfunction should always be dealt with in some fashion by the treatment provided. Using the analogy of a computer, the nervous system can be viewed as the software and the musculoskeletal system as the hardware. Altered function of the nervous system (the software) does not allow the musculoskeletal system (hardware) to function appropriately. Some manual medicine practitioners view the effectiveness of manual medicine treatment as being the reprogramming of the software through the alteration of mechanoreceptor behavior at the joint and soft tissue levels.

A fifth theory considers changes in the biomechanical and biochemical properties of the myofascial elements of the musculoskeletal system, the capsule, the ligamentous structures, and fasciae. When these structures are altered through traumatic, inflammatory, degenerative, or other changes, reduction of normal vertebral mobility can result.

Regardless of the theory to which one might subscribe, the clinical phenomenon of restricted vertebral motion can be viewed as the influence on the paired zygapophysial joints of the segment. We speak of the capacity of facets to open and close and refer primarily to the accordion-type movement, not separation-type movement. In forward bending, the facets should normally open, and in backward bending, they should close. If something interferes with the capacity of both facets to open, forward-bending restriction will occur. Conversely, if something interferes with both facets' capacity to close, backward-bending restriction will occur. It is also possible for one facet to move normally and the other to become restricted. If, for example, the right facet does not open, but the left functions normally, right-side bending is possible, but left-side bending is restricted. Since side bending and rotation are coupled movements in the typical vertebral segments, rotation can also be affected by alteration in facet joint movement.

DIAGNOSIS OF VERTEBRAL MOTION DYSFUNCTION

Dysfunctions in the vertebral column can be described as single-segment dysfunctions involving one vertebral motion segment and group dysfunctions involving three or more vertebrae. After one completes a screening-and-scanning examination and fine-tunes the diagnostic process to segmental definition, one is particularly interested in the motion(s) lost by the vertebra(e) involved. There are many methods to accomplish the process. The most commonly used one is palpating the same bony prominence of two or more vertebrae (e.g., spinous processes or transverse processes) and actively and/or passively putting the segment(s) through successive ranges of movement into forward bending, backward bending, side bending right, side bending left, rotation right, and rotation left, comparing the motion of one segment with another. These procedures are most frequently done passively as the operator attempts to define restriction and quality of restriction of movement in one or more directions. Although this method is frequently effective, it does have two serious drawbacks. First, every time you introduce multiple-plane motion in a dysfunctional segment diagnostically, there is a therapeutic effect since you are accomplishing a mobilization without impulse (articulatory) procedure. This results in your finding being constantly under change. A second disadvantage is the difficulty in making an assessment following a treatment procedure, that is, knowing whether you have modified the amount of range present before the procedure. It is difficult to accurately remember all of the nuances of motion restriction that were present prior to the therapeutic intervention.

A second method, preferred by this author, is to follow a pair of transverse processes through an arc of forward bending and backward bending and interpret the findings on the basis of the phenomena of facets opening and closing. Regardless of the method used, one can describe vertebral motion from the perspective of the motion available, the position in which the segment is restricted, or the motion of the segment that is restricted.

In Table 6.1, a suffix is used in each term, either a static suffix representing the position of the segment, or a motion suffix, which describes the motion available or the motion lost. The current convention of describing vertebral dysfunction is either the position of the restricted segment or the motion that is lost in the restricted segment. Therefore, a segment that is backward bent (extended), right rotated, and right-side bent has forward bending (flexion), left-side bending, and left rotation restrictions. A plea is made for the use of appropriate terminology either to describe position or motion restriction. One should learn to translate between the two systems of positional and motion restriction diagnosis but clearly a statement of terms is necessary for accurate communication between examiners.

DYSFUNCTIONS OF SINGLE VERTEBRAL MOTION SEGMENT

Single vertebral motion segment dysfunctions in all areas of the spine can be easily identified by the finding of hypertonicity of fourth-layer vertebral muscle in the medial grove adjacent to the spinous processes. In the cervical spine, this hypertonicity is best appreciated with the patient in the supine position, and in the lumbar spine with the patient in the prone position; in each instance when paravertebral musculature is quiet. Palpable fourth-layer muscle hypertonicity is not present in normal vertebral motion segments. When fourth-layer hypertonicity is palpable at a vertebral level, the practitioner should identify the motion characteristics of that vertebra in relation to the one above and the one below.

A second clue to the possibility of a single vertebral motion segment dysfunction is the scanning examination finding of prominence overlying one transverse process suggesting the possibility of rotation of the vertebra to that side (Fig. 6.1).

TABLE 6.1	*Factors That Describe Vertebral Motion*		
	Position	**Motion Restriction**	**Motion Available**
T3 flexed on T4	Flexed	Extension	Flexion
	Left rotated	Right rotation	Left rotation
	Left-side bent	Right-side bending	Left-side bending
	Extended	Flexion	Extension
	Right rotated	Left rotation	Right rotation
	Right-side bent	Left-side bending	Right-side bending

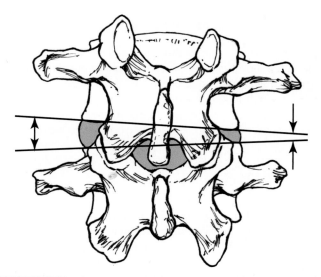

FIGURE 6.1 **Single segment right prominent transverse process.**

This can be easily accomplished in the thoracic or lumbar spine with the patient seated. In the cervical spine, prominence of a posterior articular pillar is suggestive of rotation to that side; this is best appreciated with the patient in the supine position.

The segmental definition diagnostic process of the thoracic and lumbar spine is performed by placing the thumbs over the posterior aspect of the transverse processes of a segment that is suspected of being dysfunctional. The patient then is put through a forward-to-backward bending movement arc either actively or passively. In the upper thoracic spine, the active movement of the head on the trunk is frequently used, whereas in the lower thoracic and lumbar regions, the patient is examined in three different positions: prone neutral on the table, fully backward bent (prone prop position), and seated fully forward bent (Figs. 6.2–6.4). In the cervical spine, vertebral motion segment dysfunction is performed with the patient supine by placing the index fingers over the posterior aspect of the articular pillar and laterally translating or side bending the cervical segment passively in each direction.

CLINICAL PEARL

Using this evaluation of the cervical spine, one is assessing side bending and assuming rotation, whereas in the thoracic and lumbar spine, one is assessing rotation and assuming side bending.

In determining segmental definition, one assesses the behavior of the superior segment in relation to the inferior segment that has been determined to be nondysfunctional and level against the coronal plane. For the purpose of description, assume that something interferes with opening of the right zygapophysial joint of a thoracic segment. Hypertonicity of the fourth-layer

musculature will be present. In the neutral position, the right transverse process appears to be more posterior than the left. As the patient increases the amount of forward bending, the right transverse process becomes more prominent compared with that of the left. The restricted right zygapophysial joint holds the right half of the posterior arch of that vertebra in a posterior or extended position. The free-moving zygapophysial joint on the left side allows the left half of the posterior arch to move forward and superior with the left transverse process, seeming to become less prominent. In backward bending, both transverse processes appear to become more symmetric because the right transverse process is already held posterior by the restricted right zygapophysial joint, whereas the left zygapophysial joint closes in backward bending, thus allowing the left transverse process to move posteriorly and inferiorly, becoming more symmetric in appearance.

Now let us assume that something interferes with the left thoracic zygapophysial joint's ability to close. Hypertonicity of the fourth-layer musculature will be present. In this instance, we usually find the right transverse process a little more prominent in the neutral position. In asking the patient to move into backward bending, the right transverse process appears to become more prominent. This is the result of normal closure of the right zygapophysial joint, allowing the transverse process to move posteriorly, while the left zygapophysial joint is restricted in its capacity to close and holds the left transverse process in a more anterior or flexed position. Upon forward bending, both transverse processes become more symmetric. The left transverse process is already held in an anterior position by the restricted left zygapophysial joint, and the motion of the right zygapophysial moving into an open position carries the right transverse process more anteriorly.

These single vertebral motor unit dysfunctions are also described as nonneutral dysfunctions because the restricted movement results from facet motion loss which alters the anterior or posterior (flexion or extension) curvature at that vertebral segment such that the facets control motion, coupling side bending with rotation to the same side. Historically, they have been described as type II dysfunctions. The characteristics are as follows:

1. Single vertebral motion unit involved
2. Include either flexion or extension restriction component
3. Motion restriction of side bending and rotation to the same side

We have described the phenomenon that occurs if one or the other zygapophysial joint loses the capacity to open or close. If there is a single vertebral motion segment involved in which both zygapophysial joints are restricted, the transverse processes remain in the same relative position throughout forward and backward-bending movement. One can determine the case of bilateral zygapophysial joints being closed or bilaterally being open by monitoring the interspace between the spinous process during forward and backward bending. If the z-joints are able to open, the interspinous distance will increase during forward bending. If the z-joints are able to close in a bilaterally

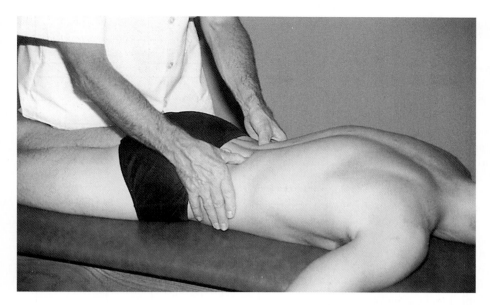

FIGURE 6.2 Vertebral motion testing, prone neutral.

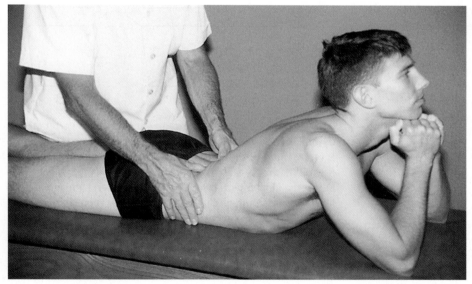

FIGURE 6.3 Vertebral motion testing, backward bent.

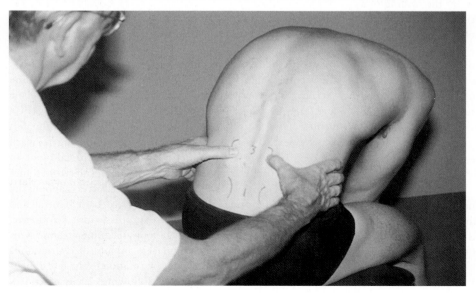

FIGURE 6.4 Vertebral motion testing, forward bent.

symmetric fashion, the interspinous distance becomes smaller during backward bending.

There are several reasons why this method of vertebral motion testing is recommended. First, this method remains consistent and reproducible over time. The challenge to the motion segment is in only one plane of movement. No multiaxial changes in movement characteristics are introduced, as in the procedure described earlier. This method does not put the segment through an articulatory procedure and thus is not changing the vertebral mechanics to any appreciable amount. This makes it possible for the examiner to be more confident in the posttreatment evaluation of a segment to be sure that, in fact, some change has occurred in the motion present before and after treatment.

Second, this procedure is easier for multiple examiners to apply because of the nontreatment aspect of the method. This allows more consistent student teaching and evaluation of vertebral diagnostic procedures. If five separate examiners tested a given segment by putting it through multiple ranges of movement, by the time the fifth examiner described the findings, the first examiner would think it was a different patient. Using this single-plane movement challenge, the findings remain much more consistent across examiners and across time.

A third reason to recommend this process is the examiner's capacity to differentiate between structural and functional asymmetry of a vertebral segment. Structural asymmetries occur frequently, and palpation of a posterior transverse process cannot distinguish asymmetric development from actual dysfunction of a rotational nature. If the prominent transverse process is due to nonneutral (type II) single vertebral motion segment dysfunction, the prominence of the transverse process will change during a forward and backward-bending arc. In one position, it will become worse, and in the other position, it will become more symmetric. If the transverse process is prominent because of asymmetric development and the segment is functional, the transverse process will retain the same amount of prominence throughout the forward-to-backward bending movement arc. There is a third possibility for the finding of a transverse process being more prominent on one side than the other. This can occur when one zygapophysial joint does not open and the other does not close. This bilateral restriction retains the same amount of prominence of the posterior transverse process throughout the movement arc. One can distinguish this bilateral restriction from a structural asymmetry by evaluating the forward-to-backward-bending capacity while monitoring at the interspinous space. One may become suspicious of a bilaterally dysfunctional vertebral segment when the fourth-layer tissue changes are greater than would be expected, given the limited asymmetry of motion observed at the transverse processes.

Figure 6.5 shows an example of the findings in the presence of nonneutral dysfunctions identified within the lumbar spine. A fundamental principle of the use of this diagnostic process is the importance of relating the behavior of the superior vertebra to the one below. The inferior segment is the plane of orientation against which the superior segment is related. The base

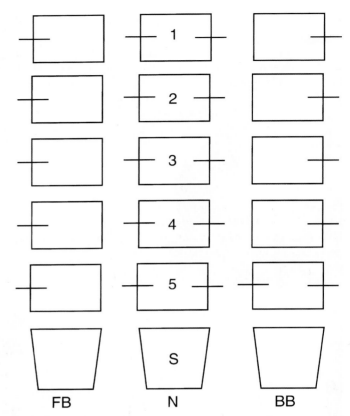

FIGURE 6.5 **L5 and L4 single-segment nonneutral vertebral dysfunction example. Oriented from posterior, the arc of motion is represented by the three columns; forward bending (FB), neutral (N) and backward bending (BB). Each box represents a numbered lumbar vertebrae, L1-L5. The unilateral horizontal lines that pass through the sides of the boxes represent prominent transverse process, side bending is assumed. The sacrum is represented by the trapezium shaped structure on the bottom of each column (S).**

reference plane is the coronal plane. If the inferior segment is rotated to the left, and the superior is level against the coronal plane, the superior vertebra in relation to the inferior segment is rotated to the right. Remember to always relate the behavior of the superior segment to that of the inferior. In this example, the sacrum (S) is nondysfunctional, level against the coronal plane and freely mobile in all three positions of forward bending (FB), neutral (N), and backward bending (BB). At L5, the left transverse process becomes more prominent during forward bending whereas it is symmetric against the coronal plane in neutral and backward bending. This finding results from something interfering with the capacity of the left zygapophysial joint to open during forward bending. In both neutral and backward bending, the transverse processes are symmetric, indicating the capacity of the zygapophysial joints to close symmetrically in backward bending. The amount of restriction is not great because it is not evident by rotation to the left in neutral. The diagnosis would be the following: L5 is extended, rotated, and side bent left (ERS$_{left}$), with motion restriction of forward bending, right-side bending, and right rotation. Also, note that in forward bending, the left transverse processes of L1, L2, L3, and L4 are also more prominent on the left. This finding is a result of the fact that L5 has rotated left during forward bending and the other four lumbar vertebrae have followed in a normal fashion with symmetric opening of their zygapophysial joints during forward bending. At L4, we have a different observation. At this level in backward bending, the right transverse process becomes more prominent in relation to the symmetric transverse processes at L5. In both neutral and forward bending, L4 follows the behavior of L5. In backward bending, it does not. In backward bending something has interfered with the capacity of the left zygapophysial joint to close. During backward bending, the normal closure of the right zygapophysial joint carries the vertebra into right rotation, right-side bending, and backward bending on the right side. In this case, the diagnosis is as follows: L4 is flexed, right rotated and right-side bent (FRS$_{right}$)with motion restriction of backward bending, left-side bending, and left rotation. Again, note that the transverse processes of L1, L2, and L3 are also posterior on the right in backward bending. This is a normal finding because they follow the right rotation of L4. Their zygapophysial joints have the capacity to close symmetrically and follow the right rotation at L4.

NEUTRAL (GROUP) DYSFUNCTION

The characteristics of a neutral group dysfunction are

1. A group of segments (three or more)
2. Minimal flexion or extension component of restriction
3. Restriction of the group to side bending in one direction and rotation in the opposite (Fig. 6.6)
4. The segments never become symmetric, maybe a little better or worse, but not symmetric

With three or more vertebral segments involved in motion restriction, a lateral curvature results to one side. There is prominence on the side of convexity of the group of segments due to rotation of the vertebrae to that side. On palpatory examination, one finds a fullness overlying the transverse processes of three or more adjacent vertebrae. This finding is frequently misdiagnosed as muscle hypertonicity or spasm because the muscle overlying the posterior transverse processes is more prominent and the impression is that the muscle is spastic, hypertonic, or tight. It is true that the muscle is more prominent, but it is the result of the rotation of the vertebrae that the transverse process is taking the muscle mass posteriorly.

During the diagnostic process of trunk, neutral, forward bending, and backward bending, the palpable fullness over the transverse processes on one side is maintained. It may get a little better or a little worse in its deformity during the movement arc, but there is no position in which the transverse processes on each side become symmetric. The forward or backward-bending motion restriction found in this group of segments will be minimal; instead there will be major restriction of side bending to the side of convexity and rotation to the side of

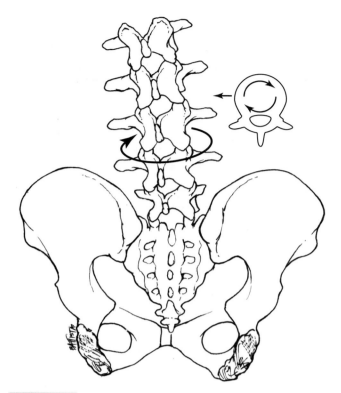

FIGURE 6.6 Neutral group vertebral dysfunction.

concavity. This motion restriction is maintained by a long restrictor on the side of the concavity. The long restrictor is typically a shortened muscle or tight fascia's influencing the position of the vertebral bodies' position without influence on the motion of the facets.

Neutral group dysfunctions are also called type I restrictions with a restricted coupled movement being side bending to one side and rotation to the opposite. These dysfunctions are present in compensatory scoliotic mechanisms and are frequently found above or below a single vertebral motion segment dysfunction. They are frequently secondary to change elsewhere, but because they involve a large number of vertebral segments they receive a lot of diagnostic attention. Because these dysfunctions are secondary to other findings, their treatment should follow appropriate treatment for the cause of the dysfunction, either a nonneutral dysfunction or unleveling of the sacral base.

Figure 6.7 portrays the findings in a group dysfunction likely maintained by nonneutral behavior of the segments below. Again, note that L5 shows a nonneutral single segment dysfunction that is ERS$_{left}$ as in Fig. 6.5 and an FRS$_{left}$ at L4. In this example, the left transverse processes are prominent from L1-L4 in both forward bending, neutral, and backward bending. No matter what position the patient assumes, there is rotation of L1 through L4 to the left. This dysfunction is a neutral group dysfunction of L1 through L4 with the positional diagnosis being neutral, side bent right, and rotated left. Another diagnostic description for this group dysfunction is L1 through

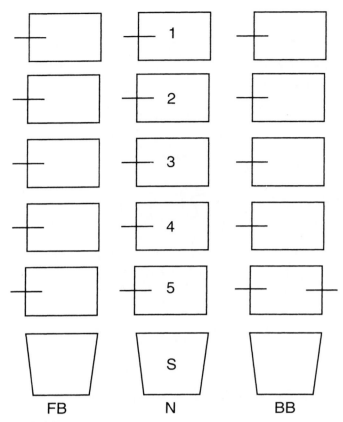

FIGURE 6.7 Neutral group dysfunction example. Oriented from posterior, the arc of motion is represented by the three columns; forward bending (FB), neutral (N) and backward bending (BB). Each box represents a numbered lumbar vertebrae, L1-L5. The unilateral horizontal lines that pass through the sides of the boxes represent prominent transverse processes, side bending is assumed. The sacrum is represented by the trapezium-shaped structure on the bottom of each column (S).

L4 EN (easy normal) left (indicating left convexity). In the therapeutic process, the practitioner identifies and treats all nonneutral dysfunctions first, and if any group dysfunctions remain, they are addressed separately. In the example portrayed in Fig. 6.7, had the ERS$_{left}$ at L5 and the FRS$_{left}$ at L4 been treated first, the neutral group dysfunction may not need further attention.

Adaptation Versus Compensation

It is common to see an adaptive side bending to one side and rotation to the other in a group of vertebrae superior to a nonneutral dysfunction or an unleveled sacrum while the patient is in the neutral posture. This adaptation is the body's desire to remain in an upright position. The finding is reversible when the nonneutral dysfunction is corrected or the sacral base made level.

Compensation occurs over time with change in the anatomy and the curve remains despite correction of the underlying problem. It is not reversible.

HYPERMOBILITY

Manual medicine procedures are appropriate for restriction of articular structures (hypomobility), but if used on hypermobile segments, they could be detrimental, enhancing the hypermobility. In structural diagnosis, we are concerned with three types of hypermobility: (a) hypermobility due to disease such as Ehlers–Danlos syndrome, Marfan syndrome, the marfanoid hypermobility syndrome, and others even more rare[3]; (b) physiologic or generalized hypermobility seen in certain body types (ectomorphic) and frequently observed in gymnasts, ballet dancers, and other athletes[4]; and (c) compensatory hypermobility due to hypomobility elsewhere in the musculoskeletal system.

The pathologic hypermobilities are a group of conditions in which there is alteration in the histology and biochemistry of the connective tissues.[3] In Ehlers–Danlos syndrome, there is articular hypermobility, dermal extensibility, and frequent cutaneous scarring. This condition has been noted in circus performers who are classified as "elastic people." The classic Marfan syndrome demonstrates long slender (Lincolnesque) limbs; ectopic lentis, dilatation of the ascending aorta, and mitral valve prolapse. While the severity of each of the components of the Marfan syndrome vary from patient to patient, all exhibit joint hypermobility. Following joint injury, the hypermobility is increased and it is very difficult to treat patients with this condition who have somatic dysfunction superimposed on their musculoskeletal anatomy. The marfanoid hypermobility syndrome has the same musculoskeletal system findings but seems not to demonstrate either the eye or the vascular changes.

The physiologic or generalized hypermobility group comprises hypermobility of fingers, thumbs, elbows, and knees and trunk forward bending. The Beighton score[5] is a 9-point scale devised for the paired fingers, thumbs, elbows, and knees, with one point assigned to trunk forward bending. Patients with this trait find it easy to become gymnasts and ballet dancers, and increased mobility can result from training and exercise. In healthy individuals, joint mobility reduces rapidly during childhood and then more slowly during adulthood. Patients with increased generalized hypermobility are at risk for increased musculoskeletal system symptoms and diseases, particularly osteoarthritis.[6]

It is in the secondary or compensatory hypermobility states that the manual medicine practitioner becomes more involved. Empirically, compensatory hypermobility appears to develop in areas of the vertebral column as a secondary reaction to hypomobility within the complex. The segments of compensatory hypermobility can be adjacent to, or some distance from, the area(s) of major joint hypomobility. Clinically, there also appears to be relative hypermobility on the opposite side of a segment that is restricted. The major difficulty encountered with these areas of secondary compensatory hypermobility is that they are frequently the ones that are symptomatic. Because they attempt to compensate for restricted motion elsewhere, they receive excess stimulation from increased mobility and frequently become painful and tender. As the painful areas, they receive a great deal of attention from the manual medicine practitioner, who can become trapped into treating the hypermobile segment because it is symptomatic, not realizing that the symptom is secondary to restricted mobility elsewhere. In most instances of compensatory hypermobility, the condition requires little or no direct treatment but responds nicely to appropriate treatment of hypomobility elsewhere in the vertebral column. Many practitioners of musculoskeletal medicine use proliferent-type injection into the ligaments of a hypermobile segment as part of treatment. This system was used empirically for many years; however, recent findings from clinical and animal studies support the observation that proliferent therapy enhances joint stability and reduces nociception.[7] In this author's experience most areas of secondary, compensatory hypermobility are self-correcting once the hypomobility areas are adequately treated and the total musculoskeletal system is restored to functional balance.

One cannot discuss hypermobility without referring to instability. Instability occurs when the degenerative changes or ligamentous damage is sufficient and the opposing joint structures lose their anatomic integrity. The dividing line between extensive hypermobility and instability is very hard to define. In actual instability, the appropriate treatment is either a stabilizing surgical procedure or a restraining orthopedic device.

Diagnosing Hypermobility

The diagnosis of hypermobility in the Ehlers–Danlos and Marfan syndrome group is not difficult as long as the index of suspicion is present and the other physical findings are identified. The 9-point Beighton Score mentioned in the previous section helps give an overall assessment of relative hypermobility. It is in the evaluation of local compensatory hypermobility that the difficulty exists. The diagnostic procedures are variations on regional segmental motion testing. In these procedures, one attempts to hold one segment and move the other in relation to it, comparing it with the perceived normal of the segments above and below the segment suspected of hypermobility. Translatory motion challenges have been found to be the most effective. With the lumbar spine, the patient can be in the lateral recumbent position while the operator monitors each vertebral segment. By grasping two spinous processes with the thumb and index finger, a to-and-fro lateral translatory movement can be introduced and compared above and below (Fig. 6.8). Using the same lateral recumbent position with the knees and hips flexed, the operator can monitor a given segment holding the superior segment and introducing an anteroposterior translatory movement by movement of the operator's thigh against the patient's knees (Fig. 6.9). Combined side bending and rotation challenge can occur in the same position with the operator grasping the feet and ankles and lifting the extremities off the table (Fig. 6.10), and dropping them down below the table (Fig. 6.11), while monitoring the posterior elements of the lumbar vertebrae. Another hypermobility test builds on the fact that in backward bending, as the zygapophysial joints symmetrically close, there is reduction in available lateral translatory movement. With the patient in the prone prop, backward bent position on the table (Fig. 6.12), the operator places thumbs on each side of the spinous

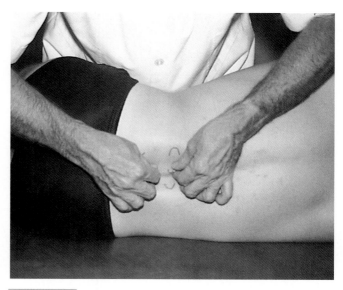

FIGURE 6.8 **Hypermobility testing, lateral translation.**

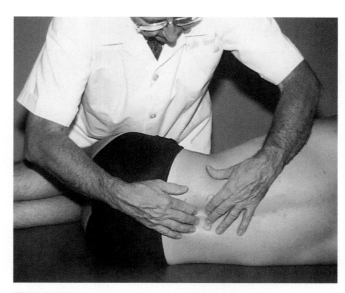

FIGURE 6.9 **Hypermobility testing, anteroposterior translation.**

process overlying the transverse processes of the vertebrae and translates from left to right (Fig. 6.13) and from right to left. Comparing the translatory mobility from segment to segment gives the operator an impression of whether one is more mobile than the other. Testing for hypermobility requires a great deal of practice and the judgment is highly individualistic. If one suspects significant segmental hypermobility, stress X-ray procedures in the flexion–extension and right- and left-side bending modes should be used to assist in the diagnosis.

CONCLUSION

While there is still a need for more research into the biomechanics of vertebral segmental motion and pathologies that might restrict vertebral motion, the concepts and methodologies

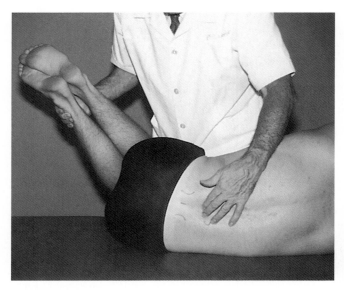

FIGURE 6.10 | Hypermobility testing, side bending rotation.

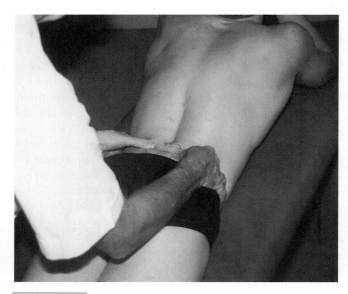

FIGURE 6.12 | Hypermobility testing beginning with thumb contact of spinous and transverse processes while backward bent.

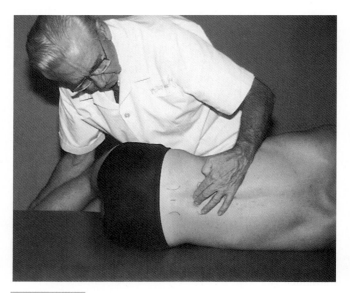

FIGURE 6.11 | Hypermobility testing, side bending rotation.

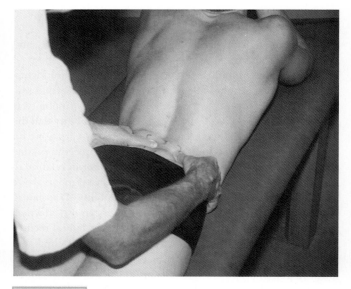

FIGURE 6.13 | Hypermobility testing translation from left to right while backward bent.

described here will provide the practicing manual medicine clinician with sufficient accurate diagnostic information for treatment purposes, for accurate records, and for communicating with a colleague. The hallmarks of structural diagnosis of restricted vertebral function are practice and experience.

REFERENCES

1. Bogduk N, Jull G. The theoretic pathology of acute locked back: A basis for manipulative therapy. *Man Med* 1985;1:78–82.
2. The International Classification of Diseases: Clinical Modification: ICD-9-CM. Dept. of Health and Human Services, Public Health Service, National Center for Health Statistics; Washington, DC; 1991.
3. Malfait F, Hakim AJ, De Paepe A, et al. The genetic basis of the joint hypermobility syndromes. *Rheumatology* 2006;45(5):502.
4. Simmonds JV, RJ Keer. Hypermobility and the hypermobility syndrome. *Man Ther* 2007;12(4):298–309.
5. Beighton P. Hypermobility scoring. *Br J Rheumatol* 1988;27(2):163.
6. Remvig L, Jensen DV, Ward RC. Epidemiology of general joint hypermobility and basis for the proposed criteria for benign joint hypermobility syndrome: Review of the literature. *J Rheumatol* 2007;34 (4):804–809.
7. Dagenais S, Haldeman S, Wooley JR. Intraligamentous injection of sclerosing solutions (prolotherapy) for spinal pain: A critical review of the literature. *Spine J* 2005;5(3):310–328.

7

PRINCIPLES OF SOFT-TISSUE AND OTHER PERIPHERAL STIMULATING TECHNIQUES

Several techniques can be classified as peripheral stimulation therapies. They include soft-tissue technique procedures, Travell trigger points, Chapman reflexes, acupuncture, and others. The soft-tissue procedures to be described have had long acceptance and use in the field of manual medicine. Many of the procedures are the same as, or similar to, those found in traditional massage. Most of the research done in this area is based on traditional massage.

DEFINITION

Soft-tissue technique is defined as a procedure directed toward tissues other than the skeleton while monitoring response and motion changes using diagnostic palpation. It usually involves lateral stretching, linear stretching, deep pressure, traction, and/or separation of muscle origin and insertion (Ward RC (ed.). *Foundations for Osteopathic Medicine*. Baltimore, MD: Williams & Wilkins, 2003: 1229–1253.).

PURPOSE OF SOFT-TISSUE TECHNIQUE

Soft-tissue procedures are widely used in a combined diagnostic and therapeutic mode. They are frequently a prelude to other more definitive manual medicine procedures to the underlying articular structures. They prepare the soft tissues for other technique procedures. They are also used as the only manual medicine intervention to achieve a specific therapeutic goal.

Mechanisms

Fibroblasts are the cellular key component of fascia and soft tissue as it synthesizes collagen, elastin, and the proteoglycans which make up the extracellular matrix (ECM) of our connective tissues. The ECM is the substrate to which cells adhere and on which they grow, migrate, and differentiate. Mechanical forces, such as gravity or movement, are essential for this synthesis and maintenance of connective tissue homeostasis.[1] The ECM is highly specialized in structure and composition to bear different types of mechanical stress; tension or shear. Under the influence of normal mechanical force, the fibroblast secretes growth factors which stimulate cell proliferation and differentiation. The mechanism by which mechanical strain is transmitted into proliferative chemical signals (mechanotransduction) is facilitated by cell surface mechanoreceptors called integrins.[2] Integrins have a signaling as well as mechanical function; they link the ECM to the cytoskeleton and hence are responsible for establishing a mechanical continuum by which forces are transmitted between the outside and the inside of cells.[3]

Transmission and dissipation of this force is one of the key roles of our connective tissues, allowing for efficacy of muscle function for the purpose of movement. This is certainly demonstrated at the muscular level where the force generated from muscle contraction is transmitted to the tendon or the bone via the connective tissue sleeves of the endomysium, perimysium, and epimysium. This mechanism has been named myofascial force transmission.[4] An example is the thoracolumbar fascias role in transferring of forces from the spine to the legs.[5]

In normal connective tissues, the ECM helps to maintain homeostasis by stress shielding the fibroblast. Following tissue damage or repetitive or static high tension states, the ECM environment allows for the differentiation of fibroblasts into myofibroblasts.[6,7] Myofibroblasts are characterized by the expression of α-smooth muscle actin which adheres to collagen within the ECM and promotes local connective tissue remodeling and fibrosis. As a result, the increase in mechanical stress is placed on local peripheral nociceptors, vessels, and muscle fibers; potentially leading to Myofascial pain type symptoms.[8,9]

Mechanical stretching of connective tissue occurs with soft-tissue techniques and acupuncture. Applying brief 10 minute static mechanical stretch to soft tissues, following an acute injury, has shown to have the potential to prevent the myofibroblast differentiation that leads to connective tissue remodeling.[10] In addition, connective tissue fibroblasts have been reported to respond to short-term mechanical stretch with reversible cytoskeletal remodeling and as such these procedures may have mechanical, circulatory, and neurologic effects which are useful in both acute and chronic conditions.[11–15]

Soft-tissue procedures are useful in encouraging circulation of the fluid in and around the soft tissues of the musculoskeletal system, enhancing venous and lymphatic return, and decongesting parts of the body compromised by injury or a disease process.[16–22] These same procedures can have a neurologic effect, particularly modifying muscle physiology to overcome hypertonicity and spasm.[23,24] These neurologic effects can be stimulatory or inhibitory depending on how the procedure was applied. Another neurologic effect is the relief of musculoskeletal pain. This may result from the release of endogenous opioids and other neurohumoral substances.[25–28] Another possible mechanism is the modulation of the spinal reflex pathways by the stimulation of mechanoreceptors, proprioceptors, and nociceptors in the soft tissues.[29,30]

Tonic Effect

Soft-tissue procedures are also useful for their general "tonic" effect on patients, particularly those who have been bedridden for any period due to illness or injury.[31] They seem to enhance the general physical tone and the level of well-being.[32–39] Since many of these procedures seem general in application and result

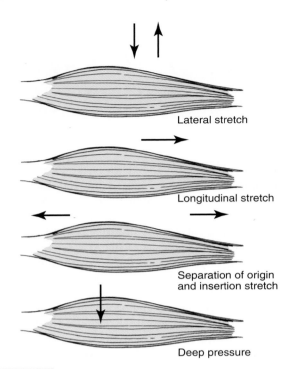

FIGURE 7.1   Soft-tissue procedures.

in various outcomes, the manual medicine practitioner must have a specific therapeutic goal in mind before instituting any soft-tissue procedure. Once the objective is clear, the procedure can be adapted to fit the patient's condition, patient's location, and the operator's strength and ability.

TYPES OF SOFT-TISSUE PROCEDURES

Soft-tissue procedures are oriented toward the direction of a force being applied to the underlying muscle(s) (Fig. 7.1). A force at right angles to the long axis of the muscle is called lateral stretch. The force applied in the direction of the long axis of the muscle is called linear or longitudinal stretch. By applying a force in both directions along the long axis of a muscle, we achieve separation of origin and insertion. If steady, deep pressure is applied to a muscle close to its attachment to the bone, the procedure is called deep pressure. Although these procedures are described in relation to muscle and its fiber direction, remember that application of external force to the muscle area also involves skin, subcutaneous fascia, and the deep fascia surrounding the muscle. All of these tissues are affected by soft-tissue procedures.

THERAPEUTIC PRINCIPLES OF SOFT-TISSUE TECHNIQUE

As in all appropriate manual medicine procedures, the operator's body should be held in a posture that is comfortable and balanced to avoid undue strain or fatigue. The treatment table or bed should be at the appropriate height so that the operator need not bend forward unnecessarily (Fig. 7.2). The operator's stance should be relaxed with one foot slightly in front of the other so that the to-and-fro rocking of the operator's body mass provides the force, not the operator muscle activity.

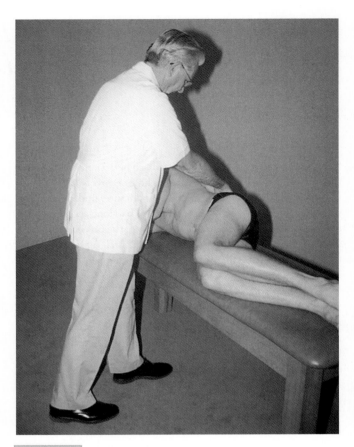

FIGURE 7.2   Operator's stance.

The patient should be in a comfortable and relaxed position. If the prone position is used, the head should be turned toward the operator so that lateral force does not put undue strain on the cervicothoracic junction. If a lateral recumbent position is used, an appropriate pillow height should maintain the head and the neck in the long axis of the trunk. It is useful to have the patient's feet and knees together, with the knees and hips slightly flexed. This provides both comfort and stability for the patient. It is most important that the relationship of the patient and the operator be relaxed and synergistic.

The placement and use of the hands in soft-tissue procedures become most important. These procedures use mainly the finger pads, the thenar eminence of the hand, and the palmer aspect of the thumb. When the operator uses the finger pads to engage the tissues, the distal interphalangeal joint flexion that occurs is a function of the flexor digitorum profundus (Fig. 7.3). Beginners in manual medicine have to practice strengthening the profundus tendon flexor action in order to maintain appropriate application of force to soft tissues. The thenar eminence and palmer surface of the thumb can be laid along the long axis of the muscle and used singly (Fig. 7.4), paired (Fig. 7.5), or with one hand reinforcing the other (Fig. 7.6). Hand placement and control become most important.

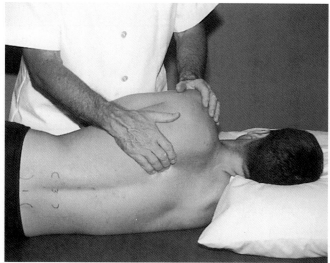

FIGURE 7.3 Soft-tissue, finger-pad contact.

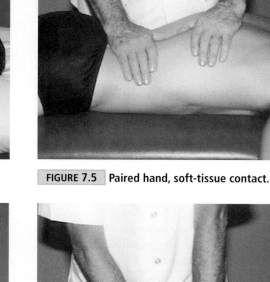

FIGURE 7.5 Paired hand, soft-tissue contact.

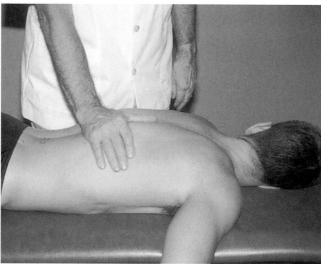

FIGURE 7.4 Single hand, soft-tissue contact.

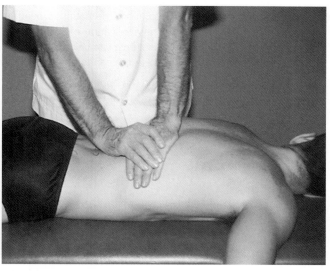

FIGURE 7.6 Combined hand, soft-tissue contact.

CLINICAL PEARL

It is very important that the soft tissues be adequately and accurately engaged at the appropriate layer. In treating the erector spinae mass, there are two common errors to be avoided. The first is pressure toward the spinous processes instead of away from the spinous processes on the side being treated. This causes compression of the erector spinae mass against the lateral side of the spinous process, is painful to the patient, and is counterproductive. The second error is allowing the therapeutic hand to "snap over" an area of hypertonic muscle through failure of control at the muscle layer.

The dosage of soft-tissue procedures is modified by the rate, rhythm, and length of time of application and, most important, by the constant feedback of the tissues to the response obtained.

Constant reassessment of the response is the hallmark of soft-tissue procedures. The operator should continue until the desired response is obtained or should stop as soon as it has been achieved. If the tissue response is not as anticipated, the procedure should be stopped and reassessment of the diagnosis and status of the patient should be made. Slow and steady soft-tissue procedures appear to have inhibitory effects on the tissues. More rapid and vigorous applications of force appear to be stimulatory. The goal to be achieved and the response of the tissues modify the application of force. The operator must also be aware of other reactions within the patient in addition to those of the tissue being treated. Sometimes patients become quite agitated and at other times, they become very relaxed and almost euphoric. It must be remembered that although these procedures are passive, they are still fatiguing, and the length of treatment might be modified by the response of the patient.

SOFT-TISSUE TECHNIQUES

Cervical Spine

Procedure: Unilateral lateral stretch

1. Patient is supine on the table with the operator on the side of the table facing the patient (example left side) (Fig. 7.7).

2. Operator's right hand stabilizes the patient's forehead.

3. Operator's left hand grasps the patient's right cervical paravertebral musculature with the fingertips medial to the muscle mass and just lateral to the spinous processes.

4. Lateral stretch is placed on the cervical musculature by the operator's left hand pulling laterally and somewhat anteriorly, with the operator's right hand maintaining the stability of the patient's head.

5. Lateral stretch is applied and released rhythmically throughout the cervical musculature with particular reference to areas of increased muscle tone and soft-tissue congestion.

6. The procedure can be varied to allow the patient's head to rotate toward the left during the application of force by the operator's left hand and a counterforce can be applied by the operator's right hand in a "push–pull" manner.

7. The procedure can be repeated on the opposite side by having the operator stand on the patient's right now.

SOFT-TISSUE TECHNIQUES

Cervical Spine

Procedure: Bilateral–lateral stretch

1. Patient is supine on the table with the operator standing at the head of the table (Fig. 7.8).

2. Operator's finger pads contact the medial side of the cervical paravertebral musculature bilaterally.

3. Operator puts simultaneous lateral stretch on both sides of the cervical musculature, moving from above downward or below upward and focusing on the side of greater tissue reaction and muscle hypertonicity.

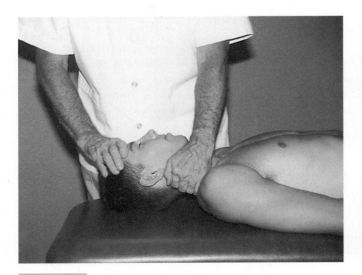

FIGURE 7.7 Soft-tissue, unilateral lateral stretch.

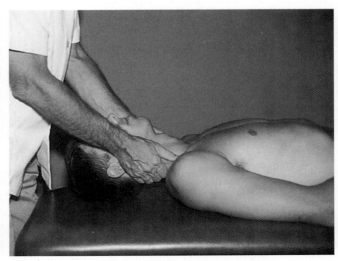

FIGURE 7.8 Soft-tissue, bilateral lateral stretch.

SOFT-TISSUE TECHNIQUES

Cervical Spine

Procedure: Long axis longitudinal stretch

1. Patient is supine with the operator standing or sitting at the head of the table.

2. Operator's one hand cradles the skull with the index finger and thumb in contact with the insertion of the cervical musculature into the occiput, and the chin is held by the other hand (Fig. 7.9).

3. By the use of body weight, the operator puts long-axis extension (traction) in a cephalic direction and then releases.

4. Repeat as necessary.

Caution: Too much traction is frequently counterproductive.

SOFT-TISSUE TECHNIQUES

Cervical Spine

Procedure: Suboccipital muscle deep pressure

1. Patient is supine with the operator standing or sitting at the head of the table.

2. Operator's fingertips of each hand contact the bony attachment of the deep cervical musculature at the suboccipital region.

3. By flexing the distal interphalangeal joints, the operator puts sustained deep pressure over the muscular attachment to the occipital bone (Fig. 7.10).

4. Pressure is applied on each side to achieve balance in tension and tone.

5. Pressure is released when bilateral relaxation occurs.

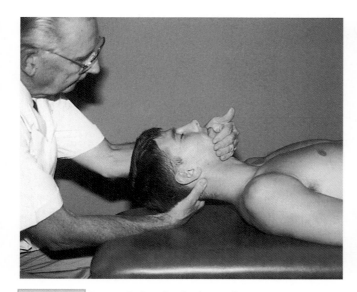

FIGURE 7.9 | Long axis, longitudinal stretch.

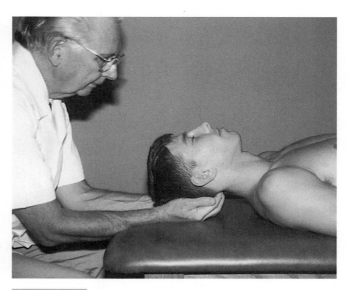

FIGURE 7.10 | Suboccipital muscle, deep pressure.

SOFT-TISSUE TECHNIQUES

Cervical Spine

Procedure: Separation origin and insertion (example: right upper trapezius)

1. Patient is supine with the operator standing at the head of the table.

2. Operator's left hand is placed over the patient's occiput and the operator controls the head and neck position.

3. Operator's right hand is placed over the patient's right acromion process (Fig. 7.11).

4. Operator's left hand side bends the head and the neck to the left with some left rotation while the right hand puts counterforce on the acromion process, separating the origin and the insertion of the upper fibers of the trapezius.

5. By reversal of hand position, the opposite side can be treated with the goal of symmetry of length and tone of each trapezius.

SOFT-TISSUE TECHNIQUES

Thoracic Spine

Procedure: Lateral stretch

1. Patient is in lateral recumbent position lying with the involved side uppermost and the operator standing and facing the patient.

2. For upper thoracic region, the patient's left arm is draped over the operator's right arm and the finger pads contact the medial side of the paravertebral musculature (Fig. 7.12).

3. Operator pulls thoracic paravertebral musculature laterally and releases in a rhythmic fashion.

4. A counterforce can be applied by the operator's left arm against the patient's left shoulder for additional leverage.

5. For rhomboid stretch, use the same body position as for upper thoracic spine but now the finger pads are in contact with the vertebral border of the scapula (Fig. 7.13). The scapula is swept anterolaterally around the chest wall with stretch in the direction of the fibers of the rhomboid muscle.

6. Repeat as necessary.

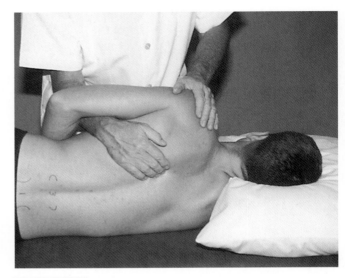

FIGURE 7.12 **Lateral stretch, upper thoracic region.**

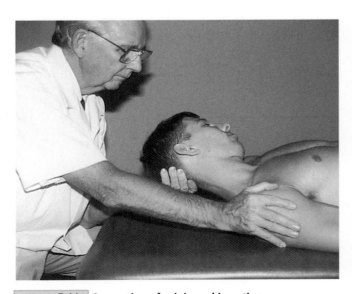

FIGURE 7.11 **Separation of origin and insertion.**

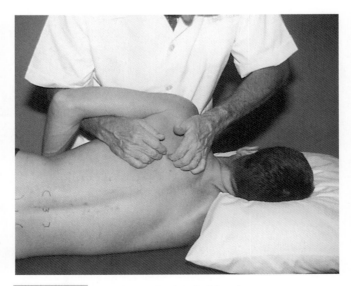

FIGURE 7.13 **Lateral stretch, rhomboid region.**

SOFT-TISSUE TECHNIQUES

Thoracolumbar Spine

Procedure: Lateral stretch

1. Patient lies in lateral recumbent position with the involved side uppermost. The operator faces the patient.

2. Operator's right hand grasps the thoracolumbar paravertebral muscle mass on the involved side with the left hand stabilizing the patient's left shoulder (Fig. 7.14).

3. An alternative hand position has the operator's left hand grasping the thoracolumbar paravertebral muscle mass with the right hand stabilizing the patient's pelvis over the left ilium (Fig. 7.15).

4. Operator's hand in contact with the paravertebral musculature stretches laterally against the counterforce applied at the pelvis or the shoulder girdle.

5. Repeat as necessary throughout the thoracolumbar muscle region.

6. Variation sometimes allows the patient's left arm to be flexed at the elbow and the operator's left hand to be threaded through before application to paravertebral musculature.

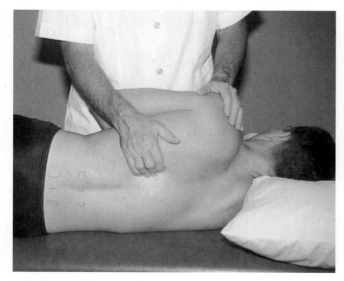

FIGURE 7.14   Lateral stretch, thoracolumbar region.

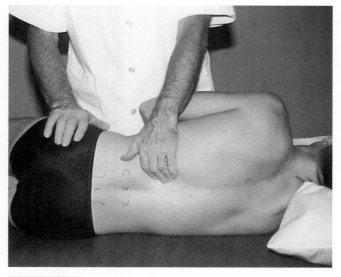

FIGURE 7.15   Lateral stretch, thoracolumbar region.

SOFT-TISSUE TECHNIQUES

Thoracolumbar Spine

Procedure: Lateral and longitudinal stretch

1. Patient is in lateral recumbent position with the involved side uppermost. The operator faces the patient.

2. Operator's left forearm is threaded through the patient's left axilla and the left hand in contact with the left paravertebral muscle mass.

3. Operator's right forearm is in a superior aspect of the patient's left ilium with finger pads in contact with the left paravertebral musculature.

4. Finger-pad contact of both the hands stretches paravertebral musculature laterally (Fig. 7.16).

5. Simultaneously with lateral stretch, the operator's forearms are separated with the right arm going caudally and the left cephalically applying a longitudinal stretch (Fig. 7.17).

6. Repeat as necessary throughout the lumbar and thoracic paravertebral musculature.

SOFT-TISSUE TECHNIQUES

Thoracolumbar Spine

Procedure: Prone lateral stretch

1. Patient lies prone on the table with arms at the side and the face turned toward the operator.

2. Operator stands at the side of the table.

3. Operator's thumbs and thenar eminences are placed on medial side of the involved paravertebral musculature. Lateral stretch is applied rhythmically throughout the involved areas (Fig. 7.5).

4. A variation is applying lateral stretch using one hand on top of the other as reinforcement (Fig. 7.6).

5. Another variation is for the operator's right hand to grasp the patient's right anterior superior iliac spine while the left thumb and thenar eminence put lateral stretch on the paravertebral musculature (Fig. 7.18). Lifting the patient's right ilium provides a counterforce.

6. Repeat as necessary.

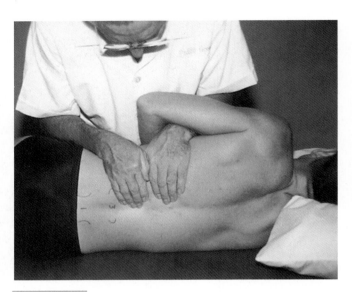

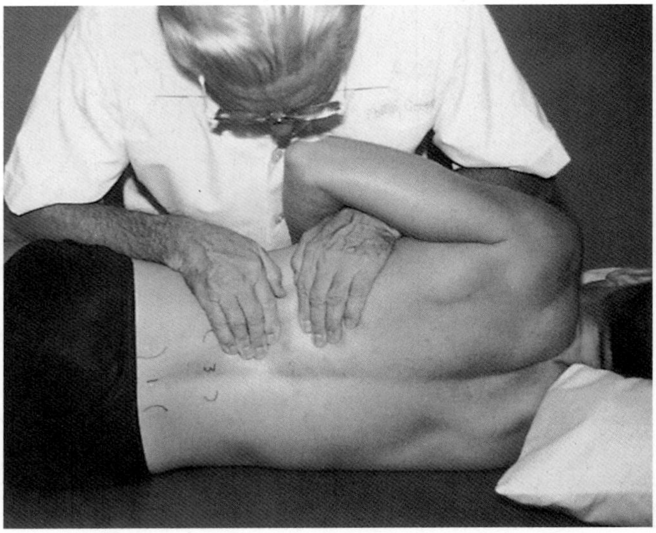

FIGURE 7.16   Lateral recumbent, lateral stretch with counterforce.

FIGURE 7.17   Separation of origin and insertion.

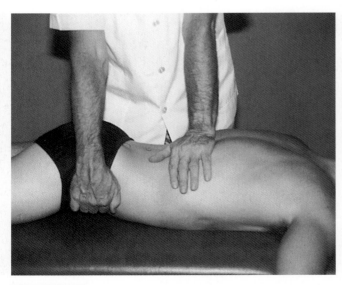

FIGURE 7.18   Prone, lateral stretch with counterforce.

SOFT-TISSUE TECHNIQUES

Thoracolumbar Spine

Procedure: Deep pressure

1. Patient is prone on the table.

2. Operator places thumbs, or thumb reinforced by hand, over the area of hypertonic muscle (Fig. 7.19). This is most effective in the medial groove between the spinous process and the longissimus, overlying the hypertonic fourth-layer vertebral muscle.

3. Steady pressure is applied in a ventral direction and sustained until muscle release is felt.

4. A variation is the placement of the operator's olecranon process of the elbow overlying the hypertonic muscle. Body weight can be used to provide ventral compressive force against the hypertonic muscle (Fig. 7.20).

5. Repeat as necessary.

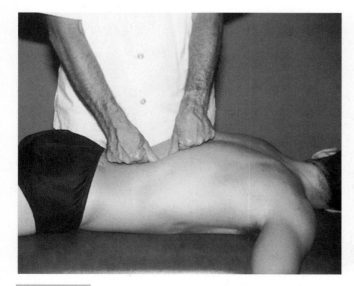

FIGURE 7.19 **Deep inhibitory pressure with thumbs.**

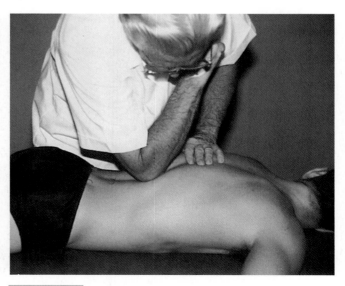

FIGURE 7.20 **Deep inhibitory pressure using elbow.**

SOFT-TISSUE TECHNIQUES

Gluteal Region

Procedure: Deep pressure

1. Patient is in prone or lateral recumbent position with the involved side uppermost.

2. Operator can stand at the side or in front of the patient.

3. Reinforced thumbs are placed over hypertonic areas of gluteal musculature either near the origin on the ilium, within the belly, or at the insertion in the greater trochanter (Fig. 7.21).

4. Deep pressure is maintained until relaxation is felt.

5. Variation can be the use of the olecranon process of the elbow as the contact point and body weight being applied against the hypertonic muscle (Fig. 7.22).

6. Repeat as necessary.

To this point, the soft-tissue techniques have been directed toward the skin, fascia, and muscle in a biomechanical or postural–structural model. Other soft tissues of the body respond well to appropriate soft-tissue techniques using different models, particularly the respiratory–circulatory model and the visceral model.

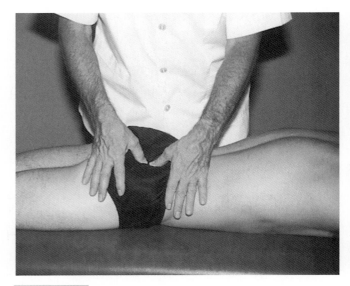

FIGURE 7.21 Deep pressure gluteal region.

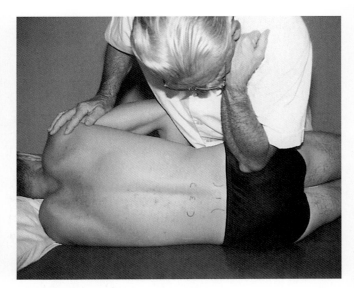

FIGURE 7.22 Deep pressure using olecranon process.

LYMPHATIC PUMP TECHNIQUES

Lymphatic pump techniques are an application of the respiratory–circulatory model. The therapeutic goal is to enhance venous and lymphatic flow throughout the body and respiratory exchange.[40,41] An underlying principle of the respiratory–circulatory model is to work from central to distal. Because all of the lymph flow of the body empties into the venous system through the subclavian veins at the thoracic inlet, the thoracic inlet is the place to start. The most effective thoracic inlet technique in this author's hand has been the necklace technique in the myofascial release technique system (see Chapter 11). The thoracoabdominal diaphragm is the most important "pump" of the venous and lymphatic systems. It is but one of several diaphragms in the body that must work synergistically for maximum total body efficiency. In addition to the thoracoabdominal diaphragm, there are three others from the functional perspective. One is in the cranium (see Chapter 12) and is the diaphragmatic function of the tentorium cerebelli. The aforementioned thoracic inlet also functions as a diaphragm exerting pumping action on the structures that pass through it. For the thoracic inlet to function effectively, there must be good biomechanics of T1 and the first ribs. The fourth is the pelvic diaphragm, which exerts a strong influence on the pelvic viscera in both males and females. The pelvic diaphragm is intimately related to the biomechanics of the pelvis, the sacrum, and the pubes. All four of these diaphragms need to function as a coordinated unit. Most of the lymph pump techniques focus on the chest wall and primarily address thoracoabdominal diaphragmatic function.

DIAPHRAMATIC TECHNIQUES

Thoracic Inlet

See thoracic inlet (necklace technique), Chapter 11.

Pectoral Release

1. Patient is supine with the operator at the head of the table.

2. Operator's two hands, particularly the middle fingers, grasp the patient's inferior border of the pectoral muscles (Fig. 7.23).

3. Operator applies bilateral cephalic traction on the inferior aspect of the pectoral muscles.

4. The response elicited is the release of muscle tension.

5. Observe thorax and abdomen for change from thoracic to abdominal breathing.

Thoracoabdominal Diaphragm

Procedure: Diaphragmatic release, supine

1. Patient is supine on the table with the operator standing at the side.

2. Operator's fingertips contact the inferior surface of the diaphragm below the costal arch on each side. Operator's other hand stabilizes the lower anterior rib cage (Fig. 7.24).

3. Operator maintains cephalic pressure on the inferior aspect of the diaphragm. Inhalation is resisted and exhalation encouraged. Fingertip compression is maintained until diaphragm is released.

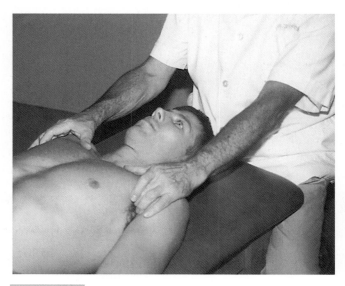

FIGURE 7.23 Pectoral release.

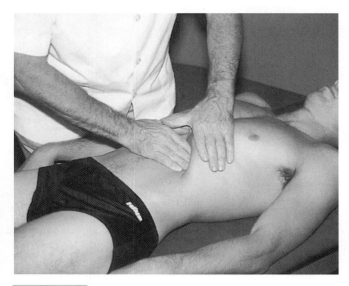

FIGURE 7.24 Diaphragmatic release, supine.

Diaphragmatic Release Sitting Technique

1. Patient sits on the table with the operator behind.

2. Operator's fingertips bilaterally contact the inferior surface of the diaphragm below the costal arch (Fig. 7.25).

3. Patient slumps against the operator by forward bending the trunk (Fig. 7.26).

4. Operator maintains cephalic compression on the inferior aspect of the diaphragm during the patient's inhalation effort.

5. Several applications may be necessary with fine-tuning of the operator's fingers on specific areas of the diaphragmatic tension.

6. A variation finds the operator sitting in front of the patient with the thumbs in contact with the inferior surface of the diaphragm below the costal arch (Fig. 7.27). Patient slumps forward on the operator's thumbs. Exhalation effort is followed by upward pressure by the operator against points of the diaphragmatic tension. Repeat until diaphragmatic release is obtained (Fig. 7.28).

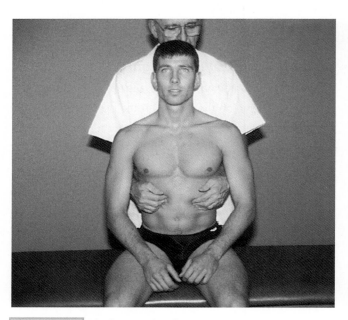

FIGURE 7.25 Diaphragmatic release, sitting.

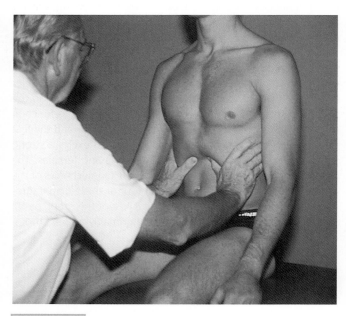

FIGURE 7.27 Diaphragmatic release, sitting.

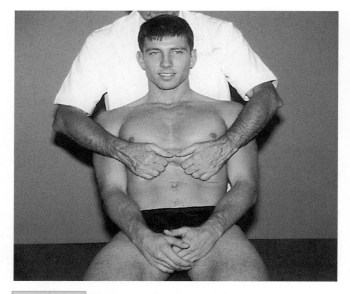

FIGURE 7.26 Diaphragmatic release, sitting.

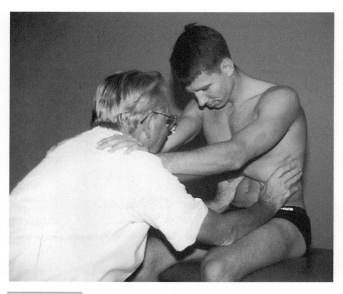

FIGURE 7.28 Diaphragmatic release, sitting.

Pelvic Diaphragm

Procedure: Pelvic diaphragm release, lateral recumbent

1. Patient is in lateral recumbent position with hips and knees flexed and the involved side uppermost.

2. Operator stands in front of the patient with the extended fingers of the right hand placed on medial side of the left ischial tuberosity (Fig. 7.29).

3. Fingers move cephalad along the ischium to the lateral side of the ischiorectal fossa until the fingertips contact the pelvic diaphragm.

4. During the patient's exhalation, the operator's fingers move cephalad and hold against pelvic diaphragm as the patient performs deep inhalation.

5. With the release of diaphragmatic tension, the palpating fingers observe the diaphragm to move freely into the fingers during inhalation and away during exhalation.

6. Repeat on both sides until symmetric balance is achieved.

Pelvic Diaphragm

Procedure: Pelvic diaphragm, supine

1. Patient is supine on the table with the hips and the knees flexed.

2. Operator stands or sits at the side of the patient facing toward the head.

3. Operator's fingers contact the medial side of the right ischial tuberosity and move cephalad to contact the pelvic diaphragm at the superior aspect of the ischiorectal fossa (Fig. 7.30).

4. During the patient's inhalation, the diaphragm should descend against the operator's fingers and during exhalation ascend away from the fingers.

5. The most common dysfunction is the inability to fully ascend. Treatment consists of maintaining cephalic pressure on the diaphragm as the patient inhales. During the patient's exhalation, the operator follows the diaphragm cephalad as far as possible and repeats the respiratory action.

6. The procedure can be combined by having the operator's other hand contact the lower right costal cage to monitor the thoracoabdominal diaphragm to be sure the two diaphragms are working synchronously.

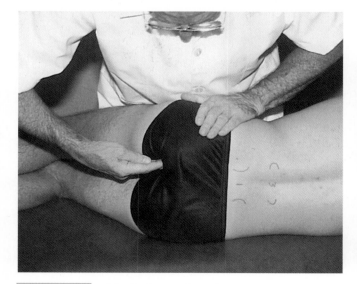

FIGURE 7.29 Pelvic diaphragm, lateral recumbent.

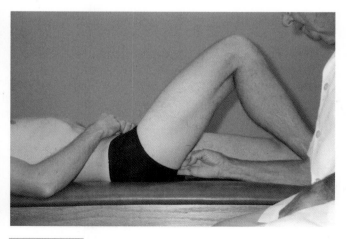

FIGURE 7.30 Pelvic diaphragm, supine.

RIB RAISING TECHNIQUES

Rib raising techniques influence rib cage mechanics to enhance venous and lymphatic flow and respiratory exchange. They also have another benefit. The lateral chain ganglia of the sympathetic division of the autonomic nervous system lie on the posterior chest wall overlying the rib heads. Increased mobility of the rib heads appears to have a positive effect on the segmental function of the sympathetic nervous system. Rib raising in the upper thorax above T5 affects the intrathoracic viscera. Below T5, the effect is on the intra-abdominal viscera. It is beneficial to maximize thoracic cage function before instituting lymph pump treatment.

Rib Raising Supine

1. Patient is supine with the operator standing or sitting at the side.

2. Operator's hands slide under the patient with finger contact medial to the rib angles and with the forearms in contact with the table (Fig. 7.31).

3. Operator's fingers put lateral traction on the rib angles while lifting the rib cage by pushing down on the forearms. Do not try to lift the rib cage by wrist flexion.

4. Move up and down the rib cage on both sides. If a second operator is available, bilateral rib raising can be done.

Rib Raising Sitting

1. Patient sits with the operator standing in front.

2. Patient crosses the forearms grasping the opposite elbow and places them on the operator's chest. An alternate position places the patient's extended arms over the operator's shoulder.

3. Operator contacts medial to the rib angles bilaterally and pulls laterally while pulling the patient toward him (Fig. 7.32).

4. Operator moves from above downward or below upward while the patient inhales when the operator pulls the patient forward and exhales on relaxation.

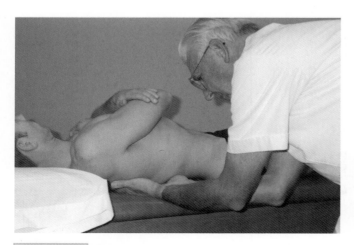

FIGURE 7.31 Rib raising, supine.

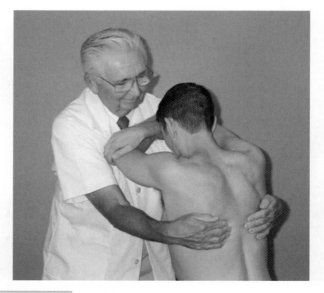

FIGURE 7.32 Rib raising, sitting.

Lymphatic Pump

Procedure: Thoracic lymphatic pump

1. Patient is supine on the table with the operator at the head of the table.

2. Operator has both hands in contact with the anterior aspect of the thoracic cage with the heel of the hand just below the clavicle (Fig. 7.33).

3. Operator repetitively and rhythmically oscillates the chest at a rate of approximately 100 to 110 times per minute.

4. A preferred alternate technique has the patient inhale deeply and then exhale.

5. During the exhalation phase, the operator puts oscillatory compression on the chest cage.

6. At the end of exhalation, the patient is instructed to breathe in while the operator holds the chest wall in the exhalation position for a momentary period.

7. Operator rapidly releases compression on the chest during the patient's inhalation effort.

8. Repeat steps 4 through 7 several times.

Lymphatic Pump

Procedure: Unilateral thoracic lymphatic pump

1. Patient is supine with the operator at the side of the table.

2. Operator's left arm grasps the patient's right upper extremity.

3. Operator's right hand is in contact with the right thoracic cage of the patient (Fig. 7.34).

4. During the patient's inhalation, the operator puts traction on the patient's right upper extremity.

5. During the exhalation phase, traction on upper extremity is released, and the operator puts oscillatory force against the thoracic cage during exhalation.

6. Operator's right hand maintains compression on the chest wall during initial phase of inhalation and gives rapid release, simultaneously cephalically lifting on the patient's right upper extremity.

7. Repeat steps 2 through 6 several times.

8. A lateral recumbent variation has the patient with the treated side being uppermost. The operator's left arm grasps the patient's right upper extremity while the operator's right hand is applied to the patient's right thoracic cage (Fig 7.35). Steps 2 through 6 are repeated several times.

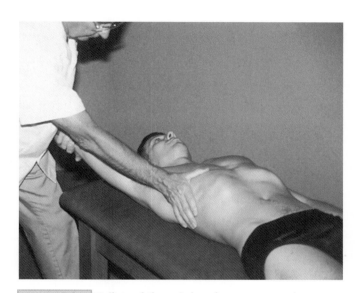

FIGURE 7.34 Unilateral thoracic lymph pump.

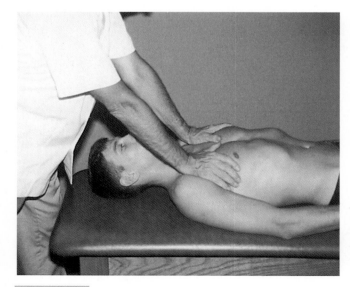

FIGURE 7.33 Bilateral thoracic lymph pump, supine.

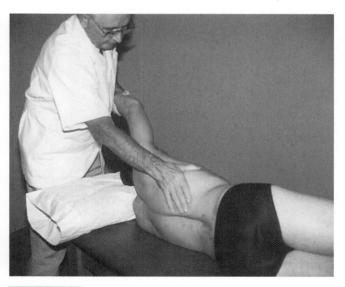

FIGURE 7.35 Unilateral thoracic lymph pump.

Lymphatic Pump

Procedure: Lymphatic pump, lower extremity

1. Patient is supine with the operator at the end of the table.

2. Operator grasps the dorsum of both the feet with each hand and introduces plantar flexion (Fig. 7.36).

3. Operator applies oscillatory movement in a caudad direction and notes oscillatory wave of lower extremities up to trunk.

4. Operator grasps the toes and the ball of the patient's foot and takes the foot into dorsi flexion (Fig. 7.37).

5. Cephalic oscillatory movement is applied to the dorsiflexed feet.

6. Repeat in the dorsiflexed and plantar-flexed directions several times.

Lymphatic Pump

Procedure: Lymphatic pump, upper extremity

1. Patient is supine with the operator at the head of the table.

2. Patient raises both the hands above the head and the operator grasps each wrist (Fig. 7.38).

3. Operator applies intermittent cephalic oscillatory traction to the patient's upper extremities noting response in the thoracic cage.

4. Repeat as necessary.

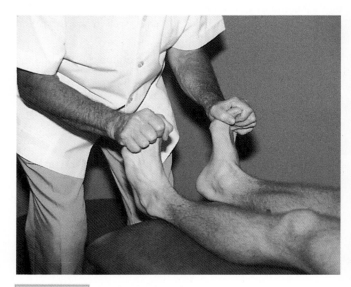

FIGURE 7.37   Lymphatic pump, lower extremity.

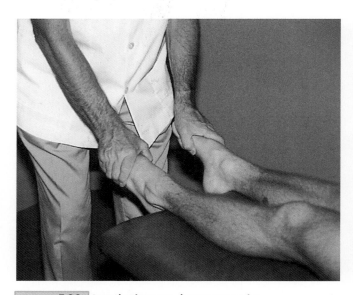

FIGURE 7.36   Lymphatic pump, lower extremity.

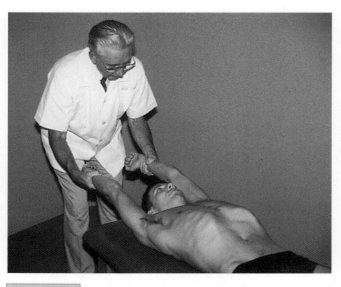

FIGURE 7.38   Lymphatic pump, upper extremity.

VISCERAL TECHNIQUE

The internal viscera are specialized soft tissues encased and suspended in specialized fasciae. As such they are subject to fascial drag, twisting, and compression. Visceral techniques are designed to enhance visceral mobility, reduce passive congestion, and increase drainage of hollow organs. In addition to direct approaches to the viscera, it is important to recall the innervation to the viscera under treatment. All internal viscera receive parasympathetic and sympathetic innervation. The best approach to the parasympathetic division is through the craniosacral technique (see Chapter 12) giving particular attention to the cranial base and the jugular foramen. The vagus nerve has some connection with the C2 root. Therefore, good function of the cranial base and the upper cervical spine seems to enhance good parasympathetic nerve function. The pelvic organs receive parasympathetic innervation from the sacral nerves. Normalization of sacral function from the craniosacral and biomechanical perspectives appears to have a beneficial effect on parasympathetic innervation to pelvic viscera. The sympathetic division innervation of the viscera is segmentally related with all of the viscera above the diaphragm having preganglionic origin in the spinal cord above T5 and all of the viscera below the diaphragm below T5. Rib raising described above is one way to positively influence sympathetic nervous system function. Visceral techniques need to be applied gently and with an appreciation of their structural anatomy. Visceral techniques found useful in this author's experience are as follows.

Visceral Technique

Procedure: Supine mesenteric release

1. Patient is supine on the table with the operator standing at the side.
2. Operator places both the hands on each side of the anterior abdomen (Fig. 7.39).
3. Operator applies clockwise and counterclockwise rotations to the anterior abdominal wall with some abdominal compression. The operator senses the mobility of the small and the large intestines and follows their directions of motility.
4. Sensation of release of the underlying abdominal contents is the end point.

Visceral Technique

Procedure: Mesenteric release, prone

1. Patient is prone on the table in knee–chest position.
2. Operator stands at the side or head of the table.
3. Operator places both the hands over the lower abdomen just above the pubic bones (Fig. 7.40).
4. Operator's hands lift the abdominal contents out of the pelvis in a slow oscillatory fashion until release is felt.
5. Operator localizes lifting force in the right lower quadrant for the cecum, the left lower quadrant for the sigmoid colon, and the suprapubic area for the pelvic organs.

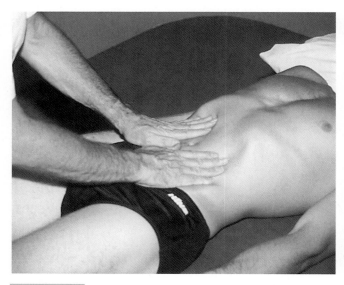

FIGURE 7.39 **Supine mesenteric release.**

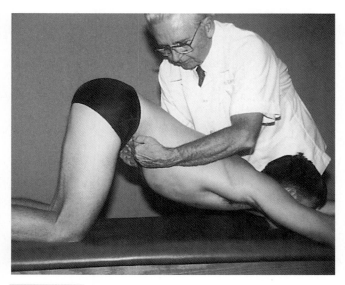

FIGURE 7.40 **Prone mesenteric release.**

Visceral Technique

Procedure: Cecum and sigmoid lifts, lateral recumbent

1. Patient is in right lateral recumbent position for the cecum.

2. Operator stands behind and reaches across the abdomen to pick up the cecum and carry it cephalad and medially (Fig. 7.41).

3. Operator follows ascending colon to the hepatic flexure reducing restrictions.

4. Patient is in left lateral recumbent position for the sigmoid colon.

5. Operator stands behind and reaches across the abdomen to pick up the sigmoid colon and carry it cephalad and medially (Fig. 7.42).

6. Operator follows descending colon to splenic flexure reducing restrictions.

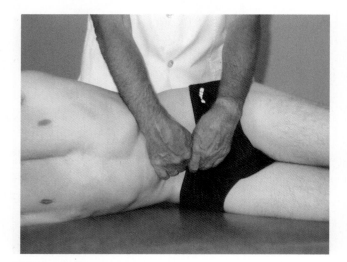

FIGURE 7.41 Lift of cecum.

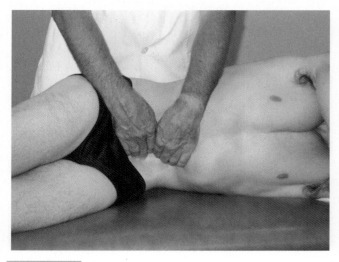

FIGURE 7.42 Lift of sigmoid colon.

Visceral Technique

Procedure: Liver and gallbladder drainage

1. Operator begins by releasing tension around the liver and the gallbladder area by modifying the supine diaphragmatic release localizing to the liver margin and the gallbladder under the right diaphragm (Fig. 7.24).

2. Patient is supine and the operator is standing at the right side.

3. Operator places one hand behind the lower right rib cage and the other over the right costal arch (Fig. 7.43).

4. Operator alternately compresses and releases the liver and the gallbladder between the two hands.

5. A variation has the patient in the left lateral recumbent position with the operator behind with the hands in front and behind the right costal arch and the lower rib cage (Fig. 7.44).

6. Operator alternately compresses and relaxes pressure over the liver and the gallbladder.

7. A second variation is a repetitive percussive application of force through the forearm contact over the right costal arch (Fig. 7.45).

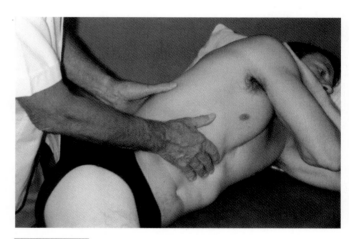

FIGURE 7.44 Liver pump, lateral recumbent.

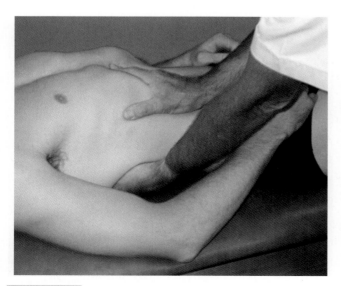

FIGURE 7.43 Liver pump, supine.

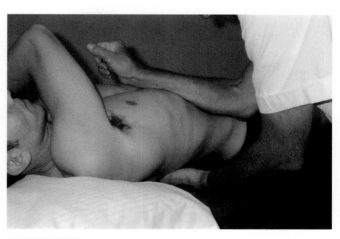

FIGURE 7.45 Liver percussion.

Visceral Technique

Procedure: Splenic drainage

1. Operator releases tension around spleen by modifying the diaphragmatic release under the left costal margin (Fig. 7.24).

2. Patient is supine on the table with the operator standing at the left side.

3. Operator places posterior hand over the left lower rib cage and the anterior hand over the left costal arch (Fig. 7.46).

4. Operator alternately compresses and releases over the spleen.

5. An alternative has the patient in the right lateral recument position and the operator behind with the hands in front and behind the spleen providing alternating pressure and relaxation (Fig. 7.47).

6. An alternative has the operator applying a percussive force over the left costal arch stimulating splenic drainage (Fig. 7.48).

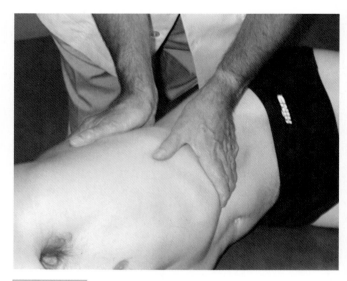

FIGURE 7.47   **Splenic pump, lateral recumbent.**

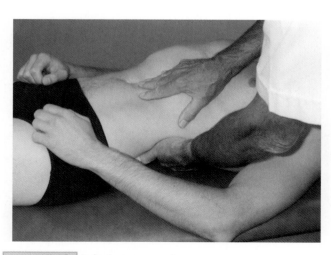

FIGURE 7.46   **Splenic pump, supine.**

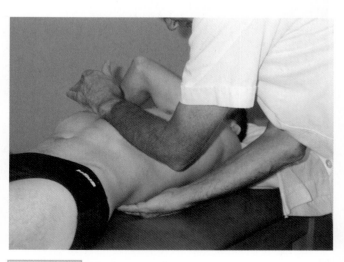

FIGURE 7.48   **Splenic percussion.**

Soft-tissue techniques can be quite helpful in treating a patient with any number of upper respiratory infections, otitis media, colds, flulike symptoms, and so forth. They are designed to assist in the drainage of the lymphatic channels from the head and the neck. Again, the thoracic inlet should be examined and treated first to allow better drainage into the mediastinum.

Soft-tissue Technique

Procedure: Mandibular drainage

1. Patient is supine with the operator standing opposite the side to be treated.

2. Operator places one hand over the frontal area to stabilize the head and the other hand grasps the ramus of the mandible as far as the angle (Fig. 7.49).

3. Patient relaxes the jaw and the operator puts rhythmic caudal and medial traction on the mandible stimulating drainage of the eustachian tube.

4. The procedure is applied bilaterally.

Soft-tissue Technique

Procedure: Hyoid mobilization

1. Patient is supine on the table with the operator standing at the side.

2. Operator's one hand holds the frontal area stabilizing the head and the thumb and the index finger of the other hand gently grasp the hyoid bone (Fig. 7.50).

3. Operator gently rocks the hyoid bone from side to side, relaxing tension in the suprahyoid and infrahyoid muscles.

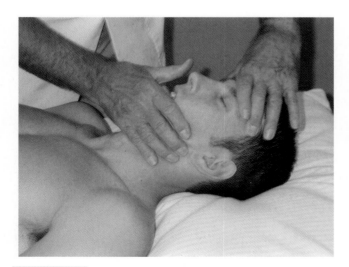

FIGURE 7.49 Mandibular drainage.

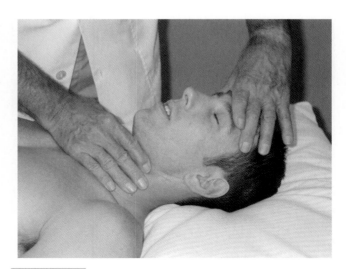

FIGURE 7.50 Hyoid mobilization.

Soft-tissue Technique

Procedure: Cervical lymphatic drainage

1. Patient is supine on the table with the operator standing at the side.

2. Operator stabilizes the head with one hand on the frontal area and the other hand placed on the cervical lymphatic chain, first in front of (Fig. 7.51) then posterior to the sternocleido-mastoid muscle (Fig. 7.52).

3. Operator gently and rhythmically "milks" the cervical lymphatic chain from above downward on each side, enhancing lymph drainage.

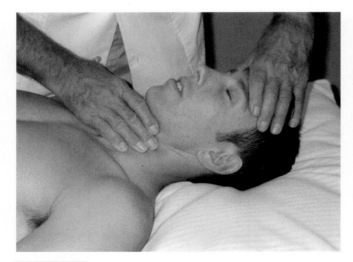

FIGURE 7.51 **Cervical lymphatic drainage.**

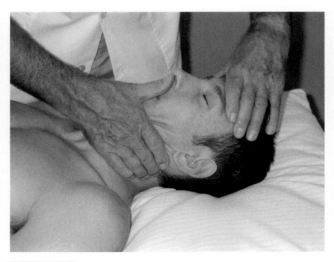

FIGURE 7.52 **Cervical lymphatic drainage.**

OTHER SOFT-TISSUE TECHNIQUES

There are a variety of peripheral stimulating techniques that have been described as beneficial. They include Chapman reflexes and Travell trigger points.

Chapman Reflexes

In the 1920s, Frank Chapman, D.O., originally described Chapman reflexes. The first definitive publication of the work was by Charles Owens, D.O., in cooperation with Chapman's widow, Ada Hinckley Chapman, D.O., and W.F. Link, D.O., in 1937. Chapman reflexes are found on the anterior and posterior surfaces of the body as small (2 to 3 mm), round, shotty, tender nodules in remarkably consistent locations usually near bony or cartilaginous structures. They have been correlated with disease or dysfunction of the internal organs. It has been postulated that they are related in some fashion to the lymphatic system and operate through the sympathetic nervous system. Attempts at histologic study of these reflexes have been disappointing, but many clinicians have corroborated the clinical observation of these reflex points. They have been deemed useful in the differential diagnosis of a patient with a difficult presentation, and their inclusion in the physical examination can be helpful. The anterior points are used more for diagnosis and the posterior points for treatment. Most clinicians find them more useful diagnostically. Finding the reflex point in the appropriate area that is exquisitely tender while other reflex areas are silent makes the diagnosis. Treatment of both anterior and posterior reflexes is by rotary pressure for 10 to 30 seconds until the reflex point becomes less tender and appears to be less well localized. Addressing the Chapman reflexes as part of the management may assist in treatment of the patient (Figs. 7.53 and 7.54).[42]

Travell Trigger Points

Another system of soft-tissue peripheral stimulation technique was developed by Janet Travell, M.D. She observed the presence of tender "taut band" points in muscles that usually had specific referred pain patterns. Travell and her colleague, David Simons, M.D., have mapped out these localized areas of muscle irritability throughout the body. She originally treated these trigger points by the injection of local procaine. Subsequently, it was found that these trigger points responded to dry needling and localized cooling and stretching. These points are also similar to those subjected to sustained compression by "acupressure." Travell identified many of these trigger points as the cause of suspected visceral disease, particularly in the pectoral muscles simulating coronary heart disease. Autonomic nervous system effects have also been associated with the presence of trigger points.[43] Identifying a trigger point in a muscle and observing its referral pattern on stimulation make the diagnosis. The exact mapping of the myriad of trigger points in the system is found in the two-volume text, Myofascial Pain and Dysfunction. Jay Shah, M.D., Ph.D., using micoanalytical techniques to measure the in vivo biochemical milieu of muscle, in near real time at the subnanogram level of concentration, within an active trigger point established unequivocally that at least nine components of the myofascial trigger point milieu were well-known sensitizers of muscle nociceptors.[44,45] His work strongly substantiates Simons and Travell's hypothesis (hypoxia and ischemia are related to local release of inflammatory substances, which may sensitize muscle nociceptors) as a valid explanation for the pain associated with myofascial trigger points.[46]

Through experience, this author has found that there is relationship between the presence of myofascial trigger points and levels of vertebral segmental dysfunction. Many times, an identified trigger point will disappear when a manual medicine procedure has been applied to a vertebral dysfunction in a dermatomal relationship to the muscle trigger. Sometimes the trigger does not respond. Likewise, treating a trigger point, particularly with needling, will result in the resolution of the vertebral somatic dysfunction. There is currently no explanation for this particular observation. It is also interesting to note that myofascial trigger points are more commonly found in postural muscles than in dynamic muscles, with the exception of the levator scapulae and quadratus lumborum muscles. This author previously injected trigger points regularly but has recently experienced the need to only inject those that do not respond to treatment of the rest of the musculoskeletal system. The most common muscles still requiring injection are the levator scapulae and the quadratus lumborum. The reader is encouraged to study this system through the work of Travell and Simons as well as Shah. It will be found very worthwhile.

CONCLUSION

Soft-tissue procedures are useful in a wide variety of acute to chronic patient conditions. They are applicable to all regions of the body. They are useful as independent procedures or can be combined with other manual medicine procedures. Experience in palpating the tissue response to the soft tissue is necessary to properly use them for the appropriate diagnosis.

FIGURE 7.53 Chapman reflexes: anterior points.

(From Kuchera ML, Kuchera WA, eds. *Osteopathic Considerations in Systemic Dysfunction*. Columbus, OH: Greyden Press, 1994, with permission.)

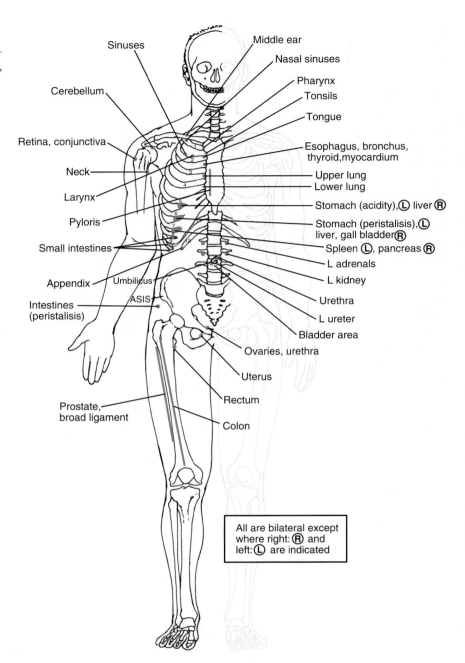

Sinuses
Middle ear
Nasal sinuses
Cerebellum
Pharynx
Tonsils
Tongue
Retina, conjunctiva
Esophagus, bronchus, thyroid, myocardium
Neck
Upper lung
Lower lung
Larynx
Stomach (acidity), Ⓛ liver Ⓡ
Pyloris
Stomach (peristalisis), Ⓛ liver, gall bladder Ⓡ
Small intestines
Spleen Ⓛ, pancreas Ⓡ
L adrenals
L kidney
Appendix
Umbilicus
Urethra
ASIS
L ureter
Intestines (peristalisis)
Bladder area
Ovaries, urethra
Uterus
Rectum
Prostate, broad ligament
Colon

All are bilateral except where right: Ⓡ and left: Ⓛ are indicated

FIGURE 7.54 **Chapman reflexes: posterior points.**
(From Kuchera ML, Kuchera WA, eds. *Osteopathic Considerations in Systemic Dysfunction.* Greyden Press, 1994, with permission.)

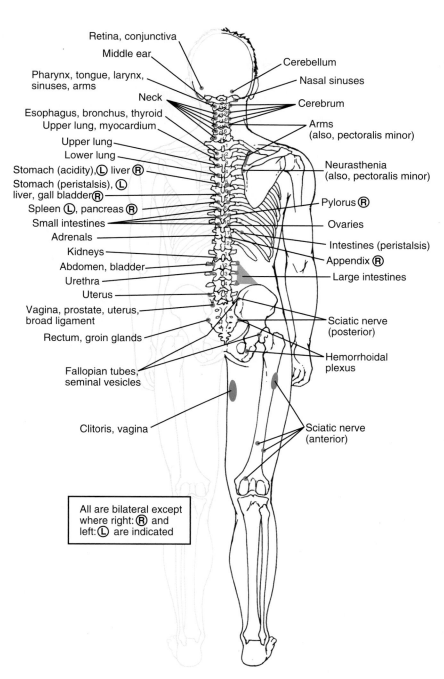

Retina, conjunctiva

Middle ear

Pharynx, tongue, larynx, sinuses, arms

Neck

Esophagus, bronchus, thyroid
Upper lung, myocardium

Upper lung

Lower lung

Stomach (acidity),(L) liver (R)

Stomach (peristalsis), (L)
liver, gall bladder(R)

Spleen (L), pancreas (R)

Small intestines

Adrenals

Kidneys

Abdomen, bladder

Urethra

Uterus

Vagina, prostate, uterus, broad ligament

Rectum, groin glands

Fallopian tubes, seminal vesicles

Clitoris, vagina

Cerebellum

Nasal sinuses

Cerebrum

Arms
(also, pectoralis minor)

Neurasthenia
(also, pectoralis minor)

Pylorus (R)

Ovaries

Intestines (peristalsis)

Appendix (R)

Large intestines

Sciatic nerve
(posterior)

Hemorrhoidal
plexus

Sciatic nerve
(anterior)

All are bilateral except
where right: (R) and
left: (L) are indicated

SUGGESTED READINGS

Sandoz R. Some physical mechanisms and effects of spinal adjustments. *Ann Swiss Chiro Assoc* 1976;6:91–141.

Travell J, Simons D. *Myofascial Pain and Dysfunction, the Trigger Point Manual.* Baltimore, MD: Williams & Wilkins, 1983.

Tucker C, Deoora T. *Fundamental Osteopathic Techniques.* Melbourne: Research Publications, 1995.

Ward RC, ed. *Foundations for Osteopathic Medicine.* Baltimore, MD: Williams & Wilkins, 2003:1229–1253.

REFERENCES

1. Chiquet M, Tunç-Civelek V, Srasa-Renedo A. Gene Regulation by Mechanotransduction in fibroblasts. *Appl Physiol Nutr Metab* 2007;32(5):967–973.
2. Schwartz MA, Ingber DE. Integrating with integrins. *Mol Biol Cell* 1994;5(4):389–393.
3. Chiquet M. Regulation of extracellular matrix gene expression by mechanical stress. *Matrix Biol* 1999;18:417–426.
4. Huijing PA. Muscle as a collagen fiber reinforced composite: A review of force transmission in muscle and whole limb. *J Biomech* 1999;32:329–345.
5. Vleeming A, Pool-Goudzwaard AL, Stoeckart R, et al. The posterior layer of the thoracolumbar fascia. Its function in load transfer from spine to legs. *Spine* 1995;20(7):753–758.
6. Tomasek JJ, Gabbiani G, Hinz B, et al. Myofibroblasts and mechanoregulation of connective tissue remodeling. *Nat Rev Mol Cell Biol* 2002;3:349–363.
7. Hinz B. Masters and servants of the force: The role of matrix adhesions in myofibroblast force perception and transmission. *Eur J Cell Biol* 2006;85:175–181.
8. Khalsa PS. Biomechanics of musculoskeletal pain: Dynamics of the neuromatrix. *J Electromyogr Kinesiol* 2004;14:109–120.
9. Gerwin RD, Dommerholt J, Shah JP. An Expansion of Simons' Integrated Hypothesis of Trigger Point Formation. *Curr pain Headache Rep* 2004;8:468–475.
10. Bouffard NA, Cutroneo KR, Badger GJ, et al. Tissue stretch decreases soluble TGF-β1 and Type-1 procollagen in mouse subcutaneous connective tissue: Evidence from ex vivo and in vivo models. *J Cell Physiol* 2008;214:389–395.
11. Dodd JG, Good MM, Nguyen TL, et al. In vitro biophysical strain model for understanding mechanisms of osteopathic manipulative treatment. *J Am Osteopath Assoc* 2006;106(3):157–166.
12. Eagan TS, Meltzer KR, Standley PR. Importance of strain direction in regulating human fibroblast proliferation and cytokine secretion: A useful in vitro model for soft tissue injury and manual medicine treatments. *J Manipulative Physiol Ther* 2007;30:584–592.
13. Howe AK. Dynamic fibroblast cytoskeletal response to subcutaneous tissue stretch ex vivo and in vivo. *Am J Physiol Cell Physiol* 2005;288:747–756.
14. Langevin HM, Storch KN, Copolla MJ, et al. Fibroblast spreading induced by connective tissue stretch involves intracellular redistribution of alpha- and beta-actin. *Histochem Cell Biol* 2006;125(5):487–495.
15. Langevin HM, Bouffard NA, Badger GJ, et al. Dynamic fibroblast cytoskeletal response to subcutaneous tissue stretch ex vivo and in vivo. *Am J Physiol Cell Physiol* 2005;288(3):C747–C756.
16. Leduc O, Bourgeois P, Leduc A. Manual lymphatic drainage: Scintigraphic demonstration of its efficacy on colloidal protein reabsorption. In: Partsch H, ed. *Progress in Lymphology.* Amsterdam, The Netherlands: Elsevier Science, 1988:551–554.
17. Francois A, Richaud C, Bouchet JY, et al. Does medical treatment of lymphedema act by increasing lymph flow? *Vasa* 1989;18:281–286.
18. Badger C, Preston N, Seers K, Mortimer P. Physical therapies for reducing and controlling lymphoedema of the limbs. *Cochrane Database Syst Rev* (Online). 2004;4:CD003141.
19. Hwang JH, Kwon JY, Lee KW, et al. Changes in lymphatic function after complex physical therapy for lymphedema. *Lymphology* 1999;32:15–21.
20. Kurz W, Kurz R, Litmanovitch YI, et al. Effect of manual lymphdrainage massage on blood components and urinary neurohormones in chronic lymphedema. *Angiology 1981;* 32(2):119–127.
21. Hamner JB, Fleming MD. Lymphedema therapy reduces the volume of edema and pain in patients with breast cancer. *Ann Surg Oncol* 2007;14(16):1904–1908.
22. Koul R, Dufan T, Russel C, et al. Efficacy of complete decongestive therapy and manual lymphatic drainage on treatment-related lymphedema in breast cancer. *Int J Radiat Oncol Biol Phys* 2007;67(3):841–846.
23. Hernandez-Reif M, Field T, Krasnegor J, Theakston H. Lower back pain is reduced and range of motion increased after massage therapy. *Int J Neurosci* 2001;106(3–4):131–145.
24. Tsao JC. Effectiveness of massage therapy for chronic, non-malignant pain: A review. *Evid Based Complement Altern Med* 2007;4(2):165–179.
25. Field T, Hernandez-Reif M, Diego M, Fraser M. Cortisol decreases and serotonin and dopamine increase following massage therapy. *Int J Neurosci* 2005;115(10):1397–1413.
26. Fogaça Mde C, Carvalho WB, Peres Cde A, et al. Salivary cortisol as an indicator of adrenocortical function in healthy infants, using massage therapy. *São Paulo Med J* 2005;123(5):215–218.
27. Kaada B, Torsteinbø O. Increase of plasma beta-endorphins in connective tissue massage. *Gen Pharmacol* 1989;20(4):487–489.
28. McPartland JM. Expression of the endocannabinoid system in fibroblasts and myofascial tissues. *JBodywork Movement Ther* 2008;12(2):169–182.
29. Langevin HM, Sherman KJ. Pathophysiological model for chronic low back pain integrating connective tissue and nervous system mechanisms. *Med Hypotheses* 2007;68(1):74–80.
30. Goats GC. Massage—the scientific basis of an ancient art: Part 2. Physiological and therapeutic effects. *Br J Sports Med* 1994;28(3):153–156.
31. Ironson G, Field T, Scafidi F, et al. Massage therapy is associated with enhancement of the immune system's cytotoxic capacity. *Int J Neurosci* 1996;84(1–4):205–217.
32. Diego MA, Field T, Sanders C, et al. massage therapy of moderate and light pressure and vibrator effects on EEG and heart rate. *Int J Neurosci* 2004;114(1):31–44.
33. Delaney J. The short-term effects of myofascial trigger point massage therapy on cardiac autonomic tone in healthy subjects. *J Adv Nurs* 2002;37(4):364–371.
34. Field TM. Massage therapy effects. *Am Psychol* 1998;3(12):1270–1281.
35. Field T, Diego M, Hernandez-Reif M. Massage therapy research. *Dev Rev* 2007;27:75–89.
36. Wilkinson S, Love S, Westcombe AM, et al. Effectiveness of aromatherapy massage in the management of anxiety and depression in patients with cancer: A multicenter randomized controlled trial. *J Clin Oncol* 2007;25(5):532–539.
37. Wu P, Fuller C, Liu X, et al. Use of Complimentary and alternative medicine amoung women with depression: Results of a national survey. *Psychiatr Serv* 2007;58(3):349–356.
38. Sharpe P, Williams H, Granner M, et al. A randomized study of the effects of massage therapy compared to guided relaxation on well-being of and stress perception among older adults. *Complement Ther Med* 2007;15:157–163.
39. Hamre H, Witt C, Glockmann A, et al. Rhythmical massage therapy in chronic disease: A 4-year prospective cohort study. *J Altern Complement Med* 2007;13(6):635–642.
40. Hodge LM, King HH, Williams AG Jr, et al. Abdominal lymphatic pump treatment increases leukocyte count and flux in thoracic duct lymph. *Lymphat Res Biol* 2007; 5(2):127–133.
41. Knott EM, Tune JD, Stoll ST, et al. Increased lymphatic flow in the thoracic duct during manipulative intervention. *J Am Osteopath Assoc* 2005;105(10):447–456.
42. Caso ML. Evaluation of Chapman's neurolymphatic reflexes via applied kinesiology: A case report of low back pain and congenital intestinal abnormality. *J Manipulative Physiol Ther* 2004 ;27(1):66.
43. Delaney JP, Leong KS, Watkins A, et al. The short-term effects of myofascial trigger point massage therapy on cardiac autonomic tone in healthy subjects. *J Adv Nurs* 2002;37(4):364–371.
44. Shah JP, Phillips TM, Danoff JV, et al. An in vivo microanalytical technique for measuring the local biochemical milieu of human skeletal muscle. *J Appl Physiol* 2005;99:1980–1987.
45. Shah JP, Danoff JV, Desai MJ, et al. Biochemicals associated with pain and inflammation are elevated in sites near to and remote from active myofascial trigger points. *Arch Phys Med Rehabil* 2008;89:16–23.
46. Simons D, Travell J, Simons L. *Myofascial Pain and Dysfunction: The Trigger Point Manual, the Upper Extremities.* Vol. 1, 2nd Ed. Baltimore, MD: Lippincott, Williams & Wilkins, 1999.

Chapter

8

PRINCIPLES OF MUSCLE ENERGY TECHNIQUE

The heritage of the "bonesetters" gave all practitioners of manual medicine the aura of "putting a bone back in place." The muscle component of the musculoskeletal system did not receive as much attention. Early techniques did speak of muscle relaxation with soft-tissue procedures but specific manipulative approaches to muscle appear to be a 20th-century phenomenon. In osteopathic medicine, Dr T.J. Ruddy developed techniques that he described as resistive duction. The patient with a tempo approximating the pulse rate accomplished a series of muscle contractions against resistance. He used these techniques in the cervical spine and around the orbit in his practice as an ophthalmologist–otorhinolaryngologist.

Dr Fred L. Mitchell, Sr, is acknowledged as the father of the system that we now call muscle energy technique. He took many of Ruddy's principles and incorporated them into a system of manual medicine procedures that could be applicable to any region of the body or any particular articulation. Mitchell was a great student of anatomy and a gifted osteopathic physician. He was influenced by the primary role of the pelvis in Chapman reflexes (see Chapter 7). He made a comprehensive study of the pelvis, its anatomy and biomechanics known at the time, and of the muscle action associated with pelvic function. He adapted muscle contraction to restore more normal motion to dysfunctional articulations in the extremities and the vertebral column. In the late 1950s and 1960s, he and Paul Kimberly, D.O., taught a 2½ day seminar under the aegis of the American Academy of Osteopathy entitled "The Pelvis and Its Environs." Despite the popularity of these offerings, the muscle energy techniques did not become integrated into common practice. In 1970, he taught an intensive, weeklong tutorial in Ft Dodge, Iowa, for six students. Five members of this class became faculty in colleges of osteopathic medicine. He continued to teach in this tutorial fashion until his death in 1974. Upon his death, his tutorial students banded together to perpetuate and disseminate his work by developing three courses for the American Academy of Osteopathy. His son, Fred Mitchell, Jr, with P.S. Moran and N.A. Pruzzo, first published the essence of the muscle energy system in 1973 entitled *An Evaluation and Treatment Manual of Osteopathic Manipulative Procedures*. Dr Mitchell Jr has recently published a three-volume work entitled *The Muscle Energy Manual*.

Dr Mitchell, Sr, is given major credit for the muscle energy system, but his system could well be described as "Mitchell's biomechanical model of the pelvis." He believed that the pelvis is the key to the musculoskeletal system. Despite the great amount of research knowledge of the pelvis gained in the past 20 years, his concepts of pelvic function and dysfunction have stood the test of time and retain great clinical relevance.

Muscle energy technique has become incorporated into the practice of physical therapy, massage therapy, and manual medicine worldwide. The first use in Europe was the Geyman–Lewyt variation. Later, Lewyt and Bourdillon, the latter a British-trained orthopedic surgeon who became a student, practitioner, teacher, and author in manual medicine, described it as postisometric technique. The Swiss neurologist and manual medicine practitioner, Jiri Dvorak, M.D., described it as NMT (neuromuscular therapy) and described three different muscle approaches.

WHAT IS MUSCLE ENERGY TECHNIQUE?

Muscle energy technique is a manual medicine treatment procedure that involves the voluntary contraction of patient muscle in a precisely controlled direction at varying levels of intensity against a distinctly executed counterforce applied by the operator. Muscle energy procedures have wide applications and are classified as *active techniques* in which the patient contributes the corrective force. The activating force is classified as intrinsic. The patient is responsible for the dosage applied.

Muscle energy technique has many clinical uses. It can be used to

- lengthen a shortened, contractured, or spastic muscle
- strengthen a physiologically weakened muscle or group of muscles
- reduce localized edema and relieve passive congestion (the muscles are the pump of the lymphatic and venous systems)
- mobilize an articulation with restricted mobility

The function of any articulation in the body that can be moved by voluntary muscle action, either directly or indirectly, can be influenced by muscle energy procedures. The amount of patient effort may vary from a minimal muscle twitch to a maximal muscle contraction. The duration of the effort may vary from a fraction of a second to a sustained effort lasting several seconds.

TYPES OF MUSCULAR CONTRACTION

There are four different types of muscle contraction in muscle energy technique. They are

1. Isometric
2. Concentric isotonic
3. Eccentric isotonic
4. "Isolytic"

During an *isometric contraction*, the distance between the origin and the insertion of the muscle is maintained at a constant length. A fixed tension develops in the muscle as the patient contracts the muscle against an equal counterforce applied by the operator, preventing shortening of the muscle from the origin to the insertion.

A *concentric isotonic contraction* occurs when the muscle tension causes the origin and insertion to approximate.

An *eccentric isotonic contraction* is one in which the muscle tension allows the origin and insertion to separate. In fact, the muscle lengthens.

An "*isolytic*" contraction is a nonphysiologic event in which the contraction of the patient attempts to be concentric with approximation of the origin and insertion, but an external force applied by the operator occurs in the opposite direction.

With the elbow as an example, let us see how each of these contractions operates. With the patient's elbow flexed, the operator holds the distal forearm and shoulder. The patient is instructed to bring the wrist to the shoulder while the operator holds the wrist and shoulder in the same relative position. The force inserted by the patient's contracting biceps has an equal counterforce applied by the operator. This results in *isometric contraction* of the biceps brachii muscle. *Muscle tone increases but the origin and insertion do not approximate.*

A *concentric isotonic contraction* occurs during the process of holding a weight in the hand and bringing it to the shoulder by increasing the flexion at the elbow. The concentric isotonic contraction of the biceps brachii *increases muscle tone, and the origin and insertion are approximated.*

An *eccentric isotonic contraction* occurs when the weight brought to the shoulder is now returned to the starting position by increasing the amount of elbow extension. *There is tone within the biceps brachii allowing the origin and insertion to separate* in a smooth and easy fashion as the elbow extends and the weight is taken away from the shoulder.

An *isolytic contraction* occurs when the elbow is flexed at 90 degrees and the *patient attempts to increase the flexion of the elbow while the operator holding the shoulder and wrist forcefully extends the elbow against the effort of the patient* to concentrically contract the biceps brachii. An isolytic procedure must be used cautiously to lengthen a severely contractured or hypertonic muscle because rupture of the musculotendinous junction and insertion of tendon into bone or muscle fibers themselves can occur.

MUSCLE PHYSIOLOGY AND PRINCIPLES

It is beyond the scope of this volume to describe all of the elements of muscle physiology that underlie muscle energy technique. The reader is referred to a physiology text for those details. Knowledge of a few principles of muscle physiology is necessary for the manual medicine practitioner to use these techniques appropriately.

Muscles are made up of multiple fibers including intrafusal and extrafusal fibers. The alpha neurons innervate the extrafusal fibers. During normal resting tone, some extrafusal fibers are contracting while others are relaxed so that not all fibers are contracting at the same time. The intrafusal fibers, or spindles, lie in parallel with the extrafusal fibers and their function is to monitor the length and tone of the muscle. The spindle is innervated by gamma fibers that set the length and tone of the spindle. *The spindle is sensitive to change in length and in rate of change.* With stimulation of the spindle by stretch or muscle contraction, afferent type II fibers project information to the spinal cord. Through complex central control systems, the spindle is preset

for the anticipated action of the muscle. If the muscle action and the spindle are not congruent, abnormal muscle tone can result. Muscle imbalance of hypertonic muscle tone has become one of the hypothetic constructs of somatic dysfunction. *The Golgi tendon apparatus lies in series with the extrafusal fibers of the muscle and is sensitive to muscle tension.* As the muscle contracts or is passively stretched, the tension buildup in the Golgi apparatus provides afferent information to the cord through 1B fibers that inhibit alpha motor neuron output.

The control of muscle tone is a complex nervous system activity that takes information from the mechanoreceptors of the articulation and periarticular structures, the muscle spindle, and the Golgi tendon apparatus and processes this information in the spinal cord, brainstem, and higher centers. The cord processes many activities through local reflexes and propriospinal tracts that have been preprogrammed. The cord has the capacity to learn good and bad muscle behavior. Complex ascending and descending spinal pathways integrate conscious and subconscious motor behavior.

Of major significance in vertebral somatic dysfunction is hypertonicity of the muscles of the fourth layer of the erector spinae group, the multifidi, rotators, and intertransversarii. These muscles are dense in spindles and function more as proprioceptors than prime movers. When dysfunctional, they alter joint mechanics locally and alter the behavior of the larger muscles of the erector spinae group. Isometric muscle energy techniques primarily reduce the tone in a hypertonic muscle and reestablish its normal resting length. Shortened and hypertonic muscles are frequently identified as the major component of restricted motion of an articulation or group of articulations. The reflexes involved are somewhat complex (Fig. 8.1). Afferents from Golgi tendon receptors and gamma afferents from spindle receptors feed back to the cord; gamma efferents return to the intrafusal fibers resetting their resting length, and this changes the resting length of the extrafusal fibers of the muscle. There is a slight delay after the muscle isometric contraction before it can be taken to a new resting length. *Simply put, after an isometric contraction, a hypertonic muscle can be passively lengthened to a new resting length.*

When using isotonic procedures, two other muscle physiologic principles are considered. The first is the classic law of reciprocal innervation and inhibition (Fig. 8.2). When an agonist muscle contracts and shortens, its antagonist must relax and lengthen so that motion can occur under the influence of the agonist muscle. The contraction of the agonist reciprocally inhibits its antagonist, allowing smooth motion. The harder the agonist contracts, the more inhibition occurs in the antagonist, in effect relaxing the antagonist. The second principle of isotonic muscle energy technique is that a series of muscle contractions against progressively increasing resistance increases the tone and improves the performance of a muscle that is too weak for its musculoskeletal function. *Isotonic muscle energy procedures reduce hypertonicity in a shortened antagonist and increase the strength of the agonist.*

All of these muscle contractions influence the surrounding fasciae, connective tissue ground substance, and interstitial fluids and alter muscle physiology by reflex mechanisms. Fascial length and tone are altered by muscle contraction. Alteration in fasciae

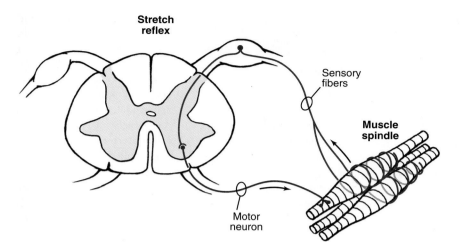

Stretch reflex

Sensory fibers

Muscle spindle

Motor neuron

FIGURE 8.1 Muscle spindle reflexes.

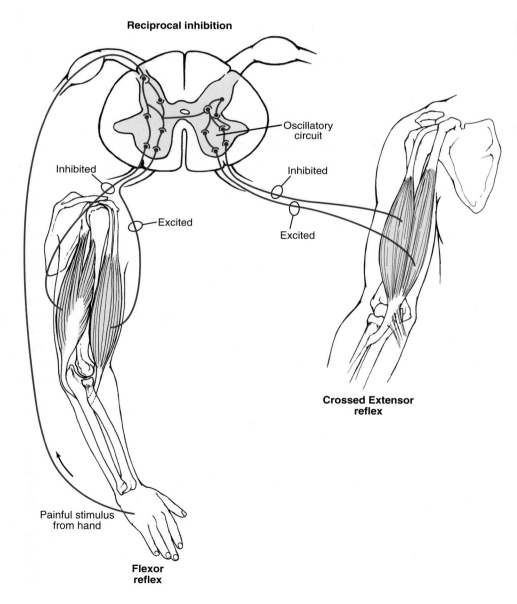

Reciprocal inhibition

Oscillatory circuit

Inhibited

Excited

Inhibited

Excited

Crossed Extensor reflex

Painful stimulus from hand

Flexor reflex

FIGURE 8.2 Reciprocal inhabitation reflex arc.

influences not only their biomechanical function, but also the biochemical and immunologic functions. The patient's muscle effort requires energy and the metabolic process of muscle contraction results in carbon dioxide, lactic acid, and other metabolic waste products that must be transported and metabolized. It is for this reason that the patient will frequently experience some increase in muscle soreness within the first 12 to 36 hours after a muscle energy technique treatment. Muscle energy procedures provide safety for the patient because the activating force is intrinsic and the patient can easily control the dosage, but it must be remembered that this effort comes at a price. It is easy for the inexperienced practitioner to overdo these procedures, and, in essence, overdose the patient.

ELEMENTS OF MUSCLE ENERGY PROCEDURES

The following five elements are essential for any successful muscle energy procedure:

1. Patient-active muscle contraction
2. Controlled joint position
3. Muscle contraction in a specific direction
4. Operator-applied distinct counterforce
5. Controlled contraction intensity

The patient is told to contract a muscle while the operator holds an articulation or portion of the musculoskeletal system in a specific position. The patient is instructed to contract in a certain direction with a specified amount of force, either in ounces or pounds. The operator applies a counterforce: one that prevents any approximation of the origin insertion (making the procedure isometric), one to allow yielding (for a concentric isotonic contraction), or one that overpowers the muscle effort (resulting in an isolytic procedure).

Patients commonly make the following errors during muscle energy procedures. They

- contract too hard
- contract in the wrong direction
- sustain the contraction for too short a time
- do not relax appropriately following the muscle contraction.

The most common operator errors are the following:

- not accurately controlling the joint position in relation to the barrier to movement
- not providing the counterforce in the correct direction
- not giving the patient accurate instructions
- moving to a new joint position too soon after the patient stops contracting

The operator must wait for the refractory period following an isometric contraction before the muscle can be stretched to a new resting length.

CLINICAL PEARL

Clinical experience has shown that three to five repetitions of muscle effort for 3 to 7 seconds each are effective in accomplishing the therapeutic goal. Experience will tell the operator when longer contraction or more repetitions are needed.

TABLE 8.1	*Comparison of Isometric and Isotonic Procedures*
Isometric	**Isotonic**
1. Careful positioning	1. Careful positioning
2. Light to moderate contraction	2. Hard to maximal contraction
3. Unyielding counterforce	3. Counterforce permits controlled motion
4. Relaxation after contraction	4. Relaxation after contraction
5. Repositioning	5. Repositioning

The *isometric contraction* need *not be too hard* (Table 8.1). It is important that it *be sustained* and that the muscle length *be maintained as nearly isometric as possible*. After the sustained but light contraction, *a momentary pause should occur before the operator stretches the shortened and contracted muscle to a new resting length*. Isotonic procedures require *forceful contraction* by the patient because the operator wants to recruit the firing of muscle fibers and make them work as hard as possible, resulting in relaxation of the antagonist. The muscle *should contract over its total range*. After any muscle energy procedure the patient should *relax before repositioning against a new resistant barrier*.

JOINT MOBILIZING MUSCLE EFFORT

There are *three different ways a muscle contraction can be used to overcome joint restriction*. Let us use as an example restriction of a segment to right rotation. The left rotator muscle is short and tight and the right rotator muscle weak.

- One approach (NMT 1) is to engage the restrictive barrier to right rotation and ask the left rotator muscle to contract isometrically. After the isometric contraction, the left rotator muscle can be stretched to a new resting length, increasing right rotation.
- A second option would be to have the right rotator muscle contract concentrically against a yielding counterforce, pulling the articulation into right rotation (NMT 2). Although this might be effective, it is infrequently used because it is painful for the patient and difficult for the operator to control.
- A third option (NMT 3) would be to engage the restrictive barrier and have the right rotator muscle contract isometrically, causing inhibition of the tight left rotator and allowing more free right rotation.

MUSCLE ENERGY TECHNIQUES

In succeeding chapters, muscle energy techniques will be described for specific regions. Here, we shall use the elbow as an example. Assume that there is a restriction of elbow movement into full extension, that is, the elbow is flexed. One cause of restricted elbow extension is hypertonicity and shortening of the biceps brachii muscle. The operator might choose an isometric muscle energy technique to treat this condition as follows:

1. Patient sits comfortably on the treatment table with the operator standing in front.
2. Operator grasps patient's elbow with one hand and distal forearm with the other hand (Fig. 8.3).
3. Operator extends the elbow until the first barrier to extension movement is felt.
4. Operator instructs the patient to attempt to bring the forearm to the shoulder using a few ounces of force in a sustained manner.
5. Operator provides equal counterforce to the patient's effort.
6. After 3 to 7 seconds of contraction, the patient is instructed to stop contracting and relax.

7. Operator waits until the patient is completely relaxed after the contracting effort and extends the elbow to a new resistant barrier (Fig. 8.4).
8. Steps 2 through 7 are repeated three to five times until full elbow extension is restored.

The restriction of elbow extension might also be the result of length and strength imbalance between the biceps muscle as the elbow flexor and the triceps muscle as the elbow extender. A weak triceps could prevent full elbow extension. The operator might choose an isotonic muscle energy technique to treat this condition as follows:

1. Patient sitting on table with operator in front.
2. Operator grasps elbow and distal forearm and takes elbow into full flexion (Fig. 8.5).

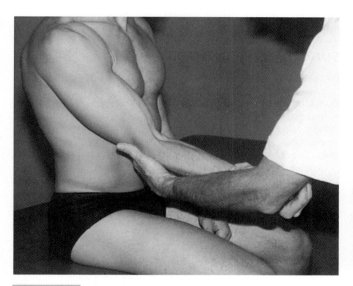

FIGURE 8.3 | Isometric muscle contraction, biceps.

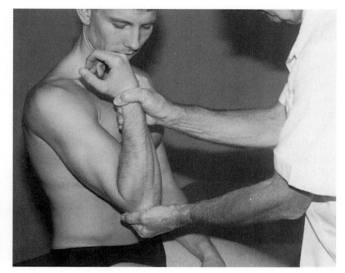

FIGURE 8.5 | Concentric isotonic contraction.

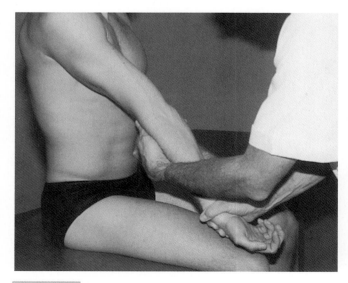

FIGURE 8.4 | Full elbow extension.

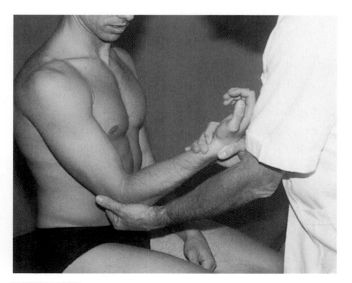

FIGURE 8.6 | Full range of elbow extension.

3. Patient is instructed to extend the elbow with as much effort as possible, perhaps several pounds.
4. The operator provides a yielding counterforce that allows the elbow to slowly but steadily extend throughout its maximal range (Fig. 8.6).
5. Operator returns elbow to full flexion and the patient repeats the contraction of the triceps to extend the elbow, but this time the operator provides increasing resistance to elbow extension.
6. Several repetitive efforts are accomplished with the operator providing increasing resistance each time and with the patient endeavoring to take the elbow through full extension with each effort.
7. Approximately three to five repetitions are usually necessary to achieve full elbow extension.

In any of these muscle energy procedures, it is important to *accurately assess the resistant barrier*. With an isometric technique, the first barrier sensed must be the point where the operator carefully holds the joint position. If the operator "crashes into" the muscle-resistant barrier in positioning the joint, an increase in the muscle hypertonicity will result, just the opposite of the desired therapeutic effect. Second, when using these procedures in a joint with multiple planes of movement available, it is important to *engage each motion barrier in the same fashion*. In the vertebral column with motion restriction around and along three different axes, precision in the engagement of the restrictive barrier is essential for therapeutic effectiveness.

Successful muscle energy technique can be ensured if the operator will constantly keep in mind the following three words:

Control
Balance
Localization

Both the operator and patient must be balanced and the operator must be in control of the localization against the resistant barrier. There must be continued control of the muscle effort by the patient and the yielding or unyielding counterforce by the operator. Each element is essential with each effort during the procedure.

CONCLUSION

In this author's opinion, muscle energy is one of the most valuable forms of manual medicine treatment because many therapeutic effects result from a single procedure and the procedures are physiologically and anatomically quite safe. It is possible to achieve increased joint movement, normalization of muscle strength and length, stretch of shortened fascia, and removal of passive congestion, all during a single procedure. Not only has muscle effort been used to move a joint, but also physiology that is more normal has been restored to the muscle.

SUGGESTED READINGS

Davidoff RA. Skeletal muscle tone and the misunderstood stretch reflex. *Neurology* 1992;42:951–963.

Dvorak J, Dvorak V. *Manual Medicine, Therapeutic*. New York, NY: Thieme-Stratton, Inc., 1983.

Korr I. Muscle spindle and the lesioned segment. In: *Proceedings of the International Federation of Orthopedic Manipulative Therapists*. Vail, CO. 1977;45:53.

Mitchell FL. *Structural Pelvic Function*. Carmel, CA: Yearbook of the American Academy of Osteopathy, 1958:71–90.

Mitchell FL. Jr, Moran PS, Pruzzo NA. *An Evaluation and Treatment Manual of Osteopathic Muscle Energy Procedures*. Valley Park, MO: Mitchell, Moran & Pruzzo Associates, 1979.

MOBILIZATION WITH AND WITHOUT IMPULSE TECHNIQUE

The field of manual medicine continues to have difficulty with the use of the term "manipulation." For many years, and continuing in many circles today, the term is used for a manual procedure resulting in the popping sound accompanying the cavitation phenomenon. *Dorland's Medical Dictionary* defines manipulation as "the skillful or dexterous treatment by the hands." The Foundations of Osteopathic Medicine text defines it as "therapeutic application of manual force." The chiropractic and much German language literature still refer to manipulation as "high-velocity, low-amplitude thrust technique." "Mobilization" is the term commonly used for a manual medicine procedure that does not include the thrusting that results in the "popping" sound. The scientific advisory committee of the International Federation of Manual Medicine, during its work in the 1980s, recommended the term "mobilization with impulse" to designate a procedure with an operator-applied extrinsic thrusting force and "mobilization without impulse" having a repetitive, graded operator-applied extrinsic force applied without a thrust. These procedures have long been deemed the treatment of choice for the "manipulable lesion." Terms such as "joint lock," "joint dysfunction," "joint blockage," and "chiropractic subluxation" all emphasize alteration in articular function.

THEORIES OF JOINT DYSFUNCTION

Many theories have been proposed for the cause of joint dysfunction and the therapeutic effect of mobilization with or without impulse. They include alteration in the relationship of the opposing joint surfaces; in particular, the articular capsules and associated meniscus and its effect on neural mechanisms from the corresponding mechanoreceptors and nociceptors and the resultant effect on segmentally related muscle function.

Theories involving opposing joint surfaces include "lack of tracking" of opposing joint surfaces and "hitching or buckling within the segment." It has been suggested that a change in the thixotropic property of the synovial fluid might make it more "sticky." It has even been postulated that a fringe of synovium from the articular capsule might be caught between the two opposing joint surfaces.[1]

Studies on the neurophysiology of spinal facet joints show there are mechanoreceptors within their fibrous articular capsule capable of detecting motion and tissue distortion.[2,3] Although small quantities were documented, each mechanoreceptor has a relatively large receptive field.[4] In particular, four types of sensory nerve fibers were documented:

- Ruffini corpuscle (type I afferent) is a slowly adapting, low-threshold receptor that responds to mechanical stress.
- Pacinian corpuscle (type II afferent) is a rapidly adapting, low-threshold receptor that responds to acceleration of a joint.

- Golgi tendon organ (type III afferent) is a slowly adapting, high-threshold receptor that responds to tensile forces and functions to feedback joint position sense or kinesthesia.
- Free nerve endings (type IV afferent) are pain responsive high-threshold nociceptors.

This proprioceptive function is more likely to play a role in modulating muscular reflexes that provide stiffness and segmental stability rather than global movement of the region.[5,6]

Interestingly, in rabbit studies, undergoing lumbar interbody fusion and immobilization of the intervertebral segment causes a reduction in the number of mechanoreceptors in the facet joint because of the reduction in mechanical stimulation. Moreover, segments above the immobilization show an increase in type IV mechanoreceptors.[7] It has been postulated that joint dysfunction also alters (corrupts) the afferent nerve traffic from the type I and type II mechanoreceptors so that central control of motion cannot determine the joint's spatial relationship. This alteration in neural control is postulated to affect the length and tone of the segmentally related muscles, further restricting normal joint movement and affecting dynamic stability.[8]

Dynamic stability of the spine relies on the interdependent relationship of active (muscular), passive (articular/ligamentous), and neural subsystems defined by Panjabi.[9] The principle active subsystem component for dynamic stabilization is the muscles which control "neutral" joint position. These "stabilizer muscles are described as having the characteristics of being monoarticular or segmental, deep, working eccentrically to control movement, and having static holding capacities."[10] The passive subsystem consists of the articular surface, ligaments, and discs. It provides structural control, movement checks, and critical afferent kinesthetic information to the spinal cord via its mechanoreceptors.[11] The neural subsystem is dependent on the central nervous feedforward motor control (anticipatory) as well as feedback (unanticipated) afferent mechanoreceptive information from the aforementioned active (muscle spindles, golgi tendon organs) and passive (mechanoreceptors) subsystems. Loss of feedback control of the joint structure during the function leaves the joint vulnerable to injury in situations where unforeseen or unanticipated movement/postural corrections are necessary; it has therefore been determined to adversely affect articular stability and lead to dysfunction.[12] This dysfunction then perpetuates ongoing joint mechanoreceptor afferent alteration to feedback control and total dynamic stability.

There has been a significant amount of research suggesting joint dysfunction is associated with inhibition of the local stabilizers leading to what Panjabi refers to as "subfailure injury" or corruption in feedforward and/or feedback mechanoreceptor signals.[13,14] The scientific question that remains to be answered is whether joint manipulation can restore or normalize these signals and improve joint function and dynamic stability. Mobilization of joint dysfunction has been shown to increase strength and control of the inhibited muscles.[15] This observation is particularly related to stacked, nonneutral (type II) dysfunctions of the extended, rotated, and side bent (ERS) type in the midscapular thoracic spine and the serratus anterior and rhomboid muscles. Much more research is needed, but clinical and scientific experience shows that joint dysfunction (somatic dysfunction) responds positively to the application of mobilization with or without impulse technique.

CLINICAL PEARL	FEEDFORWARD AND FEEDBACK CONTROL MECHANISMS

So let's say you are playing Frisbee; your partner throws the Frisbee towards you, you see where it is going, you hear and see that there is no one coming up beside you to intercept the throw, you anticipate the speed of the throw and the direction and the speed that you will need to move to make the catch, and you also anticipate how high you need to raise your arm to make the catch. Feedback control becomes important for unanticipated motor behavior that may be necessary to catch the Frisbee; for instance, as you move backwards to position your body under the Frisbee, you step in a large hole in the ground. The only way you know that there is a hole is via proprioceptive information from your foot, ankle, and knee articular and muscular mechanoreceptors. This afferent information is instantaneously fed into your motor control allowing you to alter movement, stabilize your spine, and protect your joints from injury.

CAVITATION OR "JOINT POP" PHENOMENON

Research into the mechanisms of mobilization with impulse (high-velocity, low-amplitude thrust) has demonstrated the cavitation phenomenon. Cavitation occurs at the time of the audible "joint pop." A radiographic negative shadow appears within the joint with the density of nitrogen. This gaseous density remains present for a variable period of time, usually less than 20 minutes. The cavitation phenomenon suggests that the synovial fluid changes from a liquid to a gaseous state. The exact effect on the synovial fluid is unknown at this time.[16,17,18]

MOBILIZATION WITHOUT IMPULSE

Mobilization without impulse, or articulatory, procedure is an extension of range-of-motion testing:

The technique uses a repetitively applied force at the motion barrier with the goal of increasing the range of motion in an articulation with hypomobility. The operator needs to be precise with localization with both mobilizations with and without impulse. The operator constantly monitors the end feel of the motion range and attempts to return a more normal end feel with enhanced range. A graded series of mobilizing efforts from 1 to 4 are made depending upon the amount of motion introduced (1 = limited, 4 = maximum). Some systems refer to grade 5 as mobilization with impulse.

Mobilization without impulse procedures can be applied regionally to a group of segments or individually to a single vertebral motion segment. The primary effect is a stretch of the connective tissue with mobilization of the passive congestion associated with immobility. One might also anticipate modulation of neural activity to relieve pain and discomfort and restore more normal neural activity in spinal cord segments.

Mobilizations with and without impulse are direct-action techniques and differ only in the external activating force used. They are frequently combined, beginning without impulse for several repetitions and finally applying an impulse.

Joint Play

John Mc. Mennell, M.D., is credited with contributing the concept of joint play to manual medicine. Joint play is defined as movement within a synovial joint that is independent of, and cannot be introduced by, voluntary muscle contraction. The movements are small (<1/8 in. in any plane), with a precise range that depends on the contour of the opposing joint surfaces. These joint-play movements are deemed essential for the normal, pain-free, nonrestricted, movement of the particular articulation. If these movements are absent, normal voluntary movements are restricted and frequently painful.

To exemplify the involuntary joint-play movements, extend the fingers of your right hand, now, actively flex and extend the metacarpal phalangeal joints of that hand. Using your left hand, passively rotate the metacarpal phalangeal joints of your right hand. No problem; now try to *actively rotate* the same metacarpal phalangeal joints. Active rotation of this joint cannot be accomplished, yet this passive rotational joint play is essential for pain-free active flexion and extension of those joints.

Mennell defines joint dysfunction as loss of joint-play movement that cannot be recovered by the action of voluntary muscle, that is, joint dysfunction is loss of joint play. These principles apply to all synovial joints and are applicable in the spine and the extremities. Mennell's diagnostic system tests for normal joint-play movements in each articulation and introduces therapeutic joint manipulation to restore movement and function. Mennell's 10 rules of therapeutic manipulation are as follows:

1. Patient must be relaxed.
2. Operator must be relaxed. Therapeutic grasp must be painless, firm, and protective.
3. One joint is mobilized at a time.
4. One movement in a joint is restored at a time.
5. In performance of movement, one aspect of the joint is moved upon the other, which is stabilized.
6. The extent of movement is not greater than that assessed in the same joint on opposite unaffected limb.
7. No forceful or abnormal movement must ever be used.
8. The manipulative movement is a sharp thrust, with velocity, to result in approximately 1/8 in. gapping at the joint.
9. Therapeutic movement occurs when all of the "slack" in the joint has been taken up.
10. No therapeutic maneuver is done in the presence of joint or bone inflammation or disease (heat, redness, swelling, etc.).

These 10 rules are applicable to all procedures described as high-velocity, low-amplitude thrust techniques or mobilization with impulse.[19]

MOBILIZATION WITH IMPULSE

Mobilization with impulse (high-velocity, low-amplitude thrust) is a procedure with an operator-applied extrinsic thrusting force. These procedures appear to be most effective in somatic dysfunction when the restriction is in and closely around the joint itself, the so-called "short restrictors." They are usually applied as precisely as possible to a single joint level and for specific joint motion loss. Although Mennell states that a therapeutic procedure should occur in only one plane, it is possible to influence all three planes of vertebral movement simultaneously by specific localization and leverage application. These procedures appear to be much more effective in subacute and chronic conditions than in acute somatic dysfunction. Although most are designed for a single joint and its motion loss, some of the procedures can be applied in a regional fashion. Zink advocated their use with his respiratory–circulatory model, which was designed to mobilize regions of the body to enhance fluid circulation rather than overcome specific joint restriction. The difference between specific and nonspecific mobilizations with impulse lies with the principle of localization and locking described below.

Mobilization with impulse and mobilization without impulse procedures are used in direct and exaggeration methods. The most common usage is direct, with engagement of the restrictive barrier, and applying an external activating force to the barrier to achieve joint motion that is more normal. Some authors advocate the exaggeration method (also called "rebound thrust") in which the thrust is against the normal physiologic barrier in the direction opposite the motion loss. This author uses only the direct method and would use something other than an exaggeration thrust if a direct action thrust was not possible. Other assisting forces are gravity (patient sitting or standing versus recumbent) and patient respiratory efforts, both for relaxation and for influence on joint position desired.

PRINCIPLES OF TECHNIQUE APPLICATION

Joint Gapping

All thrusting procedures result in gapping of the joint, requiring the operator to know the anatomic joint contour and the movement possible at that articulation. The gapping can be in the plane of the joint, at right angles to the plane, or with joint distraction. Any successful mobilization with impulse procedure contains an element of joint distraction and gapping. The audible joint pop or click appears to coincide with joint gapping. It must be remembered that the production of joint noise is not the therapeutic goal. In fact, Kimberly states that the goal of a successful thrusting procedure is "painless and noiseless restoration of maximum joint function."

Localization

Localization limits the thrusting procedure to the joint needing treatment but other joints receive the mobilizing impulse.

This relates to Mennell's principle of holding one bone of the articulation and moving the other bone in relation to it.

It is essential that the operator has a good understanding of vertebral mechanics, both normal and dysfunctional, before using mobilization with impulse techniques. Using impulse without appropriate localization and understanding of vertebral mechanics can result in damage to the tissues including fracture of zygapophysial joints and herniation of the intervertebral disc. One localization principle that is most useful is the introduction of convexities in two different planes localized to the segment under treatment. The first convexity introduced is into the forward-bending or backward-bending arc of movement. The objective is to engage the forward-bending (flexion) or backward-bending (extension) component of the nonneutral vertebral somatic dysfunction. The goal is to place the segment under treatment at the apex of the convexity introduced either through a forward-bending and backward-bending overturning movement or an anteroposterior or posteroanterior translatory movement. For example, if L1 has forward-bending restriction in relation to L2, forward bending of the trunk is introduced from above downward through the thoracic spine to L1. Flexion of the lower extremities, pelvis, and lumbar spine from below upward is introduced up to L2. The L1 through L2 interspace becomes the apex of the forward-bending curve introduced and is localized against the forward-bending (flexion) barrier. This localization can also be performed by translation from anterior to posterior at the L1 through the L2 level. The second convexity introduced is that of side bending, creating a convexity right or left. Introduction of side bending while forward bent (flexed) or backward bent (extended) couples the rotation to the same side (nonneutral vertebral mechanics). If in our example of L1 through L2 the side-bending and rotation restrictions are to the right, side bending to the right establishes a convexity of the thoracolumbar spine to the left with the apex of the L1 through the L2 interspace. This left convexity can be established by a right-to-left translatory movement as well as right-side bending from above or below. The introduction of two convexities, one from front to back and the other through side bending with the apex of each convexity at the segment to be treated, is the principle used for a nonneutral (type II) vertebral dysfunctions in which there is either forward-bending or backward-bending restriction, together with side bending and rotation restriction to the same side.

In the neutral group (type I), vertebral dysfunction's localization is accomplished by the introduction of side bending and rotation to the opposite sides from above downward and from below upward to the segment requiring treatment. Forward bending and backward bending are introduced only to place the joint(s) under treatment at the point of maximum ease in the forward-bending or backward-bending arc of movement that is "neutral" at that level. This is best demonstrated when using the lateral recumbent (lumbar roll) technique. With the patient in the left lateral recumbent position, the apex of the group curve is placed in the neutral position of the forward-bending and backward-bending arc. With L1 through L2 as our example, forward bending and backward bending are introduced until L1 through

L2 is in its neutral position in the anteroposterior curve. The operator pulls the patient's left upper extremity anteriorly and caudally, introducing left-side bending and right rotation of the vertebral column down to the L1 level. With the other hand, the operator rolls the patient's pelvis anteriorly, introducing rotation to the left from below upward until L2 is reached. This results in neutral group localization at L1 through L2 and any articulatory or thrusting force summates at that level. The goal is to localize so that the transverse processes of the segment under treatment are maintained in the coronal (*xy*) plane. The lower the lumbar spine localization is desired, the more movement is introduced from above downward and less from below upward. Higher in the lumbar spine and into the lower thoracic spine, less movement is introduced from above downward and more from below upward.

Levers

Levers are classified as short or long. A short lever is one in which a portion of one vertebra (spinous process) is firmly held while force is applied to a bony process of the adjacent vertebra (spinous process, transverse process, mamillary process) and the resultant applied force is sufficient to move one segment on the other. Long levers are established by using one of the extremities, or multiple segments within the vertebral column, in a "locking" maneuver. Long levers have the advantage of reducing the force required and increasing the distance the force travels. Long-lever technique requires precise localization and limitation of force. A vertebral column long lever involves the principles of ligamentous or bony lock. A ligamentous lock occurs when the spine is sufficiently forward bent to place maximum tension on the posterior ligamentous structures surrounding the zygapophysial joints. A joint lock occurs when the spine is backward bent with engagement of the zygapophysial joints. Both of these maneuvers reduce joint mobility. Levers can also be established using concept III of vertebral motion in which introduction of motion in one direction reduces vertebral motion in all others. The introduction of a neutral (type I) vertebral movement (side bending and rotation to opposite sides) limits the movement of the vertebra involved and can include as many segments of the vertebral column as desired. Long levers are used to establish localization at any specific vertebral segmental level. Segments above and below the dysfunctional vertebral segment are "locked" in a long lever while the segment to be treated is "free" to receive the activating force applied. It is not uncommon for a novice practitioner to use excessive force to a joint that is inappropriately locked through poor localization.

Fulcrum

A fulcrum is used in many mobilizations with impulse techniques, particularly in the cervical and thoracic spines. The role of the fulcrum is to assist in localization of the activating force to the appropriate segment. There are firm rubber blocks or wedges of varying sizes and shapes that some practitioners use. This author prefers the use of hand position to establish a fulcrum. The advantage of using fingers or hand combinations for a fulcrum is the ability to sense localization at the segment under treatment. In the cervical area, a finger-pad pressure against a zygapophysial joint line serves as fulcrum around which the vertebrae can be moved to overcome restriction of the opposite zygapophysial joint. In the thoracic spine, various hand positions can be used to block the lower segment of the vertebral motion segment under treatment, allowing the operator to move the superior segment in any direction necessary to engage the restrictive barrier. In rib dysfunctions, the thenar eminence above or below a dysfunctional rib can serve as an appropriate fulcrum against which an activating force can be localized.

Velocity

Velocity means the speed of application, not force. In mobilization with impulse technique, the velocity is high. The maneuver should have quickness. A common mistake made is that the maneuver is a "push" rather than a "quick thrust." The thrusting maneuver should be applied only when all of the "slack" within the joint is removed. One must engage the restriction at its elastic barrier so that the thrusting procedure reestablishes the residual joint play available until one reaches the firm anatomic barrier. Remember that additional force does not make up for poor localization and poor velocity. A novice practitioner frequently "backs off" from the barrier in an attempt to get a "running start" against the barrier. This must be avoided by careful localization against the elastic barrier of the restriction and moving with the velocity from that point in the direction of motion loss.

Amplitude

Mobilization with impulse technique attempts to create movement of 1/8 in. at the joint under treatment. The thrusting force should be applied quickly and for a short distance. With short lever technique, the amplitude of the thrust to achieve 1/8 in. at the joint is considerably less than that with the long-lever technique. When two long levers are used, a great deal of movement is introduced by the operator to the patient. What must be remembered is that the summation of all of that movement results in a thrust amplitude at the joint under treatment of 1/8 in.

Balance and Control

As in any successful manual medicine procedure, both the operator and the patient must be in body positions that are comfortable, easily controlled, and balanced. The patient can be completely relaxed so that the operator can apply the thrust with maximum efficiency. The table must be at the appropriate height for the patient's and the operator's sizes. If the table is too high, the operator's ability to control the patient is compromised. The patient should be appropriately placed on the table, not too far away, not too close to the operator, so that localization can be accurate and the patient does not fear falling. The thrust is most appropriately provided by weight transfer of the operator's body rather than by a specific muscle action. In lateral recumbent lumbar roll technique, some operators attempt to introduce the thrust by an adduction movement of the arm placed on the pelvis, rather than with a total body movement. It is most difficult to provide appropriate velocity, amplitude, and direction with an adductor muscular movement of the operator's upper extremity. It is much easier to apply the proper thrust by the weight transfer of the operator's body (with the arm contacting the patient being incorporated as part of the operator's body) or with the arm fully extended and the thrust applied by a balanced movement of the operator's body in the right direction.

Therapeutic Goals of Mobilization With or Without Impulse Technique

These procedures are useful in increasing the range of movement of an articulation that has dysfunction (loss of joint play). Although the motion loss seemed to be only in one direction, a successful thrust procedure will increase the range of movement in all possible directions. While moving the joint, one might attempt to realign the skeletal parts in his/her normal anatomic relationship, intending to restore normal joint receptor activity at that level. An additional outcome is reduction of muscle hypertonicity and/or spasm in an attempt to restore balance to the segmentally related musculature. Another therapeutic outcome might be the stretching of shortened connective tissues surrounding the articulation. The fascial connective tissues may be shortened and tightened as the result of the altered position of the articulation, the healing of the inflammatory process following injury. As suggested earlier, the therapeutic goal might be the movement of fluid, both intravascular and extravascular, by "wringing out" the tissues. One or more of these therapeutic goals might be the objective of a procedure, but many of the others would be operative simultaneously. These procedures seem most effective for subacute and chronic dysfunctions that appear to be due to short restrictors.

Contraindications

As in all forms of manual medicine, accurate diagnosis is essential, and precision and accuracy of therapeutic intervention are required. When these criteria are met for mobilization with impulse, the contraindications become fewer. However, these procedures have more contraindications, both absolute and relative, than others. Absolute contraindications for mobilization with impulse are hypermobility and instability of an articulation and the presence of inflammatory joint disease.

There are many relative contraindications and authors classify them differently. For example, in the cervical spine, there is a major concern about these procedures and the vertebral artery. The vertebral artery is anatomically at risk at the craniocervical junction, and movements of extension and rotation will narrow normal arteries. In the presence of disease of the vertebral arteries, these movements become even more potentially dangerous. The need for precision of diagnosis and application of technique becomes crucial in the presence of disease of the vertebral arteries. The cervical spine is also a site of developmental and congenital conditions that might contraindicate a thrusting procedure. These include agenesis of the odontoid process and Down syndrome. Throughout the vertebral column, there is concern for metabolic and systemic bone disease, particularly osteoporosis and metastatic carcinoma. With careful and precise localization and the appropriate amount of force, mobilization with impulse technique can restore the lost joint play despite the alteration in osseous architecture. Degenerative joint diseases of the zygapophysial and uncovertebral joints of

Luschka are also relative contraindications. Degenerative joint disease alters the capacity of the zygapophysial joints to function, and an inappropriate mobilization with impulse technique could damage these joints. However, somatic dysfunction of these joints can complicate the degenerative joint process. The joint dysfunction can be successfully treated with a mobilization with impulse procedures if the aforementioned principles are applied properly. The thrusting impulse can be appropriately applied to the elastic barrier of the joint dysfunction even in the presence of altered anatomic barrier because of degenerative joint disease.

Of major concern is the use of mobilization with impulse procedures in the presence of intervertebral disc disease, particularly in the acute phase. Some authors believe that it is the treatment of choice, whereas others believe it is contraindicated. The concern is the possibility of exacerbating the disc pathology into increased herniation and sequestration with entrapment of neural elements. This author has used mobilization with impulse procedures with successful therapeutic results in the presence of known disc herniation demonstrated by appropriate imaging. It is interesting to note that little change has occurred in the imaging of the disc by the procedure. It has been reported that an acute cauda equina syndrome has followed the use of mobilization with impulse technique in the presence of lumbar disc disease. This potential danger should always be considered.

CONCLUSION

Mobilizations with and without impulse techniques are valuable in the armamentarium of the manual medicine practitioner. They require accuracy of diagnosis and precision of therapeutic intervention. They differ only in the form of mobilizing force. In mobilization with impulse technique, the application of velocity rather than force is a necessary skill to be mastered.

SUGGESTED READINGS

Brunarski DJ. Clinical trials of spinal manipulation: A critical appraisal and review of the literature. *J Manip Physiol Ther* 1984;4:243–249.

Dorland's Medical Dictionary. 23rd Ed. Philadelphia, PA: W.B. Saunders Co., 1959.

England R, Deibert P. Electromyographic studies, I: Consideration in the evaluation of osteopathic therapy. *J Am Osteopath Assoc* 1972;72:221–223.

Ward RC, *Exec* ed. *Foundations for Osteopathic Medicine.* Baltimore, MD: Williams & Wilkins, 1997.

Grice AA. Muscle tonus changes following manipulation. *J Can Chiropractic Assoc* 1974;19:29–31.

Kimberly PE. MSU/COM Tutorial on Mobilization with Impulse Technique. Personal communication. East Lansing, MI, 1984.

Shekelle PG. Spinal update: Spinal manipulation. *Spine* 1994;19:858–861.

Walton WJ. *Osteopathic Diagnosis and Technique Procedures.* 2nd Ed. Colorado Springs, CO: American Academy of Osteopathy, 1970.

Unsworth A, Dowson D, Wright V. Cracking in the metacarpophalangeal joint. *Ann Rheum Dis* 1971;30:348–351.

REFERENCES

1. Bogduk N, Jull G. The theoretical pathology of acute locked back: A basis for manipulative therapy. *Man Med* 1985;1(3):78–82.
2. McLain RF, Pickar JG. Mechanoreceptor endings in human thoracic and lumbar facet joints. *Spine* 1998;23(2):168–173.
3. Vandenabeele F, Creemers J, Lambrichts I, et al. Encapsulated Ruffini-lime endings in human lumbar facet joints. *J Anat* 1997;191:571–583.

4. McLain RF. Mechanoreceptor endings in human cervical facet joints. *Spine* 1994;19(5):495–501.

5. Johansson H, Sjolander P, Sojka P. Activity in receptor afferents from the anterior cruciate ligament evokes reflex effects on fusimotor neurons. *Neurosci Res* 1990;8:54–59.

6. Johansson H, Sjolander P, Sojka P. Receptors in the knee joint liaments and their role in biomechanics of the joint. *Crit Rev Biomed Eng* 1991;18:341–368.

7. Onodera T, Shirai Y, Miyamoto M, et al. Effects of anterior lumbar spinal fusion on the distribution of nerve endings and mechanoreceptors in the rabbit facet joint: Quantitative histological analysis. *J Orthop Sci* 2003;8:567–576.

8. Hurley H, Young A, Stokes M, et al. Effect of joint pathology on muscle. *Clin Orthop Relat Res* 1987;219:21–27.

9. Panjabi MM. The stabilizing system of the spine. part i. function, dysfunction, adaptation, and enhancement. *J Spinal Disord* 1992;5(4):383–389 (discussion 397).

10. Mottram S L, Comerford M. Stability dysfunction and low back pain. *J Orthop Med* 1998;20(2):13–18.

11. Holm S, Indahl A, Solomonow M. Sensorimotor control of the spine. *J Electromyogr Kinesiol* 2002;12(3):219–234.

12. Falla D, Jull G, Hodges PW. Feedforward activity of the cervical flexor muscles during voluntary arm movements is delayed in chronic neck pain. *Exp Brain Res* 2004;157(1):43–48.

13. Panjabi MM. A hypothesis of chronic back pain: Ligament subfailure injuries lead to muscle control dysfunction. *Eur Spine J* 2006;15:668–676.

14. Hodges PW, Richardson CA. Inefficient muscular stabiliztion of the lumbar spine associated with low back pain. A motor control evaluation of transversus abdominis. *Spine* 1996;21:2640–2650.

15. Liebler EJ, Tufano-Coors L, Douris P, et al. The effect of thoracic spine mobilization on lower trapezius strength testing. *J Man Manipulative Ther* 2001;9(4):207–212.

16. Unsworth A, Dowson D, Wright V. 'Cracking joints'. A bioengineering study of cavitation in the metacarpophalangeal joint. *Ann Rheum Dis* 1971;30:348–358.

17. Reggars JW. The therapeutic benefit of the audible release associated with spinal manipulative therapy. *Australas Chiropr Osteopathy* 1998;7(2):80–85.

18. Mierau D, Cassidy J, Bowen V, et al. Manipulation and mobilization of the third metacarpophalangeal joint. A quantitative radiographic and range of motion study. *Manual Med* 1988;3:135–140.

19. Mennell, J McM. *Joint Pain*. Boston: Little Brown & Co., 1964.

Indirect techniques are not as well known as the direct action techniques, particularly mobilization with impulse (high-velocity thrust). There are a number of variations of indirect technique with different names and terminology, but they all seem to have a common mode of action. They all move away from, rather than into, the barrier (indirect technique). The mechanism of action seems to be through a neural reflex with reduction of aberrant afferent impulses to the spinal cord resulting in more normal motor behavior. They might well be called afferent reduction techniques. Many people view them as being highly complex, although the principles are relatively simple and straightforward. These procedures focus more on the functional than the structural aspect in the structure–function interface.

HISTORY

Indirect techniques have a rich history developing primarily within the osteopathic profession beginning in the 1940s and 1950s. William Garner Sutherland, D.O., the developer of the craniosacral concept and techniques (see Chapter 12), treated the vertebral column and extremity articulations with "balanced membranous tension." He did not address the articular restriction in a direct fashion but held the articulation in a position of balance. He believed the balance was within the ligaments, but subsequent study has found that the underlying principle is more likely through complex neural control of motor function. Several groups of osteopathic physicians in different areas of the country built on this work and developed the functional approach to technique. Hoover led one group in the Pacific Northwest and focused on the principle of the dynamic neutral point of joint motion.[1] Bowles, Johnston, and other members of the New England Academy of Osteopathy on the east coast developed a study group and refined these concepts, emphasizing "ease" and "bind" as terms for the variations of palpatory sensation. Laughlin, of Kirksville, Missouri, developed his variation of this technique building on the balanced membranous tension concepts of Sutherland.[2]

Jones developed the system he called "strain–counterstrain" in 1955 after observing relief of pain and improved function after the patient assumed a pain-free position.[3] He further observed the relation of tender points on the anterior and posterior aspects of the body with various somatic dysfunction patterns. His technique evolved by associating the behavior of the tender points and their response to a pain-free position and the subsequent slow return to normal posture.

Schiowitz and his colleague DiGiovanna developed a variation called "facilitated positional release" in 1977. This system focuses on localized tissue texture abnormalities instead of tender points and identifies body positions that facilitate reduction of the tissue tension and improved function. This system also adds compression or torsion of the part under treatment at the balanced point. The position is held for 3 to 4 seconds instead of the 90 seconds recommended for the strain–counterstrain technique of Jones.

As can be seen, there are multiple varieties of these techniques that have gained in popularity and now are included in the manual medicine practitioner's armamentarium.

STRUCTURE–FUNCTION INTERFACE

The interrelationship of structure and function in the body and the body's tendency to self-regulate are well-recognized basic principles. Indirect (functional) techniques build on these principles, particularly from the perspective of function. In viewing a dysfunctional vertebral segment, the thought is not that the bone is out of place but that it has abnormal behavior in relation to the rest of the organism. The classic structural approach would attempt to "put the bone back in place," whereas the functional approach would attempt to "integrate" or restore coordinated activity with other segments of the vertebral column and the related soft tissues.

A helpful analogy is to imagine a rank of soldiers marching in a parade. One soldier in the rank is out of step. Because he is out of step, he is easily visible. The soldier is in line in the rank, he is not out of place, but he is highly visible because he is "out of step." He does not function in a coordinated manner with his fellow soldiers. The soldier's commanding officer would not take the soldier out of the rank and put him elsewhere but would change his stride so that it matches the remaining soldiers in the rank. The practitioner using functional technique focuses on restoring coordinated activity in an involved vertebral dysfunction in a similar fashion to the change in behavior in the soldier who is out of step in the rank.

BARRIER CONCEPTS

Chapter 3 described normal and restrictive barriers. In the absence of dysfunction, there is a midrange neutral point of maximum ease or freedom within the total range of motion. In the presence of somatic dysfunction, the neutral point is no longer in midline but is found as the point of maximum ease or freedom between the restrictive barrier in one direction and the normal physiologic and anatomic barriers in the opposite direction. Direct action techniques, such as muscle energy and mobilization with and without impulse, are interested in engaging the restrictive barrier and applying an activating force in the direction of motion loss. Functional technique is more interested in the behavior of the motion present than in its specific relationship to the barrier. The practitioner is more interested in the quality of motion, rather than the quantity. More so, the practitioner is interested in how the dysfunctional segment or tissue behaves or responds when motion is introduced. Functional diagnosis looks for the normal and reasonably expected coordination of movement as well as the quality and ease of movement in any given area or segment.

NEUROLOGIC HYPOTHESIS

In order to understand the rationale for the use of indirect functional technique, it is vital that one has a keen basic understanding of how "normal" muscular proprioceptive feedback and spinal networks function. Every joint in our body has mechanoreceptors within its articular and soft tissues whose role is to detect and transmit to the spinal cord via the dorsal roots information as to where the joint is in space, how fast it is moving, and how much compression and/or stretch is occurring within its tissues.

Similarly, our muscles have a vital sensory function contributing to the appreciation and control of body position sense and movement. They are loaded with stretch and force sensitive mechanoreceptors, the muscle spindles which detect and transmit to the spinal cord information as to the change in length of muscle, speed of that change, and the dynamic tension within the musculotendonous junction. All of this "afferent" information protects the joint and allows for efficient and effective motor and postural function.[4]

In applying functional technique to treat a somatic dysfunction one might consider Denslow's hypothesis that "it represents a facilitated segment of spinal cord maintained in that state by impulses of endogenous origin entering the corresponding dorsal root. All structures receiving efferent signals from that segment are, therefore, potentially exposed to excessive excitation or inhibition."[5] Upon further consideration for the site of the endogenous origin, it is well established that the final common pathway of the alpha motor neuron to the muscle can be influenced by alteration of the mechanoreceptors in neighboring joints, muscle fatigue, and muscle inflammation.[6-9] Hypothetically, restoration of more normal afferent signals to the central nervous system returns the neural traffic at the spinal cord to more normal levels, resulting in restoration of more normal neural activity to the muscle. Functional techniques can be described as "afferent reduction techniques." The functional diagnostic process is extensive in that it searches for alteration in the behavior of all the segments within the musculoskeletal system, attempts to restore them to more normal behavior, and requires that each dysfunctional segment is given appropriate attention.

FUNCTIONAL DIAGNOSIS

Functional diagnosis begins by identifying areas of tenderness, tissue tension, and/or the areas of greatest restriction. One diagnostic process has the operator percussing with fingertips over vertebral motion segments and their paravertebral tissues. Loss of tissue resilience is identified in areas of significant dysfunction. A second diagnostic method has the operator looking for areas of tender points and localized tension points. A third method finds the operator passively introducing ranges of motion throughout the vertebral axis in a symmetric fashion

seeking for areas of resistance to the induced motion. A fourth process is to identify vertebral somatic dysfunction by the biomechanical method described in Chapter 6 and then assess the functional characteristics of the dysfunction.

EASE–BIND CONCEPT

In functional technique, the practitioner searches for the response of the tissues to initial movement rather than range. Is the tissue response to initial movement easy and free (ease), or is the tissue response to initial movement restricted and difficult (bind)? The spectrum runs from maximum ease to maximum bind with many gradations between. Functional diagnosis searches for the ease–bind interface.

The procedure to identify ease and bind is as follows. A palpating hand is placed over the suspected segmental dysfunction and is called the "listening hand." Contact is maintained in a quiet and noninvasive fashion. The joints of the contact hand are relaxed and ready to appreciate small changes that occur at the dysfunctional segment and its adnexal tissues. The listening hand seldom introduces movement or energy. It is a "receiver" of information. The operator's other hand contacts some area of the musculoskeletal system adjacent or distant from the dysfunctional segment and either introduces motion. This hand is called the "motor hand." It introduces the movement that the listening hand monitors. The process requires a motion demand and a response. The motion hand initiates the demand, and the listening hand monitors the response.

Functional technique has a constant diagnostic and treatment interaction. The motor hand introduces diagnostic and therapeutic motions, and the listening hand monitors the response, giving constant feedback as the outcome. The diagnosis–treatment can be viewed as a cybernetic loop of continuous input and output with feedback assessment throughout the process. Because of the dynamic process involved in functional technique, the practitioners may look as though they are performing many different things with little standardization. In fact, the processes are quite standard in that there is motion introduced by one hand and constantly monitored by the other.

THERAPEUTIC USE
Acute Conditions

Functional technique is particularly useful in acute conditions because it is nontraumatic and can be performed repeatedly and frequently. Functional technique does not seek a major structural change but a tissue response. Reprogramming of aberrant afferent stimulation is important in acute and chronic conditions. Acute conditions appear to respond quite favorably and rapidly to functional technique. Special equipment is not necessary and it can be performed in any location, even in an intensive care unit.

Chronic Conditions

Functional technique is also effective in chronic conditions because it overcomes the abnormally programmed neural response and not just altered position. Restoring the position of a dysfunctional vertebral segment is of little value without restoring the neuromuscular mechanisms that control its function. The diagnostic component of functional technique is useful in chronic conditions as it monitors tissue response and behavior regardless of the therapeutic intervention.

Prognostic Value

Functional diagnostic technique is of prognostic value. It assesses the therapeutic response of a dysfunctional level regardless of the therapeutic intervention. For example, lift therapy for an anatomically short lower extremity and pelvic tilt mechanism (a structural intervention) will change the functional capacity of the entire musculoskeletal system. Functional diagnosis helps to determine if the structural intervention of the lift has accomplished improvement in musculoskeletal function both locally and distantly.

TYPES OF INDIRECT TECHNIQUE

All functional techniques can be classified as afferent reduction techniques. Most functional techniques can be placed in one of the following categories: balance and hold, dynamic functional procedures, strain–counterstrain, and release by positioning.

Functional Technique using Balance and Hold

These procedures are performed in any body position: standing, sitting, supine, prone, or lateral recumbent. Each hand has a particularly important role in performing balance-and-hold functional technique. The listening hand monitors at the dysfunctional segment as the motor hand introduces motion passively, or the patient assumes body positions under the practitioner's verbal commands. Motion is sequentially introduced in six different directions seeking the balance point of maximum ease within each range. Each is then held in that position while stacking one on top of the other. The stacking sequence makes little difference. The ranges introduced are forward bending–backward bending; side bending right–side bending left; rotation right–rotation left; anteroposterior (AP) translation; translation laterally, both right and left; and translation cephalic–caudad.

The last movement introduced is respiration. Once each of the ranges within the dysfunctional segment has been "stacked" at the point of maximum ease, inhalation and exhalation effort is introduced. The phase of respiration found to be the freest is then held as long as comfortably possible. This is usually for 5 to 30 seconds. At the end of the comfortable holding of the breath, the patient is instructed to breathe normally and naturally. A new balance point is sought for each of the motion directions. The respiratory effort is repeated. The entire process is repeated until release of restriction is felt and increased mobility is obtained. The usual operator sense is that the neutral point is returning more and more toward normal and that range is increasing.

Dynamic Functional Procedures

The second category of functional technique is described as "dynamic functional." The focus is on the restoration of normality to the apparently abnormal tracking of the dysfunction.

The process follows the inherent tissue motion. Inherent tissue motion is a function of many physiologic phenomena, particularly the cranial rhythmic impulse, contraction–relaxation of muscle tone, and the dynamic effects of respiration and circulation. In dynamic functional technique the listening hand monitors the response to motion introduced by the motor hand and directs the motion demand along the path of increasing ease. The goal is to restore more normal movement patterns, and the operator attempts to "ride out" the dysfunction. In doing so the operator continually seeks ease and avoids bind. These techniques look quite varied because of the dynamic motion patterns introduced. They can be standardized by the formula C–C–T–E–T.

C (1)—Contact over the adnexal tissue of the dysfunctional segment

C (2)—Control of the induced motion by the motor hand

T (1)—Test the adnexal tissue response

E—Evaluate the compliance of the segment as normal or abnormal

T (2)—Treatment by constantly monitoring the bind–ease point of the dysfunctional segment

Strain–Counterstrain Technique

"Strain–counterstrain" was originated and developed by Jones. There are three cardinal features of this system. The first is the identification and monitoring of palpable tender points on the anterior and posterior aspects of the body. They are similar in location to diagnostic points identified by other authors: Travell trigger points, Chapman reflexes, and acupuncture points (see Chapter 7). The second element has the patient assuming a body position that palpably "quiets" the tissues that make up the tender point. The position is held for 90 seconds while the operator monitors the tender point for reduction of tenderness and tension. Clinical experience has found that 90 seconds is the ideal: less is usually not effective and more does not increase the response. The third element is the slow operator-assisted movement of the patient to a normal posture. This is crucial for success.

There are more than 200 Jones tender points (Figs. 10.1 and 10.2) and each correlates with a somatic dysfunction in the musculoskeletal system. Anterior tender points seem related to flexed dysfunctions and respond best to a flexion body position. Posterior tender points relate to extended dysfunctions and respond best to extension body position. The more lateral the tender point, the more side bending and rotation are necessary in the held body position.

The diagnostic process is to systematically assess the patient for tender points in the usual locations, particularly looking for "hot" (most tender and reactive) and clusters of tender points.

The treatment by counterstrain usually involves five or six tender points. It is recommended that the most "hot" be treated first and clinical experience will show that many of the minor points will resolve spontaneously. There is a common post treatment reaction despite the apparent nontraumatic nature of the procedure. It usually occurs from 12 to 36 hours after treatment and the patient should be advised of the possibility. Caution is advisable to prevent over treatment. Counterstrain can be used

FIGURE 10.1

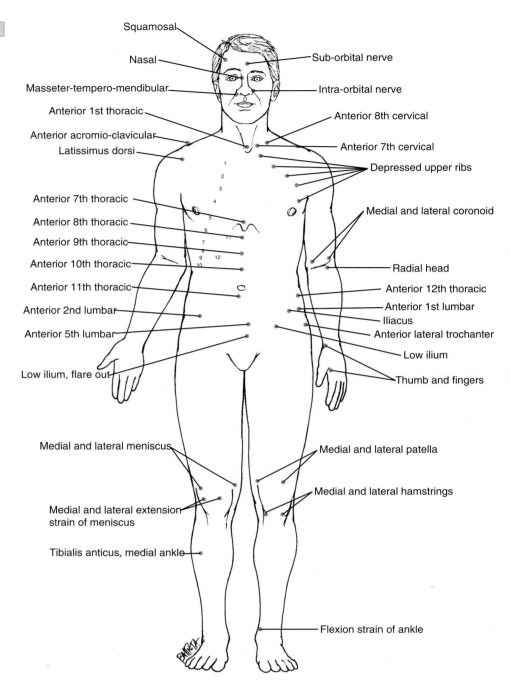

Squamosal

Nasal

Masseter-tempero-mendibular

Anterior 1st thoracic

Anterior acromio-clavicular

Latissimus dorsi

Anterior 7th thoracic

Anterior 8th thoracic

Anterior 9th thoracic

Anterior 10th thoracic

Anterior 11th thoracic

Anterior 2nd lumbar

Anterior 5th lumbar

Low ilium, flare out

Medial and lateral meniscus

Medial and lateral extension strain of meniscus

Tibialis anticus, medial ankle

Sub-orbital nerve

Intra-orbital nerve

Anterior 8th cervical

Anterior 7th cervical

Depressed upper ribs

Medial and lateral coronoid

Radial head

Anterior 12th thoracic

Anterior 1st lumbar

Iliacus

Anterior lateral trochanter

Low ilium

Thumb and fingers

Medial and lateral patella

Medial and lateral hamstrings

Flexion strain of ankle

in combination with other techniques. It is recommended that a text specific to this system be studied before attempting to use this technique.[10]

Release by Positioning

This system has many similarities to the strain–counterstrain approach. The diagnosis of a somatic dysfunction is made by any of a variety of ways. Of particular value is the role of palpation of tissue texture change associated with the dysfunction. Once identified, the vertebral segment is started at the neutral point of flexion–extension and the part is taken to a point of ease in rotation and side bending by the operator guiding while monitoring the response of the tissue texture. When the point of ease is found, a small amount of segmental mechanoreceptive input is introduced in the form or compression or distraction. Once this additional mechanoreceptive information is introduced the monitoring hand will follow motion of the segment as it seeks a new balance. Theoretically, the positional release changes the behavior of the spindle system resulting in the change of cord-level control of muscle hypertonicity. It is nontraumatic, quickly applied, and can be combined with other procedures.

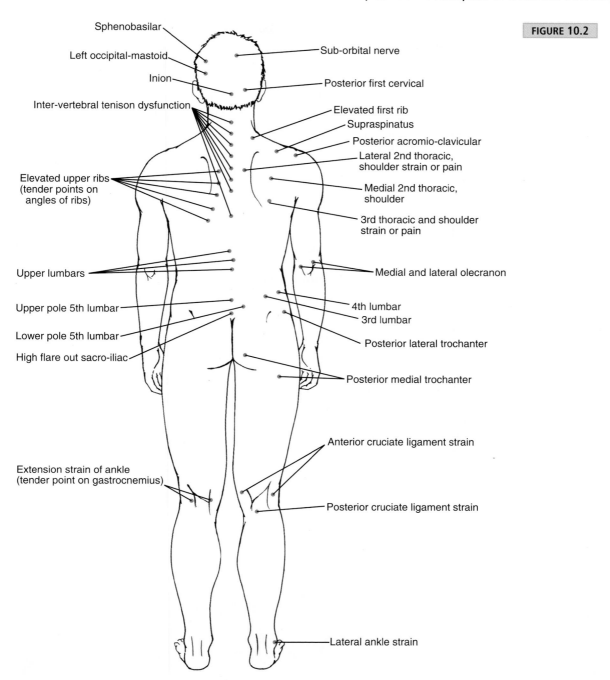

FIGURE 10.2

- Sphenobasilar
- Left occipital-mastoid
- Inion
- Inter-vertebral tenison dysfunction
- Elevated upper ribs (tender points on angles of ribs)
- Upper lumbars
- Upper pole 5th lumbar
- Lower pole 5th lumbar
- High flare out sacro-iliac
- Extension strain of ankle (tender point on gastrocnemius)

- Sub-orbital nerve
- Posterior first cervical
- Elevated first rib
- Supraspinatus
- Posterior acromio-clavicular
- Lateral 2nd thoracic, shoulder strain or pain
- Medial 2nd thoracic, shoulder
- 3rd thoracic and shoulder strain or pain
- Medial and lateral olecranon
- 4th lumbar
- 3rd lumbar
- Posterior lateral trochanter
- Posterior medial trochanter
- Anterior cruciate ligament strain
- Posterior cruciate ligament strain
- Lateral ankle strain

PALPATION EXERCISE

The following exercise is useful in learning the principles of functional diagnosis and treatment.

1. Patient sits on the examining table in an erect position with arms folded across the chest, each hand holding the opposite shoulder.
2. Operator stands behind and to the side of the patient placing a listening hand over the upper thoracic region. The listening hand should be as relaxed and quiet as possible in order to appreciate subtle movements.
3. Operator's other hand becomes the motor hand and is placed on top of the head. This hand leads the patient through certain movements in the fashion of the use of the reins on the bridle of a horse. The motor hand introduces passive movement as the listening hand monitors the tissue response.
4. Operator introduces forward bending *in a slow and smooth fashion* attempting to identify (with the listening hand) changes in ease and bind from maximum ease to maximum bind. Operator reverses the procedure into backward bending. Several repetitions are made, constantly evaluating the range of ease to bind motion in both directions.

5. With the patient in the neutral starting position, the motor hand introduces side bending to the right and rotation to the left of the head and the neck on the trunk. This introduces neutral (type I) vertebral motion. The operator monitors the range of this coupled movement through the ease and bind phenomena. Reverse the movement to side bending left and rotation right. Is there symmetry to the ease and bind? As you modulate side bending and rotation, is there difference in the ease and bind of each component of the motion?

6. Beginning at the neutral position, the operator introduces a small amount of forward bending, right-side bending, and right rotation of the head and the neck on the trunk. This introduces nonneutral (type II) coupled movement. The listening hand monitors for ease and bind of this motion. Repeat to the left side. Are they symmetric in the quality of ease and bind and in each component of the motion?

This exercise can be repeated throughout the vertebral axis in a number of positions. Diagnostically, the operator is attempting to classify each segment as normal, marginally dysfunctional, or significantly dysfunctional. The normal segment has a wide range of minimal signaling throughout the procedure. A significantly dysfunctional segment has a narrow range of rapid signaling in the ease–bind range. It is not uncommon to find a segment that is marginally dysfunctional, and it is important to decide how significant it is within the total musculoskeletal complex. This decision can only be achieved through experience that is the only and the best teacher.

FUNCTIONAL TECHNIQUES

The following techniques demonstrate the system of functional technique attributed to Laughlin, of Kirksville, Missouri. These techniques have been refined and standardized by Stiles, who had the opportunity to study extensively with Laughlin. There are many systems of functional (indirect) technique. These techniques are examples of the balance-and-hold and the dynamic functional principles. The diagnosis attributed to these techniques follows the postural structural model for terminology purposes, but to successfully use these techniques, the principles identified previously need to be implemented.

FUNCTIONAL TECHNIQUE

Lumbar Spine

Sitting

Diagnosis: Nonneutral dysfunctions: extended, rotated, side bent (ERS) and flexed, rotated, and side bent (FRS)

1. Patient sits on the table.

2. Operator sits behind the patient.

3. Operator's listening hand is placed over the dysfunctional segment with the index finger on the superior vertebra and the thumb on the inferior vertebra (Fig. 10.3).

4. Operator's motion hand placed on the patient's shoulder to control side bending and rotation from above (Fig. 10.4).

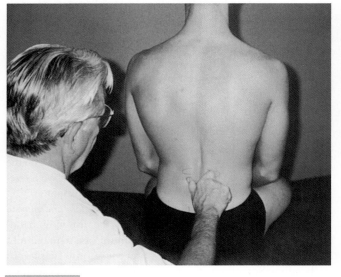

FIGURE 10.3

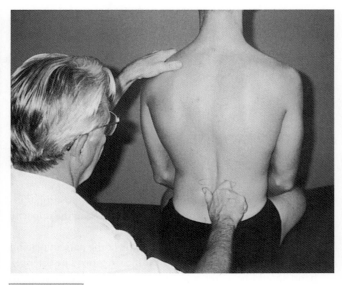

FIGURE 10.4

5. Operator places his head at the patient's thoracolumbar region to control flexion and extension through AP translation (Fig. 10.5).

6. Operator introduces side bending and rotation through the motion hand and flexion–extension through AP translation to the balance point of ease in all six degrees of freedom (Fig. 10.6).

7. Inhalation/exhalation efforts are used to find the point of maximum ease and are held until release occurs (balance and hold).

8. A dynamic indirect approach can be implemented by applying a compressive load from the motion hand to the listening hand at step 6 and following the unwinding inherent motion in the tissues as they seek balance.

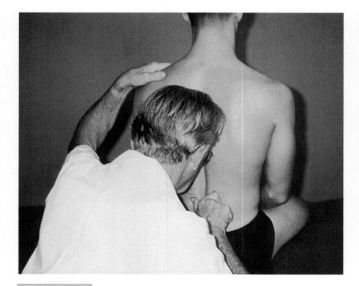

FIGURE 10.5

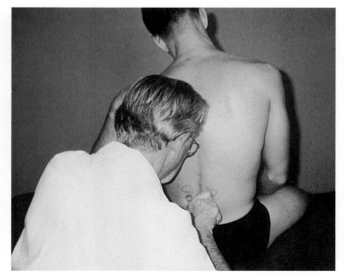

FIGURE 10.6

FUNCTIONAL TECHNIQUE

Pubes

Supine

Diagnosis: Superior or inferior pubes

1. Patient supine with the knees flexed and dropped into abduction with the soles of the feet together.

2. Operator stands at the side of the table and palpates the right and the left sides of the pubic symphysis with the index fingers of each hand above and the thumbs below (Fig. 10.7).

3. Operator introduces cephalic-to-caudad motion to the point of maximum ease (Fig. 10.8).

4. Balance-and-hold approach uses respiratory force assist until balance of symmetric position and motion occurs.

5. A dynamic approach introduces motion in the direction of ease and follows the inherent motion until balance of function is achieved.

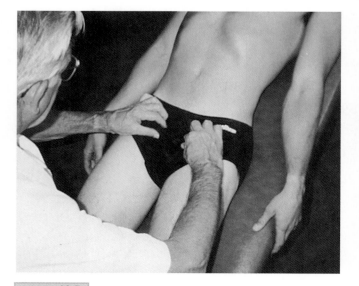

FIGURE 10.7

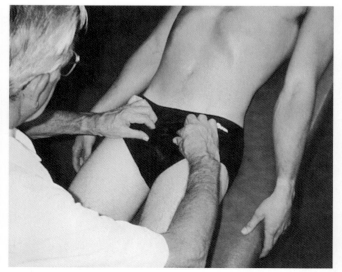

FIGURE 10.8

FUNCTIONAL TECHNIQUE

Sitting

Sacroiliac

Diagnosis: Left-on-left torsion

1. Patient sits on the table.

2. Operator sits behind the patient with the right hand over the right sacral base as the listening hand (Fig. 10.9) and the left hand on the left shoulder as the motion hand (Fig. 10.10).

3. Operator's head is placed in the thoracolumbar region to assist and control flexion–extension by AP translation (Fig. 10.11).

4. Operator's right thumb is over the sacral base while the flexed right index finger exerts lateral distraction on the medial side of the posterior superior iliac spine (PSIS) sensing for ease at the upper pole of the right sacroiliac joint.

5. Using his/her head, the operator introduces AP translation (flexion and extension) to ease at the listening hand.

6. Operator's (left) motion hand introduces left-side bending and right rotation of the patient's trunk to ease at the listening hand (Fig. 10.12).

7. The balance-and-hold approach fine-tunes ease at the listening hand and then introduces respiratory effort to achieve release of tension and return of function. Several repetitions may be necessary with fine-tuning after each respiratory assist.

8. The dynamic indirect approach initiates motion in the direction of ease and follows the inherent tissue response as the tissues "unwind." The thumb of the right hand may be moved to the left inferior lateral angle to initiate and assist the process.

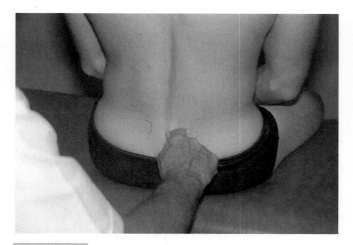

FIGURE 10.9

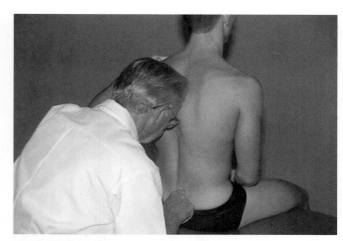

FIGURE 10.11

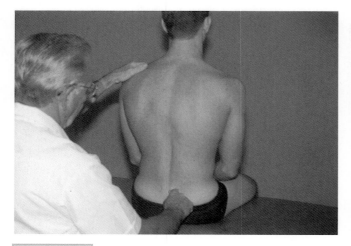

FIGURE 10.10

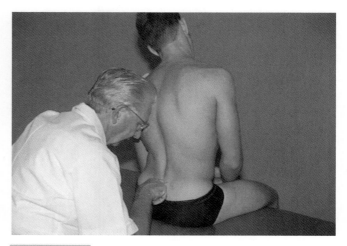

FIGURE 10.12

FUNCTIONAL TECHNIQUE

Sacroiliac

Sitting

Diagnosis: Left sacrum (flexed) anterior nutated

1. Patient sits on the table.

2. Operator sits behind the patient with the left hand over the left sacral base as the listening hand with the thumb over the sacrum and the index finger medial to the left PSIS (Fig. 10.13).

3. Operator's right hand is placed on the patient's right shoulder as the motion hand (Fig. 10.14).

4. Operator's head is placed at the thoracolumbar junction.

5. Using his/her head, the operator introduces AP translation (flexion and extension) until ease is felt at the listening hand (Fig. 10.15).

6. Operator's motion hand introduces right-side bending and left rotation until ease is felt at the listening hand (Fig. 10.16).

7. The balance-and-hold approach maintains the point of ease and uses respiratory action to achieve release of restriction in the tissues.

8. The dynamic indirect approach initiates motion in the direction of ease through the motion hand and follows the inherent tissue motion as it seeks ease and balance of tension. The operator's left thumb can be moved to the left inferior lateral angle to assist in release. The motion hand controls the trunk as ease is sought in all dimensions.

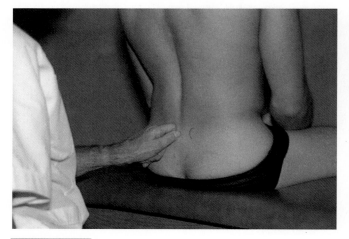

FIGURE 10.13

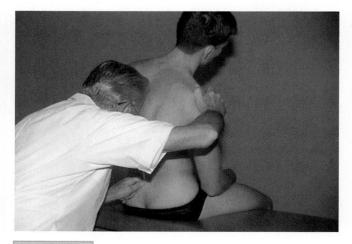

FIGURE 10.15

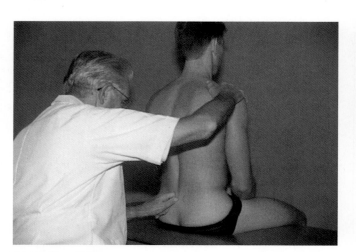

FIGURE 10.14

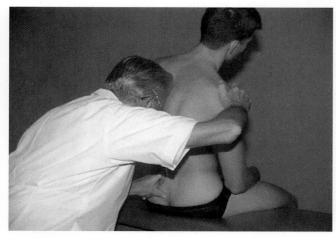

FIGURE 10.16

FUNCTIONAL TECHNIQUE

Sacroiliac

Sitting

Diagnosis: Right sacrum (extended) posterior nutated

1. Patient sits on the table.

2. Operator sits behind the patient with the right hand over the upper pole of the right sacroiliac joint as the listening hand. The thumb is over the right sacral base and the right index finger provides lateral distraction on the right PSIS.

3. Operator's left hand is on the patient's left shoulder as the motion hand (Fig. 10.17).

4. Operator's head is at the thoracolumbar junction.

5. Operator introduces a little flexion, posterior translation, and right-side bending/rotation until ease is felt at the listening hand. The patient's weight is shifted to the right ischial tuberosity (Fig. 10.18).

6. The balance-and-hold approach maintains the point of maximum ease at the right sacral base by fine-tuning and then using respiratory effort to achieve balance of tissue tension.

7. The dynamic indirect approach initiates motion at the right sacral base through the motion hand and follows the balance point until tissue release occurs and function is restored.

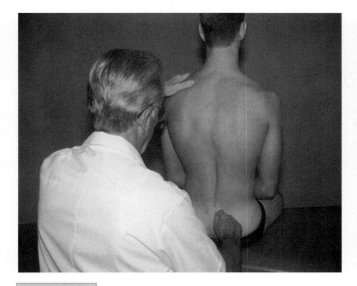

FIGURE 10.17

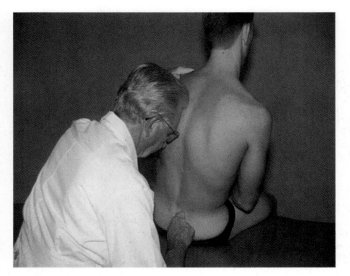

FIGURE 10.18

FUNCTIONAL TECHNIQUE

Sacroiliac

Sitting

Diagnosis: Left-on-right torsion

1. Patient sits on the table.

2. Operator sits behind the patient with the left hand over the upper pole of the left sacroiliac joint as the listening hand. The thumb is on the sacral base and the index finger gives lateral distraction on the left PSIS.

3. Operator's right hand is placed on the patient's right shoulder as the motion hand (Fig. 10.19).

4. Operator's head is placed at the thoracolumbar junction.

5. Operator introduces flexion and posterior translation to localize to the listening hand.

6. Operator's motion hand introduces side bending and rotation to the left to balance at the left sacral base. The patient's weight is usually on the left ischial tuberosity (Fig. 10.20).

7. The balance-and-hold approach localizes ease in all dimensions at the left sacral base and initiates respiratory action to achieve tissue balance.

8. The dynamic indirect approach initiates motion through the motion hand in the direction of ease at the listening hand and follows the inherent tissue motion in the direction of ease to tissue balance.

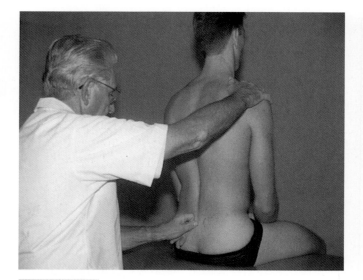

FIGURE 10.19

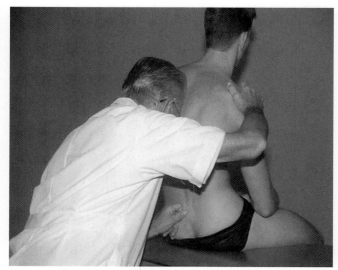

FIGURE 10.20

FUNCTIONAL TECHNIQUE

Iliosacral

Sitting

Diagnosis: Right anterior ilium

1. Patient sits on the table.

2. Operator sits behind the patient.

3. Operator's right hand lies over the right iliac crest with the thumb over the sacrum at the lower pole of the sacroiliac joint as the listening hand.

4. Operator's left hand contacts the patient's left shoulder as the motion hand (Fig. 10.21).

5. Operator's head is placed at the thoracolumbar junction.

6. Operator introduces AP translation until the right ilium starts to move forward and then introduces left-side bending and rotation until ease is felt over the upper pole of the right sacroiliac joint. The patient's weight is usually on the left ischial tuberosity (Fig. 10.22).

7. The balance-and-hold approach seeks ease in all dimensions, adds respiratory effort, and fine-tunes until balance of tissue tension occurs.

8. The dynamic indirect approach is initiated by loading through the motion hand in the direction of the listening hand and following the inherent tissue motion until tissue balance is achieved.

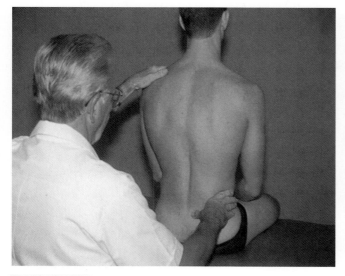

FIGURE 10.21

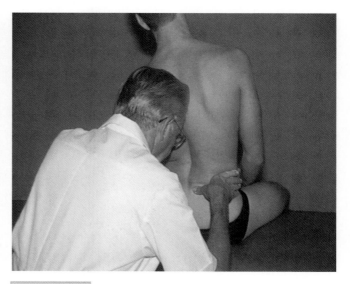

FIGURE 10.22

FUNCTIONAL TECHNIQUE

Iliosacral

Sitting

Diagnosis: Left posterior ilium

1. Patient sits on the table.

2. Operator sits behind the patient.

3. Operator's left hand contacts the left iliac crest with the thumb over the sacrum at the lower pole of the left sacroiliac joint as the listening hand.

4. Operator's right hand contacts the patient's right shoulder as the motion hand (Fig. 10.23).

5. Operator's head is at the thoracolumbar junction.

6. Operator introduces AP translation to localize to the lower pole left sacroiliac joint (Fig. 10.24) and then introduces left-side bending until the left ilium moves to ease in the posterior rotation (Fig. 10.25).

7. The balance-and-hold approach seeks ease in all dimensions and adds respiratory effort to achieve balanced tissue tension.

8. The dynamic indirect approach introduces motion through the motion hand toward the left sacroiliac joint and follows the inherent tissue motion until balanced tissue tension is achieved.

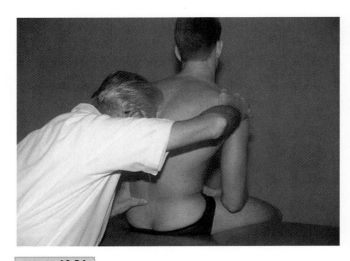

FIGURE 10.24

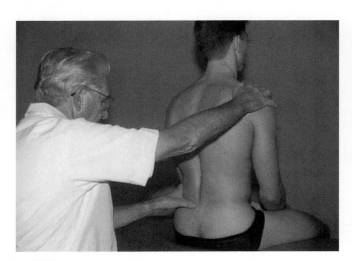

FIGURE 10.23

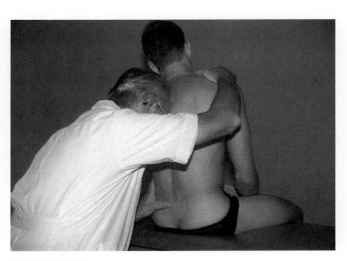

FIGURE 10.25

FUNCTIONAL TECHNIQUE

Pelvis

Sitting

Diagnosis: Pelvic compression

1. Patient sits on the table.

2. Operator sits behind the patient.

3. Operator's hands grasp the ilia with the thumbs over the sacral base and the fingers along the iliac crests (Fig. 10.26).

4. Operator's head contacts the thoracolumbar junction.

5. Operator introduces AP translatory motion until ease is felt at the two sacroiliac joints (Fig. 10.27).

6. Operator's hands compress the pelvis and rotate anteriorly and posteriorly on each side to the point of ease (Fig. 10.28).

7. The balance-and-hold approach holds the two ilia at the point of maximum ease and using respiratory effort seeks release and balance of tissue tension.

8. The dynamic indirect approach introduces motion through both hands and follows the inherent tissue motion until balance in three dimensions is achieved.

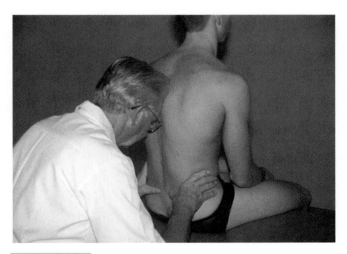

FIGURE 10.27

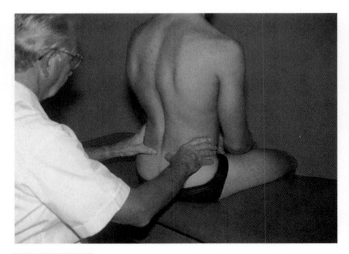

FIGURE 10.26

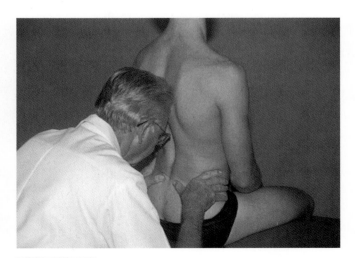

FIGURE 10.28

FUNCTIONAL TECHNIQUE

Thoracolumbar Spine

Sitting

Diagnosis: Vertebral dysfunction either ERS or FRS

1. Patient sits on the table, arms folded across chest.

2. Operator sits behind the patient.

3. Operator's right hand contacts the thoracolumbar spine as the listening hand.

4. Operator's left hand grasps the patient's left elbow as the motion hand (Fig. 10.29).

5. Operator's listening hand introduces flexion and extension through AP translation and adds cephalic distraction to the point of ease.

6. Operator's motion hand introduces side bending and rotation of the trunk, plus cephalic distraction, to the point of maximum ease (Fig. 10.30).

7. The balance-and-hold approach introduces motion to maximum ease in all dimensions and adds respiratory effort until balance in tissue tension is achieved.

8. The dynamic indirect approach introduces motion through the motion hand in the direction of ease and follows the inherent tissue motion until balance of tissue tension is achieved.

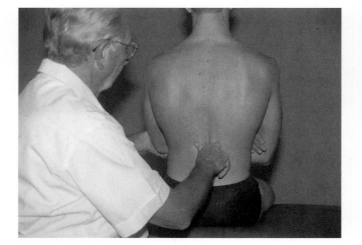

FIGURE 10.29

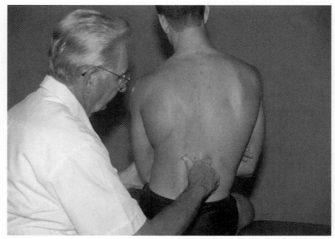

FIGURE 10.30

FUNCTIONAL TECHNIQUE

Upper Thoracic Spine

Sitting

Diagnosis: Vertebral dysfunction either ERS or FRS

1. Patient sits on the table.

2. Operator stands behind the patient with the patient's trunk against the operator for control.

3. Operator's left hand contacts the dysfunctional segment as the listening hand with the fingers on each vertebra.

4. Operator's right hand contacts the top of the patient's head as the motion hand (Fig. 10.31).

5. Operator introduces flexion (Fig. 10.32) and extension (Fig. 10.33) through AP translation to maximum ease at the listening hand.

6. Operator's motion hand introduces side bending and rotation to the dysfunctional segment, seeking maximum ease at the listening hand (Fig. 10.34).

7. The balance-and-hold approach seeks balance in all dimensions and then adds respiratory effort until tissue tension balance is achieved.

8. The dynamic indirect approach introduces motion through the motion hand in the direction of the listening hand and follows the inherent tissue motion until tissue tension balance is achieved.

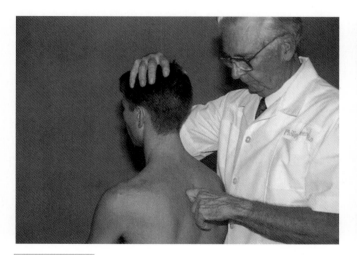

FIGURE 10.31

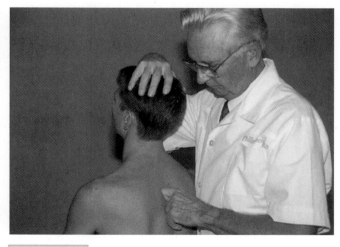

FIGURE 10.33

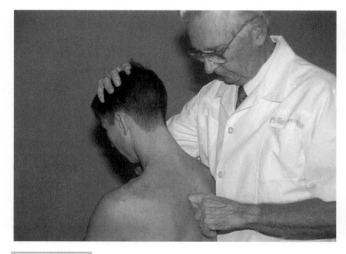

FIGURE 10.32

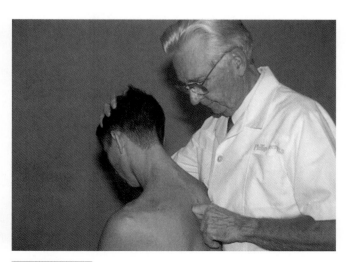

FIGURE 10.34

FUNCTIONAL TECHNIQUE

Middle and Lower Thoracic Spine

Sitting

Diagnosis: Vertebral dysfunction, either ERS or FRS

1. Patient sits on the table.

2. Operator stands behind the patient with the patient's trunk against the operator's torso for control.

3. Operator's left hand contacts the dysfunctional segment with a finger contact on each of the two vertebrae as the listening hand.

4. Operator's right hand lies over the patient's right shoulder with the hand behind the patient's neck as the motion hand (Fig. 10.35).

5. Operator introduces flexion (Fig. 10.36) or extension (Fig. 10.37) through AP translation to ease at the listening hand.

6. Operator's motion hand introduces side bending and rotation to ease at the listening hand (Fig. 10.38).

7. The balance-and-hold approach seeks ease in all dimensions and adds respiratory effort until balance of tissue tension is achieved.

8. The dynamic indirect approach initiates motion through the motion hand in the direction of ease at the listening hand and follows the inherent tissue motion until balance of tissue tension is achieved.

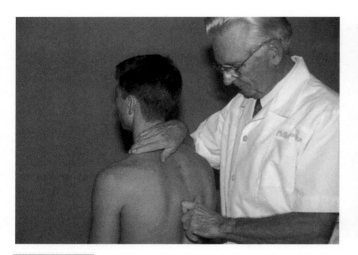

FIGURE 10.35

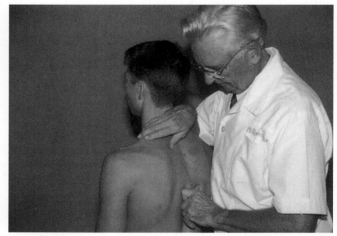

FIGURE 10.37

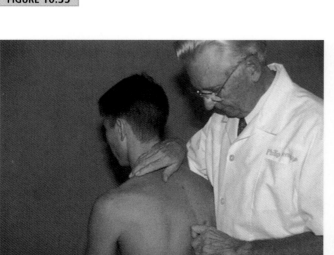

FIGURE 10.36

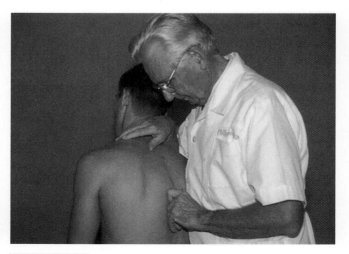

FIGURE 10.38

FUNCTIONAL TECHNIQUE

Thoracic Spine and Ribs

Sitting

Diagnosis: Combined vertebral and rib dysfunction

1. Patient sits on the table with the left hand on the back of the neck.

2. Operator stands behind the patient with the left hand grasping the patient's left elbow as the motor hand (Fig. 10.39).

3. Operator's right hand is placed in the medial groove adjacent to the spinous processes over the restricted segments and serves as the listening hand. The thumb lies over the zygapophysial joints and the palm over the costotransverse articulation of the rib (Fig. 10.40).

4. Operator introduces flexion (Fig. 10.41) and extension (Fig. 10.42) through AP translation to ease at the listening hand.

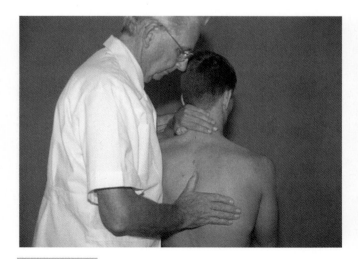

FIGURE 10.39

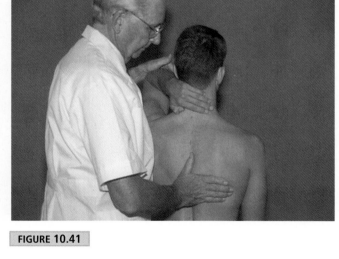

FIGURE 10.41

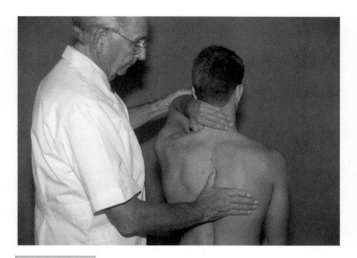

FIGURE 10.40

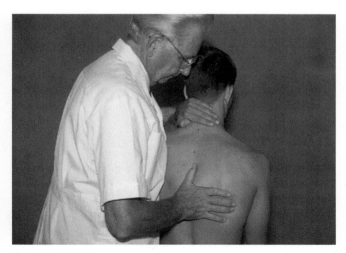

FIGURE 10.42

5. Operator introduces side bending and rotation to ease at the listening hand (Fig. 10.43).

6. The balance-and-hold approach seeks ease in all dimensions and adds respiratory effort until balance in tissue tension is achieved.

7. The dynamic indirect approach initiates motion through the motion hand to ease at the listening hand and follows the inherent tissue motion until three-dimensional tissue tension balance is achieved.

8. A variant of this technique has the patient's left hand grasping the right shoulder, the operator's left hand becoming the listening hand over the thoracic vertebra and ribs, and the operator's right hand grasping the patient's left elbow as the motion hand (Fig. 10.43). The rest of the procedure follows as above. This variant allows for different combinations of flexion–extension and side bending/rotation to the listening hand (Fig. 10.44).

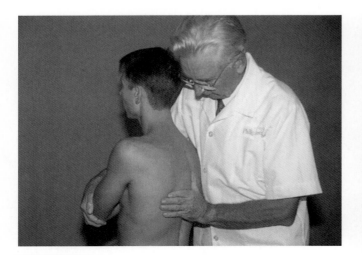

FIGURE 10.43

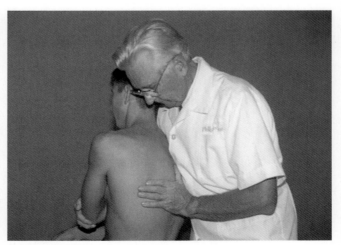

FIGURE 10.44

FUNCTIONAL TECHNIQUE

Mid and Lower Ribs

Sitting

Diagnosis: Structural or respiratory rib dysfunction

1. Patient sits on the table.

2. Operator stands behind the patient with the trunk supporting the patient's torso.

3. Operator's right hand is placed over the medial side of the rib angle with the fingers along the rib shafts of the dysfunctional rib(s) as the listening hand (Fig. 10.45).

4. Operator's left arm reaches across the patient's upper trunk and grasps the right shoulder as the motion hand.

5. Flexion–extension is introduced through AP translation to ease at the listening hand.

6. Operator's motion hand introduces side bending and rotation to ease at the listening hand (Fig. 10.46).

7. The balance-and-hold approach localizes ease in all dimensions at the listening hand and uses respiratory effort until balance of tissue tension is achieved.

8. The dynamic indirect approach introduces movement through the motion hand in the direction of ease at the listening hand and follows the inherent tissue motion until balance in tissue tension is achieved. Occasionally, compression is useful in initiating the inherent tissue motion.

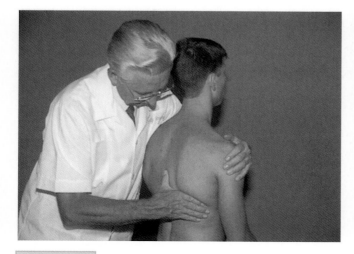

FIGURE 10.45

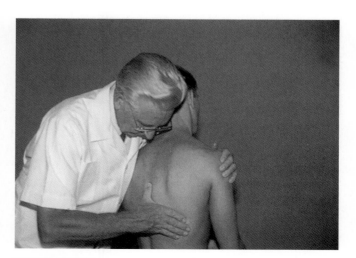

FIGURE 10.46

FUNCTIONAL TECHNIQUE

First Rib

Sitting

Diagnosis: Respiratory dysfunction, first rib

1. Patient sits on the table with the right hand grasping the back of the neck.

2. Operator stands behind the patient with the listening left hand palpating the patient's right first rib with the thumb on the posterior aspect and the fingers on the anterior aspect (Fig. 10.47).

3. Operator's motion right hand grasps the patient's right elbow.

4. Operator introduces AP trunk translation and internal–external rotation of the patient's right arm localizing ease at the listening hand (Fig. 10.48).

5. The balance-and-hold approach localizes ease in all directions and adds respiratory effort until balance of tissue tension occurs.

6. The dynamic indirect approach initiates a compressive action in the direction of ease through the motion hand and follows the inherent tissue motion until tissue tension is relieved and motion is reestablished.

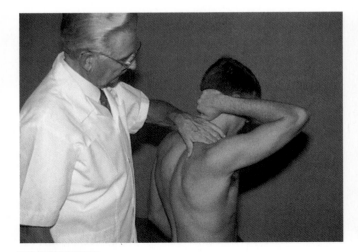

FIGURE 10.47

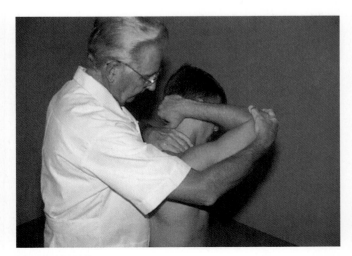

FIGURE 10.48

FUNCTIONAL TECHNIQUE

Upper Ribs

Sitting

Diagnosis: Respiratory rib dysfunction

1. Patient sits with the left hand grasping the right shoulder.

2. Operator stands behind the patient with the thorax supporting the patient's torso.

3. Operator's left listening hand contacts the upper left ribs (Fig. 10.49) with the thumb behind and the fingers over the anterior aspect.

4. Operator's right motion hand controls the patient's left upper extremity through the elbow.

5. Operator's body introduces AP translation; the motion hand introduces flexion, adduction, and abduction of the patient's upper arm to maximum ease at the listening hand (Fig. 10.50).

6. Additional ease may be obtained by the patient side bending and rotating the head to the right.

7. The balance-and-hold approach maintains ease in all dimensions and adds respiratory effort until tissue balance and motion is restored.

8. The dynamic indirect approach initiates motion through the motion hand in the direction of ease at the listening hand and follows the inherent tissue motion until tissue tension is relieved and motion is restored.

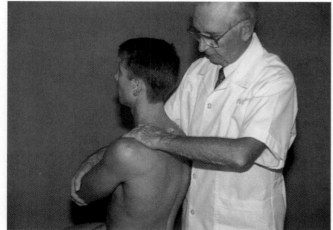

FIGURE 10.49

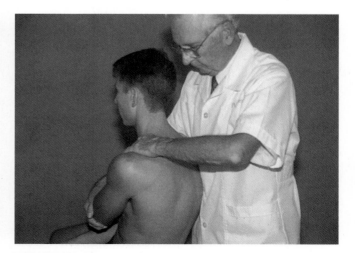

FIGURE 10.50

FUNCTIONAL TECHNIQUE

Single Rib (Variation 1)

Sitting

Diagnosis: Respiratory or structural rib dysfunction

1. Patient sits on the table.
2. Operator stands or sits at the side of the patient and identifies the dysfunctional rib (Fig. 10.51).
3. Operator places both thumbs at the midaxillary line of the dysfunctional rib with the middle fingers spanning and holding the rib shaft anteriorly and posteriorly (Fig. 10.52).
4. Patient is instructed to lean toward the operator's hands and gently side bend and rotate the trunk away (Fig. 10.53).
5. Operator translates the patient until the rib appears to "float" and then initiates respiratory effort until release of tissue tension and restoration of motion occur.

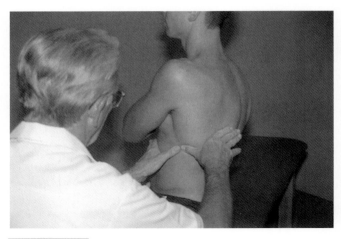

FIGURE 10.52

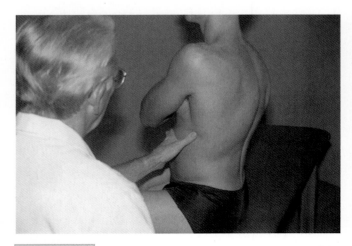

FIGURE 10.51

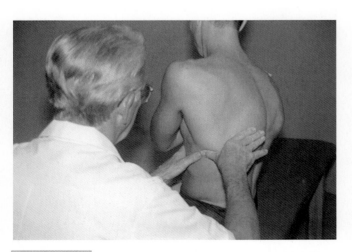

FIGURE 10.53

FUNCTIONAL TECHNIQUE

Single Rib (Variation 2)

Sitting

Diagnosis: Respiratory or structural rib dysfunction

1. Patient sits on the table.

2. Operator stands behind the patient with the thorax supporting the patient's torso.

3. Operator's listening hand is placed over the posterior aspect of the dysfunctional rib with the thumb near the costotransverse articulation and the fingers along the rib shaft.

4. Operator's motion hand reaches across anterior upper thorax of the patient and grasps the shoulder on the side of the dysfunction (Fig. 10.54).

5. Operator introduces translation of the patient's body and moves the shoulder through elevation, depression, and anterior and posterior rotations until ease is felt at the listening hand (Fig. 10.55).

6. The balance-and-hold approach seeks ease in all dimensions and adds respiratory effort until release of tissue tension and restoration of motion are achieved.

7. The dynamic indirect approach initiates motion in the direction of ease and follows the inherent tissue motion until tissue tension is released and motion is restored.

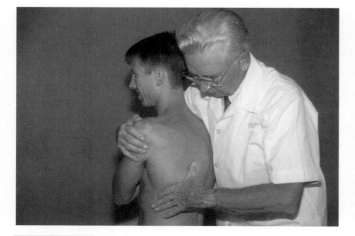

FIGURE 10.54

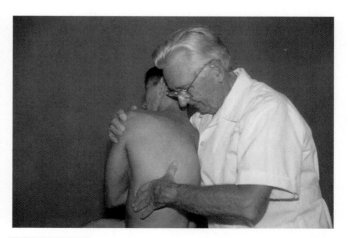

FIGURE 10.55

FUNCTIONAL TECHNIQUE

Single Typical Rib Dysfunction

Supine

Diagnosis: Respiratory or structural rib dysfunction

1. Patient supine on the table.

2. Operator sits at the side of the dysfunction (hand position shown with patient sitting [Fig. 10.56]).

3. Operator's posterior hand slides under the patient and contacts the posterior shaft while the anterior hand contacts the anterior shaft of the dysfunctional rib (Fig. 10.57).

4. Operator introduces AP compression and seeks point of maximum ease.

5. The balance-and-hold approach adds respiratory effort to achieve tissue tension balance and restore function.

6. The dynamic indirect approach initiates motion through both hands in the direction of ease and follows the inherent tissue motion until tissue tension is relieved and motion is restored.

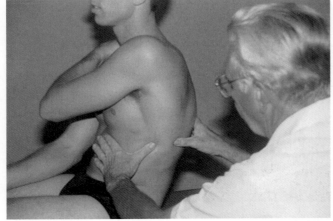

FIGURE 10.56

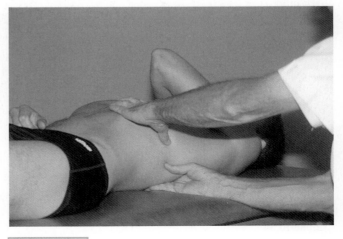

FIGURE 10.57

FUNCTIONAL TECHNIQUE

Sternum

Supine

Diagnosis: Manubriosternal dysfunction

1. Patient supine on the table.

2. Operator stands at the side of the patient.

3. Operator places one hand over the sternum (Fig. 10.58) with the other hand overlying the first and pointed in the opposite direction (Fig. 10.59). A variant of the hand position has one hand over the body of the sternum pointed vertically and the other horizontally across the manubrium with the two hands adjacent to the angle of Louis (Fig. 10.60).

4. Operator introduces slight compression followed by cephalic–caudad, clockwise, (Fig. 10.61) and counterclockwise compressions (Fig. 10.62), shifting side to side, with AP rocking movements seeking point of maximum ease.

5. The balance-and-hold approach seeks the point of maximum ease and introduces respiratory effort until balanced motion is achieved.

6. The dynamic indirect approach initiates motion by added compression and follows the inherent tissue motion until tissue tension is relieved and motion is restored.

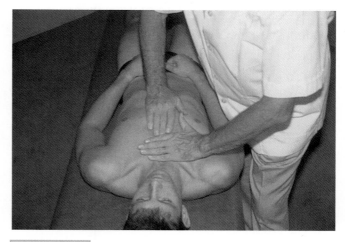

FIGURE 10.60

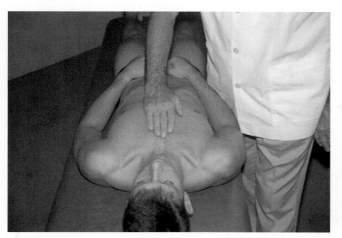

FIGURE 10.58

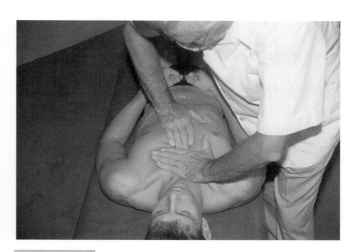

FIGURE 10.61

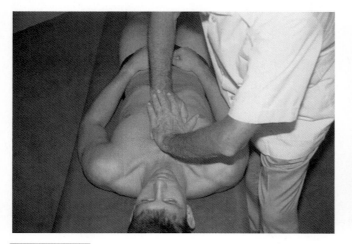

FIGURE 10.59

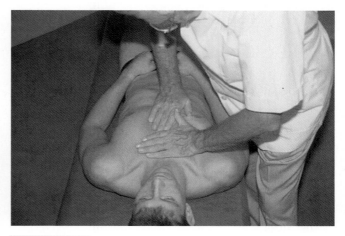

FIGURE 10.62

FUNCTIONAL TECHNIQUE

Occipitoatlantal Junction (C0-C1)

Sitting

Diagnosis: Flexion–extension C0-C1 dysfunction

1. Patient sits on the table.
2. Operator stands behind the patient with the chest wall and abdomen supporting the patient's posterior torso.
3. Operator's hands grasp the skull with the thumbs along the occipital protuberance (Fig. 10.63).
4. Operator's arms contact the patient's shoulders and a cephalic lift to the head is applied until ease is felt.
5. Operator fine-tunes ease with head flexion–extension, rotation, and side bending to maximum (Fig. 10.64).
6. The balance-and-hold approach holds ease in all dimensions and adds respiratory effort until tissue tension is relieved and motion is restored.
7. The dynamic indirect approach initiates motion in the direction of ease and follows the inherent tissue motion until release is felt and motion established.

FUNCTIONAL TECHNIQUE

Upper Cervical Spine (C1-C2)

Sitting

Diagnosis: Dysfunction at C1-C2

1. Patient sits on the table.
2. Operator stands behind the patient with the chest wall and the abdomen supporting the patient's posterior torso.

3. Operator's left hand is placed over the front of the skull and the right hand under the occiput with the thumb and index fingers in contact with the atlas/axis region (Fig. 10.65).
4. Operator introduces cephalic distraction followed by flexion–extension and side bending/rotation seeking the point of maximum ease.
5. The balance-and-hold approach would hold the point of maximum ease and would apply respiratory effort until tissue tension is released and motion is restored.
6. The dynamic indirect approach initiates motion in the direction of ease through combined motion of both hands and follows the inherent tissue motion until tissue tension is released and motion is restored.

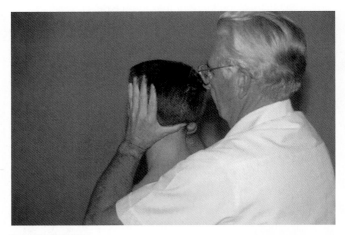

FIGURE 10.64

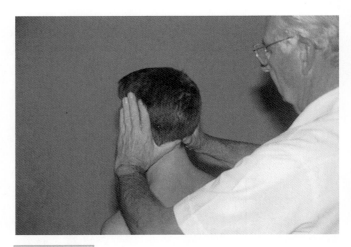

FIGURE 10.63

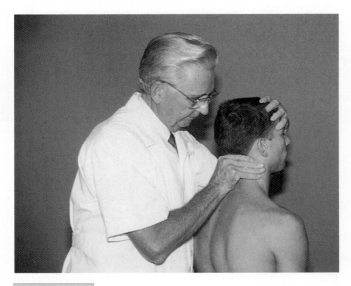

FIGURE 10.65

FUNCTIONAL TECHNIQUE

Occiptitoalantal Junction (C0-C1)

Supine

Diagnosis: Flexion–extension dysfunction

1. Patient supine on the table with the arms at the sides.

2. Operator sits at the head of the table.

3. Operator's left hand cradles the occiput with the thumb and index finger in contact with the posterior arch of the atlas (Fig. 10.66).

4. Operator's right hand contacts the frontal area (Fig. 10.67).

5. Operator introduces small AP nodding movements of the skull until the atlas is at maximum ease.

6. Operator applies compression\distraction through the occiput and right–left translation through the atlas to the point of maximum ease (Fig. 10.68).

7. The balance-and-hold approach holds the point of maximum ease and applies respiratory effort until tissue tension is released and motion is restored.

8. The dynamic indirect approach initiates motion in the direction of ease through both hands and follows the inherent tissue motion until tissue tension is released and motion is restored.

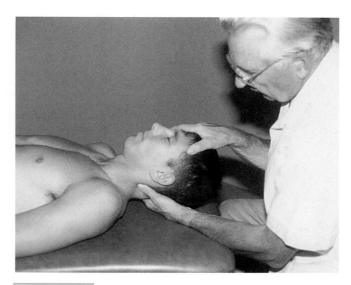

FIGURE 10.67

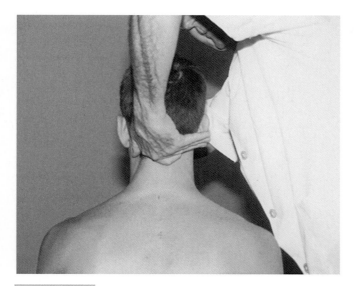

FIGURE 10.66

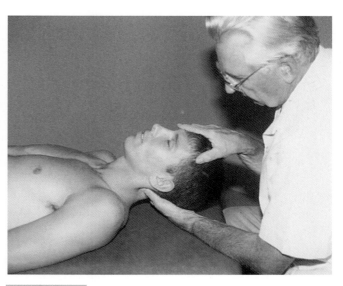

FIGURE 10.68

FUNCTIONAL TECHNIQUE

Typical Cervical Spine

Sitting

Diagnosis: ERS or FRS

1. Patient sits on the table.

2. Operator stands behind the patient with the chest and the abdomen supporting the patient's posterior torso.

3. Operator's listening left hand is placed over the dysfunctional segment of the lower cervical spine. The thumb and index finger span the posterior pillars or the transverse processes (Fig. 10.69).

4. The motion right hand is placed on the patient's forehead.

5. Operator introduces flexion–extension, side bending, and rotation through the motion hand to maximum ease at the listening hand (Fig. 10.70). AP translatory movement can be introduced through the operator's trunk. Cephalic-to-caudad translation can be introduced through combined movement of both hands.

6. The balance-and-hold approach maintains the point of maximum ease and applies respiratory effort until tissue tension is released and motion is restored (Fig. 10.71).

7. The dynamic indirect approach introduces motion through the right hand in the direction of ease and follows the inherent tissue motion until tissue tension releases and motion is restored.

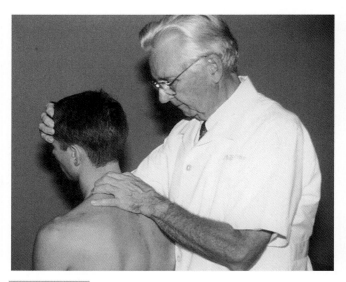

FIGURE 10.70

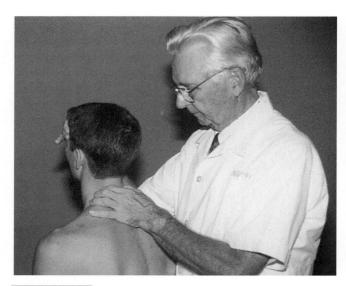

FIGURE 10.69

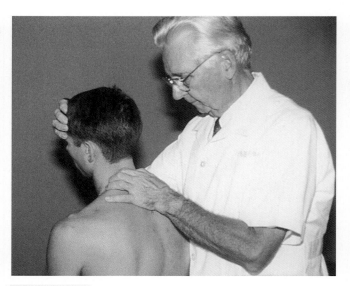

FIGURE 10.71

FUNCTIONAL TECHNIQUE

Typical Cervical Spine

Supine

Diagnosis: ERS or FRS

1. Patient supine on the table.

2. Operator sits at the head of the table.

3. Operator's hands support the patient's head and upper cervical spine with the index and middle fingers over the articular pillar of the dysfunctional segment (Fig. 10.72).

4. Operator introduces flexion–extension, AP translation, side bending, and rotation through combined movement of both hands seeking point of maximum ease under finger tips (Fig. 10.73).

5. The balance-and-hold approach maintains the point of maximum ease and applies respiratory effort until tissue tension is released and motion is restored (Fig. 10.74).

6. The dynamic indirect approach initiates motion in the direction of ease and follows the inherent tissue motion until tissue tension is released and motion is restored.

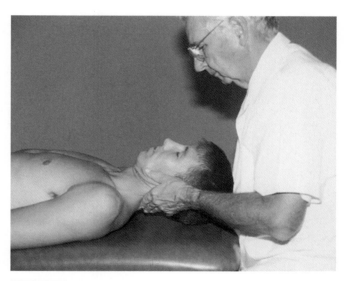

FIGURE 10.73

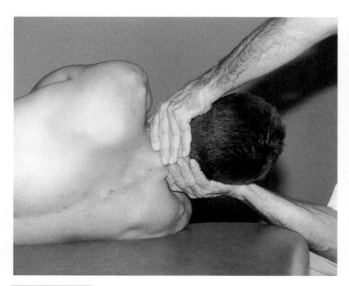

FIGURE 10.72

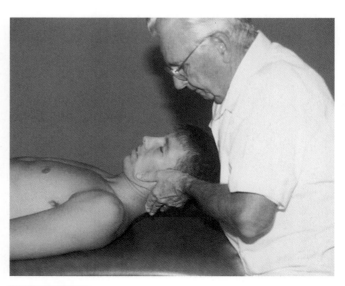

FIGURE 10.74

FUNCTIONAL TECHNIQUE

Shoulder Girdle

Step 1

1. Patient is supine on the table.

2. Operator sits at the side of the shoulder to be treated.

3. Operator's listening hand is placed over the patient's clavicle with the little finger along the shaft and the fourth and fifth finger pads over the sternoclavicular joint. The heel of the hand is over the acromioclavicular joint (Fig. 10.75).

4. Operator's motion hand grasps the patient's arm either above or below the elbow and abducts to about 90 degrees (Fig. 10.76).

5. Operator's motion hand introduces adduction–abduction, internal–external rotation, and compression–distraction along the humerus to ease at the listening hand.

6. The balance-and-hold approach maintains the point of ease and adds respiratory effort until release of tissue tension occurs.

7. The dynamic indirect approach introduces motion in the direction of ease and follows the inherent tissue motion until tissue tension is relieved.

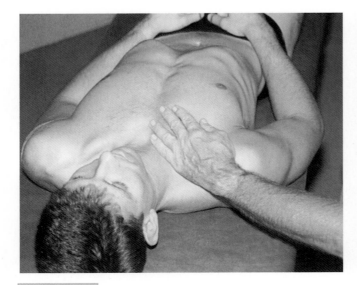

FIGURE 10.75

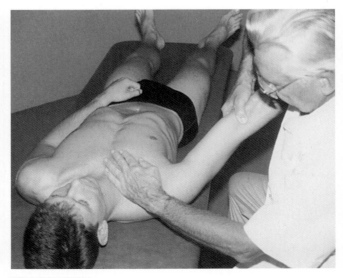

FIGURE 10.76

FUNCTIONAL TECHNIQUE

Shoulder Girdle

Step 2

1. Operator and patient position as in step 1.

2. Operator's listening hand is placed over the glenohumeral joint with the thumb behind and the fingers in front (Fig. 10.77).

3. Operator's motion hand grasps the patient's arm in the same fashion as step 1 and introduces abduction to 80 to 90 degrees and then fine-tunes through the listening hand by internal–external rotation and compression–decompression until maximum ease is obtained (Fig. 10.78).

4. The balance-and-hold approach maintains ease and adds respiratory effort until release of tissue tension is achieved.

5. The dynamic indirect approach initiates motion in the direction of ease through the motion hand and follows the inherent tissue motion until tissue tension is released and motion is restored.

FUNCTIONAL TECHNIQUE

Shoulder Girdle

Step 3

1. Operator and patient position as in steps 1 and 2.

2. Operator switches hands with the listening hand over the pectoral region in the direction of the fibers of the pectoralis minor. The motion hand controls the arm and introduces abduction so that the arm is in the direction of the pectoral muscle fibers (Fig. 10.79).

3. Operator's motion hand introduces compression–decompression, internal–external rotation, and adduction–abduction until the point of maximum ease is felt at the listening hand.

4. The tissues are balanced between the hands.

5. The balance-and-hold approach maintains the point of maximum ease and adds respiratory effort until tissue tension is relieved and motion is returned.

6. The dynamic indirect approach initiates motion in the direction of ease and follows the inherent tissue motion until tissue tension is relieved and motion is restored.

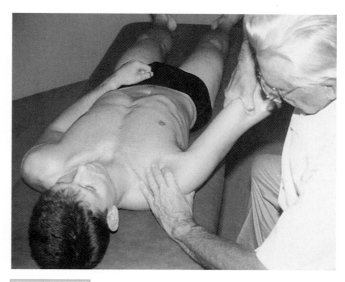

FIGURE 10.78

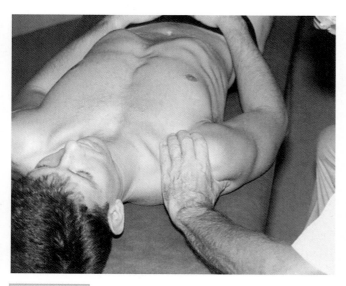

FIGURE 10.77

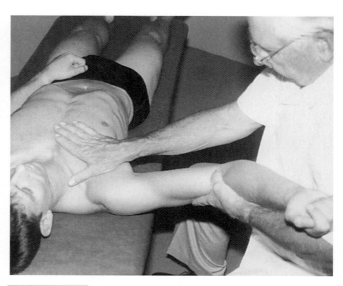

FIGURE 10.79

FUNCTIONAL TECHNIQUE

Acromioclavicular and Glenohumeral Joints

Sitting

1. Patient sits on the table.

2. Operator stands behind the patient and supports the patient's trunk against the operator's body.

3. Operator's foot is placed on the table on the side being treated and drapes the patient's relaxed arm over the knee with the medial hand placed over the patient's acromioclavicular and glenohumeral areas (Fig. 10.80).

4. Operator's lateral hand grasps the patient's elbow.

5. Operator introduces AP and medial–lateral translation and rotation of the patient to ease both at the shoulder and at the elbow (Fig. 10.81).

6. The balance-and-hold approach identifies the point of maximum ease and adds respiratory effort until tissue tension is relieved and motion is restored.

7. The dynamic indirect approach introduces motion in the direction of ease, frequently with a compression–decompression maneuver in the long axis of the arm, and follows the inherent tissue motion until tissue tension is relieved and motion is restored.

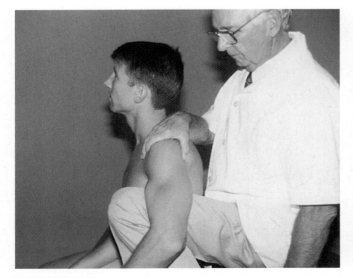

FIGURE 10.80

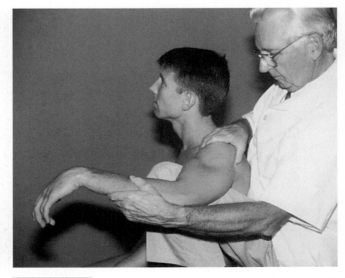

FIGURE 10.81

FUNCTIONAL TECHNIQUE

Radial Head

Sitting

1. Patient sits.

2. Operator stands in front of the patient with the listening hand over the dysfunctional elbow with the thumb over the anterior aspect and the index finger over the posterior aspect of the radial head (Fig. 10.82).

3. Operator's motion hand grasps the patient's distal forearm and introduces flexion–extension, internal–external rotation, adduction–abduction, and compression–decompression to the point of maximum ease (Fig. 10.83).

4. The balance-and-hold approach maintains the point of maximum ease and introduces respiratory effort until tissue tension is relieved and motion is restored.

5. The dynamic indirect approach introduces motion in the direction of ease and follows the inherent tissue motion until tissue tension is relieved and motion is restored.

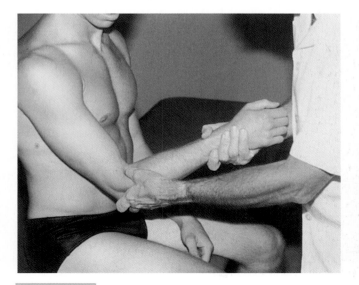

FIGURE 10.82

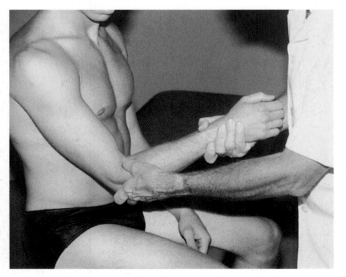

FIGURE 10.83

FUNCTIONAL TECHNIQUE

Wrist and Hand

Sitting

1. Patient sits on the table.

2. Operator stands in front of the patient grasping the dysfunctional wrist and the hand with the proximal hand over the distal forearm (Fig. 10.84).

3. Operator's distal hand grasps the patient's hand either with a handshake hold (Fig. 10.85) or with the fingers interdigitating (Fig. 10.86).

4. Operator's distal hand introduces flexion–extension, internal–external rotation, adduction–abduction, and compression–decompression to the point of maximum ease (Fig. 10.87).

5. The balance-and-hold technique maintains the point of ease and adds respiratory effort until tissue tension is relieved and motion is restored.

6. The dynamic indirect approach introduces motion in the direction of ease and follows the inherent tissue motion until tissue tension is relieved and motion is restored.

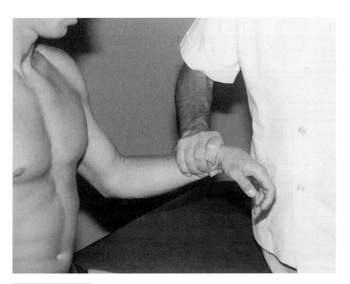

FIGURE 10.84

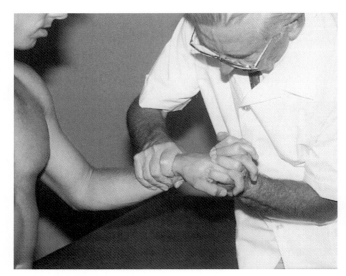

FIGURE 10.86

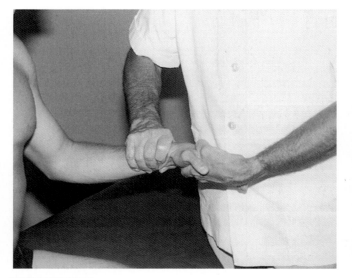

FIGURE 10.85

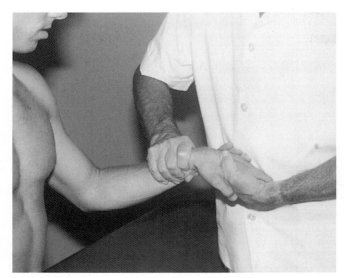

FIGURE 10.87

FUNCTIONAL TECHNIQUE

Hip and Leg

Supine

1. Patient is supine on the table.

2. Operator stands at the side of the table on the side of the dysfunctional leg and one foot on the table.

3. Operator flexes the patient's leg to about 90 degrees of hip and knee flexion with the leg draped over the operator's thigh.

4. Operator's proximal hand is on the patient's knee with the distal hand holding the patient's foot (Fig. 10.88).

5. Operator introduces compression–decompression through the thigh and/or leg until ease is obtained. Fine-tuning is done by medial–lateral rotation, adduction–abduction, and flexion–extension of the hip and the knee (Fig. 10.89).

6. The balance-and-hold approach maintains the point of maximum ease and adds respiratory effort until tissue tension is relieved and motion is restored.

7. The dynamic indirect approach initiates motion in the direction of ease and follows the inherent tissue motion until tissue tension is relieved and motion is restored.

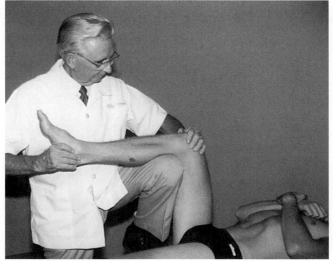

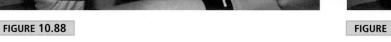

FIGURE 10.88

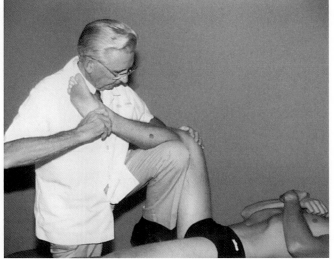

FIGURE 10.89

FUNCTIONAL TECHNIQUE

Knee and Fibular Head

Sitting

1. Patient sits on the table with the legs dangling.

2. Operator sits in front of the patient.

3. Operator's listening hand palpates the knee with the thumb over the medial meniscus and the fingers on the fibular head (Fig. 10.90).

4. Operator's motion hand holds the foot and ankle and introduces compression–decompression to loose pack the tibia on the femur.

5. Operator fine-tunes ease at the listening hand by introducing adduction–abduction, internal–external rotation, and flexion–extension (Fig. 10.91).

6. The balance-and-hold approach maintains maximum ease and adds respiratory effort until tissue tension is relieved and motion is restored.

7. The dynamic indirect approach initiates motion in the direction of ease and follows the inherent tissue motion until tissue tension is relieved and motion is restored.

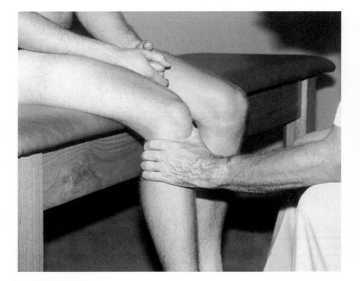

FIGURE 10.90

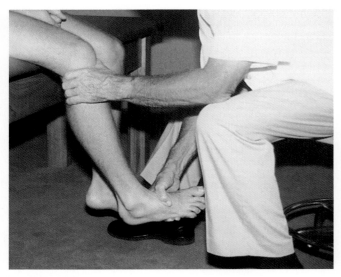

FIGURE 10.91

FUNCTIONAL TECHNIQUE

Foot and Ankle

1. Patient sits or is supine on the table.

2. Operator's listening hand grasps the heel of the patient (Fig. 10.92).

3. Operator's motion hand grasps the forefoot and initiates motion through compression (Fig. 10.93).

4. Operator fine-tunes maximum ease through the introduction of dorsi and plantar flexion, inversion–eversion, and adduction–abduction (Fig. 10.94).

5. The balance-and-hold approach maintains maximum ease and uses respiratory effort until tissue tension is relieved and motion is restored.

6. The dynamic indirect approach initiates motion primarily through compression–distraction and follows the inherent tissue motion until tissue tension is relieved and motion is restored.

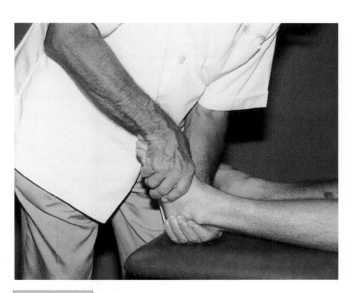

FIGURE 10.93

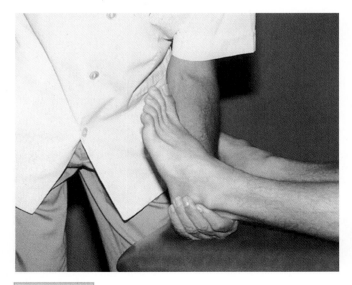

FIGURE 10.92

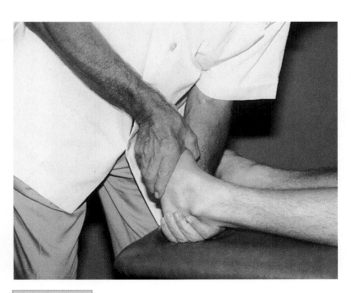

FIGURE 10.94

CONCLUSION

Indirect (functional) techniques are based on a common neurologic model in which reducing the flow of abnormal afferent impulses into the central nervous system reprograms the "central computer" to more normal function. These procedures focus on the quality of movement, particularly the quality on the initiation of motion, rather than the amount of range or the feel of its end point. They are primarily nontraumatic and are easily used in a variety of patient conditions and health care settings. They require considerable practice to educate the senses to the ease-and-bind phenomena and to the point of maximum pain-free position for the tissues of the musculoskeletal system. The value of these procedures in patient care warrants the expenditure of time and effort needed for the student to acquire proficiency.

SUGGESTED READINGS

Johnston WL, Friedman HD. *Functional Methods*. Indianapolis, IN: American Academy of Osteopathy, 1994.

Johnston WL, Robertson JA, Stiles EG. *Finding a Common Denominator for the Variety of Manipulative Techniques*. Carmel, CA: Yearbook of the American Academy of Osteopathy, 1969:5–15.

Stiles EG. Manipulative techniques: Four approaches. *Osteopathic Med* 1975;1:27–30.

REFERENCES

1. Hoover HW. *Functional Technique*. Carmel, CA: Yearbook of the Academy of Applied Osteopathy, 1958:47–51.
2. Stiles EG, Shaw HH. Functional techniques based upon the approach of George Andrew Laughlin DO. Course syllabus. Michigan State University, College of Osteopathic Medicine, Continuing Education, 1991.
3. Jones LH. *Strain and Counterstrain*. Colorado Springs, CO: American Academy of Osteopathy, 1981.
4. Korr, IM. Proprioceptors and somatic dysfunction. *J Am Acad Osteopathy: The Collected Papers of Irvin M Korr*. 1979:200–207.
5. Denslow JS, Korr IM, Krems, AD. Quantitative studies of chronic facilitation in human motoneuron pools. *Am J Physiol* 1947;150:229–238.
6. Freeman MAR, Wyke B. Articular reflexes at the ankle joint: An electromyographic study of normal and abnormal influences of ankle-joint mechanoreceptors upon reflex activity in the leg muscles. *Br J Surg* 1947;54:990–1001.
7. Schomburg ED. Spinal functions in sensorimotor control movements. *Neurosurg Rev* 1990;13:179–185.
8. Gardner E. Reflex muscular responses to stimulation of articular nerves in the cat. *Am J Physiol* 1950;161:133–141.
9. He X, Proske U, Schailble H, et al. Acute inflammation of the knee joint in the cat alters responses of flexor motoneurons to leg movements. *J Neurophysiol* 1988;59:326–340.
10. Jones LH, Kusunose RS, Goering EK. *Jones Strain–Counterstrain*. Boise, ID: Jones Strain-counterstrain, Inc., 1995.

PRINCIPLES OF MYOFASCIAL RELEASE AND INTEGRATED NEUROMUSCULOSKELETAL TECHNIQUE

Robert C. Ward, D.O., F.A.A.O., is credited with developing these release techniques as one of the newer additions to the field of manual medicine.[1] He describes these myofascial release techniques as "bridging" techniques spanning the spectrum of manual medicine procedures. They combine many of the principles of soft-tissue technique, muscle energy technique, indirect technique, and inherent-force craniosacral technique. They are classified as combined procedures as they influence the biomechanics of the musculoskeletal system and the peripheral and central neural control mechanisms. There are multiple authors and teachers of myofascial release technique with many similarities and differences.

Fascia has received the attention of many individuals including William Neidner, the osteopathic physician, who used twisting forces on the extremities to restore fascial balance and symmetry.[2] Rolf[3] was famous for deep pressure and stretching of the fascia for the purpose of "Structural Integration". Rolfing requires extensive investment in time and energy, both by the patient and the operator, and the process is not always comfortable.

The fascial release technique described here can be classified as direct or indirect and is frequently used in a combined fashion. It applies the principles of biomechanical loading of soft tissue and the neural reflex modifications by stimulation of mechanoreceptors in the fascia. The resistant barrier may be engaged directly with tissue stretching, or loading can occur in the direction away from the resistant barrier in an indirect fashion. These are frequently called direct and indirect barriers. Frequently, the barriers are addressed in a combined fashion in each direction in a balanced fashion.

Fascial release technique fosters inherent tissue motion. Living tissues have an inherent motion that continues at various rates and amplitudes.[4–12] The inherent tissue motion of the musculoskeletal system is thought to be the result of rhythmic changes in tone of muscle, pulsating forces of arterial circulation, the effects of respiration, and the inherent force of the cranial rhythmic impulse. Connective tissue and fascia are primary transmitters of inherent motion throughout the body.[13,14] Loss of inherent motion of tissues can be used as a diagnostic cue as to the need for treatment.

Activating forces used in fascial release technique are both intrinsic and extrinsic. *Intrinsic activating forces* include inherent tissue motion, inherent body rhythms, respiration, muscle contraction, and eye movement. *Extrinsic activating forces* are applied by the operator and include compression, traction, and twisting to focus the appropriate tension in the soft tissues to effect biomechanical and reflex change. This technique is used for regional and local dysfunctions. It shares the common goal of all manual medicine procedures to achieve symmetric, pain-free motion of the musculoskeletal system in postural balance.

FASCIA

The clinician using fascial release technique must have a thorough working knowledge of the continuity and integration of fascia. Connective tissue, including the fasciae, surrounding all muscles and organs forms a complex continuous matrix (network) throughout the body that has mechanosensory, regulatory, and signaling functions.[15–24]

Fasciae can be described as consisting of three layers. The *pannicular or superficial fascia* is attached to the undersurface of the skin and is a loosely knit, fibroelastic, areolar tissue. Within the superficial fascia are fat, vascular structures (including capillary networks and lymphatic channels), and nervous tissues. The skin can be moved in many directions over the deeper structures because of the loosely knit nature of the superficial fascia. Within the superficial fascia is potential space for the accumulation of fluid and metabolites. Many of the palpatory changes of tissue texture abnormalities are the result of changes within the superficial fascia.

Deep fascia is tough, tight, and compact. It compartmentalizes the body. It envelops and separates muscles, surrounds and separates internal visceral organs, and contributes greatly to the contour and function of the body. The peritoneum, the pericardium, and the pleura are specialized elements of the deep fascia. The tough, resistant, and confining characteristics of the deep fascia can create problems such as the compartment syndromes. Trauma with hemorrhage in the anterior compartment of the lower leg can cause swelling that is detrimental to the sensitive nerve structures within the compartment. Frequently, surgical fasciectomy is necessary to relieve the compression on neural elements.

The *subserous fascia* is the loose areolar tissue that covers the internal visceral organs. The many small circulatory channels and fluids within this fascia lubricate the surfaces of the internal viscera.

Generally, fascia provides support for vessels and nerves throughout the body. It enables adjacent tissues to move on each other while providing stability and contour. It also provides lubricating fluid between structures for movement and nutrition. From a manual medicine perspective, this bodywide connective tissue network is not only composed of a weblike collagenous

155

matrix, but also includes a network of fibroblasts that are linked to the collagen matrix by specialized proteins, as well as to each other by abundant cell-to-cell contacts.[25,29] The fibroblast cells are chiefly responsible for manufacturing the extracellular matrix. Recent studies also suggest that they are dynamically responsive to mechanical stimulation. Short-term mechanical stress (minutes to hours) leads to α-and β-actin redistribution and rapid cytoskeletal remodeling that may play an important role in the regulation of connective tissue tension. This is in contrast to the response of fibroblasts to long-term mechanical stress (days to weeks) and/or injury causing increased α-actin synthesis and transformation into a contractile myofibroblast phenotype.[26]

Mechanoreceptors, abundant within the superficial fascia, provide afferent information for many complex reflexes involving the neuromuscular system. Continuous with specialized elements such as the extrafusal and interfusal muscle fiber, ligaments, and tendons, fascia has unique characteristics but shares some characteristics with connective tissue collagen fibers, elastic fibers, cellular elements, and ground substance. Mechanoreceptors and proprioceptors, found within these specialized elements of fascia, report information to the spinal cord and brain on body position and movement, both normal and abnormal. Sophisticated neuromuscular reflexes constantly maintain body posture and prepare for, initiate, and continue movement patterns. The function of muscles is an integrated and highly complex process; motor control through the central nervous system from the premotor cortex through the brainstem, cerebellum, spinal cord, and finally to the final common pathway, the alpha motor neuron to skeletal muscle. This control system for muscle function has voluntary and involuntary components which are highly influenced by afferent impulses coming from the mechanoreceptors within the articular and fascial systems. When this central control system is working efficiently, movement patterns are symmetric, coordinated, and free. When altered, inefficient and uncoordinated movement results. One need only contrast the performance of an Olympic-level runner and a patient with advanced Parkinson disease. Between these two extremes are gradations of hypertonicity, hypotonicity, and altered integrative coordination.

Muscle injury interferes with fascial anatomy and function. Acute trauma results in muscle tears, disturbances at the myotendinous junction, and alterations of insertion of tendon into bone. These injuries undergo fibrosis as part of the healing process similar to other injuries of soft tissues. Functional loss can result. Injury not only alters the anatomy of the muscle, but also interferes with its neuroreflexive response to motor control and contributes to persistent long-term symptoms.

Stretch-induced or stress-induced fibroblast cytoskeletal remodeling that results in changes in collagen fiber density and orientation, with resultant changes in tissue viscoelastic properties (e.g., changes in stiffness) may play an important role in connective tissue responses to injury, normal movement, posture, and exercise, as well as mechanical forces applied therapeutically.[27–30] This may explain why biochemical and immunologic changes occurring within the ground substance of the fascia have general systemic effects that seem quite far removed from the injury to the soft tissues. Scarring during the healing process frequently interferes with the functions of support, movement, and lubrication. Many detrimental symptoms result that are difficult to objectify. Soft-tissue changes lead to persistent symptoms long after there has been healing of the acute tissue injury.

Biomechanics of Fascia

Fascia's intimate connection with muscle provides the opportunity for contraction and relaxation. Fascia has elasticity that allows it to both retain its shape and respond to deformation. *Elastic deformation* is the capacity of fascia to recover its original shape when the load is removed. If the load is great and applied for a longer period, the fascia may not be able to recover its original size and shape, resulting in *plastic deformation*. When subjected to an elongation load and held constant, the fascia has the capacity to "*creep.*" The relaxation of the tissue that accompanies creep allows for less resistance to a second application of load. This phenomenon has clinical significance when the clinician observes the effects of acute and repetitive injury and long-term stress on connective tissues. Fascia has the capacity to convert mechanical stress into heat when subjected to a load. This phenomenon, called "*hysteresis,*" is used therapeutically in fascial release technique.

CONCEPTS IN FASCIAL RELEASE TECHNIQUE

The first concept is "tight–loose." Within the fascial system, tightness creates and weakness permits asymmetry. There are biomechanical and neural reflexive elements to the tight–loose concept. Increased stimulation causes an agonist muscle to become tight, and the tighter it becomes, the looser its antagonist becomes because of reciprocal inhibition. The fascia surrounding a hypertonic, contracted muscle shortens and requires loosening of the fascia in the opposite direction for adaptation. In acute conditions, the cycle can be described as continuing spasm–pain–spasm. The result is tightness that progresses from the acute condition of muscle contraction to muscle contracture, leading to chronicity. In chronic conditions, the cycle is described as pain–looseness–pain. Manual medicine practitioners are familiar with the painful symptoms of hypermobility. The practitioners using fascial release procedures apply the fundamental tight–loose concept on a continuing basis.

The second concept is the use of "palpation" and "observation." Many diagnostic and therapeutic systems build on peripheral stimulation; these include acupuncture, acupressure, Chapman reflexes, Travell trigger points, and Jones tender points. Skilled observation of movement patterns and palpation of fascial elements frequently identifies locations of dysfunction that can be therapeutically addressed by the hands. Frequently noted is the occurrence of fascial pain in areas of muscle facilitation which is the result of the loss of "dynamic stability" (see Chapter 9) somewhere else in the body. Sensitivity of the fascial elements, particularly in the chronic state, frequently has a burning quality. Recall that the sympathetic division of the autonomic nervous system is the only division that innervates the musculoskeletal system. Sympathetic nervous system reflexes probably mediate many symptoms found in myofascial pain syndromes.

CLINICAL PEARL

Having polled many manual therapists on definitive treatment of levator scapulae myofascial pain syndrome, stretching or performing specific fascial techniques on the specific muscle is not nearly as valuable as restoring dynamic stability of the ipsilateral scapulothoracic and rib cage fascial and articular mechanics.

The third concept is "neuroreflexive change" occurring with the application of manual force on the musculoskeletal system. Hands-on application of force to the musculoskeletal system results in afferent stimulation through mechanoreceptors that require central processing at the spinal cord, brainstem, and cortical levels, resulting in alpha motor neuron efferent balance change. When afferent stimulation of a stretch is applied during a fascial release procedure, the operator waits for relaxation in the tight tissues by efferent change. The neuroreflexive response is highly variable and modified by the amount of pain, the patient's pain behavior, the level of wellness, the nutritional status, the stress response, and the basic lifestyle of the individual including the use/abuse of alcohol, tobacco, and drugs, including prescription medications.

The fourth concept is the "release" phenomenon. The sensation of release occurs in other forms of manual medicine, particularly in craniosacral technique and the ease–bind of indirect (functional) technique. When using fascial release technique, appropriate application of stress on tissue results in tissue relaxation in the fascia and in the muscle. Tightness "gives way" or "melts" under the application of load. Release of tightness is sought to achieve improvement in symmetry of form and function. The release phenomenon is both an enabling and a terminal objective when applying a fascial release procedure. Release can occur in several directions and through different levels of tissue during a fascial release procedure. The release phenomenon is one that guides the practitioner through the treatment process.

CLINICAL PEARL

Students frequently have a difficult time wrapping their heads around this palpable concept of the "release" phenomenon. How does one actually learn how to feel and trust that these subtle changes occur? It is helpful to revisit some of the palpatory exercises in Chapter 2 and keep in mind that perception of the release phenomenon can only be accomplished via the cutaneous and joint mechanoreceptors of the operator's palpatory hand. Cutaneous receptors are very sensitive to stretch or skin displacement. Joint mechanoreceptors are extraordinarily sensitive to joint position sense and any finite changes that may occur in this position (see Chapter 2). It is impossible to "perceive" anything through stiff joints; it is important to never grasp or compress so hard that the joints of your palpating hand(s) cannot relax. With this in mind you will begin to use more whole hand contact rather than finger grip. Relaxing the joints of the palpating hand(s) is simply allowing them to bend a bit and meld with the contact surface.

FASCIAL RELEASE TREATMENT CONCEPTS

Ward has coined a mnemonic to describe the principles of fascial release treatment. It is P O E (T)2. P O E stands for point of entry into the musculoskeletal system. Entry may be made from anywhere in the musculoskeletal system including the lower extremity, the upper extremity, the thoracic cage, the abdomen, and the vertebral complex from the cranial cervical junction to the pelvis. The two Ts stand for traction and twist. Traction and twist are but two of the applications of load that are of assistance in the diagnostic and treatment processes. Traction produces stretch along the long axis of fascial elements that are short and tight. Stretch should always be applied in the long axis rather than transversely across fascial elements. Twisting force provides the opportunity to localize the traction, not only at the point of contact with the patient, but also at points some distance away. Compressive and shear forces are commonly used to localize to different levels of the fascial system and to provide different loads. The practitioner should develop the ability to sense change locally at the point of contact as well as at some distance away. For example, when grasping the lower extremity near the ankle, the operator should attempt to feel through the extremity to the knee, thigh, hip, sacroiliac joint, and into the vertebral column sensing compliance of tissue throughout. This is all perceived through the contact point at the ankle.

The practitioner grasps the ankles, gently leans backward, straightens the arms, and slowly and consistently tractions the tissues (no tugging). This gentle constant traction allows the proprioceptors in the wrists and elbows to perceive loss of tissue compliance. Timing has a good deal to do with perception of the location of fascial asymmetry; if the asymmetrical load is perceived with initial traction of the ankles, it is likely that the dysfunction is distal. If the asymmetrical load is perceived after a long interval of traction at the ankles, it is likely that the dysfunction is proximal. This skill requires concentration, practice, and an appreciation for the three-dimensional aspects of the musculoskeletal system.

The treatment process includes assessment of tightness and looseness throughout the system and the application of loads, both into the direct and indirect barriers, seeking the release phenomena. Tightness and looseness can be different between the superficial and deep layers of the musculoskeletal system. Frequently, tightness in the superficial layers is found overlying the looseness in the deeper structures surrounding the articular elements. This may be compensatory in nature, but the superficial tightness and the deep-level looseness should both be approached appropriately so that the result is more symmetric function throughout the system.

Patient activity during the treatment process can assist in the achievement of the therapeutic goal. These enhancers include muscle contraction, joint motion of the upper and lower extremities, respiration, and eye movement. Any activity that increases the central nervous system processing, particularly of the cranial nerves, seems to enhance the effectiveness of the practitioner-applied loading forces. One or more enhancers may be used throughout the treatment process. The process of adding enhancers has led Ward to call this "integrated neuromuscular release." The enhancers add the neural-challenging component to the biomechanical challenge of the soft tissues.

Following treatment by these techniques, patients are given specific exercises that are individualized for their problem. Stretching exercise maintains the added length of the tight tissues and strengthening exercise restores the functional capacity of the weaker inhibited muscles. In treatment of muscle imbalance, first stretch the short, tight muscle groups and follow with strengthening exercise for the weaker, loose muscle groups. Exercise programs should also enhance the integrative function of muscle balance. Such exercises as cross-pattern pep walking, swimming, square dancing, rebounding, and so forth can be used. The goal is to increase mobility and strength and enhance muscular coordination.

These procedures are more than biomechanical and neuroreflexive. They address the total patient. General health issues such as lifestyle, coping mechanisms, appropriate use of alcohol and other medications, discontinuance of tobacco, adequate and appropriate nutrition, and weight control are all issues that need to be addressed concurrently with the fascial release treatment program.

EXERCISES IN PALPATION

Fascial release procedures require skill at palpating the musculoskeletal system for something other than one bone moving on the other. One must learn to "read the tissues" for their tightness–looseness, their inherent mobility, and the usual soft tissue texture abnormalities of hard–soft, cool–warm, smooth–rough, and so forth (see Chapter 2). One needs to develop increased sensitivity to the patient's tissues both at the point of contact and at some distance. There are many exercises in palpation that can be useful and the following are but a few.

Place the fingertips of all five fingers together without contact with the rest of the hand. Introduce force from one hand to the other and then reverse. Sense what goes on with the hand generating the force and the one receiving the force. Are they different from side to side? Now take one hand and stroke with the finger pads down the volar surface of the fingers and palms, first with light stroking and then with increased pressure. Repeat using the other hand as the motor hand. Sense the difference in the sensitivity of the hand being stroked, as well as the sensation of touch by the finger pads of the motor hand. To properly sense what goes on in the patient, you must have an awareness of your own palpatory skills and sensations and your own self-body awareness.

Fold your hands together, interlacing all your fingers. You will find that either the right or the left second metacarpophalangeal joint is on top. Now reverse the position so that the other metacarpophalangeal joint is on top. Sense the difference, with one appearing to be more comfortable than the other does and with the less comfortable one feeling tighter.

Stretch your arms out ahead of you, crossing them at the wrist and pronating both hands until the palmer surfaces meet. Interlace your fingers and raise the extended arms over your head. As you reach toward the ceiling, feel the difference in tension between the right and left sides of your body. Return to the starting position, reverse the way in which your wrists are crossed, and repeat the procedure. Again, note the difference in tension from side to side and the difference introduced by altered crossing of the wrists.

Working with a patient partner, return to the forearm palpatory exercise described in Chapter 2. This time, start with your palpating hand some distance from the forearm and slowly move toward the forearm until you begin to feel radiant energy from the patient. This is usually sensed as heat. Repeat the procedure several times with your eyes closed to see if you can repeatedly stop at the point where you first feel the sensation and if the distance from your palpating hand to the forearm is consistent. Continue to approach the forearm until you are palpating just the superficial hair, and course up and down over the forearm, attempting to sense what is going on under your hand. See if you can identify differences in the proximal forearm, distal forearm, wrist, and hand. Place the palmer surface of your hand in contact with the skin, relax the joints of your wrist and hand and concentrate, applying no motion of your own, but attempt to sense the inherent movement of the patient's tissues under your hand. It takes several seconds to several minutes to begin to sense an inherent oscillatory movement within the forearm.

When you have mastered the ability to apply pressure but not movement and the ability to sense inherent movement within your patient, place the palm of your hand in contact with the bony sacrum. This should be done both in the supine and prone positions. The contour of the sacrum fits nicely in the palm of your hand. In the prone position it is sometimes necessary to use a slight compressive "melding" force to begin to feel the inherent motion of the sacrum. In a supine position the patient's body weight on your hand is sufficient to initiate inherent sacral movement. Try to follow the sacrum in the directions in which it wishes to move. Do not attempt to direct it. What are the rhythm, amplitude, and direction of the sacrum moving in space? When you have been able to identify inherent soft-tissue and bony movement, you are well on your way to being able to use fascial release technique.

CLINICAL PEARL

A simple exercise to begin with is to perform the old "Indian burn" to your partner's forearm. Grasp your partner's forearm with both hands close together, apply enough pressure to control the skin and superficial fascia down to the deep fascia, twist each hand in opposite directions sensing for the initial barrier, and then reverse the direction of your hand-twisting to sense the difference. Is one direction tight and the other loose? Twist into the tight direction and hold it there (joints of the hand relaxed, whole hand contact). Now ask your partner to add an enhancing maneuver by having him/her gently make a fist, squeezing only until you palpate that the internal forces of his/her contraction "match" your external load. Do you feel it begin to loosen? That is the sensation of hysteresis and creep. It occurs very quickly if the appropriate internal matching load is used as an enhancer. If your partner squeezes too hard, the internal load will push you off your initial external twist.

USING ENHANCING MANEUVERS

Enhancing maneuvers define the difference between fascial release techniques and "integrated neuromusculoskeletal technique." Oftentimes, our students will comment that using fascial release techniques is hard on the hands because of the perceived amount of compression and load that is necessary to hold or engage in order to achieve the release. The enhancer has two major benefits; first it speeds up the release by allowing afferent information from muscle and joint proprioceptors, and the fascias that surround them, to join the afferent information generated from your load upon the superficial and deep fascias. Secondly, using enhancers allows one to use less compression and external load, so the joints within the operator's hands can relax such that their proprioceptors can perceive the restoration or tissue resiliency, inherent motion, and the sense of release.

The problem that students have is that there is very little "structure" in the use of the enhancing maneuver. The key is to have your patients do whatever is necessary to internally enhance the load that you have imposed externally. If you ask them to push their right knee into the table and it decreases the external load that you have placed onto the barriers of the sacrum, then have them stop and use the left knee. It is trial and error, constantly sensing the effect on the barrier. If the enhanced load is too much and it pushes your hands off the engaged system, then communicate to have your patients decrease their load.

EXAMPLES OF FASCIAL RELEASE TECHNIQUE

Wide varieties of fascial release techniques are in use by many practitioners. They are highly individualized to the skill of the practitioner and to the needs of the patient at the treatment visit. The following examples are those taught by Ward but have been found most effective in this author's hands. They provide the reader with only a small sample of the total system.

FASCIAL RELEASE TECHNIQUE

Lumbosacral Spine

Prone with longitudinal traction

1. Patient is prone with arms off the sides of the table and feet over the end, with the head turned to the most comfortable side.

2. Operator stands at the side of the patient, facing the foot of the table; if right-handed, on the patient's left, if left-handed, on the patient's right.

3. Operator places the distal hand over the sacrum with the heel of the hand at the lumbosacral junction. Operator's proximal hand is placed in the midline over the thoracolumbar junction with the fingers pointing caudally (Fig. 11.1).

4. Operator introduces gentile compression and separates both hands in a longitudinal fashion, first sensing for a loss of tissue resiliency and/or inherent tissue motion, then sensing (within this area of loss) direct and indirect barriers, constantly searching for balance of tightness and looseness (Fig. 11.2).

5. Operator applies a longitudinal load necessary to initially engage the direct barrier while the patient is asked to add an enhancing maneuver.

6. After release is achieved, reassess the patient for enhanced motion and balance.

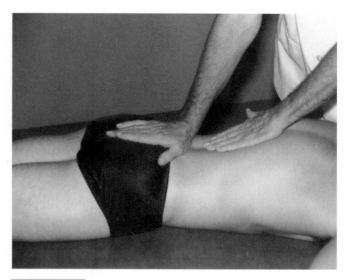

FIGURE 11.1 Longitudinal compression.

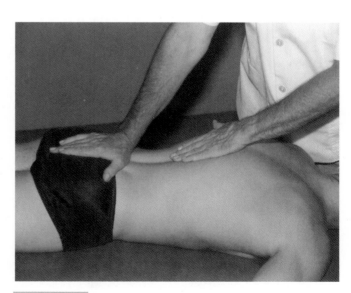

FIGURE 11.2 Longitudinal distraction.

FASCIAL RELEASE TECHNIQUE

Thoracolumbar Junction and Posterior Diaphragm

Prone

1. Patient is prone with arms off the sides of the table, feet off the end, and head turned to the most comfortable side.

2. Operator stands at the side of the patient, facing toward the head.

3. Operator's hands are placed on each side of the thoracolumbar junction with the thumbs vertical along the spinous processes and the remainder of the hand along the lower ribs, overlying the posterior diaphragm (Fig. 11.3).

4. Operator's whole hand introduces compressive load and the left moves clockwise while the right moves counterclockwise in a lateral and superior direction (Fig. 11.4).

5. Operator assesses direct and indirect barriers three dimensionally, from superficial to deep, superior to inferior, and right to left, sensing for loss of tissue resiliency and then engaging the initial direct barrier within this loss, while the patient performs enhancing maneuvers.

6. Redness of the skin is frequently seen after this technique and is described as the "blush" phenomenon.

7. After release is achieved, reassess the patient for enhanced motion and balance.

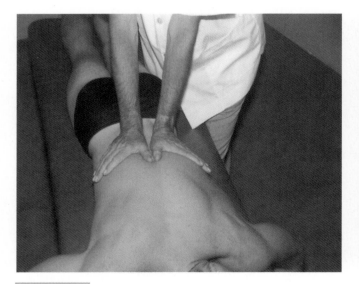

FIGURE 11.3

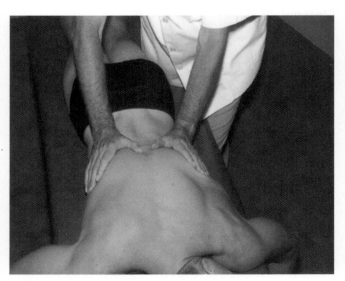

FIGURE 11.4

FASCIAL RELEASE TECHNIQUE

Prone

Sacral release

1. Patient is prone with arms off the sides of the table, feet off the end of the table, and head turned to the most comfortable side.

2. Operator places a hand over the sacrum with the heel over the base and the fingers over the apex including the inferior lateral angles (Fig. 11.5).

3. Operator's other hand is placed on top (Fig. 11.6).

4. Operator gently compresses the soft tissues overlying the sacrum, sensing for loss of tissue resiliency.

5. Operator engages, in an additive fashion, the initial direct barriers of nutation and counternutation, gentile left and right rotation of the whole pelvis, and twist along an antero-posterior (AP) axis at around S2, in no specific order.

6. Engaging the barriers in this fashion allows the operator to sense for a focus of increased fascial restriction in one pole or arm (left, right, upper, or lower) of the sacrum.

7. Operator communicates to the patient to perform enhancing maneuvers for the specific pole of sacral restriction.

8. Treatment goal is the balance of the sacrum between the innominates.

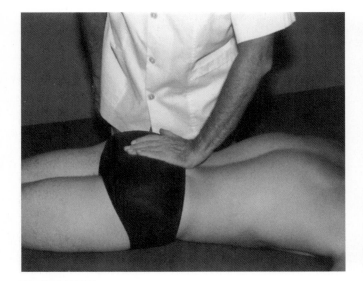

FIGURE 11.5

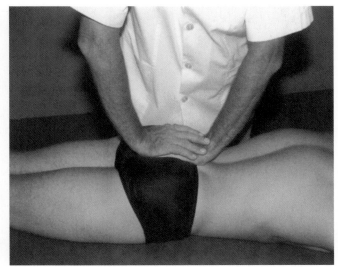

FIGURE 11.6

FASCIAL RELEASE TECHNIQUE

Prone

Sacrotuberous ligament and urogenital diaphragm release

1. Patient is prone with arms off the sides of the table, feet off the end of the table, and head turned to the most comfortable side.

2. Operator at the side of the table facing cephalad places the hands over the buttocks area with the thumbs in contact with the medial aspect of the sacrotuberous ligament. This may be at the attachments at the inferior lateral angles of the sacrum or midbody of the ligament (Fig. 11.7).

3. Tension in the sacrotuberous ligaments is tested for symmetric balance.

4. Operator's hands and arms twist in clockwise and counterclockwise directions, sensing for tightness and looseness (Fig. 11.8).

5. Operator applies a load to balance the tension in the sacrotuberous ligament, three dimensionally, while communicating to the patient to perform an enhancing maneuver.

6. Treatment goal is the balance of the sacrotuberous ligaments and urogenital diaphragm.

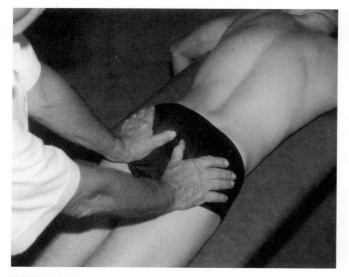

FIGURE 11.7

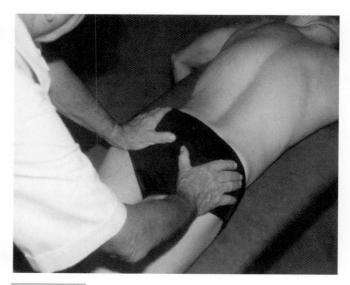

FIGURE 11.8

FASCIAL RELEASE TECHNIQUE

Thoracic Inlet (Necklace) Technique

1. Patient is supine on the table with the operator sitting at the head of the table, hands in contact with the thoracic inlet with palms over the trapezius and fingers contacting the medial end of the clavicle and upper sternum (Fig. 11.9).

2. Operator introduces alternating hand inferior compression followed by very slight alternating hand lateral to medial (toward midline) load, seeking direct and indirect barriers along the deep cervicothoracic and mediastinal columns of fasciae.

3. Operator loads into the inferior and medial direct barriers with both hands and communicates to the patient to add an enhancing maneuver.

4. A wonderful enhancer is to have the patient pull his/her tongue back into the back of his/her throat and breathe gently. This maneuver fires the deep cervical flexors, which are the dynamic stabilizers of the neck and often inhibited, and reflexly inhibits the SCM and Scalenus hold on the cervicothoracic junction.

These are but a few examples of fascial release technique. They can be used as the primary manual medicine intervention or as a terminal technique to assess the success of other manual medicine interventions to ensure that fascial balance has been achieved. Some practitioners find these techniques fatiguing and time-consuming, whereas others find them easy and efficient.

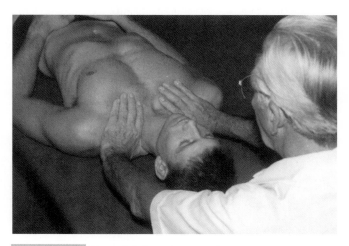

FIGURE 11.9 Thoracic inlet release supine.

CONCLUSION

Fascial release and integrated neuromuscular release techniques use direct and indirect actions with activating forces that are extrinsic and intrinsic. They influence the biomechanics of the musculoskeletal system and the reflexes that direct, integrate, and modify movement. The goal is restoring functional balance to all of the integrative tissues in the musculoskeletal system, and the techniques are useful in acute, subacute, and chronic conditions, with simple and complex problems. The techniques can be used in multiple patient positions. They usually consist of symmetric placement of the operator's hands, introducing some twisting force to engage the tissues, and following directly or indirectly along fascial planes to sense areas of tightness and looseness. Traction is placed on the tight area awaiting the sensation of release. Release is hypothesized as following reflex neural efferent inhibition and biomechanical hysteresis within the tissues. The techniques are highly individualized to the patient's needs and the operator's training and experience.

REFERENCES

1. Ward RC. Integrated neuromusculoskeletal release and myofascial release: An introduction to diagnosis and treatment. In: Ward RC, et al., eds. *Foundations for Osteopathic Medicine*. Baltimore, MD: Williams & Wilkins, 1997.

2. Manheim C. *The Myofascial Release Manual*. 4th Ed. Thorofare, NJ: Slack Inc., 2008, p. 8.

3. Rolf I. *Rolfing: Reestablishing the Natural Alignment and Structural Integration of the Human Body for Vitality and Well-Being*. Rochester, VT: Healing Arts Press, 1989, pp. 199–204.

4. Hering E. About the influence of respiration to the circulation. I. About respiratoric movements of the vessels system. [Über den Einfluss der Athmung auf den Kreislauf I. Über Athembewegungen des Gefäss-systems.] Sitzungsbericht der mathematisch-naturwissenschaftlichen. *Classe Wien* 1869;60:829–856.

5. Traube L. About periodic actions of the vasomotor and inhibitory nerve center. [Üeber periodische Thätigkeits-Aeusserungen des vasomotorischen und Hemmungs-Nervencentrums]. Centralblatt für die medicinischen Wissenschaften, Berlin, 1865, 3:881–885.

6. Mayer S. Studies about the physiology of heart and blood vessels. [Studien zur Physiologie des Herzens und deg Blutgfässe]. Sitzungsbericht der mathematisch-naturwissenschaftlichen. *Classe Wien* 1876;74:281–307.

7. Julien C. The enigma of Mayer waves: Facts and models. *Cardiovasc Res* 2006;70:12–21.

8. Nilsson H, Aalkjaer C. Vasomotion: Mechanisms and physiological importance. *Mol Interv* 2003;3(2):79–89.

9. Haddock RE, Hill CE. Rhythmicity in arterial smooth muscle. *J Physiol* 2005;566(3):645–656.

10. Van Helden DF, Zhao J. Lymphatic vasomotion. *Clin Exp Pharmacol Physiol* 2000;27(12):1014–1018.

11. Aalkjær C, Nilsson H. Vasomotion: Cellular background for the oscillator and for the synchronization of smooth muscle cells. *Br J Pharmacol* 2005;144:605–616.

12. Strik C, Klose U, Erb M, et al. Intracranial oscillations of cerebrospinal fluid and blood flows: Analysis with magnetic resonance imaging. *J Magn Reson Imaging* 2002;15(3):251–258.

13. Langevin HM. Connective tissue. A body-wide signaling network? *Med Hypotheses* 2006;66(6):1074–1077.

14. Chiquet M. Regulation of extracellular matrix gene expression by mechanical stress. *Matrix Biol* 1999;18(5):417–426.

15. Langevin HM, Rizzo DM, Fox JR, et al. Dynamic morphometric characterization of local connective tissue network structure in humans using ultrasound. *BMC Syst Biol* 2007;1:25.

16. Abu-Hijleh MF, Roshier AL, Al-Shboul Q, et al. The membranous layer of superficial fascia: Evidence for its widespread distribution in the body. *Surg Radiol Anat* 2006;28(6):606–619.

17. Singer E. *Fasciae of the Human Body and Their Relations to the Organs They Envelop*. Baltimore, MD: Williams & Wilkins, 1935:1–34.

18. Tobin CE, Benjamin JA. Anatomic and clinical re-evaluation of Camper's, Scarpa's, and Colles' fasciae. *Surg Today* 1949;88:545–559.

19. Congdon ED, Edson J, Yanitelli S. Gross structure of the subcutaneous layer of the anterior and lateral trunk in the male. *Am J Anat* 1946;79:399–429.

20. Nash LG, Phillips MN, Nicholson H, et al. Skin ligaments: Regional distribution and variation in morphology. *Clin Anat* 2004;17:287–293.

21. Ghassemi A, Prescher A, Riediger D, et al. Anatomy of the SMAS revisited. *Aesthetic Plast Surg* 2003;27:258–264.

22. Lockwood TE. Superficial fascial system (SFS) of the trunk and extremities: A new concept. *Plast Reconstr Surg* 1991;87(6):1009–1018.

23. Markman B. Anatomy and physiology of adipose tissue. *Clin Plast Surg* 1989;16:235–244.

24. Markman B, Barton FE Jr. Anatomy of the subcutaneous tissue of the trunk and lower extremity. *Plast Reconstr Surg* 1987;80:248–254.

25. Langevin HM, Cornbrooks CJ, Taatjes DJ. Fibroblasts form a body-wide cellular network. *Histochem Cell Biol* 2004;122:7–15.

26. Langevin HM, Bouffard NA, Badger GJ, et al. Dynamic fibroblast cytoskeletal response to subcutaneous tissue stretch ex vivo and in vivo. *Am J Physiol Cell Physiol* 2005;288:C747–C756.

27. Langevin HM, Bouffard NA, Badger GJ, et al. Subcutaneous tissue fibroblast cytoskeletal remodeling induced by acupuncture: Evidence for a mechanotransduction-based mechanism. *J Cell Physiol* 2006;207:767–774.

28. Langevin HM, Storch KN, Cipolla MJ, et al. Fibroblast spreading induced by connective tissue stretch involves intracellular redistribution of alpha- and beta-actin. *Histochem Cell Biol* 2006;125:487–495.

29. Giancotti FG, Ruoslahti E. Integrin signaling. *Science* 1999;285:1028–1032.

30. Cummings GS, Tillman LJ. Remodeling of dense connective tissue in normal adult tissues. In: Currier DP, Nelson RM, eds. *Dynamics of Human Biologic Tissues Contemporary Perspectives in Rehabilitation*, Vol. 8. Philadelphia, PA: F.A. Davis, 1992:45–73.

Section

TECHNIQUE PROCEDURES

William G. Sutherland, D.O., is credited with extending the osteopathic concept, and osteopathic manipulative treatment, above the craniocervical junction. His curiosity was raised when viewing the temporoparietal suture in the anatomy laboratory and thought it resembled the gills of a fish. He further reasoned that it might relate to respiration in some fashion. Thus began many years of study, research, and self-manipulation. Sutherland began to teach the principles of craniosacral technique in the mid-1940s.[1] Craniosacral technique procedures were initially not readily received in the professional community but have become increasingly popular through the work of Sutherland and his many students.

Sutherland extended the principles of Andrew Taylor Still to the articulations of the skull. He reasoned that the sutures functioned as joints between the bones of the skull and were intricately fashioned for the maintenance of motion. The sutures are present throughout life and consistently have similar areas of bevel change. Skulls can be disarticulated by "explosion" (filling with beans through the foramen magnum, then immersing in water), and the bones consistently separate at the sutures. The bone does not fracture, the sutures separate. Sutherland reasoned that the skull would have normal mobility during health and show restrictions in response to trauma or systemic disease.[2] Clinical observations were consistent with his hypothesis. Since Sutherland's time, there has been an increasing body of clinical evidence and research supporting some of the basic premises of his concept.[3] Craniosacral technique requires the practitioner to make an intense study of the osseous cranium, sutures, and meninges and to finely tune the palpatory sense necessary to perceive inherent mobility within the craniosacral mechanism. Application of manual medicine procedures to the cranium and sacrum requires precision and dexterity.

ANATOMY

The skull can be divided into three elements: (a) the vault, consisting of portions of the frontal bone, the two parietal bones, the occipital squama, and the temporal squama that develop from membrane; (b) the base, consisting of the body of the sphenoid, the petrous and mastoid portions of the temporals, and the basilar and condylar portions of the occiput that form in cartilage; and (c) the facial bones. The bones of the skull can be further divided into those that are paired and unpaired. The unpaired midline bones are the occiput, sphenoid, ethmoid, and vomer. The paired bones include the parietals, temporals, maxillae, zygoma, palatines, nasals, and frontal. The frontal is viewed as a paired bone because of the functional characteristics it provides, and the fact that the metopic suture frequently remains open during life. The mandible has both paired and unpaired characteristics. It is bilaterally related to the temporal bones, but when the teeth are present and approximated, they serve as a long suture between the mandible and the two maxillae.

MOTION

The sphenobasilar junction appears to fuse after the late teens[4] but the motions perceived from contact on the skull exterior can be best described as having taken place at the sphenobasilar junction. There appears to be residual pliability of bone at the sphenobasilar junction throughout life similar to the pliability of bone in the remaining bones of the skeleton.[5] The motion of the midline bones is primarily flexion and extension with an overturning movement around a transverse (x) axis. Flexion–extension movement is described as occurring when the sphenoid and occiput rotate in opposite directions. During sphenobasilar flexion, the sphenoid rotates anteriorly with the basisphenoid being elevated and the pterygoid processes moving inferiorly. Concurrently, the occiput rotates posteriorly with the basiocciput being elevated, and the squamous portion and condylar parts being depressed caudally. During sphenobasilar flexion, the ethmoid rotates in the opposite direction to the sphenoid and in the same direction as the occiput. During sphenobasilar flexion, the vomer is carried caudad as the anterior portion of the sphenoid moves in that direction. During sphenobasilar extension, all of the motions are reversed. The paired bones move into internal and external rotations as they accompany sphenobasilar flexion and extension. During sphenobasilar flexion, there is external rotation of the paired bones. During sphenobasilar extension, the paired bones move into internal rotation.

The combination of flexion–extension of the midline unpaired bones and the internal–external rotation of the paired bones causes observable change in cranial contour. With flexion, the transverse diameter of the skull increases, the anteroposterior (AP) diameter decreases, and the vertex flattens. With sphenobasilar extension, the transverse diameter decreases, the AP diameter increases, and the vertex becomes more prominent. The facial bones can be viewed as being suspended from the frontal bone. The paired bones consist of the parietal, temporal, frontal, zygoma, maxilla, palatine, and nasal bones. Their motion is described as internal and external rotation and is normally synchronous with sphenobasilar flexion and extension. During sphenobasilar flexion, there is external rotation of the paired bones. The sphenoid determines the motion characteristics of the paired facial bones. Dysfunction of the front half of the cranium, particularly of the facial bones, is related to altered function of the sphenoid. Dysfunction of the posterior half of the cranium relates to dysfunction of the occipital bone.

MENINGES

The dura is attached at the foramen magnum, continues down the spinal canal with attachment to the upper two or three cervical vertebrae, and continues freely within the spinal canal until attachment at the second segment of the sacrum. This membrane attachment appears to link the sacral component with the occiput in the craniosacral mechanism. As one of many movements, the sacrum has an involuntary nutation–counternutation movement that is synchronous with flexion–extension at the sphenobasilar junction. During sphenobasilar flexion, the foramen magnum is elevated and the tension on the dura causes the base of the sacrum to move posteriorly and the apex anteriorly. This counternutational movement is described as craniosacral flexion. During sphenobasilar extension, the foramen magnum moves inferiorly, reducing tension on the dura, resulting in the sacral base moving anteriorly and the apex posteriorly. This nutational movement is called "craniosacral extension." The terms "flexion" and "extension" are the reverse of that used in a postural–structural model for sacral mechanics. Despite the terminology confusion, the concept to be understood is the relationship of the movement of the occiput and the sacrum that normally occurs in synchronous directions (Table 12.1).

The dura also is continuous with the spinal nerve roots as they emerge from the spinal canal, and it forms the perineurium. Traction on peripheral nerves can influence the central dura as well.

SUTURES

The sutures are joints that join the bones of the skull. At birth, there are no sutures and the vault bones are separate plates on the dura. The skull is like a bag filled with fluid and under tension. As the skull bones grow and mature, they develop the sutures as articulations. The sutures develop their shape and contour depending on the motion occurring at the area during growth. It is fascinating to see the marked similarity of sutures and their beveling across a number of different specimens. There are many different types of sutures that are designed to permit and direct specific types of movement between opposing cranial bones. The sutures contain extensions of the dura and other connective tissue, primarily Sharpey fibers. Anatomic and histologic studies of the sutures demonstrate that fiber direction is not haphazard and random, but specific at each sutural level. The sutures contain blood vessels with accompanying nerves for vasomotor control.[6] Free nerve endings with unmyelinated C-fibers are found within the sutures suggesting the possibility of pain perception and transmission.[7] A detailed description of the cranial sutures is beyond the scope of this text. The reader is strongly urged to study the classical anatomic work as well as the sutures found on each bone of a disarticulated skull.

SUTURE PALPATION EXERCISE

The following palpation exercise identifies palpable sutures in a living subject and the location of anatomic parts used in diagnosis and treatment of cranial dysfunctions (Fig. 12.1).

1. Palpate the depression at the base of the nose and between each orbit. This is the junction of the two nasal bones and the frontal bone and is called "nasion."
2. Proceed laterally over the upper margin of the orbit and follow it laterally and inferiorly to the upper outer portion and feel the frontozygomatic suture.
3. Continuing inferiorly along the lateral aspect of the orbit and beginning to move medially one feels the zygomaticomaxillary suture.
4. Continuing medially along the inferior aspect of the orbit and up its medial way, palpate the suture of the maxillonasal junction and the maxillofrontal suture.
5. Returning to the nasion, move upward between the two supraorbital ridges of the frontal bone, the midline of which is a point called "glabella." Moving superiorly from glabella along the midline the palpator may feel the remnant of the metopic suture as a depression or a ridge.
6. Continuing toward the vertex of the skull in the midline, one strikes a depression approximately one third of the way posteriorly on the vertex. This depression is the junction of the sagittal and coronal sutures and is the remnant of the anterior fontanel and is called "bregma."
7. Moving posteriorly from bregma along the midline, the sagittal suture is palpable and by moving the finger pads from side to side one can feel the serrated sutural contour (Fig. 12.2).
8. Starting from bregma, palpate bilaterally along the coronal suture feeling the junction of the frontal and the parietal bones on each side. At the lower extremity of the coronal suture, the palpating finger moves somewhat deeper and palpates the junction of the sphenoid, frontal, parietal, and temporal bones. This junctional area is called "pterion." The inferior aspect of this junction is the palpable tip of the great wing of the sphenoid, which is used extensively for craniosacral diagnosis and treatment.
9. From the pterion, follow the suture line posteriorly along the junction of the parietal and temporal squama. This suture courses over the top of the ear in a circular fashion and ends just posterior to the ear.
10. Moving straight posteriorly from the posterior inferior aspect of the suture between the parietal and the temporal squama is a short suture between the parietal bone and the mastoid portion of the temporal. At the posterior aspect of this suture is a slight depression at the junction

TABLE 12.1	*Various Models of Sacral Motion*	
Sacral Motion	**Biomechanical Model**	**Craniosacral Model**
Nutation	Flexion	Extension
Counternutation	Extension	Flexion

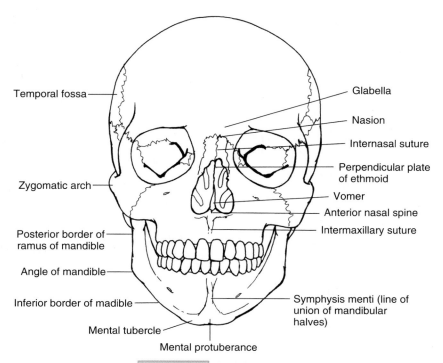

FIGURE 12.1 Skull, frontal view.

Temporal fossa

Glabella

Nasion

Internasal suture

Zygomatic arch

Perpendicular plate of ethmoid

Vomer

Anterior nasal spine

Posterior border of ramus of mandible

Intermaxillary suture

Angle of mandible

Inferior border of madible

Symphysis menti (line of union of mandibular halves)

Mental tubercle

Mental protuberance

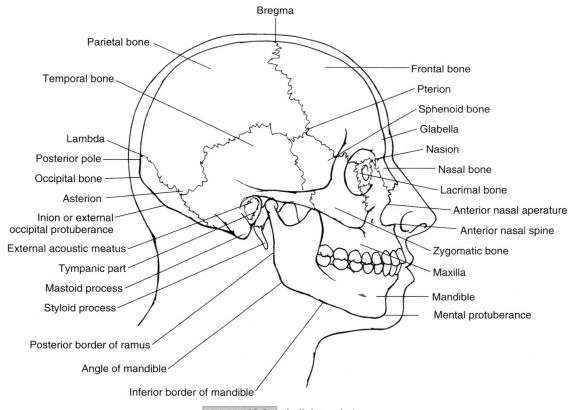

FIGURE 12.2 Skull, lateral view.

Bregma

Parietal bone

Frontal bone

Temporal bone

Pterion

Sphenoid bone

Glabella

Nasion

Lambda

Nasal bone

Posterior pole

Lacrimal bone

Occipital bone

Asterion

Anterior nasal aperature

Inion or external occipital protuberance

Anterior nasal spine

External acoustic meatus

Zygomatic bone

Tympanic part

Maxilla

Mastoid process

Styloid process

Mandible

Mental protuberance

Posterior border of ramus

Angle of mandible

Inferior border of mandible

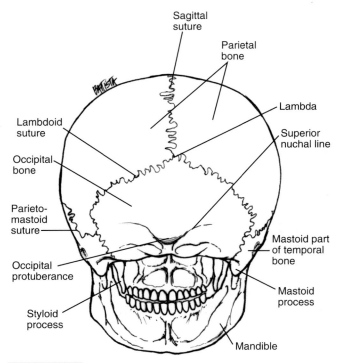

FIGURE 12.3 Skull, posterior view.

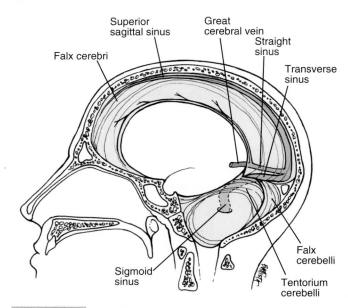

FIGURE 12.4 Cranial meninges.

of the parietal bone, mastoid portion of the temporal, and the occiput called the "asterion."

11. From the asterion, move inferiorly along the posterior aspect of the mastoid process following the occipital mastoid suture. The lower portion of this suture is lost in the soft tissues of the muscular attachment of the head to the neck (Fig. 12.3).

12. From the asterion on each side, course medially and superiorly along the lambdoidal suture separating the parietal bone from the occipital squama. The point at which the two sutures join with the sagittal suture is called "lambda." The lambdoidal sutures are frequently asymmetric and occasionally contain extra bony structures called "wormian bones."

This exercise should be repeated on multiple patients until the examiner is confident of his or her ability to palpate the sutures of the skull and identify landmarks used to control the bones of the skull during the examination and the treatment process. The pterion and asterion are the two most frequently used in the craniosacral technique system.

CRANIAL MENINGES

The meninges are divided into three layers: the pia, the arachnoid, and the dura. The external layer of the dura is continuous with the periosteum and the cranium. The internal layer has several duplications that separate segments of the brain and encircle the venous sinuses (Fig. 12.4).

There are three duplications of the dura with intricate fiber directions in each and are named the falx cerebri, tentorium cerebelli, and falx cerebelli. The falx cerebri is attached anteriorly to the crista galli of the ethmoid, the frontal bone, both parietal bones, and the occipital squama. It encloses the superior sagittal sinus at

its osseous attachment. At its free border is found the inferior sagittal sinus. The falx cerebri separates the two cerebral hemispheres. The tentorium cerebelli separates the cerebrum and cerebellum and attaches to the sphenoid, occiput, both parietals, and temporal bones. It attaches to the petrous ridges of the temporal bones and along the occipital squama where it encloses the transverse sinus. It is attached to the posterior inferior corner of each parietal bone where the transverse sinus starts into sigmoid sinus. At the junction of the falx cerebri and the tentorium cerebelli is found the straight sinus. This junction is of significance as the location of the reciprocal tension membrane is called the "Sutherland fulcrum." The falx cerebelli is a posterior continuum of the falx cerebri. Attached to the posterior aspect of the occiput, it separates the two hemispheres of the cerebellum and contains the occipital sinus. The diaphragm sellae is a fold of dura that covers the sella turcica of the sphenoid and is penetrated by the stalk of the pituitary. These dural membranes are under constant dynamic tension so that increased tension in one requires relaxation in another and vice versa. During sphenobasilar flexion, there is shortening of the falx cerebri from before backward because of the overturning of the sphenoid and occiput in opposite directions. This is accompanied by flattening of the tentorium cerebelli resulting from external rotation of the two temporal bones. During sphenobasilar extension, the reverse occurs, with the lengthening of the AP diameter of the skull by rotation of the sphenoid and the occiput and elevation of the tentorium cerebelli because of internal rotation of the temporal bones. Craniosacral motion combines articular mobility and change in tension within the membranes. The membranous attachment at the foramen magnum of the occiput and at S2 of the sacrum determines the synchronous movement of the cranium and the sacrum. This dural attachment allows the examiner to influence the cranium through the sacrum and the sacrum through the cranium.

RESPIRATION AND THE THREE DIAPHRAGMS

Sphenobasilar flexion and extension are related to and influenced by voluntary respiratory activity. Inhalation enhances sphenobasilar flexion, and exhalation enhances sphenobasilar extension. The tentorium cerebelli can be viewed as the diaphragm of the craniosacral mechanism. It descends and flattens during inhalation similar to the thoracoabdominal diaphragm. The pelvic diaphragm is intimately related to the sacrum within the osseous pelvis. The pelvic diaphragm also descends during inhalation. One can then view the body from the perspective of the three diaphragms: the tentorium cerebelli, the thoracoabdominal diaphragm, and the pelvic diaphragm. In health, these diaphragms should function in a synchronous fashion. If dysfunction interferes with the capacity of any of the three, it is reasonable to assume that the other two will be altered as well. This observation has been made in clinical practice. The thoracic inlet can also be viewed as a diaphragm as it participates in respiration and could be described as a fourth diaphragm.

PRIMARY RESPIRATORY MECHANISM

By placing both hands over the superior and lateral aspects of the skull and allowing the hands to relax, the examiner can experience the palpatory sensation of widening and narrowing of the skull. This motion sensation occurs at a normal rate of 8 to 14 times per minute and is of relatively low amplitude. This sensation, called the "cranial rhythmic impulse" (CRI), is interpreted by Sutherland as the result of the five components of the Primary Respiratory Mechanism[2]:

1. Inherent mobility of the brain and spinal cord.
2. Fluctuation of the cerebrospinal fluid (CSF).
3. Motility of intracranial and intraspinal meninges.
4. Articular mobility of cranial bones.
5. The involuntary mobility of the sacrum between the ilia.

Sutherland reasoned that the skull would have normal mobility during health and show restrictions in response to trauma or systemic disease; his premise was that the Primary Respiratory Mechanism was critical for cellular respiration and metabolism.[1] The existence of the motion of the CRI is a very controversial aspect of osteopathic medicine. The motion is very subtle, often overlooked and considered existent only amongst the believers of cranial osteopathy. Significant evidence of rhythmic oscillations with frequencies consistent in timing with the CRI has been described in the literature. These oscillations were first described during arterial blood pressure monitoring by Hering, Traube, and Mayer as early as the 19th century.[8–10] Measured at a rate of 0.1 Hz or 10 cycles per minute, they are considered sympathetic nervous discharges or a reflection of efferent sympathetic vasomotor tone. Since that time, similar physiological fluctuations have been observed in arterial, venous, and lymphatic vessel diameters.[11–16] The term vasomotion describes the latter; observed since the invention of the microscope, it is characterized as rhythmic oscillations in vascular tone caused by local changes in smooth muscle constriction and dilatation.

Vasomotion appears to be dependent on synchronization of a multitude of individual cellular oscillators. These oscillations differ from the Hering, Traube, and Mayer waves in that neural influence is not required for vasomotion to occur. Slow oscillations or low-frequency fluctuations with frequencies similar to the 0.1 Hz Traube-Hering waves have been described in the brain using intercranial pressure measurements, Doppler, and MRI.[17–22] Measured in CSF flow, venous blood flow, arterial blood flow and brain parenchyma, it was initially suggested that these oscillations are native to those tissues. Razavi et al.,[23] using functional MRI phase analysis, contend that the primary physiologic source of native low-frequency fluctuations is initiated from cerebral blood vessel vasomotion and that fluctuation in the other structures may be due to passive transmittal of these vessel oscillations. CSF in interventricular and subarachnoid space of the spinal cord has also been shown to have low-frequency fluctuations. Contrary to the low-frequency arterial pulsations of the brain, motion of CSF is greatly enhanced by respiration; in spinal CSF, expiration encourages downward motion, whereas inspiration encourages upward motion.[20,21,24]

Sutherland believed inherent motion was necessary for tissue cellular respiration, metabolic function, and well-being. In fact, low-frequency fluctuations and vasomotion have been linked to tissue oxygenation and neuronal function and shown to be altered in persons with known disease states such as hypertension, atherosclerosis and diabetes.[25–30]

Inherent motion and the CRI are palpable and perceptible by the human hand. Kenneth Nelson, D.O., and Nicette Sergueef, D.O.,[31,32] (France) simultaneously recorded palpable CRI and the 0.10 to 0.15 Hz Traube-Hering-Mayer (THM) oscillation (6 to 9 cycles per minute) using laser-Doppler flowmetry in humans. They concluded that the CRI is palpably concomitant with the THM oscillations at a 1:2 ratio; a flexion event perceived coincident with one THM oscillation, and an extension event perceived coincident with the next THM oscillation. They subsequently demonstrated that cranial manipulation specifically affects the THM rate.[33] Moskalenko and Kravchenko, using cranial and lumbosacral bioimpedance plethysmography, recorded changes in blood/CSF volume which was synchronous with the THM oscillations at a rate of 6 to 10 cycles per minute.[34] Although much more research is necessary, it is plausible, in this author's mind, that reflections of multiple physiological sources of low-frequency oscillations passively distributed throughout the body's fascias are indeed palpable not only on the cranium but throughout the body.

CRANIOSACRAL DIAGNOSIS

The diagnostic process begins with observation and palpation in a screening examination. The examiner looks for skull symmetry from the anterior, posterior, superior, and both lateral views. Observation is made for symmetry of the frontal bosses, orbits, nose, zygoma, maxillae, mandible, level of the ears, and overall cranial contour. The screening examination proceeds by palpation of the skull contour in all dimensions and, in particular, palpation of the sutures as previously described. Palpation of the sutures

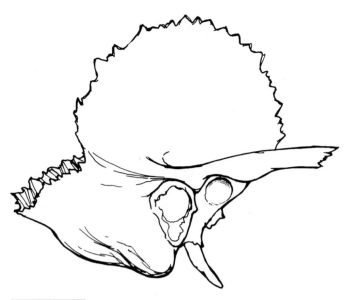

FIGURE 12.5 Temporal bone, lateral view.

looks for widening, narrowing, tension and other tissue texture changes, and tenderness. The skull is assessed by palpation for resiliency to see if it is harder and less resilient than normal. Normal bone has a pliability that is lost in the presence of motion restriction. Craniosacral diagnosis using the presence of the CRI (Fig. 12.6) is accomplished by placing the hands and fingers over the skull in a position that is called the "vault hold." There are several variations of the vault hold, but each includes control of the greater wings of the sphenoid at the pterion and the occiput at the asterion. The classic vault hold has the index finger on the sphenoid at the pterion and the little finger at the asterion, with the ear between the middle and ring fingers (Fig. 12.7). The motion of the CRI is very subtle and can only be perceived through the operator's hand joint capsule proprioceptors, so it is imperative that the operator allows the joints in the hands to relax. The operator's forearms should be in contact with the table. The pressure of the hands on the vault is such that the operator cannot determine where his/her hands end and the patient's head begins; it is a melding contact. Using the vault hold with a melding contact and relaxed hand joints, the operator will begin to feel the widening and narrowing of the cranium and ascertain the rate, rhythm, and amplitude of the CRI.

Another screening examination helpful for determining if there is asymmetric loss of cranial motion is the temporal lift (Fig. 12.5).

A five-finger hold for the temporal lift has the examiner grasp each temporal bone with the middle finger in the external auditory meatus, the thumb and index fingers on the superior and inferior aspects of the zygomatic process, and the ring and little finger in front and behind the mastoid process. With the patient supine on the table, the examiner pulls both temporal bones in a direction toward the vertex. Each temporal bone is then allowed to settle back to its neutral position. The examiner assesses the symmetry or asymmetry of the small amount of joint play motion available in each temporal bone. The horizontal

portions of the sphenosquamous suture, the horizontal portion of the occipital mastoid suture, and the zygomaticotemporal sutures are beveled such that the temporal bone sits on top of the sphenoid, zygoma, and occiput. The temporal lift procedure assesses the presence or absence of mobility of the temporal bones on each side.

The sacrum is screened for its anterior and posterior nutational movements between the two ilia in either prone or supine position. The examiner cradles the sacrum in the palm of the hand and assesses the sacral movement and its relation to the CRI palpated at the skull. A finding of exaggerated, depressed, or irregular movements instead of the normal anterior and posterior nodding movements requires additional diagnostic assessment. If the screening examination provides evidence of craniosacral dysfunction, additional scanning and segmental definition examinations are necessary.

ASSESSMENT OF SPHENOBASILAR MOTION

Evaluation of sphenobasilar mechanics (Fig. 12.6) is accomplished using the "vault hold" (Fig. 12.7). A second vault hold uses the thumbs on the sphenoid at the pterion with the little finger on the occiput at the asterion and the ear between the index and middle fingers (Fig. 12.8). A third vault hold finds the examiner cradling the occiput in the palm of one hand holding posterior to the occipitomastoid suture and the other hand spanning the front of the skull with the thumb on one great wing of the sphenoid and the long finger on the opposite great wing (Fig. 12.9). Each of these vault holds has its uses. The beginning student should use the first vault hold described.

Sphenobasilar flexion and extension are described as occurring around two parallel transverse axes with each moving in the opposite direction. With sphenobasilar flexion, the index and little fingers separate as they move in the caudad direction. With sphenobasilar extension, the fingers on each side move closer together as the hands move cephalically.

Sphenobasilar side bending–rotation is described as motion of the sphenoid and occiput along two different axis systems. They both rotate in the same direction around an AP axis and in opposite directions around two parallel vertical axes. With sphenobasilar side bending–rotation to the right, the fingers of the right hand separate and move in a caudad direction while the fingertips on the left side narrow and move cephalically, resulting in the right side of the skull appearing to become more convex. Sphenobasilar left-side bending–rotation results in similar findings on the opposite side.

Sphenobasilar torsion movement is described as movement of the sphenoid and occiput in opposite directions along an AP axis. The motion is introduced through the four-point vault hold contact, by alternately turning one hand forward while the other turns backward. The hand moving anteriorly carries the sphenoid caudad and elevates the occiput on that side. The hand that rotates posteriorly carries the sphenoid high and the occiput low on the same side. This torsional movement should be bilaterally symmetric, but if restricted, the dysfunction is named for the side in which the sphenoid is held in a cephalic (high) position.

FIGURE 12.6 Sphenobasilar junction from above.

Pterion

Squamous part

Petro-squamous fissure

Petrous part

Mastoid part

Dorsum sellae

Basi-occipital

Foramen magnum

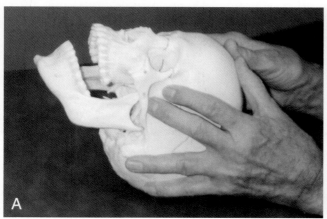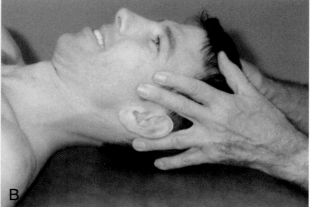

A   B

FIGURE 12.7 Vault hold, index and little finger.

Sphenobasilar flexion–extension, side bending–rotation, and torsion are all present physiologically. Other altered movements of the sphenobasilar junction usually resulting from trauma include lateral strain, vertical strain, and sphenobasilar compression. Traumatic episodes can include birth trauma, childhood falls, sports injuries, motor vehicle collisions, industrial accidents, altered muscle balance from chronic postural deficit, abnormal chewing from poor dental hygiene, and many others.

Sphenobasilar compression can be anterior–posterior resulting from injury to the skull from before backward and behind forward. If present, the compression restricts the midline sphenobasilar movement patterns. The skull usually compensates for this restriction by increased internal and external rotation of the paired lateral bones. Lateral compression can occur with trauma from right to left or left to right resulting on impaction of the temporal bone on that side.

Sphenobasilar lateral strain results from trauma from left to right or right to left in front of, or behind, the sphenobasilar junction altering the relation of the sphenoid and occiput in the horizontal plane. **Lateral strain is described as movement of the sphenoid and occiput in the same direction around two parallel vertical axes.** To test for a lateral strain with the patient supine using the vault hold, one hand lifts one side of the head toward the ceiling, allows it to return, and reverses it on the opposite

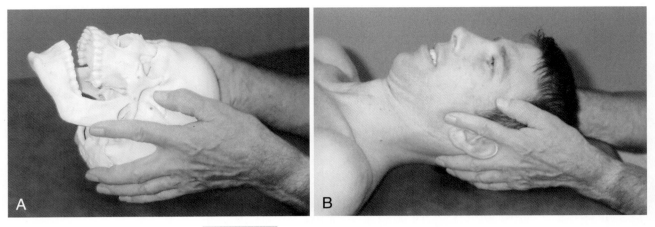

FIGURE 12.8 Vault hold, thumb and little finger.

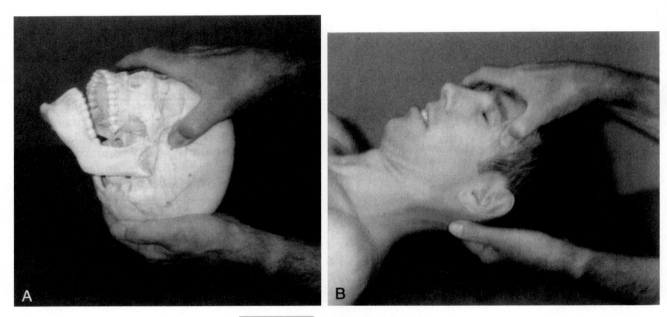

FIGURE 12.9 Two-handed vault hold.

side. This introduces side-to-side translatory movement. If this motion test is asymmetric, it is described as a lateral strain to the side in which the basisphenoid moves freely. A skull with a lateral strain pattern has a quadrilateral appearance.

Vertical strain results with trauma from above or below, in front or behind, the sphenobasilar junction altering the relation of the sphenoid and occiput in the sagittal plane. **Vertical strain is described as rotation of the sphenoid and occiput in the same direction around two parallel transverse axes.** If asymmetric, a vertical strain is named for the position of the basisphenoid and is superior or inferior. To test for vertical strain, both hands of the vault hold rotate forward and backward symmetrically. As both hands rotate forward, they carry the sphenoid into flexion with elevation of the basisphenoid and the occiput into extension. As both hands rotate backward, they carry the sphenoid into extension with depression of the basisphenoid and flexion of the occiput. Both of these strain mechanisms alter the central axis through the sphenobasilar

junction. Traumatic lateral and vertical strains and compressions significantly alter the craniosacral mechanism. Sphenobasilar compression is identified by reduction in the rate and amplitude of the CRI and the overall reduction of cranial mobility.

Interference with symmetric sphenobasilar function leads the operator to assess articular causes of the restriction. After assessment of abnormal sphenobasilar mechanics, the operator needs to decide whether the restriction is in the anterior or posterior aspects of the skull and whether it is more on the right or left. This leads to "four-quadrant" diagnosis. The decision is based on the operator's judgment of the location of the major restrictor while assessing the sphenobasilar strain patterns. The operator also makes an assessment of the nature of the restriction. Is it articular? Is it membranous from the meninges? Is it reduced fluid fluctuation? The answers to these questions determine the therapeutic strategy. Comprehensive specific sutural motion testing is beyond the scope of this volume and the reader is referred to standard texts in the field. However, the major, more common articular restrictor of the anterior and posterior quadrants will be subsequently described.

PRINCIPLES OF CRANIOSACRAL TECHNIQUE

The goals of craniosacral technique are to improve motion in sphenobasilar mechanics, remove articular restrictions, reduce membranous tension restrictions, improve circulation (particularly of the venous system), reduce potential neural entrapment from exit foramen at the base of the skull, and increase the vitality of the CRI. These techniques have local effects within the head and neck region, distal effects throughout the body, and all are directed toward enhancing the level of wellness of the patient. All of these goals can be accomplished by the restoration of balanced membranous tension. Normal dynamic reciprocal tension of the falx cerebri and tentorium cerebelli is absent in the presence of restriction or alteration in relationship of cranial bones and their sutures. Alteration in membranous tension affects the venous sinuses within the skull resulting in the reduction of venous drainage and overall intracranial congestion. The dura is intimately attached to the periosteum on the internal surface of the skull and at each exit foramen. Abnormal dural tension might contribute to neural entrapment and result in altered neural function. Restoring maximum mobility to the osseous cranium restores balanced membranous tension, enhances venous flow, reduces neural entrapment, and permits normal CRI rate, rhythm, and amplitude.

Treatment of the craniosacral system can begin at either the sacrum or the cranium or can be done concurrently. A sequence for treatment that has proven to be clinically effective begins by screening the cranium and identifying if the skull is rigid or nonrigid. If rigid, the approach may be used to decongest the head by venous sinus release and enhance the CRI by compression of the 4th ventricle (CV4) procedures. Following the reduction of rigidity within the skull, the sphenobasilar mechanics are assessed and appropriately treated. If sphenobasilar compression is identified, it should be addressed so that the remaining sphenobasilar motions can be more efficient. Treatment of sphenobasilar strain patterns may include approaches both from the cranial and sacral ends of the system. Temporal bone rotational capability is then assessed, and, if asymmetric, appropriate sutural evaluation and treatment are performed to restore symmetry of internal and external temporal rotations. The facial component is then assessed and treated as appropriate. Successful craniosacral treatment restores functional balance to the cranial and sacral limbs of the mechanism, enhances mobility of the cranial bones, balances membranous tension, and enhances the vitality of the CRI.

METHODS OF CRANIOSACRAL TECHNIQUE

Craniosacral technique shares with other forms of manual medicine the approach to barriers. In addition to the usual methods of direct action, indirect, and exaggeration technique, there are two others, namely disengagement and molding.

- Direct action method: the barrier is engaged and an activating force is applied in the direction of motion loss.

- Exaggeration method: the barrier is moved in the opposite direction to motion loss against the physiologic barrier and applies an activating force.
- Indirect method: the neutral point between the area of normal motion in one direction and restricted motion in the opposite is determined and held while activating forces are applied. This is described as "balanced membranous tension."
- Disengagement method: an activating force is applied to separate sutures particularly at pivot areas.
- Molding technique: resiliency and contour of bone are modified by the application of external force while waiting for intrinsic activating forces to alter the contour and resiliency of bone.

The most commonly applied procedures in craniosacral technique are indirect balanced procedures and exaggeration. Direct action technique is used more commonly in infants and children prior to the full development of the sutural components to the cranial bones. Direct action technique in adults can be helpful but requires very precise indication and localization.

ACTIVATING FORCES

The primary activating force in craniosacral technique is the inherent primary respiratory mechanism. Fluctuation of CSF is a potent intrinsic activating force that is easily directed from the exterior of the skull. The normal fluid fluctuation is in an anterior-to-posterior midline direction, but can be altered for intrinsic activating force purposes by being directed with finger contact exactly opposite the area of skull restriction. This principle is frequently used in V-spread technique. As an example, in the presence of restriction of the left occipitomastoid suture, the operator's left index and middle fingers are placed on each side of the occipitomastoid suture. The index finger of the right hand is placed over the right frontal bone directly opposite the left occipitomastoid suture (Fig. 12.10). Following separation of the two fingers of the left hand, an attempt is made to direct the fluid from the right frontal to the left occipitomastoid regions. Minimal compression on the right frontal area results in a sensation of surflike pounding against the restricted joint until release occurs. The same fluid-fluctuation activating force is used in some of the molding method techniques.

Respiratory assistance is a second activating force. Voluntary inhalation enhances flexion and external rotation movements of the craniosacral mechanism and voluntary exhalation enhances extension and internal rotation movements. The use of forced inhalation or exhalation, and holding respiration at the extreme of movement, can be used as an activating force to enhance motion in any direction.

A third activating force is enhancement of dural tension by application of effort at the sacrum and from the feet. Enhancement of flexion and extension movement can be made directly from the sacrum by the operator's hand in either direction as desired. Dorsiflexion and plantar flexion of the foot, either voluntarily by the patient or passively by an operator, enhances the intrinsic activating force. Dorsiflexion appears to enhance

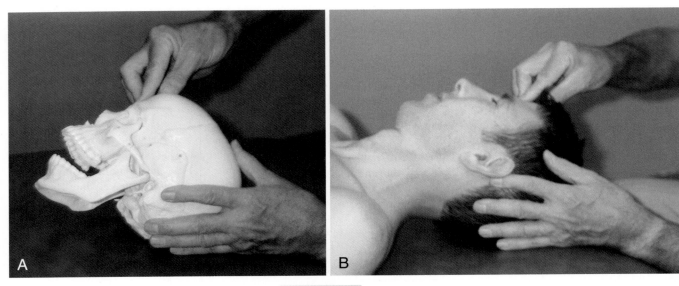

FIGURE 12.10 V spread.

flexion at the sphenobasilar junction, whereas plantar flexion enhances extension. Dorsiflexing or plantar flexing the right foot when working on the left side of the skull and using the left foot when working on the right side use the principle of the longest diagonal.

The fourth activating force is the procedure called "CV4." This procedure is performed by the operator cradling the skull in the hands with the thenar eminence of the palms against the occiput just medial to the occipitomastoid suture (Fig. 12.11). During normal craniosacral flexion, this portion of the occipital bone appears to become fuller and wider, and during exhalation less full and more narrow. After tuning into the CRI, the operator follows the occiput into its extension phase and resists the occiput during its flexion phase until a "still point" is reached. The sensation experienced is that no motion is felt. The operator holds the occiput in this position for several cycles, awaiting the return of fluid fluctuation that is perceived by the inherent force pushing the hands away. The operator then allows restoration of the normal flexion and extension movement through the occipital bone. The outcome seems to be the enhancement of fluid movement, change in the rhythm of the diaphragms, and increased temperature in the suboccipital region. A still point can be achieved by a similar process of compression in places other than the occiput that results in a temporary period of reduced motion in the CRI.

CRANIOSACRAL TECHNIQUES

The preceding are all methods of enhancing activating forces in craniosacral technique. The main activating force continues to be the inherent mobility of the brain, meninges, and CSF. This can be termed "inherent force technique" and is intrinsic in nature. Enhanced fluctuation of the CSF by respiratory assistance, sacral or extremity force applications, or by the CV4 maneuver all ultimately depends on the intrinsic inherent force reestablishing normal mobility. The other main activating force

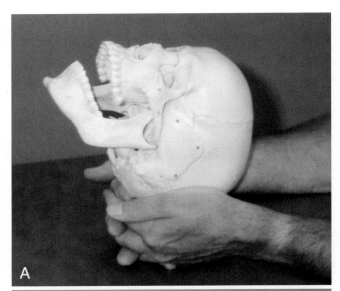

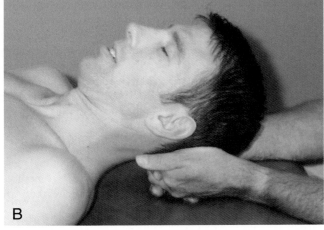

FIGURE 12.11 CV4.

is operator guiding where the operator applies external force to the skull by directing action to a suture, membranous tension, or the sphenobasilar junction. Another ancillary activating force can be through dural mobilization of the upper or lower extremities.

The operator needs to make a decision about the major restrictor in order to choose the appropriate technique. Is the restrictor articular? If so, a direct action articular technique is indicated. Is the restrictor membranous? If so, a membranous technique, such as, a frontal or parietal lift, temporal rocking, sacral technique, or the use of extremity dural mobilization technique is in order. Is the restrictor lack of fluid fluctuation? If so, V spread, CV4, or venous sinus release technique is indicated. In most instances, a combination of techniques is required to reach the therapeutic goal.

Venous Sinus Technique

The goal of venous sinus technique is to enhance the flow of venous blood through the venous sinuses to exit from the skull through the jugular foramen. It is particularly useful when the initial palpatory screening examination reveals a hard, rigid skull with loss of resiliency. Venous congestion is believed to contribute to this hard, rigid sensation and the operator attempts to enhance venous return to the central venous circulation. This is considered by some to be a myofascial release technique applied to the cranium.

The operator performs this procedure by sitting at the head of a supine patient and placing fingertip contact with the middle fingers over the external occipital protuberance of the occipital bone. The weight of the head is carried on these finger pads spreading the fascias laterally as the operator awaits a softening sensation of bone and beginning of a sensation of freer mobility. The fingers are moved sequentially along the midline of the occiput in the direction of the foramen magnum, awaiting the same softening sensation. The examiner returns to the external occipital protuberance and applies firm pressure with the pads of all four fingers along the superior nuchal line with increasing pressure from medial to lateral until softening is felt. This reduces congestion within the transverse sinus. Returning to the external occipital protuberance, the examiner places a thumb on each side of the occiput addressing the superior sagittal sinus while applying a pressure with the palmar surface of the thumb in a separation manner. The operator continues from posterior to anterior along the superior sagittal sinus working one thumb breadth at each application until reaching the bregma. From the bregma forward, the operator places the pads of four fingers on each side of the midline of the frontal bone and applies compression and lateral distraction waiting for the sensation of softening and release. Venous sinus technique is frequently used before approaching specific articular restrictions.

Condylar Decompression

The patient lies supine with the operator sitting at the head of the table cradling the skull in the palms of the hands. The middle finger pads are placed along the inferior aspect of the occiput beginning at the inion and sliding forward as far as possible. By flexing the distal interphalangeal joints of the middle fingers, the operator applies cephalic and posterior traction on the occiput. The operator's elbows are brought together, resulting in supination of both hands and separation of the middle fingers. The resultant force vector is cephalic and posterolateral on each side of the occiput posterior to the foramen magnum. This pressure is continued until release of tension is felt, particularly the sensation of equal softening on each side of the occipital bone (see description in Chapter 13).

CV4: Bulb Compression

This technique has been previously described under activating forces. It is used independently or in combination with other approaches to restore function to the craniosacral mechanism. CV4 technique is particularly valuable in the enhancement of the amplitude of the CRI.

Sphenobasilar Symphysis

Dysfunctions at the sphenobasilar symphysis, both physiologic and traumatic, are addressed by one of the vault holds. The operator controls the greater wings of the sphenoid at the pterion and the occiput at the asterion and determines the sphenobasilar strain patterns present. Addressing the sphenobasilar strain pattern that appears to be the most restricted is frequently a valuable first approach. The operator addresses the dysfunction in either a direct, exaggeration, or indirect method. The most commonly used is the indirect method of balanced membranous tension. The operator finds the point of maximum ease within the range of the strain pattern and holds the mechanism at a balanced point until some release is achieved. Respiratory assistance and membranous enhancement from the sacrum and lower extremities are frequently concurrently used. Finding the balanced point of each of the strain patterns in a stacked fashion and applying a distraction force by separating the finger contact on the sphenoid and occiput in an AP direction accomplish decompression of the sphenobasilar symphysis.

Temporal Rocking

With the patient supine on the table and the operator sitting at the head, the skull is supported in the palms of the hand with each thumb behind the ear in front of the mastoid process with the interphalangeal joint at the apex and the metacarpophalangeal at the mastoid portion. This thumb placement allows control of the temporal bones on each side. Pressure by the distal phalanx of the thumb in a posteromedial direction on the inferior aspect of the mastoid process introduces external rotation. Compression in a posteromedial direction with the base of the thumb on the mastoid portion of the temporal bone enhances internal rotation. Movement of the thumbs can rock the temporal bones into internal and external rotations either synchronously (both temporals into internal rotation or external rotation) or asynchronously (one temporal moving into internal rotation and the other into external rotation). Asynchronous rocking of the temporals through several cycles appears to change the fluid fluctuation from an AP to-and-fro movement to a side-to-side to-and-fro movement. Once asynchronous rocking is symmetric on each side, synchronous

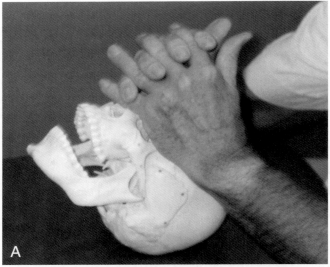

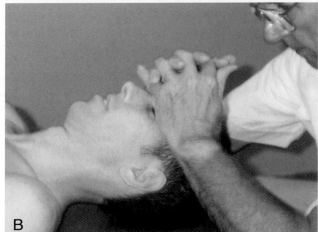

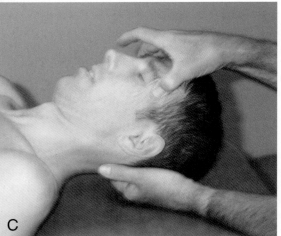

FIGURE 12.12   Frontal lift.

rocking is reintroduced to restore the normal AP to-and-fro fluid fluctuation. The operator should never leave a patient with asynchronous motion of the temporals because an adverse reaction of dizziness and nausea can result. Enhancement of synchronous rocking of the two temporals appears to have a beneficial effect on membranous balance. It is also of value in the temporomandibular joint function because asymmetric relationship of temporal movement interferes with symmetric temporomandibular joint function.

V SPREAD

This procedure is useful to separate restricted and impacted sutures wherever present. The principle is to place two fingers on each side of the restricted suture with distraction and separation using fluid fluctuation as the activating force by applying pressure with the opposite hand at a point of greatest distance and opposite to the suture under treatment. The occipitomastoid suture is one frequently treated by means of V spread ("Activating Forces"), but the principles can be applied to any suture within the skull or face.

Lift Technique

Frontal and parietal lift techniques are commonly used to aid in the balance of membranous tension. To perform a frontal lift, the patient is supine on the table with the operator sitting at the head. The operator grasps the inferior and lateral corners of the frontal bone on each side with one hand spanning the frontal bone or with two hands interlaced with the pisiforms on the frontal bone (Fig. 12.12). The hands apply a medial compression force to disengage the frontal, which is then lifted toward the ceiling sensing for a release. A frontal lift puts longitudinal traction on the falx cerebri as it lifts the frontal from the sphenoid. When the frontal bone appears to be in the midline and has been released anteriorly, it is slowly allowed to settle back to its normal relationship. It is not uncommon during this procedure to have the sensation that the frontal bone is wobbling from side to side when being distracted.

A parietal lift is performed by a four-finger contact on the two anteroinferior and posteroinferior corners of the parietal bones (Fig. 12.13). Compressive force is applied through the tips of the

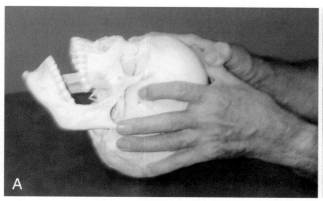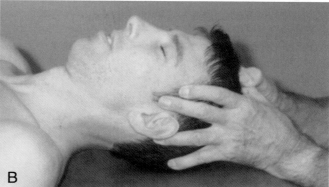

FIGURE 12.13 Parietal lift.

four fingers and each parietal bone is lifted toward the vertex. The four-corner compression disengages the parietal bone, allowing for the lift that results in external rotation of the two parietal bones. The parietal lift places a transverse stress on the tentorium cerebelli balancing its tension from right to left. As with the frontal lift, when balance is achieved, the operator reduces the lifting force and allows the parietals to settle back into the skull. Lift techniques distract one bone from the other and apply loads to the meninges to achieve membranous balance.

SEQUENCE OF TREATMENT

Sequence of treatment varies from practitioner to practitioner, from patient to patient, and from one treatment to the next. There are several general principles that can be useful, applied, and adapted individually for the patient need. First and foremost, the craniosacral mechanism must be viewed within the context of the total musculoskeletal system. Craniosacral dysfunction may be primary, secondary, or of little significance in the patient's overall status. Secondary cranial dysfunction resulting from altered functional capacity elsewhere in the system will not respond well until the primary dysfunction is identified and appropriately treated. Conversely, continued treatment to dysfunction of the musculoskeletal system elsewhere in the system, without addressing the craniosacral dysfunction, will lead to less than satisfactory results.

Treatments that the craniosacral mechanism can follow are noted on page 181 (principles of craniosacral treatment). The goal should be to reduce venous congestion, mobilize articular restrictions, balance the sphenobasilar symphysis, and enhance the rate and amplitude of the CRI.

Craniosacral treatment, like all manual medicine, needs to be prescribed in the dosage appropriate for the individual patient's need. These procedures do not appear to be aggressive and forceful, but are powerful and if inappropriately applied can result in a poor outcome for the patient.

COMPLICATIONS AND CONTRAINDICATIONS

Complications to craniosacral treatment are fortunately quite rare, but do occur. The brainstem with its many control functions for the total body is intimately related to the sphenobasilar junction. Craniosacral treatment, particularly that which addresses sphenobasilar strain patterns, might lead to alteration in nervous system control of systemic function resulting in symptom exacerbation. This may include alterations in heart rate, blood pressure, or respiration and gastrointestinal irritability with nausea, vomiting, and diarrhea. These exacerbated symptoms appear to result from an alteration in autonomic nervous system control. A second area of potential symptom exacerbation and complications comprises the cervicocranial syndromes with headache, dizziness, and tinnitus. The vestibular system is highly sensitive to balance or imbalance of the temporal bones. Overly aggressive or improperly applied temporal rocking of the synchronous and asynchronous nature may exacerbate symptoms of dizziness, vertigo, nausea, and vomiting. Care must be exercised in using craniosacral technique in individuals with psychological and psychiatric problems. These procedures can cause significant emotional change in response to the patient's environment. Neurologic complications and symptom exacerbation can occur in patients with seizure states and dystonia of the central nervous system. Traumatic brain injury is a common, but frequently unrecognized, patient problem. Great care must be used in applying craniosacral technique to patients with traumatic brain injury, because it is difficult to predict the outcome of craniosacral treatment in these patients. The practitioner must be aware of and be prepared to deal with symptom exacerbation or onset of new symptoms in the patient under craniosacral treatment.

Contraindications are few but include suspicion for acute intracranial bleed or increase in intracranial pressure. These should be evaluated by appropriate diagnostic testing before implementing craniosacral treatment. Skull trauma requires adequate investigation to rule out fractures of the cranial base, depressed fractures of the vault, or subarachnoid hemorrhage. Seizure states are not an absolute contraindication but are relative, depending upon the control of the seizure status.

Although the complications and contraindications are few, the admonition of primum non nocere (first do not harm) applies when using craniosacral technique.

CRANIAL TECHNIQUES

Condylar Compression (CV4)

1. Patient is supine on the table with the operator sitting at the head.

2. Operator's two hands cradle patient's occiput with the thenar eminences in contact with the occipital squama, palpating cranial rhythm (Fig. 12.11).

3. Operator resists occipital flexion movement until motion temporarily ceases (still point).

4. Operator gradually releases compression on occiput when cranial rhythm begins again until returned to normal.

5. Operator observes for a change in respiration and an increased perspiration of the cervical area and forehead.

Frontal Lift

1. Patient is supine on the table with the operator sitting at the head.

2. Operator interlaces the fingers of the hands and grasps the frontal bone with each pisiform in contact with the inferior lateral angle (Fig. 12.12).

3. Operator lifts the frontal bone anteriorly, following any side-to-side fluctuation until the lift appears to be midline.

4. Operator allows the frontal to return to neutral.

Parietal Lift

1. Patient is supine on the table with the operator sitting at the head.

2. Operator applies each index finger on the anteroinferior corner and each little finger on the posteroinferior corner of the parietal bone (Fig. 12.13).

3. Operator interlaces thumbs over the vertex of the skull without touching and compresses medially with all four fingers.

4. Traction is applied toward the vertex until tension is felt to be symmetric in all four corners.

5. Operator gently releases traction allowing the parietals to return to neutral.

The following are the four most commonly found restrictors of the four quadrants of the skull: two posteriorly, the occipitomastoid and parietal notch, and two anteriorly, the sphenosquamous and palatines. There are numerous other sutural restrictions in the vault, base, and face that may need attention. The reader should pursue further study of these in a comprehensive text of the craniosacral system.

Occipitomastoid Suture

1. Operator sits at the head of the supine patient and controls the occiput in the right hand, and the left hand controls the left temporal bone with the five-finger hold (Fig. 12.14).

2. Operator introduces external and internal rotations of the temporal and monitors the response in the occiput. If the occiput moves into extension rather than flexion when the temporal is externally rotated, there is restriction of the left occipitomastoid suture.

3. Treatment begins with establishing the longest diameter of dural tension by dorsiflexing the right foot.

4. The operator's right hand holds the occiput in flexion while the left hand externally rotates the temporal to the external rotation barrier while the patient fully exhales.

5. The operator instructs the patient to fully inhale rapidly or use a series of step breathing while the operator enhances temporal external rotation against the stabilized occiput.

6. The procedure may be repeated until normal motion between the temporal and occiput is restored.

7. Reassessed.

Note: This dysfunction is the most common articular restriction of the posterior quadrant and is frequently related to dysfunction of the upper cervical vertebral complex.

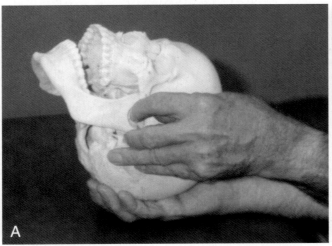
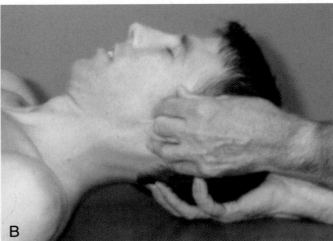

FIGURE 12.14 Occipitomastoid suture.

Parietal Notch

1. Operator sits at the head of the supine patient. Diagnosis is by medial springing of the posteroinferior corner of the parietal, sensing for loss of mobility unilaterally.

2. Operator's left thumb is in contact with the mastoid process of the left temporal and the operator's right hand lies over the parietal bone with the thumb over the posteroinferior corner of the parietal (Fig. 12.15).

3. After establishing the longest diagonal by dorsiflexing the right foot, the operator presses medially with the right thumb and rotates the right hand counterclockwise on the parietal while the left thumb externally rotates the temporal to the barrier and the patient fully exhales.

4. The patient is instructed to take a rapid deep breath, or step breathe, while the operator's left thumb increases the temporal external rotation and the right hand lifts the parietal superiorly and anteriorly, disengaging the parietal notch suture.

5. Reassessed.

Sphenosquamous Suture

1. Operator stands at the right side of the supine patient with one knee stabilizing the right side of the head.

2. Operator's left hand controls the left temporal with the thumb in front of the mastoid process.

3. Operator's gloved right hand places the little finger against the left lateral pterygoid plate of the sphenoid while the middle finger is placed on the left great wing and the right thumb on the right great wing if possible (Fig. 12.16).

4. After establishing the longest diameter by dorsiflexing the right foot, the operator engages the barrier by externally rotating the left temporal and pulling the left great wing anteriorly and having the patient fully exhale.

5. The patient takes a rapid deep breath and the operator simultaneously externally rotates the temporal while increasing the rotation of the sphenoid to the right and slightly into flexion.

6. Reassessed.

Note: Dysfunction of this suture is one of the most common restrictors of the anterior quadrant.

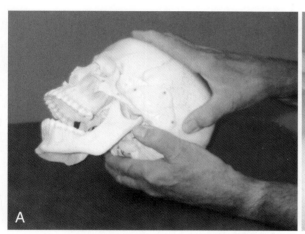
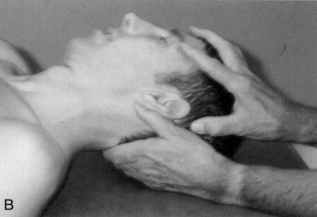

FIGURE 12.15 Parietal notch suture.

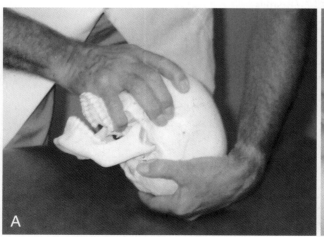
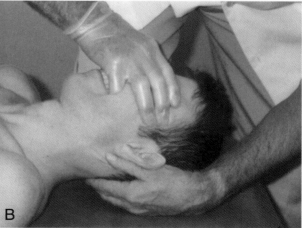

FIGURE 12.16 Sphenosquamous pivot suture.

Palatine

1. Operator stands at the side of the supine patient with the left hand grasping the sphenoid at the pterion bilaterally.

2. Operator places gloved right little finger pad against the palatine just posterior to the left second molar (Fig. 12.17).

3. Operator flexes and extends the sphenoid and monitors the response at the palatine. During flexion, the palatine should move laterally and during extension, it should move toward the vertex.

4. If restricted, the longest diameter is established and the sphenoid taken into marked flexion to disengage the pterygoid processes from the palatines.

5. If external rotation is restricted, the little finger presses laterally on the palatine as the patient takes a deep breath in.

6. If internal rotation is restricted, the little finger presses toward the vertex as the patient breathes deeply into exhalation.

7. The sphenoid is returned to neutral, recapturing the palatines by the pterygoid processes.

8. Reassessed.

Note: Palatine dysfunction is a common restrictor of the anterior quadrant.

Facial Balance

1. Operator sits at the head of the supine patient and places the palms of both hands over the frontal and facial bones (Fig. 12.18).

2. Operator follows internal and external rotation motion of the facial bones and the frontal during inhalation and exhalation.

3. If asymmetric, operator exaggerates the desired motion as patient deeply inhales and exhales.

4. Sometimes shearing motion is added to the internal and external rotational motions for enhanced mobility.

5. If still not symmetric, each facial bone needs to be assessed and treated as appropriate. Since the facial mechanics respond to the sphenoid, and are all suspended beneath the frontal, restoration of balance to the sphenobasilar symphysis and of normal motion to the frontal usually restore mobility to the face. Most commonly, dysfunction of the zygoma is present.

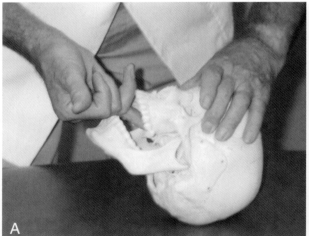
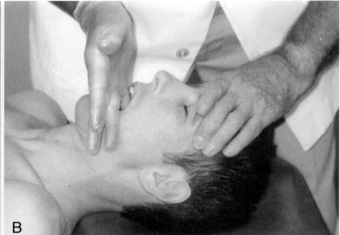

FIGURE 12.17 Palatine.

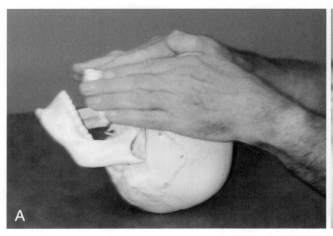
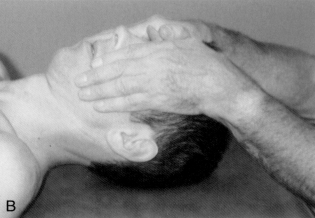

FIGURE 12.18 Facial balance.

Zygoma

1. Operator stands at the right side of the supine patient and with a gloved right hand slides the tip of the little finger inside of the cheek to contact the inferior margin of the zygoma and the thumb is placed on the outside of the cheek, grasping the zygoma.

2. The operator's left hand stabilizes the head and monitors the attachments of the zygoma to the frontal and the great wing of the sphenoid (Fig. 12.19).

3. Operator's right hand internally and externally rotates the zygoma and the left hand monitors motion at the zygomatico-frontal and zygomaticosphenoid articulations.

4. If restricted, the longest diameter is established by dorsiflexing the right foot, using inhalation to enhance external rotation and exhalation to enhance internal rotation as the zygoma is distracted from the frontal or sphenoid.

5. The zygoma can be mobilized from the maxilla by distracting the zygoma using the same thumb and little finger hold and stabilizing the maxilla by its frontal process attachment to the frontal, again using an appropriate respiratory assist.

6. Reassess.

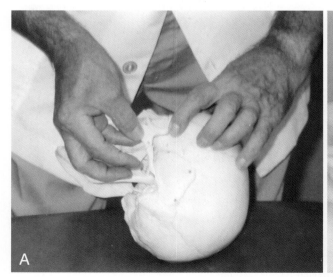 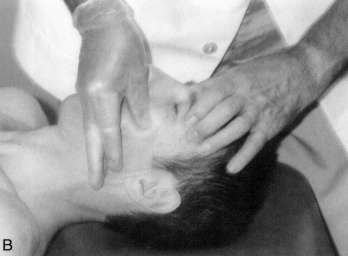

FIGURE 12.19 Zygoma.

Two-Person Decompression

1. Patient is supine and one operator sits at the head of the table with the occiput in the palms of the hands and the thumbs in front of the mastoid processes.

2. The second operator spans the front of the skull and contacts the two great wings of the sphenoid (Fig. 12.20).

3. The second operator directly engages the restrictive barrier of the sphenobasilar strain patterns of torsion, lateral strain, and vertical strain and puts anterior distraction on the sphenoid as the other operator stabilizes the occiput and temporals posteriorly.

4. Two or three applications of anterior distraction and flexion movement of the sphenoid are frequently necessary to restore mobility to the compressed head and reduce the restrictions of the strain patterns.

Note: This is a powerful technique and requires accurate direct engagement of the strain patterns before distraction is applied. It has been found most effective in the compressed skull associated with closed head injuries when indirect decompression is inadequate.

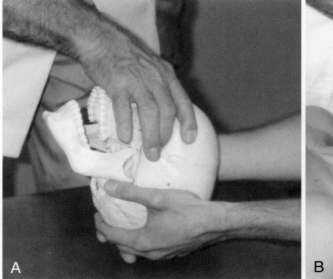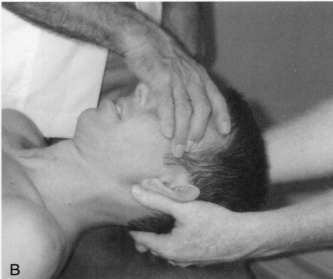

FIGURE 12.20 Two-person sphenobasilar decompression.

CONCLUSION

Craniosacral technique is a valuable addition to the armamentarium of the manual medicine practitioner. Craniosacral technique requires extensive study and practice. It should be performed within the context of total patient evaluation because of its powerful systemic effects. It influences, and is influenced by, the rest of the musculoskeletal system. This chapter includes basic and preliminary information about the craniosacral system. Students should pursue additional study from the standard texts in the field and structured courses of instruction.

SUGGESTED READINGS

Gehin A. Atlas of *Manipulative Techniques for the Cranium and Face*. Seattle: Eastland Press, 1985.

Greenman PE. Craniosacral manipulation. *Phys Med Rehab Clin N Am* 1996;7:877–896.

Hruby RJ. *Craniosacral Osteopathic Technique: A Manual*. 2nd Ed. Okemos, MI: Institute for Osteopathic Studies.

Magoun HI. *Osteopathy in the Cranial Field*. 2nd Ed. Kirksville, MO: Journal Printing Co., 1966.

Retzlaff EW, Mitchell FL Jr. *The Cranium and its Sutures*. Berlin: Spinger-Verlag, 1987.

Upledger JE, Vredevoogd JD. *Craniosacral Therapy*. Seattle: Eastland Press, 1983.

REFERENCES

1. Sutherland WG. Preamble. In: *The Cranial Bowl*. Sutherland WG, ed. Mankato, MN, 1939. (Reprinted by the Osteopathic Cranial Association, Meridian, ID: Fee Press Company, 1948.)
2. Sutherland WG. Wales AL, ed. Primary respiratory mechanism. In: *Teachings in the Science of Osteopathy*. Portland, OR: Rudra Press, 1990.
3. Herring SW. Mechanical influences on suture development and patency. *Front Oral Biol* 2008;12:41–56.
4. Sahni D, Jit I, Neelam, et al. Time of fusion of the basisphenoid with the basilar part of the occipital bone in northwest Indian subjects. *Forensic Sci Int* 1998;98:41–45.
5. Heisey SR, Adams T. Role of cranial bone mobility in cranial compliance. *Neurosurgery* 1993;33(5):869–876.
6. Pritchard JJ, Scott JH, Girgis FG. The structure and development of cranial and facial sutures. *J Anat* 1956;90:73–86.
7. Retzlaff E, Mitchell FL Jr, Upledger J, et al. Nerve fibers and endings in cranial sutures. *J Am Osteopath Assoc* 1978;77:100–101 [abstract].
8. Hering E. About the influence of respiration to the circulation. I. About respiratoric movements of the vessels system. [Über den Einfluss der Athmung auf den Kreislauf I. Über Athembewegungen des Gefäss-systems.] Sitzungsbericht der mathematisch-naturwissenschaftlichen. *Classe Wien* 1869;60:829–856.
9. Traube L. About periodic actions of the vasomotor and inhibitory nerve center. [Üeber periodische Thätigkeits-Aeusserungen des vasomotorischen und Hemmungs-Nervencentrums. Centralblatt für die medicinischen Wissenschaften, Berlin, 1865, 3:881–885.]
10. Mayer S. Studies about the physiology of heart and blood vessels. [Studien zur Physiologie des Herzens und deg Blutgfässe.] Sitzungsbericht der mathematisch-naturwissenschaftlichen. *Classe Wien* 1876;74:281–307.
11. Julien C. The enigma of Mayer waves: Facts and models. *Cardiovas Res* 2006;70:12–21.
12. Nilsson H, Aalkjaer C. Vasomotion: Mechanisms and physiological importance. *Mol Interv* 2003;3(2):79–89.
13. Haddock RE, Hill CE. Rhythmicity in arterial smooth muscle. *J Physiol* 2005;566(3):645–656.
14. Van Helden DF, Zhao J. Lymphatic vasomotion. *Clin Exp Pharmacol Physiol* 2000;27(12):1014–1018.
15. Aalkjær C, Nilsson H. Vasomotion: Cellular background for the oscillator and for the synchronization of smooth muscle cells. *Br J Pharmacol* 2005;144:605–616.
16. Jacobsen JC, Aalkjær C, Nilsson H, et al. A model of smooth muscle cell synchronization in the arterial wall. *Am J Physiol Heart Circ Physiol* 2007;293:H229–H237.
17. Lundberg N. Continuous recording and control of ventricular fluid pressure in neurosurgical practice. *Acta Psychiatr Scand Suppl* 1960;36(149):1–193.
18. Jenkins CO, Campbell, JK, White DN. Modulation resembling Traube-Hering waves recorded in the human brain. *Eur Neurol* 1971;5:1–6.
19. White DN. Early development of neurosonology: III. Pulsatile echoencephalogrphy and Doppler techniques. *Ultrasound Med Biol* 1992;18(4):323–376.
20. Strik C, Klose U, Erb M, et al. Intracranial oscillations of cerebrospinal fluid and blood flows: Analysis with magnetic resonance imaging. *J Magn Reson Imaging* 2002;15(3):251–258.
21. Strik C, Klose U, Kiefer C, et al. Slow rhythmic oscillations in intracranial CSF and blood flow: Registered by MRI. *Acta Neurochir Suppl* 2002;81:139–142.
22. Friese S, Hamhaber U, Erb M, et al. B-waves in cerebral and spinal cerebrospinal fluid pulsation measurement by magnetic resonance imaging. *J Comput Assist Tomogr* 2004;28(2):255–262.
23. Razavi M, et al. Source of low-frequency fluctuations in functional MRI signal. *J Magn Reson Imaging* 2008;27(4):891–897.
24. Friese S, Hamhaber U, Erb M, et al. The influence of pulse and respiration on spinal cerebrospinal fluid pulsation. *Invest Radiol* 2004;39(2):120–130.
25. Van Helden DF, Hosaka K, Imtiaz MS. Rhythmicity in the microcirculation. *Clin Hemorheol Microcirc* 2006;34(1–2):59–66.
26. Stücker M, Steinbrügge J, Ihrig C, et al. Rhythmical variations of haemoglobin oxygenation in cutaneous capillaries. *Acta Derm Venereol* 1998;78(6):408–411.
27. Tsai AG, Intaglietta M. Evidence of flowmotion induced changes in local tissue oxygenation. *Int J Microcirc Clin Exp* 1993;12(1):75–88.
28. Meyer MF, Rose CJ, Hülsmann JO, et al. Impairment of cutaneous arteriolar 0.1 Hz vasomotion in diabetes. *Exp Clin Endocrinol Diabetes* 2003;111(2):104–110.
29. Rossi M, Carpi A, Galetta F, et al. The investigation of skin blood flowmotion: A new approach to study the microcirculatory impairment in vascular diseases? *Biomed Pharmacother* 2006;60(8):437–442.
30. Landmesser U, Hornig B, Drexler H. Endothelial function: A critical determinant in atherosclerosis? *Circulation* 2004;109(21 Suppl 1):II27–II33.
31. Nelson KE, Sergueef N, Lipinski CM, et al. Cranial rhythmic impulse related to the Traube-Hering-Mayer oscillation: Comparing laser-Doppler flowmetry and palpation. *J Am Osteopath Assoc* 2001;101(3):163–173.
32. Nelson KE, Sergueef N, Glonek T. Recording the rate of the cranial rhythmic impulse. *Am Osteopath Assoc* 2006;106(6):337–341.
33. Sergueef N, Nelson KE, Glonek T. The effect of cranial manipulation on the Traube-Hering-Mayer oscillation as measured by laser-Doppler flowmetry. *Altern Ther Health Med* 2002;8(6):74–76.
34. Moskalenko IuE, Kravchenko TI, Bainshtein GB, et al. [Slow-wave fluctuations in craniosacral space: Hemo-liquorodynamic conception of origin.] *Ross Fiziol Zh Im I M Sechenova* 2008;94(4):441–447.

The cervical spine is an important region of the vertebral column in the field of manual medicine. It receives a great deal of attention by manual medicine practitioners. It functions as the support of the skull and biomechanically provides mobility for a number of activities of daily living. A myriad of head, neck, and upper extremity symptoms have been observed when the cervical spine is dysfunctional. Symptomatic conditions in the area can be categorized as cervicocephalic syndrome, cervical syndrome, and cervicobrachial syndrome.

The *cervicocephalic syndrome* includes pain and restriction of motion of the upper cervical spine and associated superficial and deep pain in the head. This syndrome frequently demonstrates functional alteration in vision, vertigo, dizziness, and nystagmus.

The *cervical syndrome* includes painful stiffness of the neck of varying severity from mild to an acute spastic torticollis.

The *cervicobrachial syndrome* couples painful stiffness of the cervical spine with symptoms in the shoulder girdle and upper extremity. The upper extremity symptoms result from alteration of the functional capacity in the brachial plexus or altered vascular function through the arterial, venous, and lymphatic symptoms. Associated dysfunctions of the thoracic inlet, particularly the first and the second ribs and in the thoracic spine and the rib cage as far as T5 or T6, contribute to the cervicobrachial syndrome.

The cervical spine is subjected to acute injuries, such as the flexion–extension "whiplash" injury and chronic repetitive injury from improper posture and abnormal positions of the head and neck. It is seldom that the whiplash injury is a true flexion–extension injury. Most commonly, there is a rotary torque included in the trauma which gives rise to a number of motion restriction possibilities and different vectors of soft-tissue injury.[1,2] It is common in our society to have patients with forward head carriage as a component of poor posture. Forward head posture results in an increase in the upper cervical lordosis and a flattening in the lower cervical spine. The balance of the head on the neck is altered, resulting in muscle imbalance with resulting tightness of the neck extensors and weakness of the deep neck flexors.[3,4]

The cervical spine is the area of the musculoskeletal system in which most of the reported complications of manual medicine treatment have occurred. Traumatic insult to the vertebrobasilar artery system is a rare but catastrophic event. Congenital, inflammatory, and traumatic alterations in the upper cervical region place the cervical spinal cord at risk from improper diagnostic and manual medicine treatment methods. Down syndrome, rheumatoid arthritis, agenesis of the odontoid process, and fracture of the odontoid base are but a few of these conditions.[5,6] The student and the practitioner must understand the anatomy, physiology, and biomechanics of the region to understand the therapeutic role of manual medicine and avoid potential complications.

FUNCTIONAL ANATOMY AND BIOMECHANICS

The cervical spine can be divided into the atypical segments of the upper cervical complex and the typical cervical vertebra from C3 through C7. The upper cervical complex, consisting of the occipitoatlantal (C0-C1), atlantoaxial (C1-C2), and the superior aspect of C2, functions as an integrated unit. The biomechanics of this region are complex and are under intense research and study. Although the C0 through C3 region functions as an integrated unit, it is useful to assess each level individually to identify its contribution to the overall function of the complex.

Occipitoatlantal Articulation

The occipitoatlantal junction (C0-C1) consists of two articulations formed by the occipital condyles and the superior articular facets of the atlas. The occipital condyles are convex from front to back and from side to side. The superior articular facets of the atlas are concave from the front to the back and from side to side. The two articulations are divergent from front to back. The primary movements are forward bending and backward bending (nutation and counternutation). There is a small amount of coupled side bending and rotation to opposite sides that becomes highly clinically significant when lost. During side bending, one occipital condyle slides upward on one side of the atlas and downward on the other. This side-bending component is approximately 5 degrees in each direction. Rotation couples to the opposite side of side bending and is in the range of 5 degrees to each side. The coupling of rotation to the opposite side appears to be a function of the ligamentous attachments of the occiput to the atlas and the axis, the relationship of the slope of the size of the superior facets of the atlas, and the divergence posteriorly.

Atlantoaxial Articulation

There are four articulations at the atlantoaxial junction (C1-C2). The right and the left zygapophysial joints are formed by the inferior facet of the atlas articulating with the convex superior facet of the axis. The inferior facet of the atlas is covered by an articular cartilage that is convex anteroposteriorly and from side to side. This relationship results in a unique convex-to-convex apposition of the joint surfaces. The superior articular facets of the axis are convex anteroposteriorly, and from side to side, and face superiorly and laterally giving the appearance of a pair of shoulders. The other two articulations at the atlantoaxial junction involve the odontoid process. The anterior surface of the odontoid articulates with a small facet on the posterior aspect of the anterior arch of the atlas. On the posterior aspect of the odontoid process is an articulation with the transaxial ligament. The integrated functions of these four articulations, modified by ligamentous and muscular attachments, result in a small amount of forward bending, backward bending, and side bending, with the primary motion being rotation to the right and the left. There is a small amount of cephalic-to-caudad translatory movement that accompanies rotation. This is a result of the unique convex-to-convex articular apposition of the zygapophysial joints. As the atlas turns right on the axis, the right facet of the atlas slides downward on the posterior aspect of the right facet of the axis, and the left inferior facet of the atlas slides downward on the anterior aspect of the left facet of the axis, resulting in caudad translation. On returning to neutral, the inferior facets of the atlas ascend on the articular shoulders of the facets of the axis, resulting in a cephalic translatory movement.

C2 functions as a transitional segment with its atypical superior surface articulating with the atlas and with the occiput through ligamentous and muscular attachments. The inferior surface is the same as the remaining typical cervical segments below.

Typical Cervical Articulations

The typical cervical segments from C3-C7 articulate at the vertebral bodies with an intervening intervertebral disk. The superior surface of the vertebral body is convex from before backward and concave from side to side, while the inferior surface is convex from side to side and concave from before backward. This joint configuration, with the intervening intervertebral disk, allows it to move in all directions. The uncovertebral joints of Luschka are found at the posterolateral corner of the vertebral bodies and appear to function in the gliding movements during forward and backward bending. They also seem to protect the intervertebral disk from herniation in a posterolateral direction. These joints are subject to degenerative productive change resulting in lipping, which occasionally encroaches on the anterior aspect of the lateral intervertebral canal. The zygapophysial joints of the typical cervical vertebra face backward and upward at an angle of approximately 45 degrees. The greatest load bearing is through the posterior arches instead of the vertebral bodies as in the thoracic and the lumbar spines. This loading, plus the facing of the zygapophysial joints and the characteristics of the vertebral bodies and intervening intervertebral disk, results in the motions available being forward bending, backward bending, and coupled side bending and rotation movements to the same side. This results in the typical cervical segments having only nonneutral somatic dysfunction. There are no group dysfunctions in the typical cervical segments, although several segments can become dysfunctional one on top of the other.

Vertebral Artery

The course of the vertebral artery is of major significance in the field of manual medicine. The vertebral artery begins its relationship with the cervical spine at the level of C6-C7 where it enters between the transverse processes, immediately turns cephalad, runs through the intertransverse foramen, and exits from the superior side of the transverse process of C1. Here, it turns acutely posteriorly over the posterior arch of the atlas and penetrates the posterior occipitoatlantal membrane before entering the foramen magnum. It joins the vertebral artery of the opposite side to form the basilar artery. The vertebral artery is at risk at the acute angulation at C6-C7, by productive change in and around the intertransverse foramen from C7-C1, and at the occipitoatlantal junction. *Normal vertebral arteries can narrow as much as 90% of their luminal size on the contralateral side during cervical rotation. This normal phenomenon is exacerbated when performed in the backward bending of the head on the neck.* Congenital asymmetry, and even atresia, of the vertebral arteries is not uncommon, and they are subject to degenerative vessel disease. A commonly used provocative diagnostic test for the integrity of the vertebral artery is the hanging (De Kleyn) test (Fig. 13.1). The examiner backward bends the head and the neck over the end of the table (Fig. 13.2) and introduces rotation to the right (Fig. 13.3) and to the left (Fig. 13.4), holding

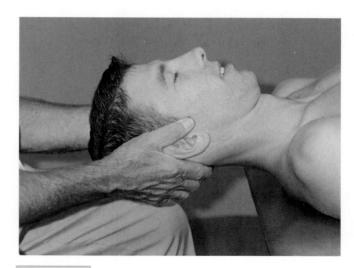

FIGURE 13.1

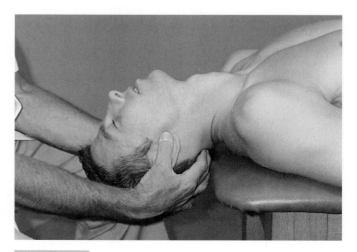

FIGURE 13.2

the head in each rotated position looking for the development of nystagmus. This author does not advocate this test as it unnecessarily puts normal vertebral arteries at risk. It also has a high false-positive rate.[7,8] A less aggressive test that provides equally valid information is the following: Have the sitting patient look up at the ceiling (Fig. 13.5), then turn the head both to the left (Fig. 13.6) and to the right (Fig. 13.7) while the operator observes for the initiation of nystagmus and adverse symptoms such as dizziness. This is a hands-off test by the practitioner and asks the patient only to introduce normal ranges of active movement. Probably, the best sign of impending cerebral anoxia is the symptom of acute anxiety and panic. If this occurs during a structural diagnostic or manual medicine procedure in the cervical spine, the operator should stop and immediately institute evaluation and treatment for potential vascular complications.

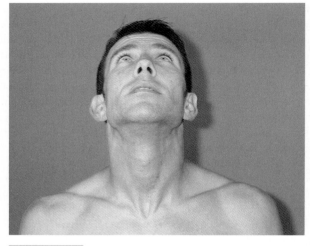

FIGURE 13.5

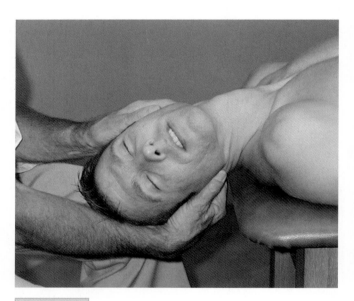

FIGURE 13.3

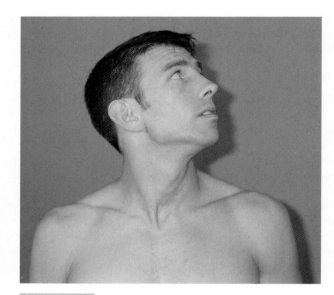

FIGURE 13.6

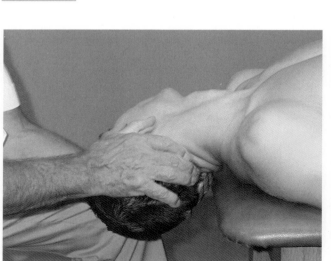

FIGURE 13.4

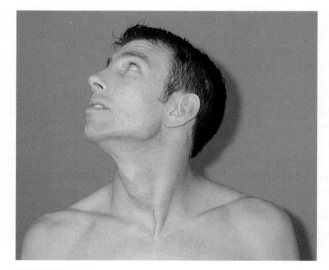

FIGURE 13.7

Mechanoreceptors and Nociceptors

The articular and periarticular structures of the cervical spine, particularly the upper cervical complex, are heavily invested by mechanoreceptors and nociceptors. Cervical spine dysfunction can result in altered afferent stimulation by these mechanoreceptors and nociceptors and influence the integrated function of the musculoskeletal system, as well as contribute to local and regional symptoms.[9] The suboccipital cervical muscles have a large number of spindles per unit mass. The proprioceptive function of these muscles must have a high level of significance. Recent magnetic resonance imaging (MRI) research in this region has demonstrated fatty replacement of the rectus capitis posterior major and minor muscles in some patients with post-traumatic cervicocranial syndromes (see Chapter 21).

Autonomic Nervous System Relationships

Sympathetic autonomic nervous system control of cerebral blood flow emanates from the superior cervical ganglion. This structure is intimately related to the longus colli muscle and the anterior surface of C2 to which it is intimately bound by deep connective fascia. Somatic dysfunction of C2 is frequently found in patients with cervicocephalic syndromes and in those with internal visceral disease. A small branch of the second cervical nerve connects with the vagus as it descends through the trunk. Hypothetically, this neural connection may account for the clinical observation of somatic dysfunction of C2 in the presence of visceral disease.[10]

STRUCTURAL DIAGNOSIS

The anatomy and biomechanics of the cervical spine result in five somatic dysfunctions. The typical cervical segments have nonneutral dysfunction with either a forward-bending or a backward-bending restriction together with a coupled side-bending and rotation restriction to the same side. At the atlantoaxial (C1-C2) junction, the primary somatic dysfunction is that of restriction of rotation to one side or the other. While there may be minor forward-bending, backward-bending, and side-bending components to the rotational restriction, adequate treatment to the rotational restriction restores the minor movement motion simultaneously. At the occipitoatlantal (C0-C1) junction, there are two dysfunctions possible. There will be either forward-bending or backward-bending restriction with coupled side-bending and rotation restrictions to opposite sides.

The structural diagnostic process begins by identifying levels of palpable deep-muscle hypertonicity. This identifies segments that need motion testing. The diagnostic and the therapeutic processes seem to be most satisfactory by beginning from below and moving cephalad.

The bony landmark of most value in the typical cervical segments is the articular pillar. They are palpated in the deep fascial groove between the semispinalis medially and the cervical longissimus laterally. The paired examiner's fingers can localize to the right and the left articular pillars of any given cervical segment and introduce motion testing. The typical cervical segment articular pillar is the size of the examiner's finger pad. The identification of the articular pillars begins by first identifying the spinous process of C2 and C7. The C2 spinous process is the first bony prominence in the midline caudad to the external occipital protuberance (inion). The spinous process of C7 (vertebra prominens) is the spinous process that remains palpable during cervical backward bending. The articular pillars of C2 and C7 are at the same level of the spinous processes. Placing the examiner's fingers between the pillars of C2 and C7 puts the finger pads in contact with C3, C4, C5, and C6. This provides the ability to localize to any specific cervical segment. The structural diagnostic process can be performed in patients in both sitting and supine positions.

CERVICAL SPINE DIAGNOSIS

Typical Cervical: Sitting

1. Patient sits on the table or a treatment stool.

2. Operator stands behind with the thumb and index finger contacting zygapophysial joints bilaterally and with the left hand on the vertex of the head to control motion (Fig. 13.8).

3. Operator's left hand introduces forward bending, right-side bending, and right rotation while monitoring left zygapophysial joint for opening movement (Fig. 13.9).

4. Operator introduces forward bending, left-side bending, and left rotation, palpating for opening of the right zygapophysial joint by the operator's right index finger (Fig. 13.10).

5. Operator's left hand introduces backward bending, right-side bending, and right rotation with the right index finger monitoring the right zygapophysial joint's capacity to close (Fig. 13.11).

6. Operator introduces backward bending, left-side bending, and left rotation with the left hand while monitoring the left zygapophysial joint's capacity to close with the right thumb (Fig. 13.12).

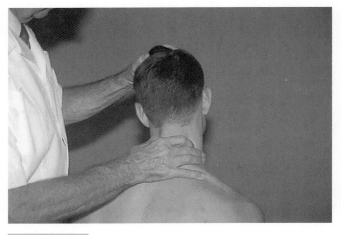

FIGURE 13.10

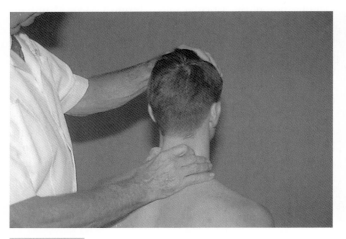

FIGURE 13.8

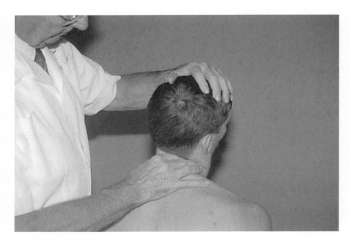

FIGURE 13.11

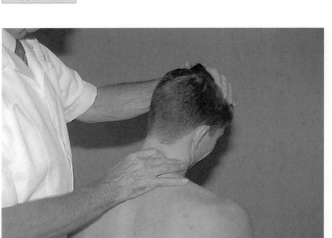

FIGURE 13.9

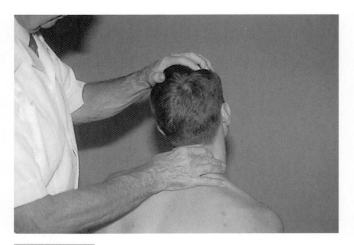

FIGURE 13.12

CERVICAL SPINE DIAGNOSIS

Atlantoaxial (C1-C2): Sitting

1. Patient sits on the table with the operator behind.

2. Operator's hands grasp the patient's head and introduce forward bending (Fig. 13.13) to reduce rotation in lower typical cervical vertebra.

3. Operator introduces right rotation sensing for resistance to movement (Fig. 13.14).

4. Operator introduces left rotation sensing for resistance to left rotation (Fig. 13.15).

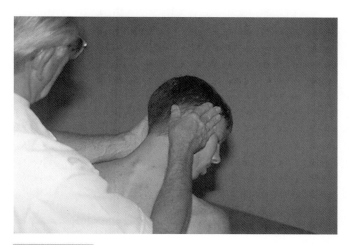

FIGURE 13.14

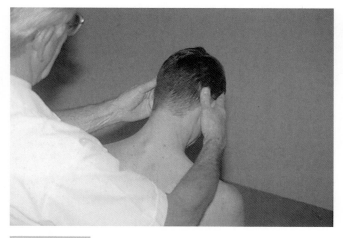

FIGURE 13.13

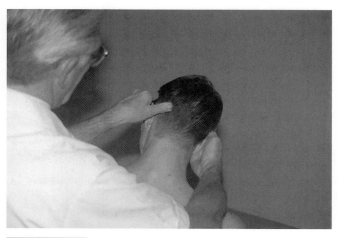

FIGURE 13.15

CERVICAL SPINE DIAGNOSIS

Occipitoatlantal (C0-C1): Sitting

1. Patient sits on the table.

2. Operator stands behind with the thumb and index finger of the right hand grasping the posterior arch of the atlas and the left hand on top of the head to introduce movement.

3. Operator's left hand introduces backward bending, left-side bending, and right rotation of the head sensing for prominent fullness under the right thumb indicating posterior rotation of the atlas on the left (Fig. 13.16).

4. Operator's left hand introduces backward bending, right-side bending, and left rotation of the head and monitors for prominence of the right posterior arch of the atlas under the right index finger, indicative of right rotation of the atlas (Fig. 13.17).

5. Operator introduces forward bending, right-side bending, and left rotation with the left hand while monitoring for prominence of the right posterior arch of the atlas under the right index finger, indicating atlas right rotation (Fig. 13.18).

6. Operator introduces forward bending, left-side bending, and right rotation of the head with the left hand while monitoring for prominence of the left posterior arch of the atlas under the right thumb, indicating left rotation of the atlas (Fig. 13.19).

Note: The right thumb and the index finger assess the rotation of the atlas in relation to the induced rotation of the occiput and not in relation to the coronal plane.

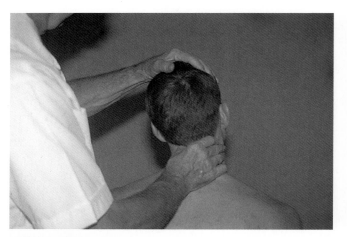

FIGURE 13.16

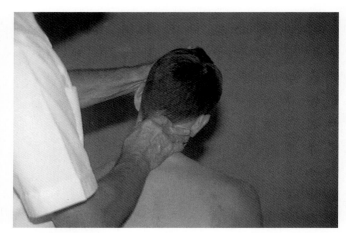

FIGURE 13.18

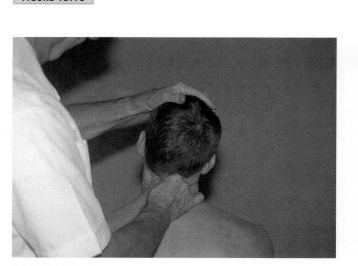

FIGURE 13.17

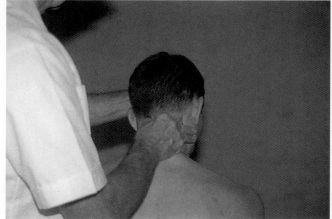

FIGURE 13.19

CERVICAL SPINE DIAGNOSIS

In the absence of dysfunction, side bending of the *typical cervical spine* to the right allows the right facet to close and the left to open. Side bending to the left allows the left facet to close and the right facet to open. In determining if a facet can close, one would bias the paired facets into extension by translating the vertebral segment anteriorly. From there, translating that segment from right to left further tests the right side's ability to close; translating that segment from left to right further tests the left side's ability to close. In determining if a facet can open, one would bias the paired facets into flexion by translating the vertebral segment posteriorly. From there, translating that segment from right to left further tests the left side's ability to open; translating that segment from left to right further tests the right side's ability to open.

Typical Cervical Segments (C3-C7) Supine for Flexed, Rotated, and Side-Bent Dysfunction

1. Patient is supine on the table with the operator sitting at the head of the table.

2. Operator's index and middle fingers of each hand contact the pillar of the superior vertebra of the motion segment being tested (Fig. 13.20).

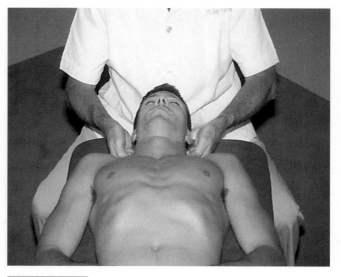

FIGURE 13.20

3. Operator's palms and thenar eminences control the patient's head and upper cervical spine (Fig. 13.21).

4. Operator's finger contacts translate the vertebra anteriorly to the backward-bending barrier (lift the fingers toward the ceiling) (Fig. 13.22).

5. With the palm and the thenar eminence controlling the patient's head and upper cervical, the operator introduces translation from right to left, sensing for resistance to movement at his index fingers (Fig. 13.23). If resistance is encountered, the motion restriction is backward bending, right-side bending, and right rotation (flexed, rotated, and side bent left [FRS$_{left}$]). Something interfered with the capacity of the right facet to close.

6. With the palm and the thenar eminence controlling the patient's head and upper cervical, the operator introduces translatory movement from left to right sensing for resistance to movement at his index fingers (Fig. 13.24). If resistance is encountered, the motion restriction is backward bending, left-side bending, and left rotation (FRS$_{right}$). Something interfered with the left facet to close.

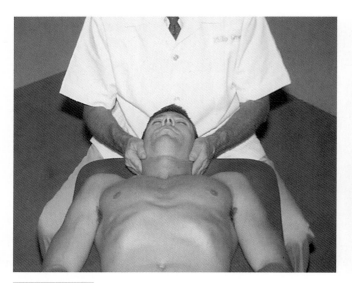

FIGURE 13.21

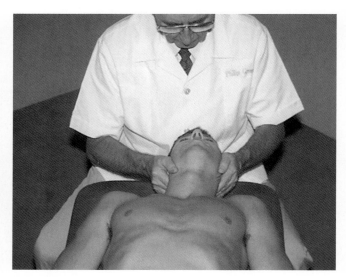

FIGURE 13.23

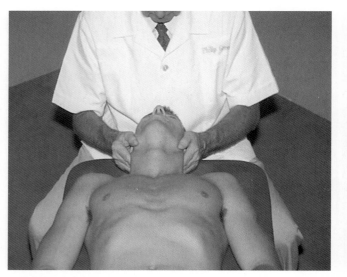

FIGURE 13.22

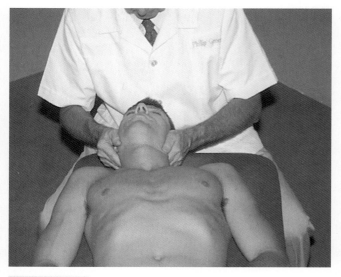

FIGURE 13.24

CERVICAL SPINE DIAGNOSIS

Typical Cervical Segment (C3-C7) Supine for Extended, Rotated, and Side-Bent Dysfunction

1. Patient is supine on the table with the operator sitting at the head of the table.

2. Operator's index and middle fingers of each hand contact the pillar of the superior vertebra of the motion segment being tested (Fig. 13.20).

3. Operator's palms and thenar eminences control the patient's head and upper cervical spine (Fig. 13.21).

4. Operator flexes the head and neck down to the segment under examination (Fig. 13.25).

5. With the palm and the thenar eminence controlling the patient's head and upper cervical, the operator introduces translation from right to left, sensing for resistance to movement at his index fingers (Fig. 13.26). If resistance is felt, the motion restriction is forward bending, right-side bending, and right rotation (extended, rotated, and side bent left [ERS$_{left}$]). Something has interfered with the capacity of the left facet to open.

6. With the palm and the thenar eminence controlling the patient's head and upper cervical, the operator introduces translation from left to right sensing for resistance to movement at his index fingers (Fig. 13.27). If resistance is encountered, the motion restriction is forward bending, left-side bending, and left rotation (ERS$_{right}$). Something interfered with the capacity of the right facet to open.

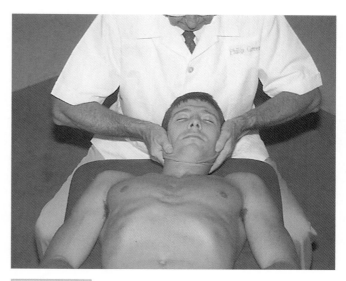

FIGURE 13.26

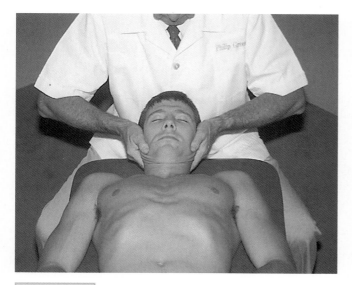

FIGURE 13.25

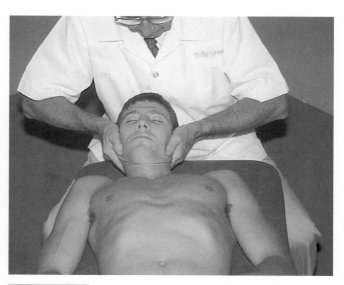

FIGURE 13.27

CERVICAL SPINE DIAGNOSIS

Atlantoaxial (C1-C2): Supine

1. Patient is supine on the table with the operator standing (or sitting) at the head of the table.

2. Operator's hands hold each side of the patient's head with index fingers monitoring the posterior arch of the atlas. The operator flexes the patient's head and neck to provide restriction of typical cervical segment rotation through ligamentous locking (Fig. 13.28).

3. Operator's hands introduce right rotation sensing for resistance to movement at his index fingers (Fig. 13.29). If resistance is encountered, the motion restriction is right rotation (atlas rotated left).

4. Operator rotates the head to the left sensing for resistance to movement at his index fingers (Fig. 13.30). If resistance is encountered, the motion restriction is left rotation (atlas rotated right).

Note: Neck flexion must be maintained throughout the procedure. Do not allow the head and the neck to go into backward bending during the rotation effort.

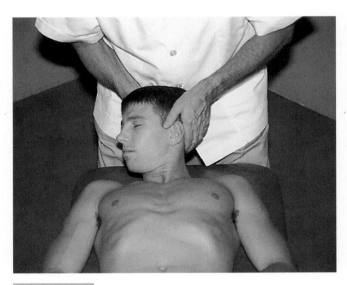

FIGURE 13.29

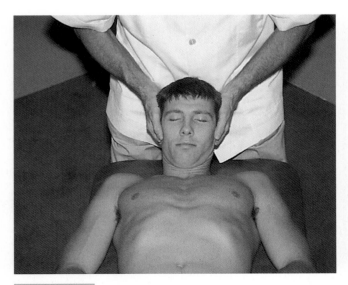

FIGURE 13.28

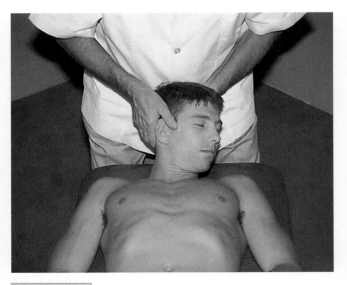

FIGURE 13.30

CERVICAL SPINE DIAGNOSIS

In the absence of dysfunction, side bending the occiput to the right (right-to-left translation) onto the superior articular facet of C1 causes the right condyle to glide anteriorly (extend) on C1 and the left condyle to glide posteriorly (flex) on C1. In determining if the condyles can symmetrically glide anterior or extend, one would bias the occiput into extension by translating the condyles anteriorly on the superior articular facets of C1 (backward bending). From there, side bending the occiput to the right further tests the right side's ability to extend; side bending the occiput to the left (left to right translation) further tests the left side's ability to extend. In determining if the condyles can symmetrically glide posterior or flex, one would bias the occiput into flexion by translating the condyles posteriorly on the superior articular facets of C1 (forward bending). From there, side bending the occiput to the right further tests the left side's ability to flex; side bending the left further tests the right side's ability to flex.

Occipitoatlantal (C0-C1), Supine Extension Restriction

1. Patient is supine on the table with the operator sitting at the head of the table.

2. Operator's hands grasp the sides of the patient's head with the lateral aspect of the index fingers monitoring along the posterior arch of the atlas and the rest of each hand controlling the head.

3. Operator introduces backward bending to the first barrier by rolling the head posteriorly around an axis of rotation through the external auditory meatus (Fig. 13.31).

4. Using the hands, the operator introduces translation of the head from right to left, maintaining the eyes parallel to the head of the table sensing for resistance to movement at his index fingers (Fig. 13.32). If resistance is felt, motion restriction is backward bending, right-side bending, and left rotation (C0 flexed [F], side bent left [S_{left}], and rotated right [R_{right}]). Something interfered with the right condyle gliding forward.

5. Using the hands, the operator introduces translation from left to right sensing for resistance to movement at his index fingers (Fig. 13.33). If resistance is encountered, the motion restriction is backward bending, left-side bending, and right rotation ($FS_{right}R_{left}$). Something interfered with the left condyle to glide forward.

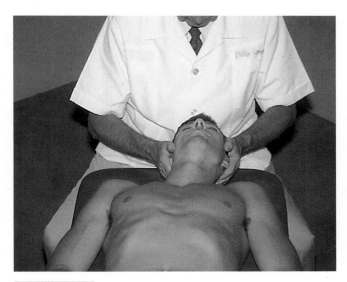

FIGURE 13.32

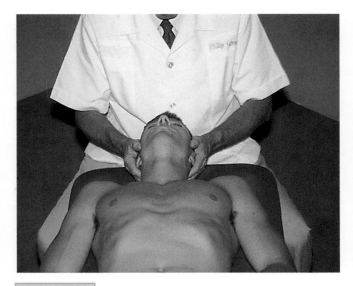

FIGURE 13.31

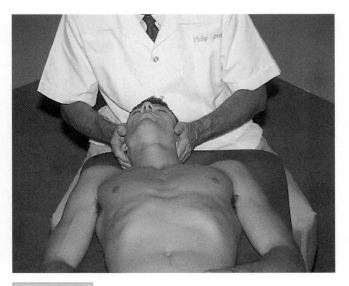

FIGURE 13.33

CERVICAL SPINE DIAGNOSIS

Occipitoatlantal (C0-C1), Supine for Flexion Restriction

1. Patient is supine on the table with the operator sitting at the head of the table.

2. Operator's hands grasp the sides of the patient's head with the lateral aspect of the index fingers monitoring along the posterior arch of the atlas and the rest of each hand controlling the head.

3. Operator forward bends the patient's head by anterior rotation around an axis through the external auditory meatus while monitoring for the first movement of the atlas (Fig. 13.34).

4. Using the hands, the operator introduces translation from right to left sensing for resistance to movement at his index fingers (Fig 13.35). If resistance is felt, the motion restriction is forward bending, right-side bending, and left rotation ($ES_{left}R_{right}$). Something interfered with the left condyle's ability to glide posteriorly.

5. Using the hands, the operator introduces translation from left to right sensing for resistance to movement at his index fingers (Fig. 13.36). If resistance is encountered, the motion restriction is of forward bending, left-side bending, and right rotation ($ES_{right}R_{left}$). Something interfered with the right condyle's ability to glide posteriorly.

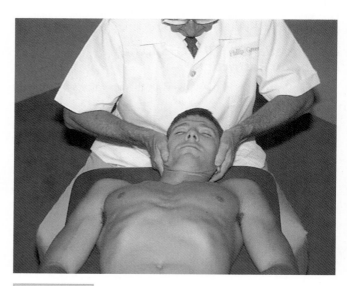

FIGURE 13.35

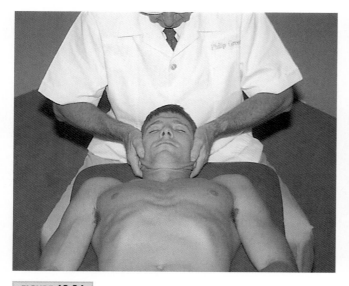

FIGURE 13.34

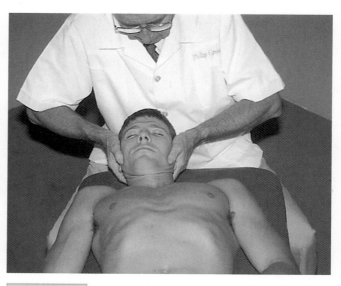

FIGURE 13.36

CERVICAL SPINE DIAGNOSIS

The articular structures of C0-C1 are unique; relative to the AP or sagittal plane, the anterior aspect of the articulating surface sits 30 degrees medial to the posterior aspect of the articular surface. Turning the occiput and C1 to the right 30 degrees places the right C0-C1 articular surface parallel to the AP plane (Fig. 13.37). Turning the occiput and C1 to the left 30 degrees places the left C0-C1 articular surface parallel to the AP plane (Fig. 13.38).

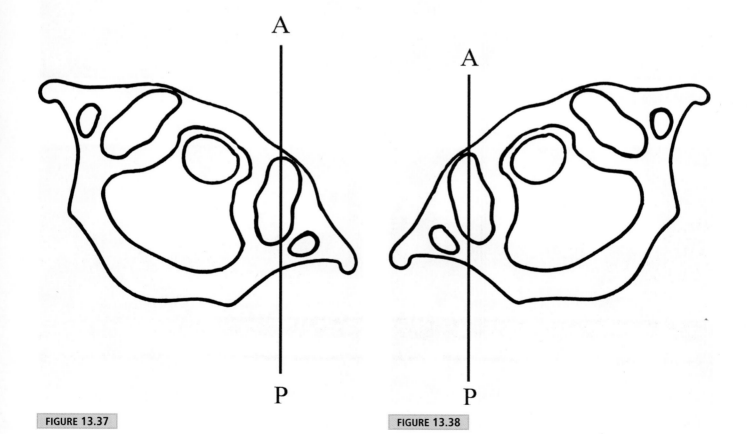

FIGURE 13.37

FIGURE 13.38

Occipitoatlantal (C0-C1) Supine Condylar Glide

Accuracy in assessing condylar glide restriction is dependent upon first biasing the condyles, anteriorly or posteriorly, into the direction which is being assessed.

1. Patient is supine on the table with the operator sitting at the head of the table.

2. Operator grasps the sides of the head with each hand and biases the condyles anteriorly by rotating the head posteriorly around an axis through the external auditory meatus while monitoring for the first movement of the atlas (Fig. 13.39).

3. Operator then rotates the head 30 degrees to the right (Fig. 13.40).

4. Operator introduces anterior translatory movement of the head, asking the right condyle to glide anteriorly while sensing for resistance (Fig. 13.41).

5. Operator rotates the head 30 degrees to the left (Fig. 13.42).

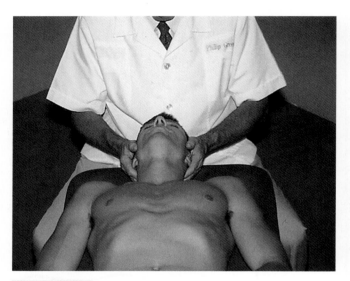

FIGURE 13.39

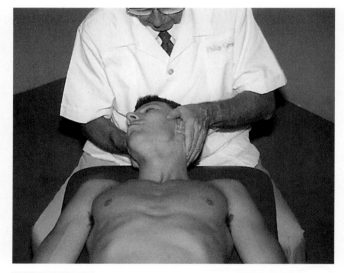

FIGURE 13.41

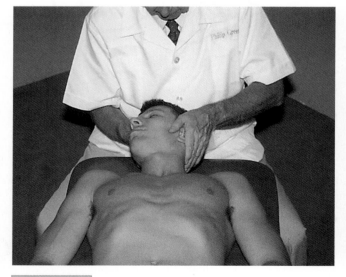

FIGURE 13.40

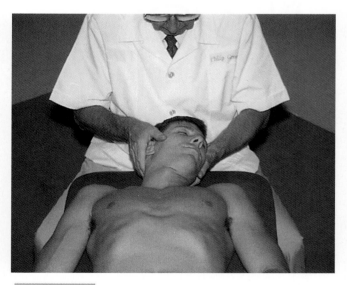

FIGURE 13.42

6. Operator introduces anterior translatory movement of the head, asking the left condyle to glide anteriorly while sensing for resistance (Fig. 13.43).

7. Operator grasps the sides of the head with each hand and biases the condyles posteriorly by rotating the head anteriorly around an axis through the external auditory meatus while monitoring for the first movement of the atlas (Fig. 13.44).

8. Operator then rotates the head 30 degrees to the right (Fig. 13.45).

9. Operator introduces posterior translation of the head, asking the right condyle to glide posteriorly while sensing for resistance to movement (Fig. 13.46).

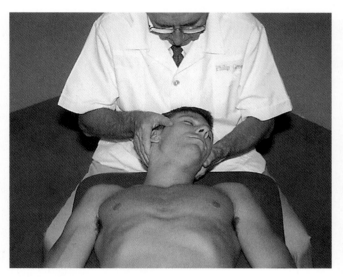

FIGURE 13.43

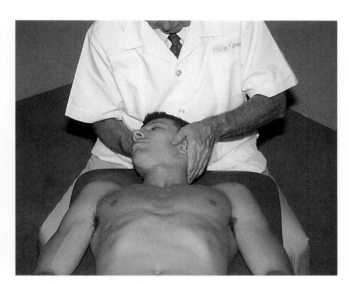

FIGURE 13.45

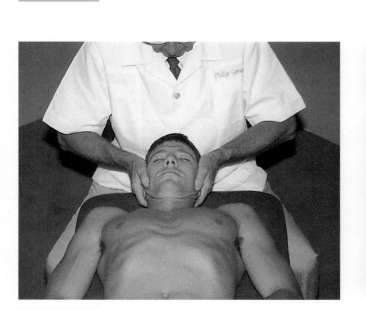

FIGURE 13.44

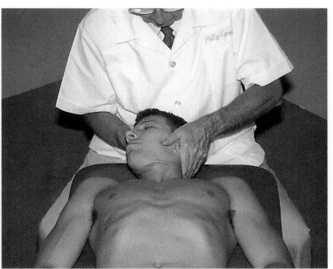

FIGURE 13.46

10. Operator rotates the head 30 degrees to the left (Fig. 13.47).

11. Operator introduces posterior translation of the head, asking the left condyle to glide posteriorly while sensing for resistance to movement (Fig. 13.48).

Note: This tests for the forward-bending and backward-bending capacity of each condyle. If resistance is encountered, there will be restriction of the side-bending and rotational motion coupled to opposite sides (the minor movements). Most often, a condyle will resist posterior glide or flexion, if this were true on the right, C0-C1 would be documented as extended right, side bent, and left rotated ($ES_{left}R_{right}$).

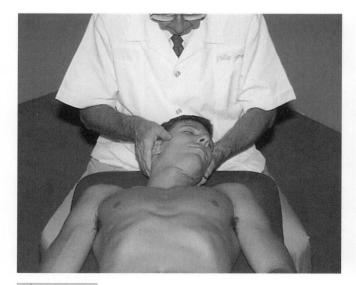

FIGURE 13.47

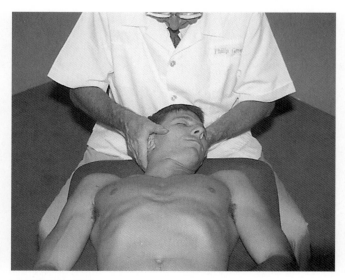

FIGURE 13.48

CERVICAL SPINE DIAGNOSIS
Stress Tests of the Upper Cervical Complex

The upper cervical complex is subject to fracture, dislocation, and ligamentous damage after trauma. Concern for fracture and dislocation is uncommon in the practice of manual medicine. Ligamentous damage may well be of concern to the manual medicine practitioner. The preceding diagnostic tests are most valuable for determining hypomobility as the result of somatic dysfunction. Early hypermobility is much more difficult to assess. Stress testing of the craniocervical junction is difficult to interpret. If the preceding diagnostic tests for the occipitoatlantal and atlantoaxial joints have full range and asymmetric loose end feel, the index of suspicion should go up for hypermobility due to ligamentous laxity.

This author uses two stress tests of the many available. The first is an anteroposterior stress of upper cervical complex: In the supine position, the operator holds the occiput (Fig. 13.49) and anteriorly translates the atlas and axis, sensing for mobility (Fig. 13.50). The thumbs are then placed on the anterior aspect of the transverse processes of the atlas and the axis, and a posterior translatory force is applied (Fig. 13.51). Abnormal anterior to posterior translatory movement may indicate some laxity of the transaxial ligament. The second test is to monitor the spinous process of C2 of the flexed head (Fig. 13.52) and introduce side bending of the head on the neck (Fig. 13.53). Left-side bending of the occiput should result in immediate left rotation of C2. Then, right-side bending is introduced and right rotation is elicited. Should this side bending be asymmetric or delayed, the possibility of alar ligament damage should be suspected.

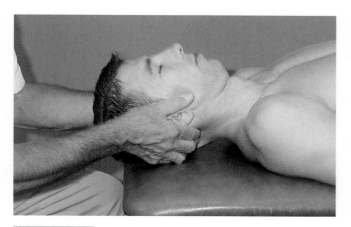

FIGURE 13.49

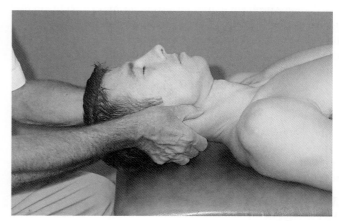

FIGURE 13.51

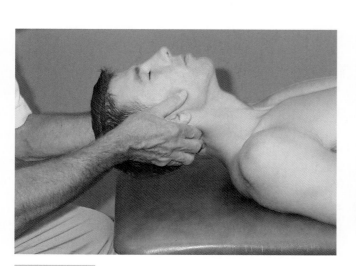

FIGURE 13.50

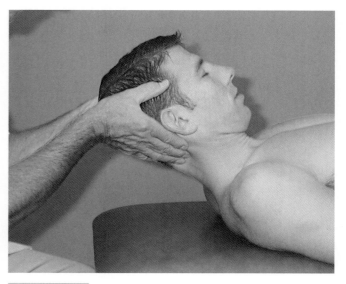

FIGURE 13.52

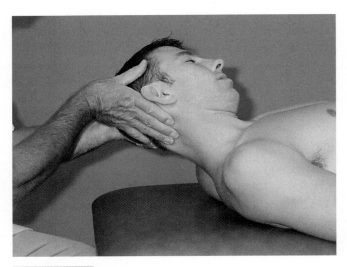

FIGURE 13.53

A major problem in motion testing for hypermobility in this region is that it may be compensatory for restricted motion in other areas of the upper cervical complex. Is the side of restriction hypomobile or is the hypermobility truly due to ligamentous damage?

If there is any question of significant ligamentous damage, it can be further evaluated by rotational stress films of the upper cervical complex using either computed tomography or MRI technology. Axial views in the right and left rotated positions provide the opportunity to assess segmental mobility and its symmetry. The MRI technology is somewhat more valuable for identifying the status of individual ligaments.

MANUAL MEDICINE THERAPEUTIC PROCEDURES

The following procedures are all direct action as they directly engage the restrictive barrier. The two activating forces will be muscle energy technique, an intrinsic activating force, and

mobilization with impulse technique, with an extrinsic activating force. The muscle energy techniques are performed initially because most of the somatic dysfunctions found within the cervical spine respond well. It is in those patients for whom muscle energy is not effective in maximizing motion that consideration should be given to the use of the mobilization with impulse technique. When the diagnostic process identifies what seems to be a deep articular or periarticular restriction, the mobilization with impulse techniques appear to be most effective.

It is recommended that the treatment sequence begin in the lower cervical spine and move upward toward the craniocervical junction. One reason is that this provides easier and more accurate diagnosis of the superior segment on the inferior throughout the diagnostic process. It is not uncommon for several typical cervical segments to demonstrate stacked nonneutral dysfunction that need to be addressed individually. The goal of any manual medicine intervention is to balance the occiput on the vertebral column. This use of the biomechanical model would suggest that the craniooccipital junction be the last treated after balancing the system below. One major exception to this rule is to approach the most restricted segment first in order to influence the system to the maximum. However, if the most restricted area is also the most acute, the practitioner might wish to work around the acute area to remove related restrictors and decongest the acute inflammatory process. In acute conditions of the cervical spine, functional (indirect) technique is the treatment of choice (see Chapter 10). Recurrent dysfunctions in the upper cervical complex and/or the craniooccipital junction imply that the primary dysfunction is in the osseous cranium.

When the diagnostic procedure reveals that several of the typical cervical segments resist translation in the same direction, the probability is high that there is asymmetric hypertonicity of the scalene muscles resulting in a long restrictor to cervical motion. Unilateral right scalene tightness is quite common and may cause the lower cervical segments to behave like stacked ERS_{left} dysfunctions or a neutral group dysfunction. The tight scalenus should be manually stretched before additional diagnosis or treatment is made to the cervical spine.

CERVICAL SPINE SCALENE MUSCLE STRETCH

1. Operator sits at the head of the table with the patient supine and the head and neck over the end of the table.

2. Operator cradles the patient's head with the left hand supporting the occiput and the upper cervical spine and the forehead in the operator's axilla (Fig. 13.54). Operator's right hand stabilizes the patient's right thoracic inlet, particularly the right first and second ribs.

3. Operator translates the head posteriorly (Fig. 13.55) to the barrier and resists patient's anterior translation of the head for 5 to 6 seconds with three to five repetitions. The operator engages a new barrier between patient contractions.

4. Occasionally, it is useful to use a series of right-side bending efforts as well as anterior translation.

5. Comparison is made with the other side and stretching is continued to symmetry.

Note: The head and upper cervical spines are not placed in extension by posterior rotation but by posterior translation. This protects the vertebral artery from the risk of acute extension of the upper cervical complex.

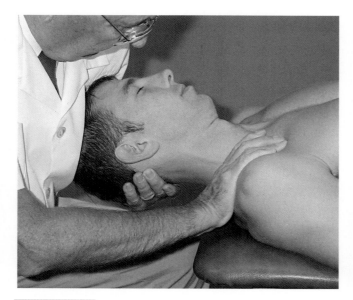

FIGURE 13.54

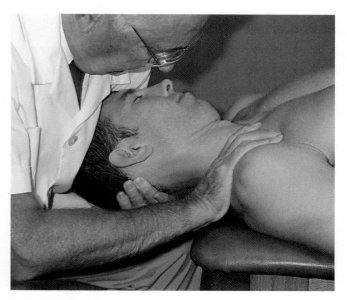

FIGURE 13.55

CERVICAL SPINE MUSCLE ENERGY TECHNIQUE

Typical Cervical Vertebra (C5-C6)

Diagnosis

Position: Flexed, rotated left, and side bend left (FRS$_{left}$)

Motion Restriction: Extension, right rotation, and right-side bending (ERS$_{right}$)

1. Patient is supine on the table with the operator sitting at the head.

2. Operator's fingertips of the right index and the middle finger are placed on the right articular pillar of C6 to hold the segment so that C5 can be moved upon it (Fig. 13.56).

3. Operator's left hand controls the left side of the patient's head and neck (Fig. 13.57).

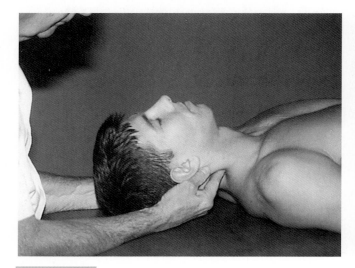

FIGURE 13.56

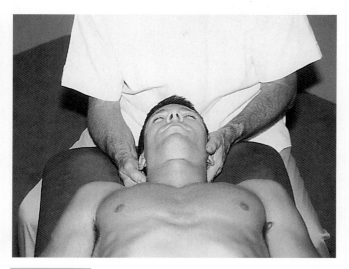

FIGURE 13.57

4. Operator's right fingers translate the segment anteriorly introducing motion to the backward-bending barrier (Fig. 13.58).

5. Operator's left hand introduces side bending and rotation of the head and neck to the right by right-to-left translation engaging the right rotation and the right-side bending barriers (Fig. 13.59).

6. Patient exerts a small isometric effort against the operator's resisting left hand into forward bending, left-side bending, or left rotation.

7. After a 3- to 5-second muscle effort, the patient relaxes and the operator increases translatory movement in an anterior and a right-to-left direction engaging the backward-bending, right-side bending, and right-rotation barriers (Fig. 13.60). The process is repeated three to five times.

8. Retest.

Note: Eye movement can be substituted for the activating force with the patient either looking down toward the feet or to the left after each localization.

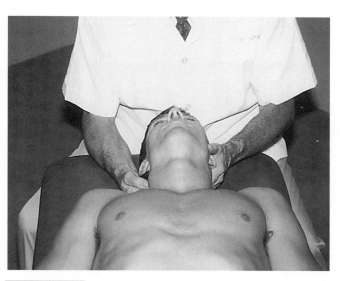

FIGURE 13.59

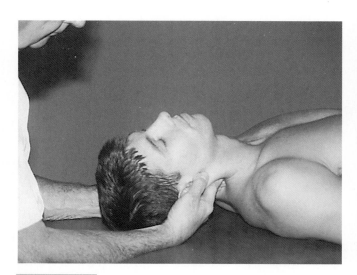

FIGURE 13.58

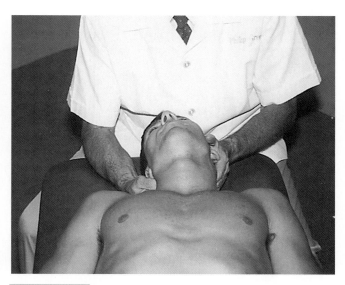

FIGURE 13.60

CERVICAL SPINE MUSCLE ENERGY TREATMENT

Typical Cervical Vertebra (Example: C2-C3)

Diagnosis

Position: Extended, left-side bent, and left rotated (ERS_{left})

Motion Restriction: Forward bending, rotation right, and side bending right

1. Patient is supine on the table with the operator sitting at the head.

2. Operator's left hand supports the occiput with the left thumb over the left C2-C3 zygapophysial joint and the left index finger blocking the right C2-C3 zygapophysial joint (Fig. 13.61).

3. Operator's right hand is placed on the patient's right frontoparietal region to control head movement (Fig. 13.62).

4. Operator's two hands roll the head and the upper neck into forward bending as far as the C2-C3 interspace (Fig. 13.63).

5. Operator introduces right-side bending and right rotation by right-to-left translation through the left index finger contact on the right zygapophysial joint of C2-C3, engaging the flexion, right-side bending, and right-rotation restriction (Fig. 13.64).

6. Patient exerts a 3- to 5-second isometric contraction into backward bending, left-side bending, or left rotation. Following relaxation, the operator engages the new flexion, right-side bending, and right-rotational barriers, and the isometric contractions are repeated three to five times.

7. Retest.

Note: Eye movement can be substituted for the activating force with the patient either looking up toward the eyebrows or to the left after each localization.

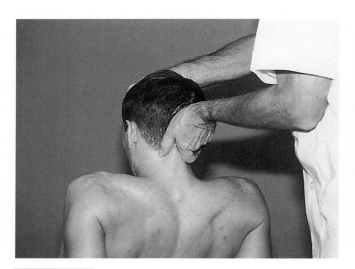

FIGURE 13.61

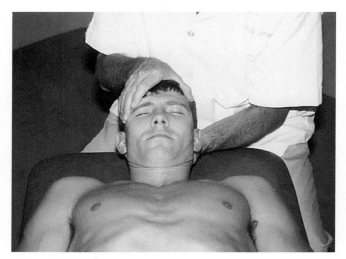

FIGURE 13.63

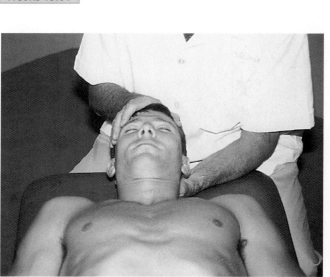

FIGURE 13.62

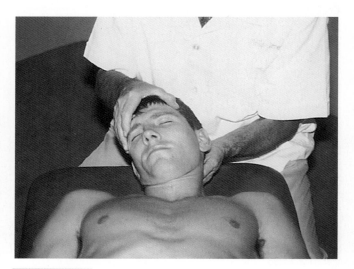

FIGURE 13.64

CERVICAL SPINE MUSCLE ENERGY TECHNIQUE

Atlantoaxial (C1-C2)

Diagnosis

Position: Atlas rotated right

Motion Restriction: Atlas resists left rotation on axis

1. Patient is supine on the table with the operator sitting or standing at the head.
2. Operator grasps the head with the palms of the hands and flexes the head to approximately 30 to 45 degrees (Fig. 13.65).
3. Operator introduces left rotation against the restricted barrier (Fig. 13.66).

4. Patient is instructed to turn the head to the right against the operator's resisting right hand with a light isometric contraction.
5. Following a 3- to 5-second contraction and subsequent relaxation, the operator increases left rotation to the next resistant barrier.
6. Patient repeats right rotational effort against resistance three to five times.
7. Retest.

Note: Eye movement activating force is looking to the right.

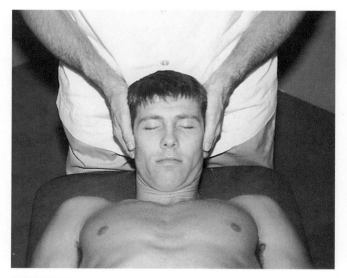

FIGURE 13.65

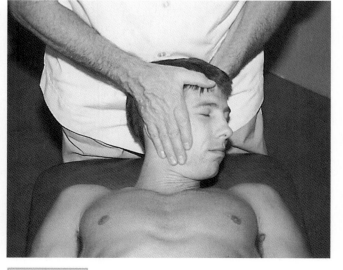

FIGURE 13.66

CERVICAL SPINE MUSCLE ENERGY TECHNIQUE

Occipitoatlantal (C0-C1)

Diagnosis

Position: $FS_{right}R_{left}$

Motion Restriction: Backward bending, left-side bending, and right rotation

1. Patient is supine on the table with the operator sitting or standing at the head.

2. Operator's left hand controls the patient's occiput with the web of the thumb and the index finger along the soft tissues at the cervicocranial junction (Fig. 13.67).

3. Operator's right hand holds the patient's chin with the index finger in front and the middle finger below the tip of the ramus and with the right forearm in contact with the right side of the patient's head (Fig. 13.68).

4. The backward-bending barrier is engaged by the operator's hands rotating the head posteriorly around a transverse axis through the external auditory meatus (Fig. 13.69).

5. Left-side bending is introduced through the operator's right forearm by slight left-to-right translation (Fig. 13.70).

   Note: Rotation is not actively introduced.

6. The patient is instructed to look down at the feet or pull the chin toward the chest against resistance offered by the operator's right hand for a 3- to 5-second light isometric muscle contraction.

7. After relaxation, the new backward-bending, left-side bending, and right-rotational barriers are engaged.

8. Operator's muscle contraction is repeated three to five times with the operator relocalizing against the resisted barrier after each effort.

9. Retest.

Note: The eye movement of looking toward the feet is usually a sufficient force for correction of this dysfunction.

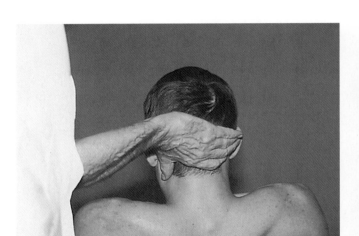

FIGURE 13.67

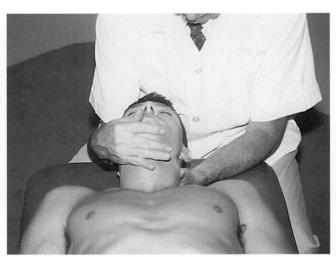

FIGURE 13.69

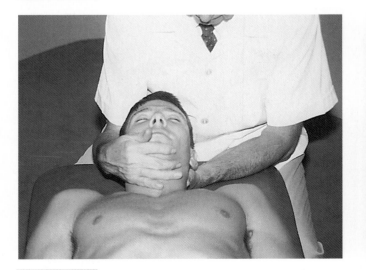

FIGURE 13.68

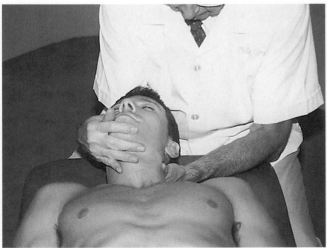

FIGURE 13.70

CERVICAL SPINE MUSCLE ENERGY TECHNIQUE

Occipitoatlantal (C0-C1)

Diagnosis

Position: ES$_{right}$R$_{left}$

Motion Restriction: Forward bending, left-side bending, and right rotation

1. Patient is supine on the table with the operator sitting or standing at the head.

2. Operator's left hand controls the occiput with the web of the thumb and the index finger along the soft tissue of the suboccipital area (Fig. 13.71).

3. The operator's right hand cups the chin with the index finger in front and the middle finger below the tip of the ramus. The operator's right forearm is placed along the right side of the patient's head (Fig. 13.72).

4. Forward bending is introduced by rotating the head forward by the operator's hands around a transverse axis through the external auditory meatus (Fig. 13.73).

5. Left-side bending and right rotation are introduced by the operator's right forearm and with slight left-to-right translation of the patient's head to engage the restrictive barrier (Fig. 13.74).

Note: Right rotation is not actively introduced.

6. Patient instruction is to push the head directly posterior toward the table into the hand offering resistance for 3 to 5 seconds of a mild isometric muscle contraction.

7. After relaxation, the operator engages the forward-bending, left-side bending, and right-rotational barriers.

8. Patient repeats the isometric contractions three to five times.

9. Retest.

Note: An eye motion activating force is to look up toward the operator or toward the eyebrows.

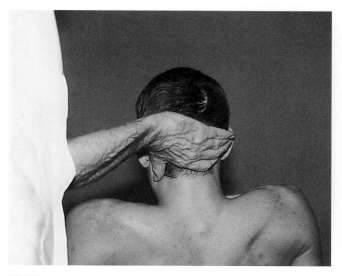

FIGURE 13.71

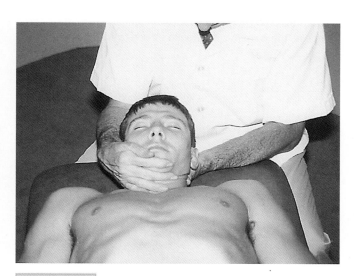

FIGURE 13.73

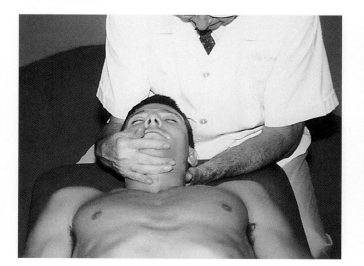

FIGURE 13.72

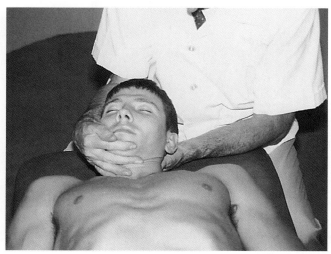

FIGURE 13.74

CERVICAL SPINE MUSCLE ENERGY TECHNIQUE

Occipitoatlantal (C0-C1)

1. Patient is supine on the table with the operator sitting at the head.

2. Operator's left thumb and index finger grasp the posterior arch of the atlas, and the occiput lies in the palm of the operator's left hand (Fig. 13.75).

3. Operator's right hand spans the frontal region of the patient's head.

4. For a dysfunction that resists forward bending, left-side bending, and right rotation ($ES_{right}R_{left}$), the operator rolls the head into forward bending and with the right hand introduces left-side bending and right rotation against the resistance of the atlas held by the operator's left hand (Fig. 13.76).

5. A 3- to 5-second slight, mild isometric contraction of the head into backward bending or right-side bending is resisted by the operator's hands.

6. After relaxation, the new barriers are engaged and the patient repeats the isometric contraction three to five times.

7. Retest.

8. For a dysfunction showing restriction of backward bending, right-side bending, and left rotation, the operator introduces backward bending through rotation, side bending to the right, and rotation to the left with the right hand (Fig. 13.77).

9. Patient provides a mild isometric contraction in the directions of forward bending or left-side bending against resistance offered by the operator's right hand and against the atlas stabilized by the operator's left hand.

10. After relaxation, the new backward-bending (extension), right-side bending, and left-rotation barriers are engaged, and the patient repeats the isometric contraction three to five times.

11. Retest.

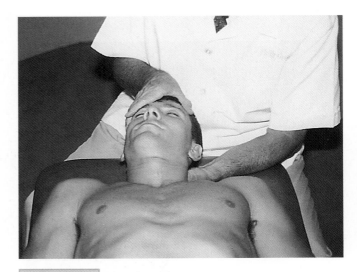

FIGURE 13.76

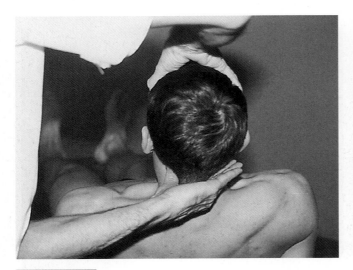

FIGURE 13.75

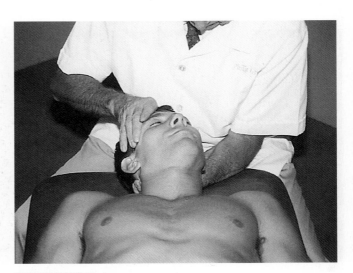

FIGURE 13.77

CERVICAL SPINE MOBILIZATION WITH IMPULSE TECHNIQUE

Typical Cervical Vertebra (Example: C5-C6)

Diagnosis

Position: FRS$_{left}$

Motion Restriction: Extension, right rotation, and right-side bending

1. Patient is supine on the table with the operator sitting or standing at the head.

2. Operator's left hand controls the left side of the patient's head and proximal neck.

3. Operator's right second proximal interphalangeal or metacarpophalangeal joint contacts the articular pillar of C5 (the superior vertebra of the dysfunctional vertebral motion segment) (Fig. 13.78).

4. Backward bending and right-side bending are introduced to the restricted barrier (Fig. 13.79).

Note: Even though the head is side bent right and rotated left through the upper cervical complex, C5 is rotating right in response to the right-side bending of C5 on C6.

5. A high-velocity, low-amplitude thrust is applied in a caudad direction toward the spinous process of T1 (Fig. 13.80).

6. Retest.

Note: Regardless of which cervical segment is dysfunctional, the thrust is always in the direction of the spinous process of T1.

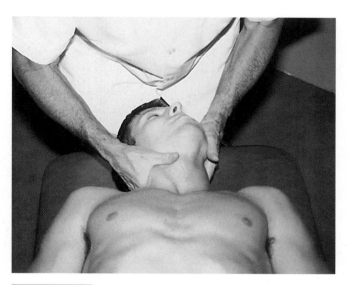

FIGURE 13.79

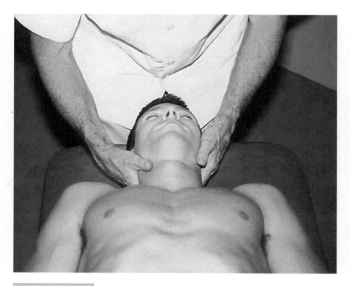

FIGURE 13.78

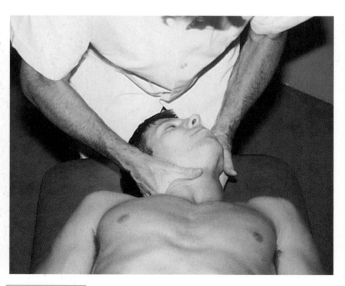

FIGURE 13.80

CERVICAL SPINE MOBILIZATION WITH IMPULSE TECHNIQUE

Example: C2-C3

Diagnosis

Position: ERS$_{left}$

Motion Restriction: Forward bending, right rotation, and right-side bending

Opening facet thrust variation 1

1. Patient is supine with the operator standing at the head of the table.

2. Operator's right second metacarpophalangeal joint contacts the right zygapophysial joint of C2 through C3. The operator's left hand controls the patient's head and neck (Fig. 13.81).

3. The head is flexed and side bent right localizing at C2-C3 (Fig. 13.82).

4. A high-velocity, low-amplitude thrust is applied horizontally in the plane of the involved C2-C3 joint resulting in a "gapping" opening of the left zygapophysial joint (Fig. 13.83).

5. Retest.

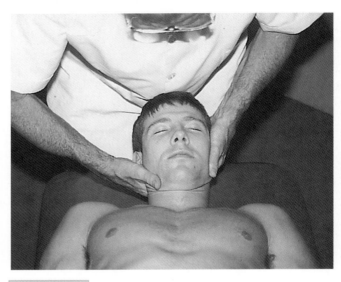

FIGURE 13.82

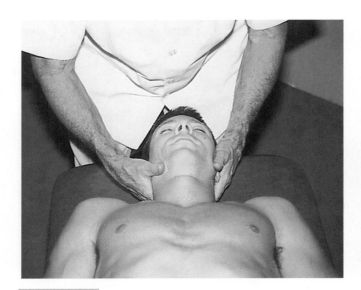

FIGURE 13.81

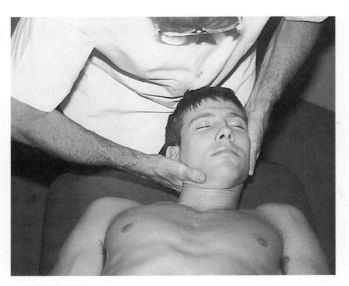

FIGURE 13.83

CERVICAL SPINE MOBILIZATION WITH IMPULSE TECHNIQUE

Typical Cervical Segments (Example: C2-C3)

Diagnosis

Position: ERS_{left}

Motion Restriction: Forward bending, right rotation, and right-side bending

Opening facet thrust variation 2

1. Patient is supine with the operator sitting or standing at the head of the table.

2. Operator controls the head through both hands with the left second metacarpophalangeal joint overlying the left pillar of C2 (Fig. 13.84). The second and third fingers of the operator's right hand contact the right zygapophysial joint of C2-C3 to serve as a blocking pivot (Fig. 13.85).

3. Using both hands, the operator forward bends the head down to the flexion barrier of C2-C3 (Fig. 13.86).

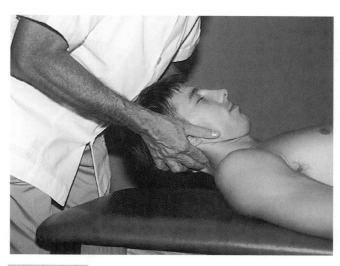

FIGURE 13.85

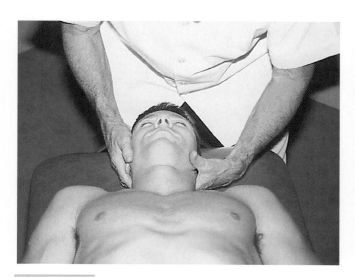

FIGURE 13.84

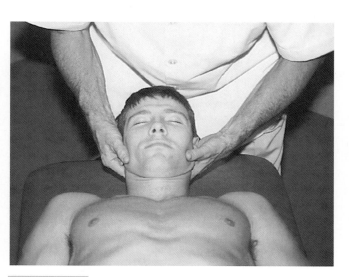

FIGURE 13.86

4. Operator's left hand rotates and right-side bends the patient's head over the fulcrum established by the right second and third fingers to the barrier (Fig. 13.87).

   Note: Be sure to maintain the right-side bending component as the left hand introduces right rotation (Fig. 13.88).

5. A high-velocity, low-amplitude rotary thrust is applied through the operator's left hand by elevating the left elbow toward the ceiling (Fig. 13.89).

6. Retest.

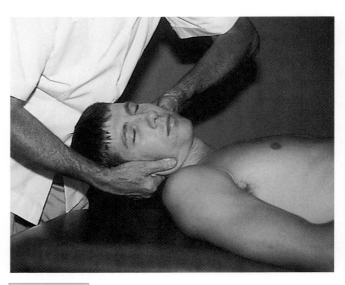

FIGURE 13.88

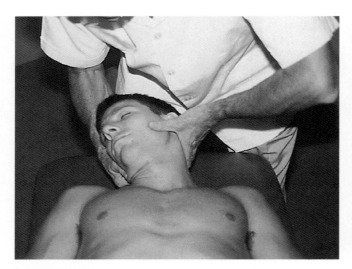

FIGURE 13.87

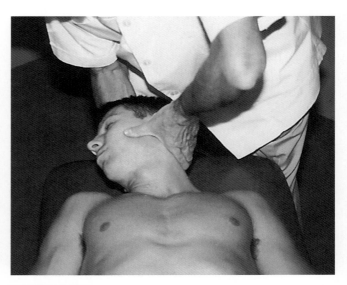

FIGURE 13.89

CERVICAL SPINE MOBILIZATION WITH IMPULSE TECHNIQUE

Atlantoaxial (C1-C2)

Diagnosis

Position: Atlas rotated right

Motion Restriction: Atlas resists left rotation on axis

1. Patient is supine with the operator sitting or standing at the head of the table.

2. Operator's right second metacarpophalangeal joint contacts the right posterior arch of the atlas. The operator's left hand controls the left side of the head and neck.

3. Patient's head is flexed approximately 30 to 45 degrees to take out the flexion mobility of the typical cervical segments below (Fig. 13.90).

4. Operator's hands rotate the atlas to the left to restrictional barrier and fine-tune the forward-bending, backward-bending, and right-side and left-side bending components to maximum ease (Fig. 13.91).

5. A rotary thrust is applied through both hands in a left rotational direction (Fig. 13.92).

6. Retest.

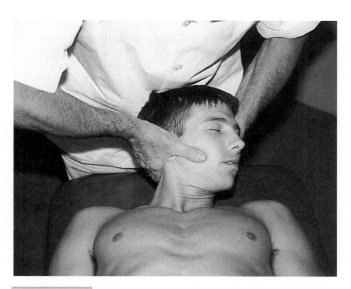

FIGURE 13.91

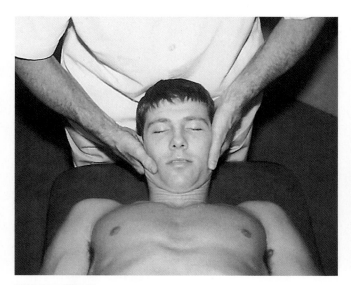

FIGURE 13.90

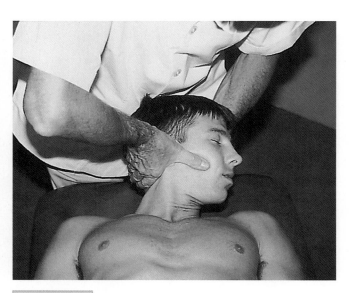

FIGURE 13.92

CERVICAL SPINE MOBILIZATION WITH IMPULSE TECHNIQUE

Occipitoatlantal (C0-C1)

Diagnosis

Position: $FS_{right}R_{left}$

Motion Restriction: Backward bending, left-side bending, and right rotation

1. Patient is supine with the operator sitting at the head of the table.

2. Operator's left hand cradles the occiput between the web of the thumb and the index finger with a bony contact at the suboccipital region. Do not compress the posterior occipitoatlantal membrane (Fig. 13.93).

3. Operator's right hand cradles the patient's chin with the right forearm along the right side of the patient's mandible and temporal regions (Fig. 13.94). Extension is introduced through both hands by posterior rotation around a transverse axis through the external auditory meatus. Left-side bending and right rotation are introduced through the operator's right forearm with a slight left-to-right translation (Fig. 13.95).

Note: Rotation is not actively introduced but follows side bending.

4. When all three barriers are engaged, a high-velocity, low-amplitude thrust is applied through the operator's hands in a cephalic, long-axis extension direction (Fig. 13.96).

Note: The left forearm is caudad to the left hand contact on the occiput for better control of the long-axis extension thrust.

5. Retest.

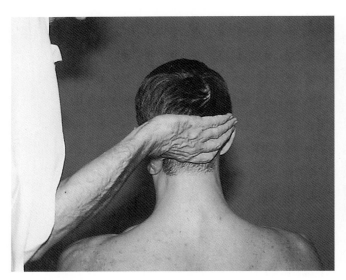

FIGURE 13.93

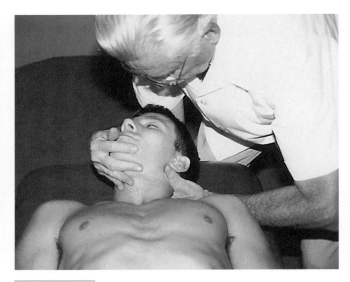

FIGURE 13.95

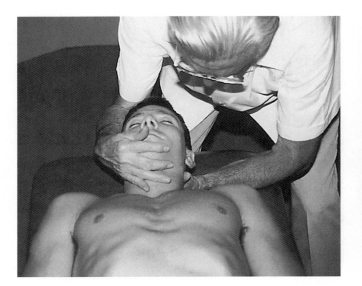

FIGURE 13.94

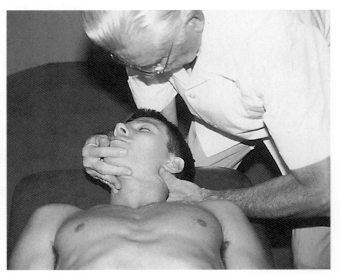

FIGURE 13.96

CERVICAL SPINE MOBILIZATION WITH IMPULSE TECHNIQUE

Occipitoatlantal (C0-C1)

Diagnosis

Position: $ES_{right}R_{left}$

Motion Restriction: Forward bending, left-side bending, and right rotation

1. Patient is supine with the operator sitting or standing at the head of the table.

2. Operator's left hand cradles the occiput with the web of the thumb and index finger on the bone to monitor suboccipital tissue tension. Do not compress the posterior occipitoatlantal membrane (Fig. 13.97).

3. Operator's right hand cradles the patient's chin with the right forearm along the right side of the patient's face and head (Fig. 13.98).

4. Operator introduces forward bending by rotating the head anteriorly around a transverse axis through the external auditory meatus.

5. Left-side bending and right rotation are introduced through the operator's right forearm and slight left-to-right translation (Fig. 13.99).

Note: Right rotation is not actively introduced.

6. When the flexion, left-side bending, and the right-rotational barriers are engaged, a high-velocity, low-amplitude thrust is applied in a cephalic, long-axis extension direction simultaneously by both hands (Fig. 13.100).

Note: The operator's left forearm to the elbow is below the occipital contact giving better control of the long-axis extension thrust.

7. Retest.

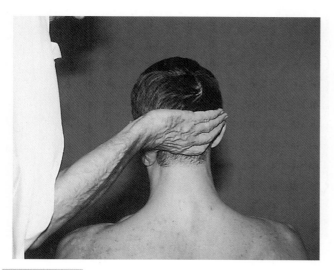

FIGURE 13.97

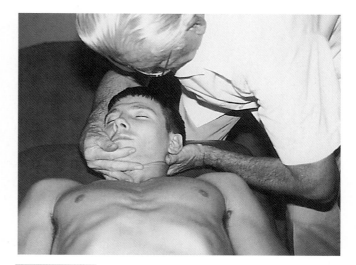

FIGURE 13.99

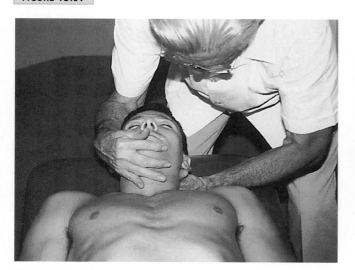

FIGURE 13.98

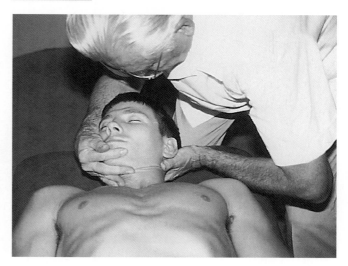

FIGURE 13.100

CERVICAL SPINE COMBINED SOFT-TISSUE INHIBITION AND CRANIOSACRAL CONDYLAR DECOMPRESSION

Cranio-occipital Junction

1. Patient is supine with the operator sitting at the head of the table.

2. Operator cradles the head in both hands with finger pads along the insertion of extensor cervical muscles in the occiput.

3. Flexion of the operator's distal interphalangeal joints place inhibitory pressure against muscle insertion in the occiput (Fig. 13.101).

4. When softening of muscle hypertonicity occurs, the operator places the two middle fingers on each side of the external occipital protuberance (inion) with the heels of the hands together.

5. With the operator's forearms on the table, the middle fingers are moved anteriorly along the bone as forward as possible with contact on the condylar portion of the occipital bone (Fig. 13.102).

6. With flexion of the distal interphalangeal joints of the middle finger putting compressive force on the occipital condylar portion, the elbows are brought together resulting in a posterolateral distraction of each condylar portion of the bone (Fig. 13.103).

7. Operator enhances the amount of compressive force on the condylar portion of the occiput that has less resilience until softening occurs.

8. The goal of the treatment is relaxation of suboccipital muscles and symmetric resiliency of bone in the occipital condylar parts.

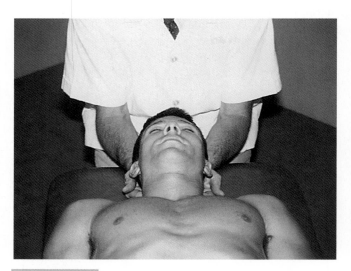

FIGURE 13.102

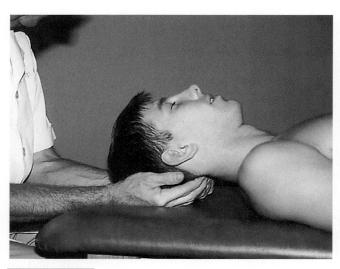

FIGURE 13.101

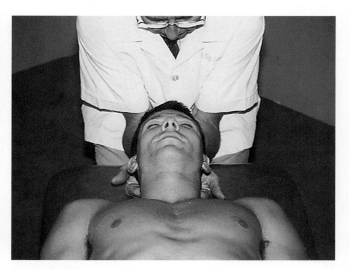

FIGURE 13.103

CONCLUSION

There are a number of structural diagnostic and manual medicine therapeutic interventions for the cervical spine. Only five somatic dysfunctions occur in the cervical spine, namely, flexion or extension restriction with coupled side bending and rotation to the same side in the typical cervical segments, rotational restriction of the atlas on the axis, and either flexion or extension with side bending and rotational restriction to opposite sides at the occipitoatlantal articulation. There are many combinations of these dysfunctions. Remember that the upper cervical complex functions as an integrative unit and dysfunctions of the occipitoatlantal, atlantoaxial, and C2 on C3 are very common. The muscle energy and mobilization with impulse techniques described in this chapter have been most effective and safe in the hands of the author. Mastery of the diagnostic and manual medicine treatment procedures for the cervical spine is useful in managing the myriad of head, neck, and upper extremity problems presenting to the manual medicine practitioner. A thorough understanding of the functional anatomy and biomechanics of the cervical spine is essential for effective and safe manual medicine technique.

REFERENCES

1. Dvorak J, Panjabi MM, Gerber M, et al. CT functional diagnostics of the rotary instability of the upper cervical spine, I: An experimental study on cadavers. *Spine* 1987;12:197–205.
2. Dvorak J, Hayek J, Zehnder R. CT functional diagnostics of the rotary instability of upper cervical spine, II: An evaluation on healthy adults and patients with suspected instability. *Spine* 1987;12:726–731.
3. Jull G. Management of cervical headache. *Man Ther* 1997;2:182–190.
4. Jull G, Bogduk N, Marsland A. The accuracy of manual diagnosis for cervical zygapophyseal joint syndromes. *Med J Austral* 1988;148:233–236.
5. Dvorak J, Orelli F. How dangerous is manipulation on the cervical spine? *Man Med* 1985;2:1–4.
6. Kleynhans AM. Complications of and contraindications to spinal manipulative therapy. In: Patijn J, ed. *Complications in Manual Medicine: A Review of the Literature*; *Man Med* 1991;6:89–92.
7. Haldeman S, ed. *Modern Developments in the Principles and Practice of Chiropractic*. New York: Appleton-Century-Crofts, 1980.
8. Haldeman S, Kohlbeck FJ, McGregor M. Risk factor and precipitating neck movements causing vertebrobasilar artery dissection after cervical trauma and spinal manipulation. *Spine* 1999;24:785–794.
9. Aprill C, Dwyer A, Bogduk N. Cervical zygapophyseal joint pain patterns, II: A clinical evaluation. *Spine* 1990;15:458–461.
10. Zhang J, Chandler MJ, Foreman RD. Cardiopulmonary sympathetic and vagal afferents excite C1–C2 propriospinal cells in rats. *Brain Res* 2003;969:53–58.

Twelve vertebrae constitute the thoracic spine and are noted for their posterior kyphosis. The thoracic spine is intimately related to the rib cage and they essentially work as a single unit. Alteration in the thoracic spine function influences the rib cage, and alteration in the rib cage function alters the thoracic spine. Hence, from the respiratory–circulatory model of manual medicine, the thoracic spine assumes major importance in providing optimal functional capacity to the thoracic cage for respiration and circulation. The thoracic spine takes on additional importance from the neurologic perspective because of the relationship with the sympathetic division of the autonomic nervous system. All 12 segments of the thoracic spinal cord give origin to preganglionic sympathetic nerve fibers, which exit through the intervertebral canals of the thoracic vertebra and either synapse in, or traverse through, the lateral chain sympathetic ganglion lying on the anterior aspect of the costovertebral articulations.

Recall that the preganglionic sympathetic nerve innervation to the soma and viscera above the diaphragm takes origin from the first four to five segments of the thoracic cord. All of the viscera and soma below the diaphragm receive their preganglionic sympathetic nerve fibers from the spinal cord below T5.

Many of the tissue texture abnormalities used in the diagnosis of somatic dysfunction appear to be manifestations of altered secre tomotor, pilomotor, and vasomotor functions of the skin viscera. Because the sympathetic nervous system is segmentally organized, skin viscera and internal viscera share many sympathetic nervous system reflexes. It has been clinically noted that the internal viscera sharing preganglionic innervation origin in the spinal cord with somatic segments demonstrating tissue texture abnormality may be involved in dysfunctional or diseased states.

FUNCTIONAL ANATOMY

The typical thoracic vertebra has a body roughly equal in its transverse and anteroposterior diameters. The vertebral bodies have demifacets, located posterolaterally at the upper and lower margins of the body that articulate with the head of the rib. These demifacets are true arthrodial joints with a capsule and articular cartilage. The posterior arch of the thoracic vertebra has zygapophysial joints on the superior and inferior articular pillars. The superior zygapophysial joints face backward, laterally, and slightly superiorly, and the inferior zygapophysial joints face just the reverse. Theoretically, this facet facing would provide a great deal of rotation to the thoracic vertebra, but rotation is restricted by the attachment of the ribs. The transverse processes are unique with the anterior surface having a small articular facet for articulation with the posterior-facing facet of the

tubercle of the adjacent rib. The relationship of the costovertebral and costotransverse articulations greatly influences the type and amount of rib motion. The posterior aspects of the transverse processes are valuable anatomical landmarks for structural diagnosis of thoracic spine dysfunction. The spinous processes project backward and inferiorly and, in the midportion, are severely shingled one on the other (see rule of 3s, Chapter 5).

Atypical Thoracic Vertebrae

The atypical thoracic vertebrae are those that are transitional between the cervical and thoracic spines, and the thoracic and lumbar spines. T1 has the broadest transverse processes in the thoracic spine and they progressively become narrower from above downward. The lateral portion of the vertebral body of T1 has a unifacet for articulation with the head of the first rib. While the inferior zygapophysial joint facing is typically thoracic, the superior zygapophysial joint facing is transitional from the cervical spine and may have typical cervical characteristics. T1 is also the junction of the change in anteroposterior curve between the cervical and thoracic spines. Dysfunction of T1 profoundly affects the functional capacity of the thoracic inlet and related structures.

T12 is the location of transition to the lumbar spine. The superior zygapophysial joint facing is usually typically thoracic, whereas the inferior zygapophysial joint facing tends toward lumbar characteristics. There is a unifacet on the lateral side of the body for articulation with the twelfth rib. The transverse processes are quite short and rudimentary and are difficult to palpate with certainty. T12 is the location for the change in the anteroposterior curve between the thoracic kyphosis and the lumbar lordosis, a location of change in mobility of two areas of the spine, and a point of frequent dysfunction.

Thoracic Kyphosis

The thoracic kyphosis is normally a smooth posterior convexity without severe areas of increased convexity or "flattening." The observation of "flat spots" within the thoracic kyphosis should alert the diagnostician to evaluate this area carefully for nonneutral, type II, vertebral somatic dysfunction. The thoracic kyphosis changes at its upper and lower extremities (at the transitional zones) to flow into the cervical and lumbar lordoses. Because of this, frequently the upper segments of the thoracic spine are viewed from the perspective of the cervical spine, while the lower thoracic segments are viewed as an extension of the lumbar spine. Many techniques for cervical dysfunction are highly appropriate and effective in the upper thoracic spine, and many lumbar techniques are effective in the lower thoracic spine.

THORACIC SPINE MOTION

Attachment of the ribs through the costovertebral and costotransverse articulations reduces the amount of mobility within the thoracic spine. Thoracic segments have forward-bending and backward-bending movements, as well as coupled movements of side bending and rotation to the same side and to opposite sides. The coupling of side bending and rotation in the thoracic spine is complex. Vertebral coupling depends on many factors, including whether the segments involved are above or below the apex of the thoracic kyphosis and whether you introduce side bending or rotation first. As a rule, if you introduce side bending with the thoracic spine in a neutral kyphosis, rotation occurs to the opposite side following neutral (type I) vertebral motion. If rotation is introduced first in the presence of a normal thoracic kyphosis, side bending and rotation occur to the same side following the rule of nonneutral (type II) vertebral mechanics. T1 through T3 most commonly follow nonneutral vertebral mechanics as a carryover from the lower cervical spine.

Despite the complexity of thoracic spine motion, clinical evaluation identifies that the thoracic spine can become dysfunctional with nonneutral single-segment (type II) dysfunctions and neutral (type I) group dysfunctions. The screening and scanning examinations can lead the examiner to pursue specific segmental diagnosis in the thoracic spine. Identification of the dysfunctional segment begins by palpating soft-tissue change of hypertonicity in the fourth layer of the erector spinae muscle mass in the medial groove between the spinous process and the longissimus. Palpable muscle hypertonicity of the deepest muscle layers including the multifidi and levator costales is pathognomonic of vertebral motion segment dysfunction at that level (Fig. 14.1).

Tissue texture changes of the skin and deeper layers of the posterior thoracic cage reflect the function of the sympathetic division of the autonomic nervous system. The changes include

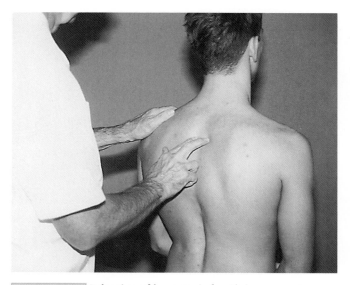

FIGURE 14.1 Palpation of hypertonic fourth-layer muscle.

"skin drag" in areas of increased skin hydration, a "red response" following stroking of the skin from above downward, reflecting change in vasomotor control, coldness or heat, bogginess, and change in thickness. Changes are seen in patients with musculoskeletal dysfunction and those with visceral disease primarily of the respiratory, cardiac, and gastrointestinal systems. It has been shown by studies of skin hydration, water evaporation loss rate, and temperature change that these palpable changes are different from those of a healthy asymptomatic population and differ between those with visceral disease or musculoskeletal disease or dysfunction. Much can be learned from judicious palpation of the soft tissues in addition to active and passive motion testing. Nonneutral dysfunctions within the thoracic spine appear to have an effect on muscle tone of segmentally related muscles, perhaps through an arthrokinetic reflex mechanism. Extended, rotated, and side-bent (ERS) dysfunctions of the midscapular region, particularly several segments stacked one on top of another, appear commonly with weakness of the serratus anterior and rhomboid muscles. Flexed, rotated, and side-bent (FRS) dysfunctions of the lower thoracic spine around T8 are associated with weakness of the lower trapezius muscle, which is essential for normal scapular control.

MOTION TESTING

Vertebral motion testing and the diagnosis of restriction of vertebral motion have been described in Chapter 6. The most useful test is to monitor change in the relationship of pairs of transverse processes through an arc of forward bending to backward bending. In the upper thoracic spine from T1-T5, the operator monitors the behavior of a pair of transverse processes during the introduction of active forward and backward bending of the head on the neck with the patient sitting. With nonneutral (type II) ERS dysfunction, the transverse process on one side will become more prominent during forward bending, and the transverse processes become symmetric during backward bending. In nonneutral (type II) FRS dysfunction, one transverse process becomes more prominent during backward bending, and the transverse processes become symmetric during forward bending. In the presence of a neutral group (type I) dysfunction, three or more vertebrae, the transverse processes are prominent on one side. During the forward-to-backward bending arc, the posterior transverse processes may change a little, but they never become symmetric.

In the mid and lower thoracic spine, the evaluation is performed in the sitting position with the patient assuming the three positions of forward bending, neutral, and backward bending, or in the three static positions of being fully forward bent, prone in neutral on the table, and in backward bending in the prone prop position.

The examiner always relates one pair of transverse processes to the segment below, asking if it is the same or different. As an example, if T8 has restriction of backward bending, left rotation, and left-side bending (FRS$_{right}$), the superior surface of T8 is not level with side bending to the right. When the patient is in the neutral position, the segments above T8 should form a neutral curve with side bending left and rotation right as an adaptive response to maintain the body erect. In the backward-bent body position, and in the absence of dysfunction above T8, all of the superior segments should follow the right rotation of T8 with their respective transverse processes being prominent on the right side. When the patient is in the forward-bent position, T8 becomes level in the coronal plane and all of the nondysfunctional segments above should follow and be straight in the coronal plane.

Structural diagnosis in the presence of a primary structural scoliosis of the thoracic spine becomes quite difficult. The segments involved in a primary scoliosis behave as a neutral group (type I) dysfunction. Patients with a primary structural scoliosis of the thoracic spine have few symptoms of back pain until a relatively minor traumatic episode occurs. Pain and restriction of motion become quite evident. A nonneutral (type II) dysfunction within the primary scoliotic curve is frequently found in this situation. The diagnosis of these nonneutral (type II) dysfunctions can be quite difficult, but if the examiner is diligent in searching from one segment to the other, he or she frequently observes a nonneutral single-segment vertebral somatic dysfunction within the curve. The usual observation is a single vertebral motion segment with rotation into the concavity. Single-segment fourth-layer muscle hypertonicity is a valuable finding in making a diagnosis of the presence and location of a nonneutral dysfunction within the primary curve. The difficulty is to identify a segment that is rotated in the opposite direction of the primary curve. The principle of relating the superior segment to the one below still holds. Also, recall that by convention we speak of the scoliotic curve as being side bent and rotated to opposite sides. This is true for the entire curve in three-dimensional space. When evaluated segment by segment, the rule of side bending and rotation to opposite sides holds below the apex of the curve, but in the segments above the apex, the rotation is to the same side as the curve gradually returns to the midline.

THORACIC SPINE DIAGNOSIS

Upper Thoracic Spine (T1-T5)

1. Patient sits on the table with the operator standing behind.

2. Operator's thumbs palpate the posterior aspect of the transverse processes of the segment under diagnosis (Fig. 14.2).

3. The operator follows the pair of transverse processes during the backward-bending arc as the patient is asked to look up toward the ceiling (Fig. 14.3).

4. The operator follows the pair of transverse processes through a forward-bending arc while asking the patient to look down at the floor (Fig. 14.4).

   Note: It is easier to follow a pair of transverse processes during backward bending than forward bending.

5. Based on the behavior of the transverse processes during the forward-bending, neutral, and backward-bending arcs, an appropriate single-segment vertebral motion somatic dysfunction diagnosis is made.

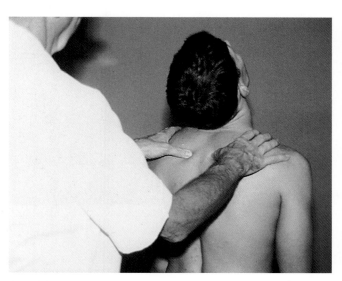

FIGURE 14.3

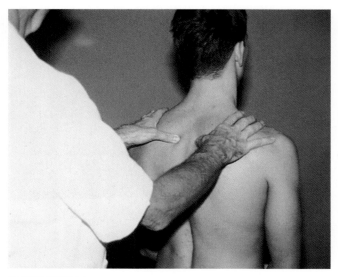

FIGURE 14.2

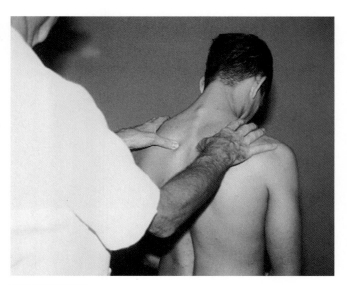

FIGURE 14.4

THORACIC SPINE DIAGNOSIS

Mid to Lower Thoracic Spine

Dynamic Process

1. The patient sits on table with the operator standing behind.

2. The operator palpates the posterior aspect of a pair of transverse processes at the segment under evaluation (Fig. 14.5).

3. Patient is asked to look up at the ceiling and arch the back by pushing the abdomen anteriorly as the operator follows the transverse processes into backward bending (Fig. 14.6).

4. Patient is asked to slump the back and forward bend the trunk as the operator follows the transverse processes into flexion (Fig. 14.7).

5. Operator evaluates the behavior of the transverse processes through the forward- and backward-bending arcs, making a diagnosis of a single-segment vertebral somatic dysfunction of the ERS or FRS type.

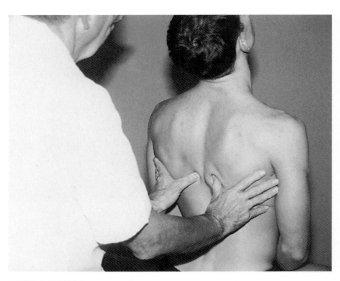

FIGURE 14.6

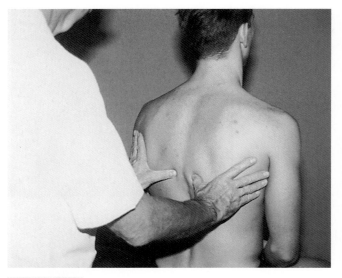

FIGURE 14.5

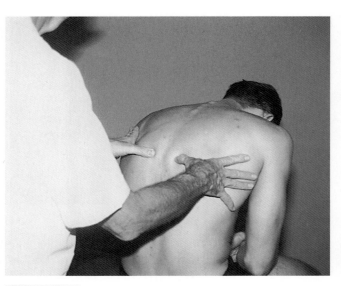

FIGURE 14.7

THORACIC SPINE DIAGNOSIS

Mid to Lower Thoracic Spine

Three Static Positions

1. Patient is prone on the table with the operator standing at the side with thumbs palpating a pair of transverse processes (Fig. 14.8).

2. Operator monitors the posterior aspect of the paired transverse processes in the backward-bent (prone prop) position (Fig. 14.9).

3. Operator evaluates the pair of transverse processes in the static forward-bent position (Fig. 14.7).

4. Evaluation of a single-segment nonneutral vertebral dysfunction is identified by comparing the behavior of the paired transverse processes through the three static positions of neutral, backward bent, and forward bent.

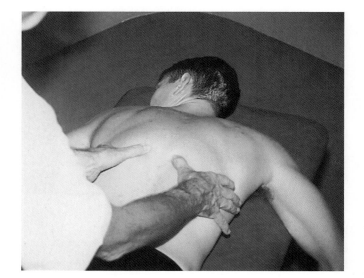

FIGURE 14.8

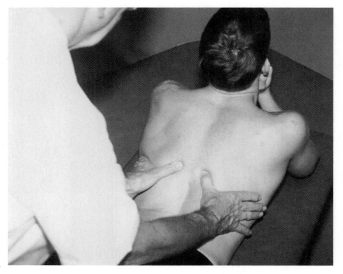

FIGURE 14.9

MANUAL MEDICINE TECHNIQUE FOR THORACIC SPINE DYSFUNCTION

In the treatment sequence of a patient presenting with multiple areas of somatic dysfunction, the thoracic spine is treated before the treatment of dysfunction of the ribs. This fundamental rule is broken only if the resolution of restriction from rib cage dysfunction assists in the treatment process of the thoracic spine dysfunction. Most muscle energy procedures for thoracic spine somatic dysfunctions are performed with the patient sitting but all can be modified for a patient in the horizontal position, either supine, lateral recumbent, or prone. As in the cervical spine, muscle energy technique is usually performed as the initial intervention. If the muscle energy procedure is ineffective and the structural diagnostic process has identified the presence of a chronic, deep motion restrictor in the articular and periarticular structures, a mobilization with impulse technique becomes indicated.

THORACIC SPINE

Muscle Energy Technique

Upper thoracic spine: T1-T5

Sitting

Diagnosis: T4-T5

Position: Extended, rotated left, and side bent left (ERS$_{left}$)

Motion Restriction: Forward bending, right rotation, and right-side bending

1. Patient sits on the table with the operator standing behind.

2. Operator's left hand monitors the T4-T5 segment with the left index finger in the interspinous space and the left middle finger overlying the posterior left transverse process of T4 (Fig. 14.10).

3. Operator's right hand is on the top of the patient's head, and the operator's trunk is against the posterior aspect of the patient's body.

4. Operator introduces forward bending to the T4-T5 segment by anterior-to-posterior translation of the patient's body (Fig. 14.11).

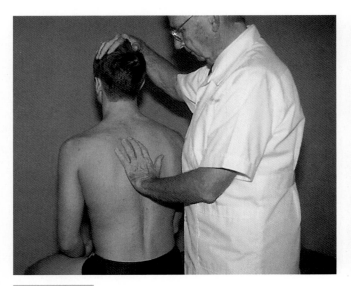

FIGURE 14.10

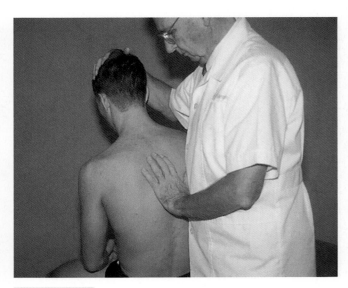

FIGURE 14.11

5. Operator engages the right-side bending and right-rotational barriers by introducing right-to-left translation through the trunk with localization at the T4-T5 level (Fig. 14.12).

6. Operator resists a backward-bending, left-side bending, or left-rotational efforts of the patient's head and neck by giving resistance with the right hand (Fig. 14.13). A 3- to 5-second isometric muscle contraction is requested.

7. After relaxation, the operator engages the new forward-bending, right-side bending, and right-rotational barriers and the patient performs three to five repetitions of the isometric muscle contraction (Fig. 14.14).

8. Retest.

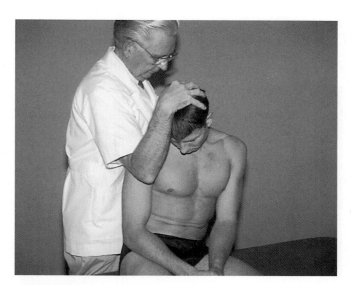

FIGURE 14.13

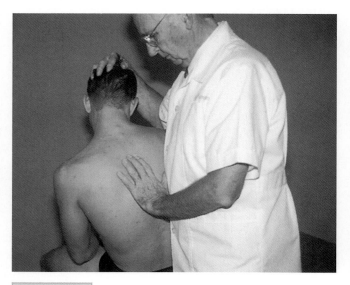

FIGURE 14.12

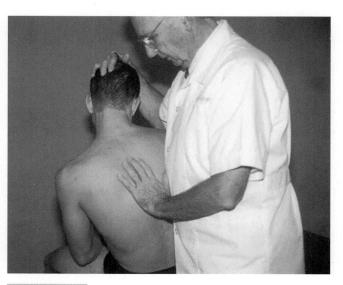

FIGURE 14.14

THORACIC SPINE

Muscle Energy Technique

Upper thoracic spine: T1-T5

Sitting

Diagnosis: T2-T3

Position: Flexed, rotated left, and side bent left (FRS$_{left}$)

Motion Restriction: Backward bending, right rotation, and right-side bending

1. Patient sits with the operator standing behind.

2. Operator's right index finger palpates the interspinous space between T2 and T3 and the right middle finger palpates over the right transverse process of T2 (Fig. 14.15).

3. Operator's left hand and forearm control the patient's head and neck with the operator's trunk against the posterior aspect of the left trunk of the patient (Fig. 14.16). Operator's left hand introduces a small amount of right rotation to gap the right zygapophysial joint at T2-T3.

4. Operator translates the trunk into extension from below upward using the thumb over the mid to lower scapular region. The patient is then asked to tuck the chin in and carry the head into posterior translation localizing extension at the T2-T3 segment (Fig. 14.17).

5. The patient is instructed to perform a mild isometric contraction of forward bending, left-side bending, or left rotation of the head and neck against the resisting left hand and forearm of the operator for a 3- to 5-second contraction.

6. After relaxation, new backward-bending, right-side bending, and right-rotational barriers are engaged, and the patient is instructed to repeat the isometric contraction three to five times (Fig. 14.18).

7. Retest.

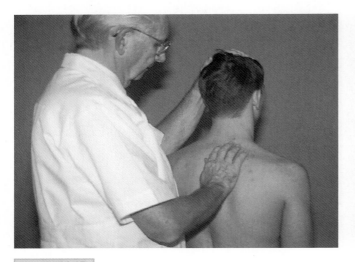

FIGURE 14.15

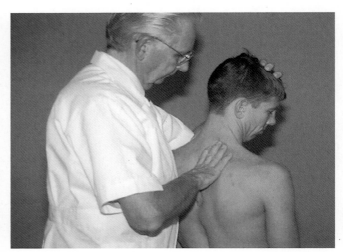

FIGURE 14.17

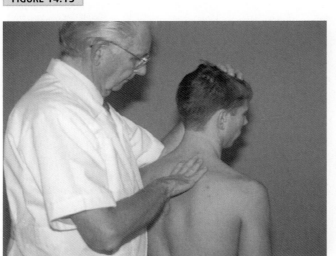

FIGURE 14.16

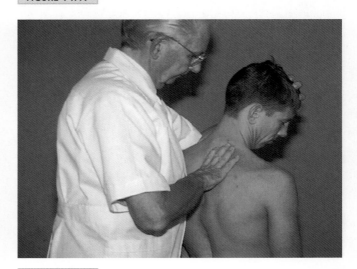

FIGURE 14.18

THORACIC SPINE

Muscle Energy Technique

Upper thoracic spine: T1-T5

Sitting

Diagnosis: T1-T3

Dysfunction: Neutral, side bent right, rotated left ($NS_{right}R_{left}$), easy normal, left convexity (EN_{left})

Motion Restriction: Side bending left, rotation right

1. Patient sits erect with the operator standing behind.

2. Operator's left thumb is localized to the apex of the left convexity (Fig. 14.19).

3. Operator's right hand controls the patient's head and stabilizes the cervical spine (Fig. 14.20).

4. Left-side bending and right rotation are introduced by translation from left to right, localized by the thumb (Fig. 14.21).

5. Patient is instructed to side bend the head to the right against the resistance offered by the operator's right hand and forearm (Fig. 14.22).

6. Following relaxation, the left-side bending and right-rotational barriers are again engaged, and the patient repeats the isometric muscle contraction of right-side bending.

7. Three to five repetitions are made of a 3- to 5-second isometric contraction.

8. Retest.

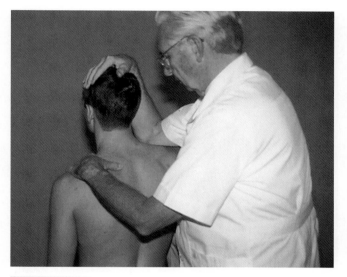

FIGURE 14.19

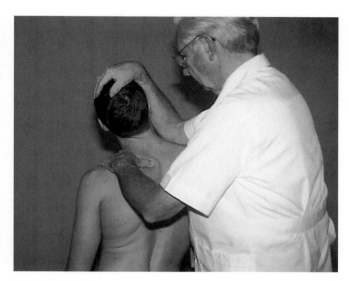

FIGURE 14.21

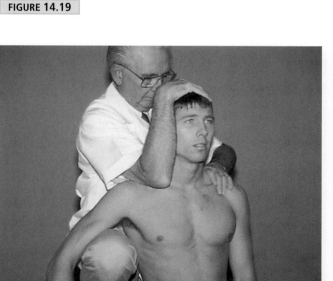

FIGURE 14.20

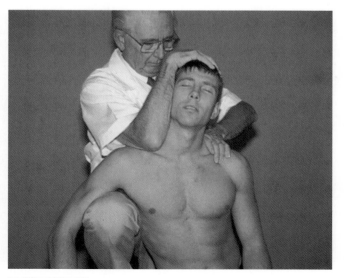

FIGURE 14.22

THORACIC SPINE

Muscle Energy Technique

Lower thoracic spine: T6-T12

Sitting

Diagnosis: T8-T9

Position: Extended (backward bent), right rotated, and right-side bent (ERS_{right})

Motion Restriction: Flexion (forward bending), left rotation, and left-side bending

1. Patient sits with the operator standing behind.

2. Patient's left hand holds the right shoulder. Operator's right arm controls the patient's trunk with the left hand grasping the right shoulder and the patient's left shoulder resting in the operator's left axilla (Fig. 14.23).

3. Operator's right index finger monitors the interspinous space at T8-T9 and right middle finger monitors the right transverse process of T8 (Fig. 14.24).

4. The forward-bending (flexion) barrier is engaged by an anterior-to-posterior translation of the trunk at the T8-T9 level (Fig. 14.25).

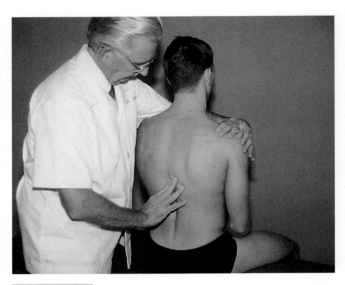

FIGURE 14.24

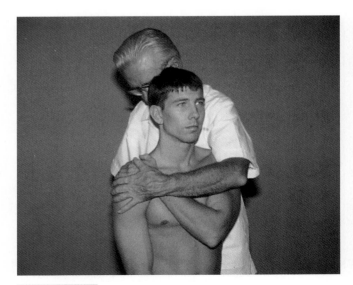

FIGURE 14.23

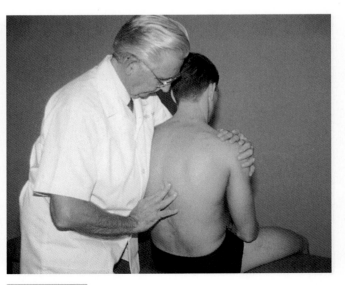

FIGURE 14.25

5. The left-side bending and left-rotational barriers are engaged by translation of the patient's trunk from left to right at the T8-T9 level (Fig. 14.26).

6. Patient is instructed to perform a right-side bending isometric contraction against resistance offered by the operator's left hand and arm for 3 to 5 seconds (Fig. 14.27).

7. Following relaxation, all three barriers are reengaged and the patient performs three to five repetitions of a 3- to 5-second isometric contraction.

8. Retest.

Note: This technique can be adapted to the upper lumbar spine.

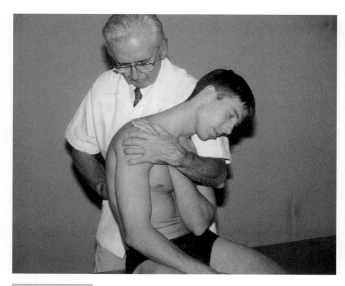

FIGURE 14.26

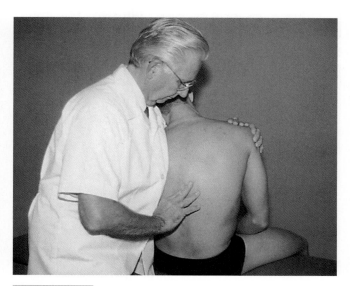

FIGURE 14.27

THORACIC SPINE

Muscle Energy Technique

Lower thoracic spine: T6-T12

Diagnosis: T8-T9

Position: Flexed (forward bent), rotated right, and side bent right (FRS_{right})

Motion Restriction: Extension (backward bending), rotation left, and side bending left

1. Patient sits with the operator standing behind.

2. Operator's left hand controls the patient's trunk through a contact on the left shoulder. Operator's right index finger monitors the interspinous space of T8-T9 and the middle finger monitors the right transverse process of T8 (Fig. 14.28).

3. With the spine in the erect *neutral position*, rotation left of T8 is introduced by right-to-left translation (right-side bending) of T8-T9 with the patient dropping the right shoulder and shifting the weight to the left buttock (Fig. 14.29). Side bending right is coupled to rotation left if the AP curve is in neutral.

4. Patient is then instructed to perform a right rotation isometric contraction against the resistance offered by the operator's left hand. This is repeated two to three times taking up the slack each time in order to enhance left rotation of T8.

Placing the superior segment into the neutral right-side bent and left rotated position initially is useful in the lower thoracic area to first back out or disengage the left inferior aspect of T8 from the superior aspect of T9 prior to closing it down or extending it into the barrier.

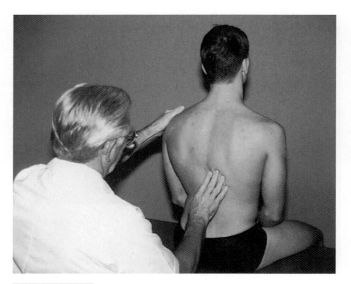

FIGURE 14.28

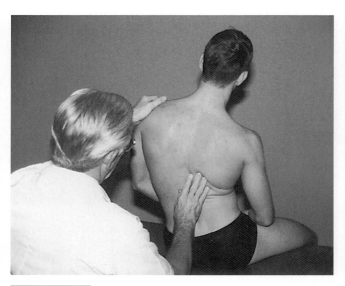

FIGURE 14.29

5. Left-side bending and extension barriers are engaged by the operator depressing the patient's left shoulder and the patient shifting the body weight to the right buttock following the operator's instruction to project the abdomen over the right knee (Fig. 14.30).

6. The patient is instructed to lift the left shoulder toward the ceiling (right-side bending effort) or pull the left shoulder forward (right-rotational effort) for 3 to 5 seconds and three to five repetitions.

7. After each effort, extension, left-side bending, and left-rotational barriers are reengaged by projecting the abdomen over the right knee and translating the trunk from left to right at T8-T9.

8. Patient's trunk is now returned to midline with operator's right hand blocking the T9 segment (Fig. 14.31).

9. Operator resists trunk forward bending by the patient's shoulders with the left arm (Fig. 14.32).

10. Retest.

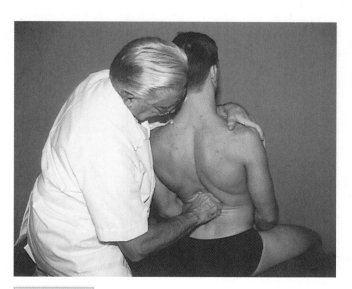

FIGURE 14.31

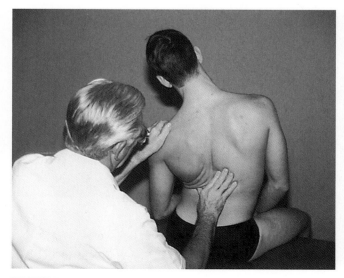

FIGURE 14.30

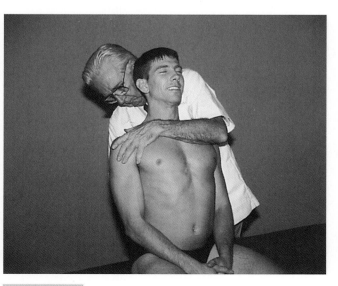

FIGURE 14.32

THORACIC SPINE

Muscle Energy Technique

Lower thoracic spine: T6-T12

Group Dysfunction

Diagnosis: T6-T9

Position: Neutral, side bent left, rotated right ($NS_{left}R_{right}$ or EN_{right})

Motion Restriction: Neutral, side bending right, and rotation left

1. Patient sits erect in neutral with the operator standing behind.

2. Operator's right thumb is localized at the apex of the right convexity with an anteromedial vector of force (Fig. 14.33).

3. Patient's left hand grasps the right shoulder and the operator places the left arm through the patient's left axilla and grasps the right shoulder (Fig. 14.34).

4. Side bending right and rotation left barriers are engaged by a right-to-left translatory movement at the apex of the convexity (Fig. 14.35).

5. Operator's left arm resists a 3- to 5-second isometric contraction of left-side bending by the patient (Fig. 14.36).

6. Following each isometric effort, new right-side bending and left-rotational barriers are engaged and the patient repeats the left-side bending isometric contraction three to five times.

7. Retest.

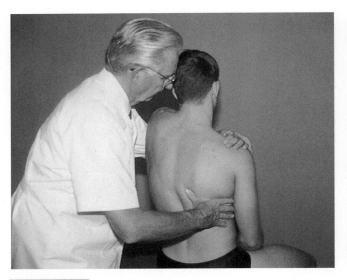

FIGURE 14.33

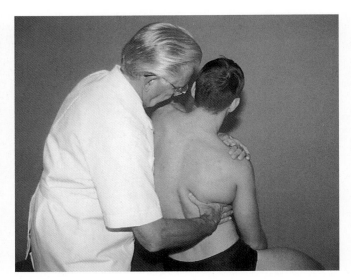

FIGURE 14.35

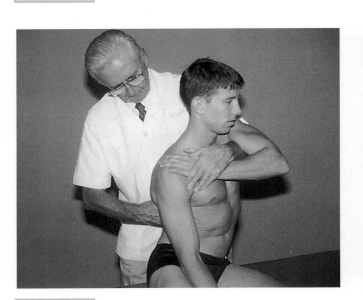

FIGURE 14.34

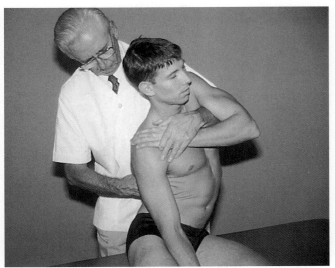

FIGURE 14.36

THORACIC SPINE

Mobilization with Impulse Technique

Upper thoracic spine: T1-T5

Sitting

Diagnosis: T3-T4

Position: Extended (backward bent), left rotated, and left-side bent (ERS$_{left}$)

Motion Restriction: Flexion (forward bending), right rotation, and right-side bending

1. Patient sits with the operator standing behind.

2. Operator's left hand and forearm control the patient's head and left-side of the neck. Operator's right hand is over the right shawl area with the thumb contacting the right side of the spinous process of T3 (the superior segment of the dysfunctional vertebral motion unit) (Fig. 14.37).

3. Operator's left hand introduces flexion, right-side bending, and right rotation of the patient's head and neck through translation from before backward and from right-to-left localizing at the T3-T4 level (Fig. 14.38).

4. When all barriers are engaged, a high-velocity, low-amplitude thrust is introduced through the operator's right thumb against the spinous process in a right-to-left translatory movement (Fig. 14.39).

5. Retest.

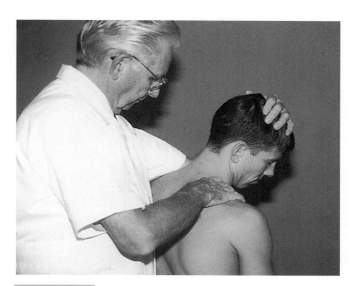

FIGURE 14.38

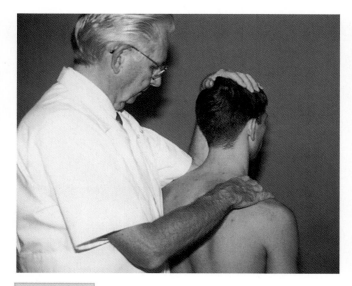

FIGURE 14.37

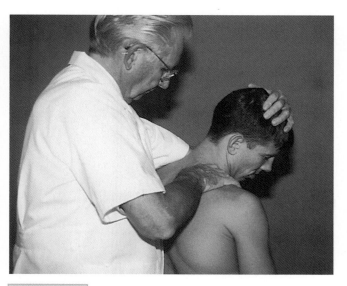

FIGURE 14.39

THORACIC SPINE

Mobilization with Impulse Technique

Upper thoracic spine: T1-T5

Sitting

Diagnosis: T3-T4

Position: Flexion, left side bending, and left rotation (FRS$_{left}$)

Motion Restriction: Extension (backward bending), right rotation, and right-side bending

1. Patient sits with the operator standing behind. Patient's left arm may be draped over the operator's left thigh with the left foot on the table.

2. Patient's head and left side of the neck are controlled by the operator's left hand and forearm. Operator's right hand overlies the patient's right shawl area with the thumb in contact with the right side of the spinous process of T3 (the superior segment of the dysfunctional vertebral motor unit) (Fig. 14.40).

3. Operator's left forearm and hand introduce extension (backward bending), right-side bending, and right rotation of the patient's head and neck to T3-T4 by translation from behind forward and from right to left (Fig. 14.41).

4. With the extension, right-side bending, and right-rotational barriers engaged, a high-velocity, low-amplitude thrust is introduced from right to left through the thumb contact with the spinous process of T3 (Fig. 14.42).

5. Retest.

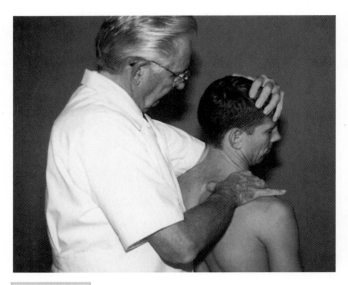

FIGURE 14.41

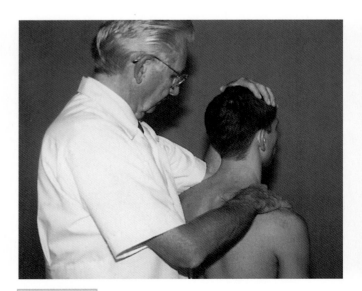

FIGURE 14.40

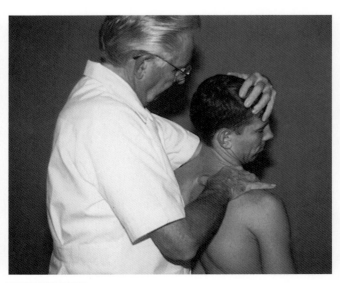

FIGURE 14.42

THORACIC SPINE

Mobilization with Impulse Technique

Upper thoracic spine: T1-T5

Sitting

Diagnosis: T1-T4

Group Dysfunction (type I)

Position: Neutral, side bent right, and rotated left ($NS_{right}R_{left}$ or EN_{left})

Motion Restriction: Side bending left, rotation right

1. Patient sits with the operator behind. Patient's right arm is draped over the operator's right leg with the right foot on the table.

2. Operator's right hand and forearm control the patient's head and right side of the neck. Operator's left hand is placed over the patient's left shawl area with the left thumb at the intertransverse space between T2 and T3 (Fig. 14.43).

3. Operator's right hand and forearm introduce left-side bending and right rotation with localization at the apex of the left convexity through the left thumb with an anteromedial vector of force (Fig. 14.44).

4. The left-side bending and right-rotational barriers are engaged by a left-to-right translatory movement of the operator's left hand and forearm (Fig. 14.45).

5. A high-velocity, low-amplitude thrust is introduced through the operator's left hand and thumb in an anteromedial direction from left to right (Fig. 14.46).

6. Retest.

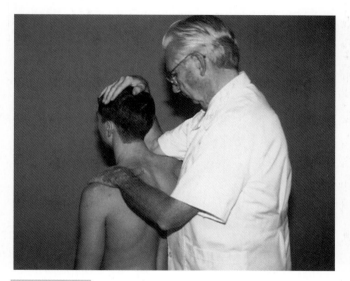

FIGURE 14.43

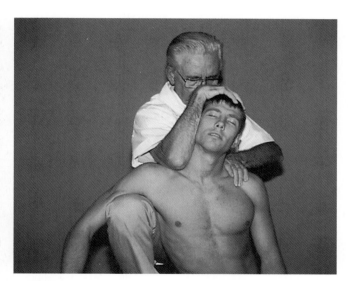

FIGURE 14.45

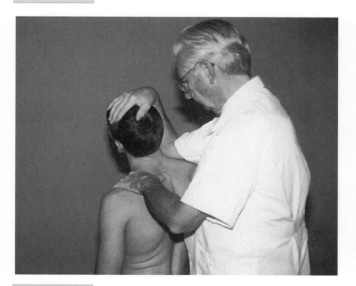

FIGURE 14.44

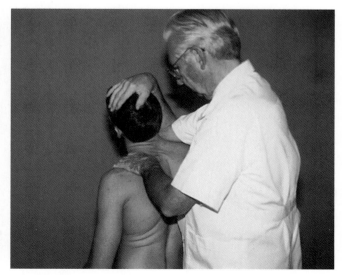

FIGURE 14.46

THORACIC SPINE

Mobilization with Impulse Technique

Upper thoracic spine: T1-T5

Prone

Diagnosis: T3-T4

Position: Flexion, left side bent, and left rotated (FRS$_{left}$)

Motion Restriction: Extension (backward bending), right rotation, and right-side bending

1. Patient is prone with the operator standing at the patient's head (Fig. 14.47).

2. Operator's hands move patient's chin to the right (introducing right-side bending) and rotating the face to the right (Fig. 14.48).

3. Operator's right pisiform is placed on the right transverse process of T4 (inferior segment of the dysfunctional vertebral motor unit) (Fig. 14.49).

4. A high-velocity, low-amplitude thrust is applied through the pisiform of the right hand with the operator's left hand stabilizing the head and neck in right-side bending and right rotation. The thrust direction is ventral, rotating T4 to the left with extension, resulting in closure of the right zygapophysial joint at T3-T4.

5. Retest.

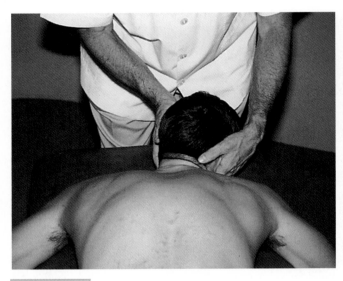

FIGURE 14.48

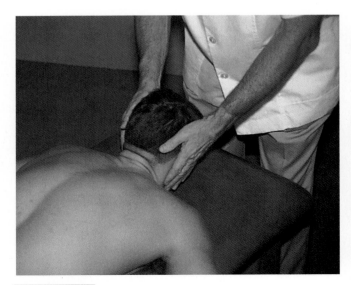

FIGURE 14.47

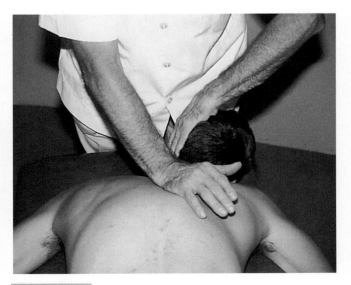

FIGURE 14.49

THORACIC SPINE

Mobilization with Impulse Technique

Upper thoracic spine: T1-T5

Prone

Diagnosis: T1-T4

    Position: Neutral, side bent right, rotated left ($NS_{right}R_{left}$) or (EN_{left})

    Motion Restriction: Side bending left, rotation right

1. Patient is prone with the operator standing with his hand controlling the patient's head (Fig. 14.50).

2. With the chin staying at the midline, operator's left hand introduces left-side bending and right rotation to the apex of the group dysfunction (Fig. 14.51).

3. With the thumb at the intertransverse space of T2-T3, a high-velocity, low-amplitude thrust is performed with an anteromedial thrust of the thumb and the left hand holding the patient's head and neck stable, or an exaggeration of the left-side bending and right rotation of the head and neck through the operator's left hand against a stable fulcrum of the right thumb.

4. An alternative contact is with the operator's right pisiform bone at the intertransverse space of T2-T3 on the left with similar thrusting force anteromedially with the right hand or exaggeration of the left-side bending and right rotation of the head and neck against the fulcrum of the right pisiform (Fig. 14.52).

5. Retest.

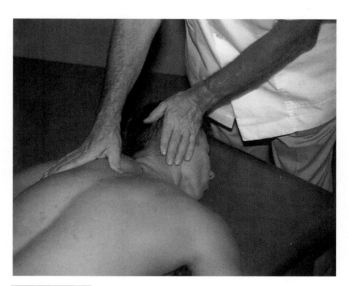

FIGURE 14.51

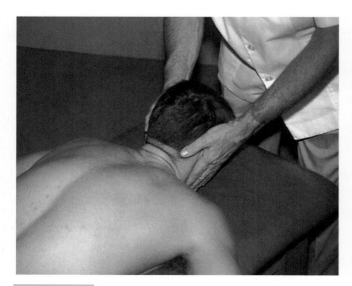

FIGURE 14.50

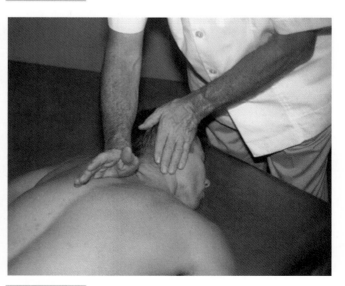

FIGURE 14.52

THORACIC SPINE

Mobilization with Impulse Technique

Limited lower thoracic spine: T6-T10

Prone

Diagnosis: T6-T7

Position: Flexed, right side bent, and left rotated (FRS$_{right}$)

Motion Restriction: Extension (backward bent), left rotation, and left-side bending

1. Patient is prone with operator standing on patient's left side.

2. Operator's left pisiform contacts the superior aspect of the left transverse process of T6 with the fingers pointing in a caudad direction (Fig. 14.53).

3. Operator's right pisiform contacts the right transverse process of T6 with anterior compression introducing left rotation of T6 (Fig. 14.54).

4. The restrictive barrier is engaged by a caudad movement with the operator's left pisiform and an anterior movement of the operator's right pisiform.

5. A high-velocity, low-amplitude thrust is made through both hands in a ventral direction introducing extension, left-side bending, and left rotation of T6 (Fig. 14.55).

6. Retest.

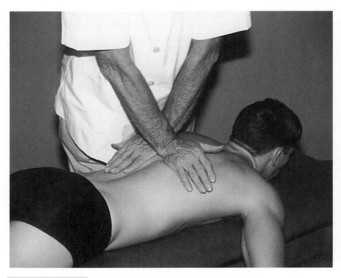

FIGURE 14.54

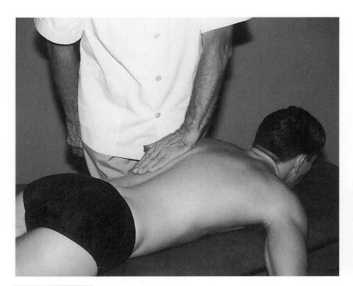

FIGURE 14.53

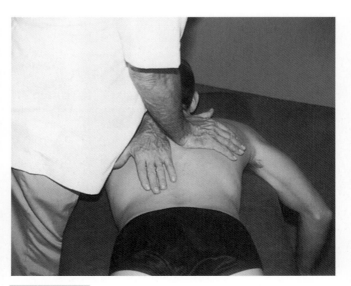

FIGURE 14.55

THORACIC SPINE

Mobilization with Impulse Technique

Limited upper and lower thoracic spine

Supine

Diagnosis: FRS Dysfunctions

Principles of the Technique

Principle 1. Establish Lever Arm

1. Patient is supine with the operator standing at the side.

2. Patient crosses arms over the chest and holds the opposite shoulder. The arm opposite the operator is the superior (Fig. 14.56).

3. A second, alternative arm position has the patient clasp the two hands together behind the cervical spine (not the head). This arm position is particularly useful in the lower thoracic region (Fig. 14.57).

4. A third, alternative arm position is unilateral, using the arm opposite the operator grasping the patient's opposite shoulder (Fig. 14.58).

5. A fourth, alternative arm position has the patient grasp the right shoulder with the left hand and the left elbow with the right hand (Fig. 14.59).

Principle 2. Establish Fulcrum

1. The hand is placed to control the inferior segment of the dysfunctional vertebral motion segment with the spinous

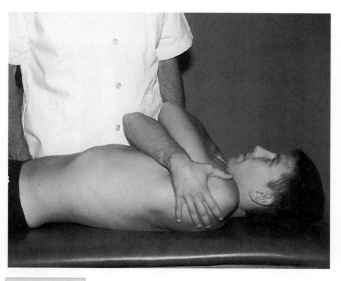

FIGURE 14.56

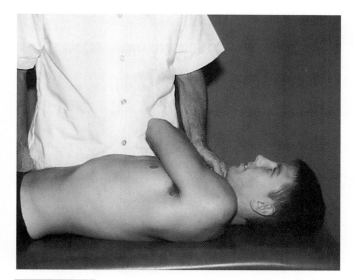

FIGURE 14.58

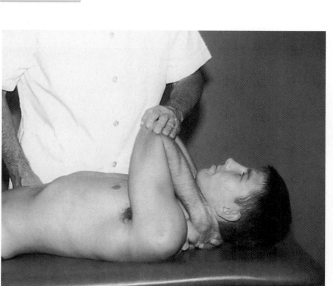

FIGURE 14.57

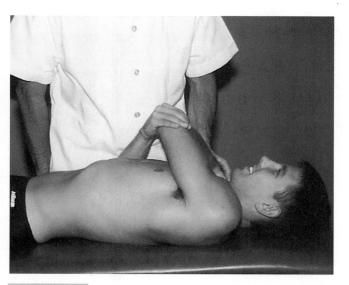

FIGURE 14.59

processes placed in the palm of the hand and with the thumb along the side of the spinous processes (Fig. 14.60).

2. A second, alternative hand position is the use of the flexed second, third, fourth, and fifth fingers on one side of the spinous process and the thenar and hypothenar eminences on the other side of the spinous process (Fig. 14.61). This hand position may be uncomfortable both to the patient and the operator.

3. A third alternative hand position uses flexion of the proximal and distal interphalangeal joints of the index finger against one transverse process of the inferior segment and the metacarpophalangeal joint of the thumb on the opposite transverse process (Fig. 14.62). This hand position is preferred as it provides for a contact of the thenar eminence against the rib shaft of a dysfunctional rib associated with nonneutral (ERS) dysfunctions of the thoracic spine.

Principle 3. Localization of the Lever Arm to the Fulcrum

1. The patient is rolled toward the operator to place the fulcrum on the inferior vertebra of the dysfunctional vertebral motor motion segment.

2. The patient is returned to the neutral position and a body contact is made with the crossed arm lever arm. This preferably is the epigastrium. Care should be taken not to put compressive force against the operator's rib cage, or in a female operator against breast tissue. A folded towel or small pillow can be used to cushion the patient's elbows against the operator's trunk (Fig. 14.63).

Principle 4. Localization of Thrust

1. The fulcrum holds the inferior segment so that the superior vertebra can be moved in the appropriate direction to engage the restrictive barrier.

2. The thrusting force is directed at the superior aspect of the fulcrum.

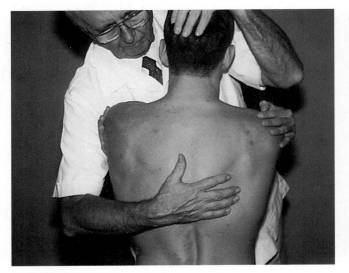

FIGURE 14.60

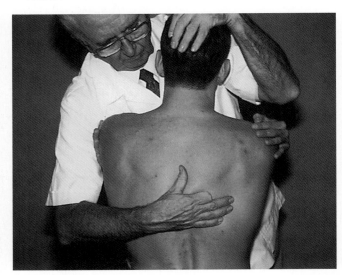

FIGURE 14.62

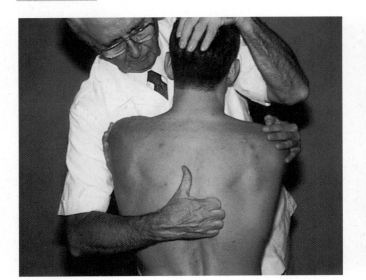

FIGURE 14.61

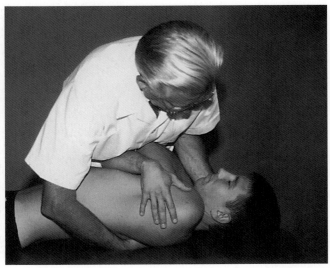

FIGURE 14.63

THORACIC SPINE

Mobilization with Impulse Technique

Limited upper and lower thoracic spine: T3-T12

Supine

Diagnosis

Position: Bilaterally extended (both facets in the closed position)

Motion Restriction: Sagittal plane flexion

1. Patient is supine with the operator standing at the side.

2. The lever arm is established by crossing both arms over the chest (or one of the alternative lever arm positions).

3. Operator places the fulcrum hand under the patient's torso localized to the inferior segment of the dysfunctional vertebral unit.

4. Patient is returned to the neutral midline position with localization of the lever arm to the fulcrum. Operator's cephalic hand controls the patient's head and neck to introduce flexion (Fig. 14.64).

5. Operator flexes the thoracic spine down to the superior vertebra of the dysfunctional vertebral motion unit (Fig. 14.65).

6. A high-velocity, low-amplitude thrust is performed by dropping the operator's body weight through the lever arm to the fulcrum with slight exaggeration of the patient's flexed position.

7. Retest.

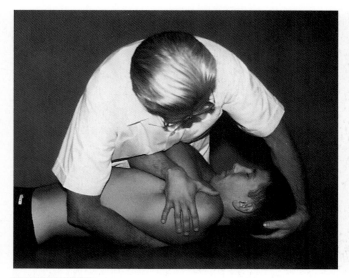

FIGURE 14.64

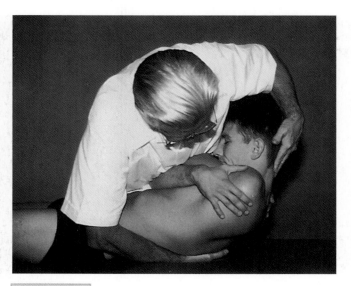

FIGURE 14.65

THORACIC SPINE

Mobilization with Impulse Technique

Limited upper and lower thoracic spine: T3–T12

Supine

Diagnosis

Position: Bilaterally flexed (both facets in the open position)

Motion Restriction: Sagittal plane extension

1. Patient is supine with the operator standing at the side.

2. Lever arm is established by crossing the arms across the patient's chest holding each shoulder.

3. Operator's hand is placed as the fulcrum on the lower segment of the dysfunctional vertebral motion unit.

4. Patient is returned to the midline with the operator controlling the patient's upper trunk, neck, and head.

5. Patient flexes the upper trunk just past the fulcrum (Fig. 14.66).

6. Operator drops the patient's head, neck, and upper trunk into extension just over the fulcrum.

7. A high-velocity, low-amplitude thrust through the operator's trunk against the lever arm takes the superior segment into extension over the fulcrum (Fig. 14.67).

8. Retest.

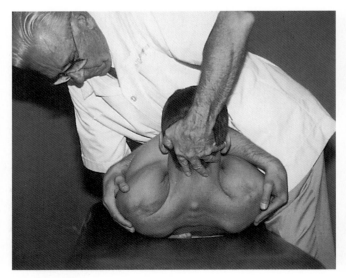

FIGURE 14.66

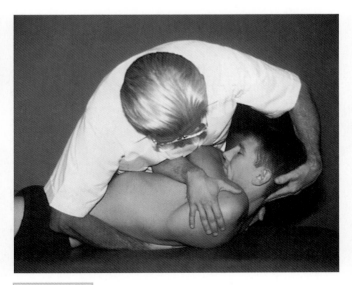

FIGURE 14.67

THORACIC SPINE

Mobilization with Impulse Technique

Limited upper and lower thoracic spine: T3-T12

Supine

Diagnosis: T4-T5

Position: Extended (backward bent), rotated left, and side bent left (ERS$_{left}$)

Motion Restriction: Flexion (forward bending), right rotation, and right-side bending

1. Patient is supine with the operator standing on the patient's right side.

2. Patient establishes lever arm by crossing hands over chest.

3. Operator's right hand establishes a fulcrum on both transverse processes of T5.

4. Patient is returned to the neutral position and the lever arm is localized to the fulcrum.

5. Operator's left hand introduces flexion, right-side bending, and right rotation of the neck and upper thoracic spine down to T4 (Fig. 14.68).

6. A high-velocity, low-amplitude thrust is made by the operator's body weight on the lever arm to the fulcrum resulting in flexion, right-side bending, right rotation of T4, and opening of the left zygapophysial joint (Fig. 14.69).

7. Retest.

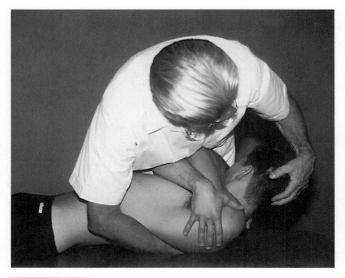

FIGURE 14.68

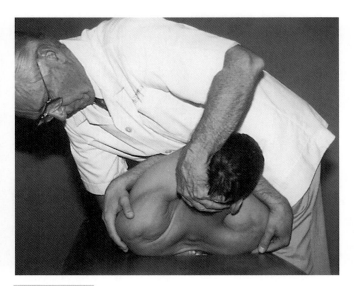

FIGURE 14.69

THORACIC SPINE

Mobilization with Impulse Technique

Limited upper and lower thoracic spine: T3-T12

Supine

Diagnosis: Group Dysfunction T3-T6

Position: Neutral, side bent right, and rotated left ($NS_{right}R_{left}$ or EN_{left})

Motion Restriction: Side bending left, rotation right

1. Patient is supine on the table with the operator standing on the right side.
2. Patient establishes the lever arm by crossing the arms over the chest.

3. Operator's right hand establishes the fulcrum with the metacarpophalangeal joint localized to the left intertransverse space of T4-T5 using the hand position shown in Figure 14.60.
4. Operator localizes lever arm to the fulcrum and with the left hand flexes and extends the head and upper trunk to ensure neutral mechanics at the dysfunctional segments (Fig. 14.70).
5. Operator's left hand introduces left-side bending and right rotation down to the dysfunctional segments (Fig. 14.71).
6. Operator's torso provides a thrusting force through the lever arm to the fulcrum, resulting in left-side bending and right rotation of the dysfunctional segments.
7. Retest.

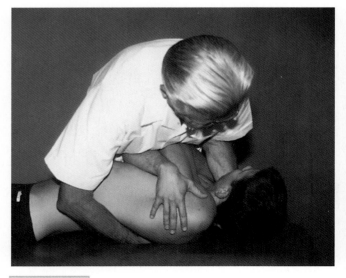

FIGURE 14.70

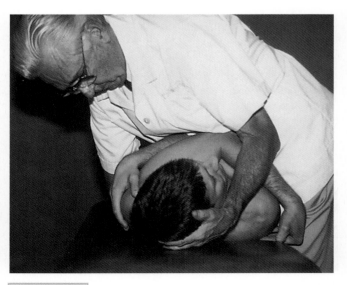

FIGURE 14.71

THORACIC SPINE

Mobilization with Impulse Technique

Lower thoracic spine: T6-T12

Sitting

Diagnosis: FRS or ERS Dysfunction

Principles of the technique

> Principle 1. Establish a Lever Arm

1. Patient sits on a stepladder treatment stool and clasps both hands together against the cervical spine (not occiput) (Fig. 14.72).

2. Operator threads both hands under the patient's axilla and grasps each forearm providing control of the patient's trunk (Fig. 14.73).

> Principle 2. Establish a Fulcrum

1. Operator places the knee on the inferior vertebra of the dysfunctional vertebral motion unit, against the spinous process or a transverse process (Fig. 14.74).

2. Operator places a foot on the appropriate step of the stepladder treatment stool to localize the knee at the dysfunctional vertebral motion unit.

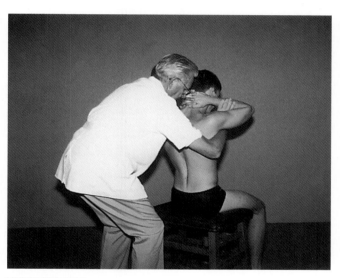

FIGURE 14.73

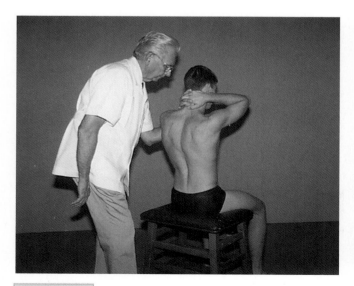

FIGURE 14.72

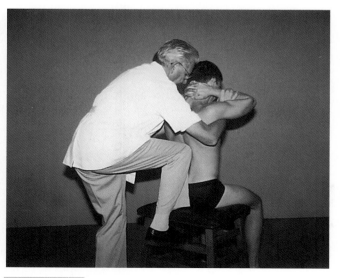

FIGURE 14.74

3. Alternatively, a rolled towel can be used as the fulcrum with the edge against the inferior segment of the dysfunctional vertebral motion unit (Fig. 14.75).

4. The operator's trunk is placed against the towel fulcrum to control the inferior vertebra (Fig. 14.76).

   Principle 3. Thrust Through the Lever Arm to the Fulcrum

1. Operator's two arms pull the patient's trunk toward the fulcrum or lift the trunk over the fulcrum depending on whether a flexion or an extension thrust is necessary.

2. The thrusting procedure occurs with the operator's arms controlling the patient's trunk through the operator's hand contact on the forearms.

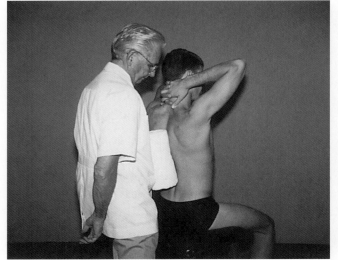

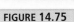
FIGURE 14.75

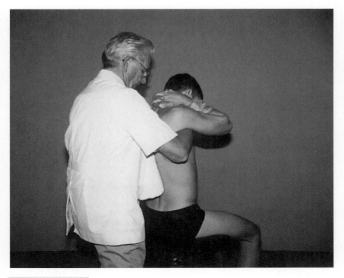

FIGURE 14.76

THORACIC SPINE

Mobilization with Impulse Technique

Lower thoracic spine: T6-T12

Sitting

Diagnosis

Position: Bilateral extended

Motion Restriction: Bilateral flexion

1. Operator is seated on a stool with the hands grasped behind the neck.
2. Operator places the knee or towel fulcrum on the spinous process of the inferior vertebra of the dysfunctional vertebral motion unit.
3. Operator threads both hands through the axilla and grasps each forearm of the patient.
4. Flexion is introduced until localized at the dysfunctional segment (Fig. 14.77).
5. Operator applies a high-velocity, low-amplitude thrust by pulling directly posteriorly toward the fulcrum, enhancing flexion from above against the fixed lower vertebra.
6. Retest.

THORACIC SPINE

Mobilization with Impulse Technique

Lower thoracic spine: T6-T12

Sitting

Diagnosis

Position: Bilateral flexed

Motion Restriction: Bilateral extension

1. Patient sits with hands clasped behind neck.
2. Operator stands behind the patient with a knee or rolled towel as fulcrum on the spinous process of the inferior vertebra of the dysfunctional vertebral motion unit.
3. Operator threads both hands under patient's axilla, grasping patient's forearms.
4. Operator localizes to the dysfunctional segment by extending the patient's trunk over the fulcrum (Fig. 14.78).
5. Operator applies a high-velocity, low-amplitude thrust by a lifting motion, extending the patient's upper trunk over the fulcrum.
6. Retest.

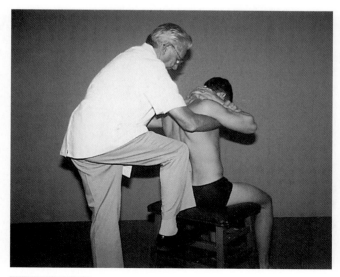

FIGURE 14.77

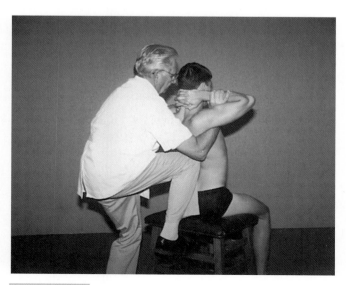

FIGURE 14.78

THORACIC SPINE

Mobilization with Impulse Technique

Lower thoracic spine: T6-T12

Sitting

Diagnosis: T8-T9

Position: Extended, rotated left, and side bent left (ERS_{left})

Motion Restriction: Flexion (forward bending), right rotation, and right-side bending

1. Patient sits with the hands clasped behind the neck.
2. Operator stands behind the patient and establishes the fulcrum against the right transverse process of T9 (the inferior vertebra).
3. Operator threads his arms through the patient's axillae and grasps each forearm.
4. Operator localizes patient's upper trunk to the barrier of flexion, right-side bending, and right rotation (Fig. 14.79).
5. Operator applies a flexion high-velocity, low-amplitude thrust by pulling the patient's upper trunk toward the fulcrum.
6. Retest.

THORACIC SPINE

Mobilization with Impulse Technique

Lower thoracic spine: T6-T12

Sitting

Diagnosis: T8-T9

Position: Flexed, rotated left, and side bent left (FRS_{left})

Motion Restriction: Extension (backward bending), right rotation, and right-side bending

1. Patient sits with the hands clasped behind the neck.
2. Operator establishes fulcrum against the right transverse process of T9 (the inferior segment).
3. Operator threads his arms through the patient's axillae and grasps patient's forearms.
4. Operator engages extension, right-side bending, and right-rotational barriers at the dysfunctional segment (Fig. 14.80).
5. Operator applies a high-velocity, low-amplitude thrust by lifting and posteriorly translating the patient's trunk over the fulcrum.
6. Retest.

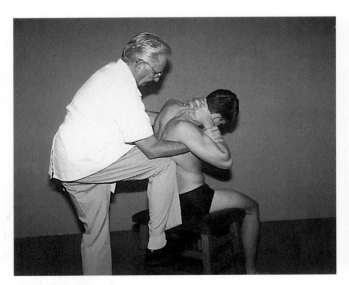

FIGURE 14.79

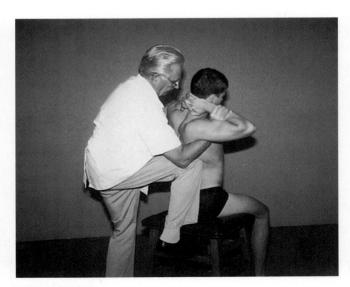

FIGURE 14.80

THORACIC SPINE

Mobilization with Impulse Technique

Lower thoracic spine: T6-T12

Sitting

Diagnosis: Group Dysfunction T7-T10

Position: Neutral, side bent left, rotated right ($NS_{left}R_{right}$) or (EN_{right})

Motion Restriction: Right-side bending, left rotation

1. Patient sits with the hands clasped behind the neck.

2. Operator establishes the fulcrum at the intertransverse space on the right of T8-T9.

3. Operator threads his arms through the patient's axillae and grasps the patient's forearms.

4. Operator flexes and extends to neutral, then introduces right-side bending and left rotation to localize at the apex of the dysfunctional segments (Fig. 14.81).

5. Operator applies a high-velocity, low-amplitude thrust by lifting and pulling the patient's upper trunk through the fulcrum, enhancing right-side bending and left rotation of the dysfunctional vertebra.

6. Retest.

CONCLUSION

In the usual treatment sequence, the thoracic spine should be evaluated and treated before evaluation and treatment of rib function. Occasionally, it is useful to treat a major rib dysfunction first to better evaluate and treat dysfunction of the thoracic spine.

In the seated mid to lower thoracic mobilization with impulse technique, this author prefers to use the knee or a rolled towel as a fulcrum on the inferior vertebra of the dysfunctional vertebral motion unit. Other practitioners and authors will occasionally apply the fulcrum against the posterior transverse process of the superior vertebra of the dysfunctional vertebral motion unit and thrust forward with the knee or the trunk through the rolled up towel to derotate the dysfunctional vertebra. In either instance, it is imperative that there be good localization of the thrusting force to the fulcrum.

It should be noted that the prone mobilization with impulse technique for T5 through T12 is best suited for FRS dysfunctions. This technique is contraindicated in an ERS dysfunction. While it is possible to adapt the supine mobilization with impulse techniques for T5 through T12 for FRS dysfunctions, they are difficult to perform. It is recommended for FRS dysfunctions in this region that the prone technique be used. In the prone and sitting mobilization with impulse techniques, it is important that the localization to the transverse processes be precise and not against the adjacent rib shaft because repetitive thrusting on a rib shaft can cause hypermobility of the costovertebral and costotransverse articulations resulting in chronic structural rib dysfunction.

SUGGESTED READING

Flynn TA, ed. *The Thoracic Spine and Rib Cage: Musculoskeletal Evaluation and Treatment*. Boston: Butterworth-Heinemann, 1996.

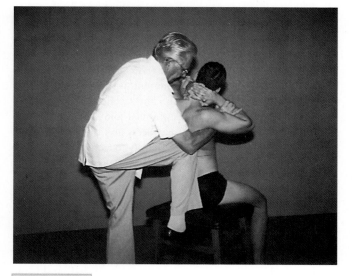

FIGURE 14.81

RIB CAGE TECHNIQUE

The thoracic cage consists of the 12 thoracic vertebra, the paired 12 ribs, the sternum, and the related ligaments and muscles. The ribs maintain the contour of the thoracic cage, much like a cylinder, and house the thoracic viscera, primarily the heart and great vessels, the lungs, trachea, and esophagus. The thoracoabdominal diaphragm (Fig. 15.1) functions as the piston within the cylinder of the thoracic cage, its contraction and descent results in relative negative "intrathoracic pressure" drawing in air for respiration. The diaphragms descent also results in a relative increase in "intra-abdominal pressure," performing as the major "pump" of the low-pressure venous and lymphatic systems. The descent of the diaphragm also allows the central tendon to become fixed by the abdominal viscera; allowing the movable ends of the diaphragm to elevate the lower ribs via its direct attachments.

FUNCTIONAL ANATOMY

Thoracic Inlet

At the cephalic end of the thoracic cage is the thoracic inlet (Fig. 15.2), which is bounded by the body of T1, the medial margins of the right and left first ribs, the posterior aspect of the manubrium of the sternum, and the medial end of the right and left clavicles. Through the thoracic inlet, pass the esophagus, trachea, and major vessels of the neck and upper extremity.

Lymphatic Drainage

The thoracic inlet is of importance in lymphatic drainage because the lymphatic system for the whole body drains into the venous system immediately posterior to the medial end of the clavicle and the first rib (Fig. 15.3).

Sympathetic Trunk

The thoracic lateral chain ganglia of the sympathetic division of the autonomic nervous system lies anterior to the capsule of the costovertebral articulations and are tightly bound down to the posterior thoracic wall by heavy, dense fascia.

Rib cage dysfunction is frequently a major component of dysfunction in the musculoskeletal system and is frequently painless. These dysfunctions are frequently described as respiratory restrictions and contribute to the persistence and recurrence of dysfunction within the thoracic spine and can contribute as long restrictors to dysfunction of the musculoskeletal system elsewhere.[1] Altered rib cage function influences respiratory activity, circulatory activity (arterial, venous, and lymphatic), and neural activity (particularly of the intercostal nerves and the brachial plexus superior to rib 1).

INTERCOSTAL NEURALGIA

Other rib dysfunctions are found in association with pain in the intercostal space, commonly described as intercostal neuralgia.

These rib dysfunctions are described as *structural rib dysfunctions.* They contribute to restriction of respiratory activity of the rib cage as well, but they primarily are found as the dysfunctions associated with the chest wall pain. Intercostal neuralgic symptoms in the absence of structural rib dysfunctions should alert the physician to search for organic causes of intercostal neuralgia (e.g., herpes zoster, cord tumor, and primary or secondary inflammatory or neoplastic disease of the thoracic viscera).

RIB ANATOMY

Ribs are described as typical or atypical. The atypical ribs are those with the numbers 1 and 2, namely ribs 1, 2, 11, and 12. The first rib is broad and flat and articulates with T1 by a unifacet. It is the lateral boundary of the thoracic inlet and has multiple types of dysfunction. The second rib articulates by two demifacets with T1 and T2. Anteriorly, it articulates by a strong cartilaginous attachment with the manubriogladiolar junction of the sternum at the angle of Louis. Ribs 11 and 12 articulate by unifacets with the 11th and 12th vertebra. They do not have typical costotransverse articulations. They are both associated with the muscles of the posterior abdominal wall. The quadratus lumborum muscle attaches to the inferior margin of rib 12. The 12th rib is frequently asymmetric in length. Neither rib attaches to the costal arch.

CLINICAL PEARL

Alteration in the function of the second rib profoundly influences the function of the sternum and frequently contributes to pain syndromes in the upper extremity (Fig. 15.4).

The typical ribs, ribs 3 through 10, have three articulations. The posterior articulations are the *costovertebral*, with the rib head attaching to demifacets of the thoracic vertebra above and below, and through a strong ligamentous attachment, to the annulus of the intervertebral disk. The second posterior articulation is the *costotransverse*. This synovial joint incorporates the anterior surface of the transverse process and the articular surface of the posterior aspect of the rib. As an example, the costovertebral articulation of rib 4 attaches to the inferior demifacet of T3 and the superior demifacet of T4, while the costotransverse articulation is at the T4 level. The anterior articulation is the costochondral. Each rib attaches either to the sternum directly or through the costal arch. *Normal rib motion requires mobility of the thoracic vertebrae and mobility at the costovertebral, costotransverse, and costochondral articulations.* The rib angle of the typical ribs is the posterior aspect of the rib shaft and is the attachment of the iliocostalis muscles.

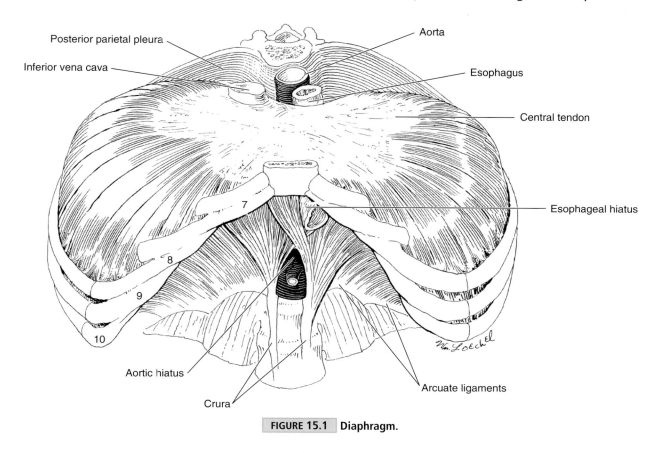

FIGURE 15.1 Diaphragm.

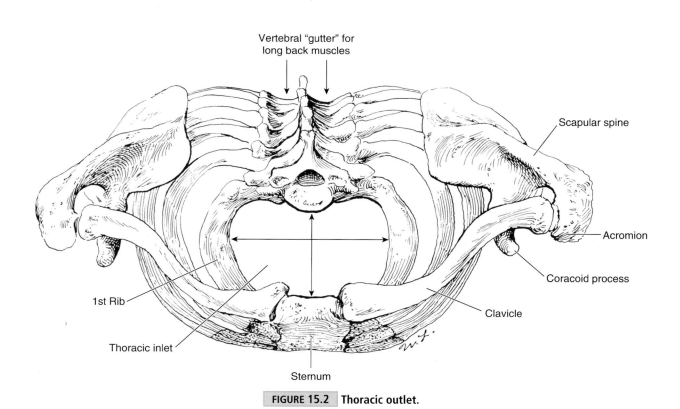

FIGURE 15.2 Thoracic outlet.

DIAPHRAGM

The diaphragm (Fig. 15.1) is the primary muscle of respiration. When it contracts it descends and increases the negative intrathoracic pressure enhancing inspiration; as it relaxes, the passive recoil of the thoracic cage results in exhalation. Other inspiratory muscles include the external intercostals, the sternocostalis, and the accessory muscles of inspiration. These include the sternocleidomastoid, scalenes, pectoralis major and minor, and occasionally, the serratus anterior and latissimus dorsi, serratus posterior superior, and the superior fibers of the iliocostalis. The primary exhalation muscles are the internal intercostals and the accessory exhalation muscles are the abdominals, lower fibers of the iliocostalis, serratus posterior inferior, and quadratus lumborum. The external and internal intercostal muscles are frequently viewed as respiratory muscles, but primarily, their function is to maintain the integrity of the contour of the thoracic cylinder and prevent invagination during increasing negative intrathoracic pressure.

RIB MOTIONS

The primary rib motion is that of inhalation and exhalation. Inhalation and exhalation are further described as *pump-handle and bucket-handle* (Fig. 15.5). During inhalation the anterior extremity of a rib moves superiorly in a pump-handle fashion, and the lateral aspect of the rib goes superiorly in a bucket-handle fashion. During exhalation both the pump-handle and bucket-handle components move in a caudad direction. *All ribs have both pump-handle and bucket-handle movements. Cephalic ribs have more pump-handle motion and Caudal ribs have more bucket-handle motion.* The major determinant of this bucket-handle or pump-handle movement is the axis of motion between the costovertebral and the costotransverse articulation. In the upper ribs, this axis is transverse providing more pump-handle activity, whereas in the lower ribs, this axis is more anteroposterior providing for more bucket-handle motion. In a true bucket-handle motion, the anterior and posterior ends of the ribs should be fixed. This is not true in the normal chest wall as the anterior extremity of the rib moves laterally and somewhat superiorly during inhalation, and medially and inferiorly during exhalation. Nonetheless, the descriptors of pump-handle and bucket-handle movements are good for describing the characteristics of the chest wall motion.

A third rib motion occurs at the 11th and 12th ribs. They have no articular attachments anteriorly and no costotransverse articulations posteriorly, resulting in their motion being primarily posterior and lateral during inhalation, and anterior and medial during exhalation. This motion has been described as *caliper motion* simulating the action of a set of ice tongs.

A fourth rib motion is that which accompanies rotation of the thoracic spine. This motion is described as *torsional movement* that results when a pair of typical ribs is attached to two thoracic vertebrae involved in a rotational movement. For example, when T5 rotates to the right in relation to T6, the posterior aspect of the right sixth rib turns externally and the

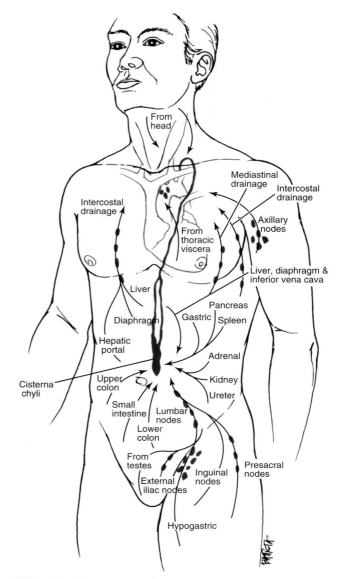

FIGURE 15.3 | **Lymphatic drainage.**

posterior aspect of the left sixth rib turns internally. The rib appears to twist on this long axis. This torsional movement continues around the rib cage to the sternal attachment with the anterior extremity of the right sixth rib being more flat with its inferior border sharp and the anterior extremity of the left sixth rib having its superior margin accentuated. As the thoracic spine returns to neutral, the rib torsional movement should return to bilateral symmetry.

Nonphysiologic Rib Motion

When the rib cage is subjected to traumatic insult resulting in costovertebral and costotransverse joint capsular sprains, abnormal rib motions can occur. Following a single traumatic episode or multiple microtraumas, one or more ribs may become subluxed anteriorly or posteriorly. These subluxations are abnormal hypermobile ribs with the rib either being carried more

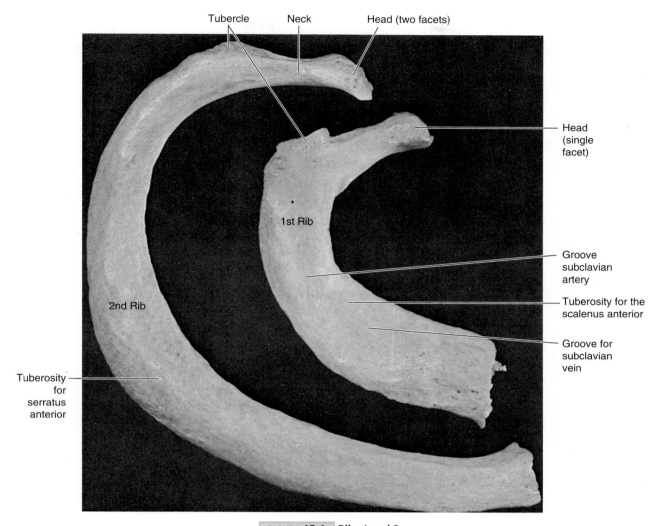

FIGURE 15.4 Ribs 1 and 2.

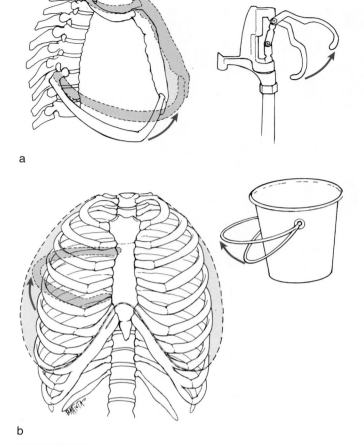

a

b

FIGURE 15.5 Pump-handle–bucket-handle motion.

anteriorly or posteriorly along the axis of motion between the costovertebral and the costotransverse articulations. A third subluxation is the possibility of rib 1 being carried cephalad at its unifacet on the lateral side of T1 resulting in the rib shaft sitting on top of the transverse process.

Rib shafts also have a great deal of pliability and are built to sustain anteroposterior and lateral compression loads as they maintain the integrity of the chest wall cylinder. Occasionally, after trauma from an anteroposterior or a lateral direction, one or more ribs lose this plasticity and become restricted in a deformed state.

STRUCTURAL DIAGNOSIS OF THE RIB CAGE

Structural diagnosis of the rib cage assesses for the diagnostic triad of asymmetry, altered range of motion, and tissue texture abnormality. The examiner assesses the symmetry or asymmetry of the chest wall by palpation anteriorly, posteriorly, and laterally. Concurrently, the examiner can assess for tissue texture abnormality, particularly *hypertonicity of the iliocostalis attachment at the rib angle and the intercostal muscles*. Symmetrically palpating ribs, both in groups and individually, and following respiratory activity of inhalation and exhalation identify motion characteristics.

RIB CAGE

Diagnosis

Sitting

Posterior Palpation

1. Patient sits with the operator standing behind.

2. Operator palpates the posterior convexity of the thorax in the upper region (Fig. 15.6), midregion (Fig. 15.7), and lower region (Fig. 15.8).

3. Assessment is made of the participation of each rib angle in the posterior convexity. Is one more prominent or less prominent than another?

4. Assessment is made of the hypertonicity and tenderness of the iliocostalis muscle at the rib angle.

5. Assessment is made of the posterior contour of the rib shaft. There is a normal posterior convexity with the lower border of the rib being somewhat more easily palpable than that of the superior.

6. Assessment is made of the width of the intercostal space and the intercostal muscle hypertonicity and tenderness. Each interspace should be symmetric with its fellow on the opposite side and with the ones above and below.

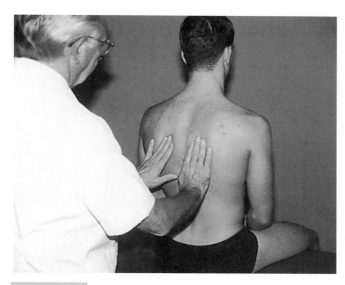

FIGURE 15.7

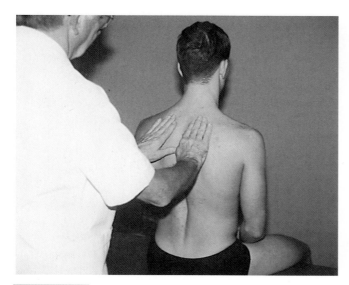

FIGURE 15.6

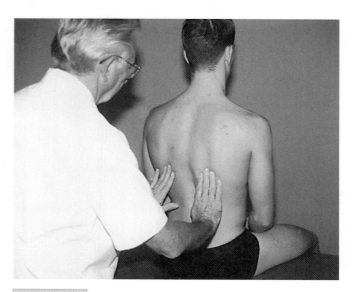

FIGURE 15.8

RIB CAGE

Diagnosis

Sitting

Anterior Palpation

1. Patient sits on the table with the operator standing in front.

2. Operator palpates the anterior contour of the chest wall and its anterior convexity beginning at the upper region (Fig. 15.9), with the longest finger palpating the costal cartilage of rib 1 under the medial extremity of the clavicle. The middle ribs (Fig. 15.10) and the lower ribs (Fig. 15.11) are palpated.

3. Assessment is made for the participation of the anterior aspect of each rib in the normal convexity. Is one more or less prominent than the one above or below?

4. Assessment is made of the symmetry of the intercostal spaces and the tissue tension and tenderness of intercostal muscles.

5. Assessment is made of the costochondral junction (Fig. 15.12) assessing for prominence, depression, tissue reaction, and tenderness.

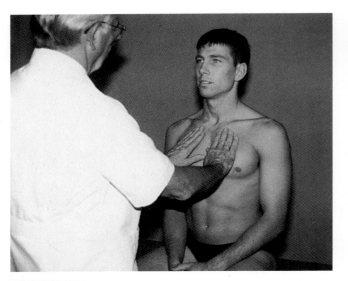

FIGURE 15.9

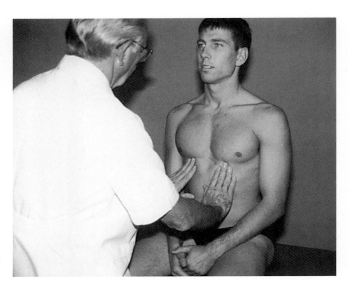

FIGURE 15.11

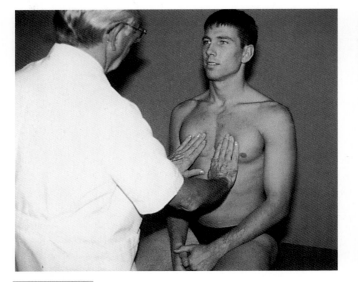

FIGURE 15.10

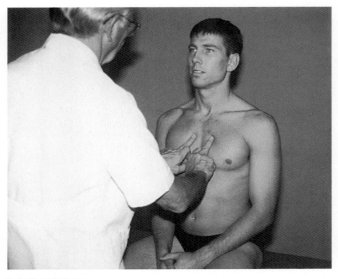

FIGURE 15.12

RIB CAGE

Diagnosis

Sitting

Lateral Palpation

1. Patient sits on the table with the operator standing in front.

2. Operator palpates the lateral contour of the chest wall from above downward assessing for the participation of all ribs in the lateral convexity (Fig. 15.13). Is one more or less prominent than the one above or below?

3. Operator assesses for symmetry of intercostal spaces and for tissue tension in intercostal muscles.

4. The ribs in the midaxillary line are noted for tenderness in the presence of rib dysfunction.

RIB CAGE

Diagnosis

Sitting

First Rib for Superior Subluxation

1. Patient sits on the table with the operator standing behind.

2. Operator grasps the anterior aspect of the superior trapezius on each side and pulls posteriorly (Fig. 15.14).

3. With posterior retraction of the upper trapezius, the long fingers are directed caudally onto the posterior shaft of the first rib.

4. Unleveling of one rib in comparison to the other by 5 mm is a positive finding (Fig. 15.15).

5. The dysfunctional rib is markedly tender on its superior aspect.

6. The dysfunctional rib has significant exhalation restriction.

7. There is usually hypertonicity of the ipsilateral scalene muscles.

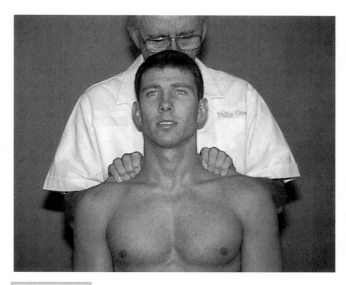

FIGURE 15.14

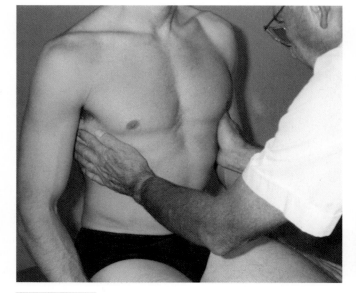

FIGURE 15.13

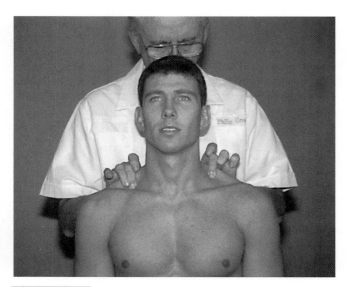

FIGURE 15.15

RIB CAGE

Diagnosis

Supine

Respiratory Motion Restriction

1. Patient is supine with the operator standing at the side with dominant eye over the midline.

2. Operator symmetrically places hands over the lateral aspect of the lower rib cage with the fingers in interspaces (Fig. 15.16).

3. Operator follows inhalation and exhalation effort looking for symmetry or asymmetry of full inhalation and exhalation excursion. Identifying which side stops moving first during the inhalation or exhalation effort makes the diagnosis of either inhalation or exhalation restriction.

4. Palpation is performed on the anterior extremity of the lower ribs (Fig. 15.17) assessing pump-handle motion.

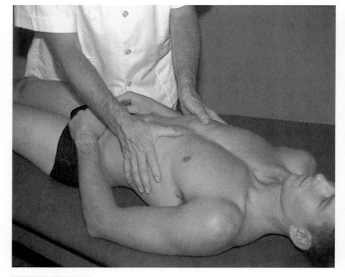

FIGURE 15.16

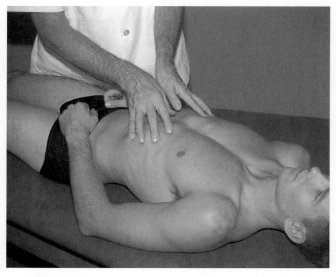

FIGURE 15.17

5. Similar assessment of bucket-handle movement (Fig. 15.18) and pump-handle movement (Fig. 15.19) is made of the middle ribs.

6. Similar assessment of the bucket-handle movement (Fig. 15.20) and pump-handle movement (Fig. 15.21) of the upper ribs is made. Note that the long finger is in contact with the anterior extremity of the first rib.

Note: It is important to challenge the end range of inhalation and exhalation for accurate diagnosis.

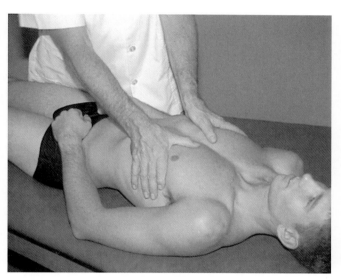

FIGURE 15.18

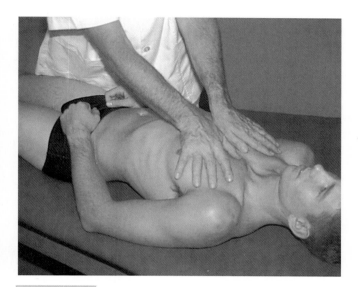

FIGURE 15.20

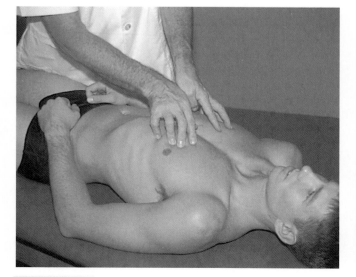

FIGURE 15.19

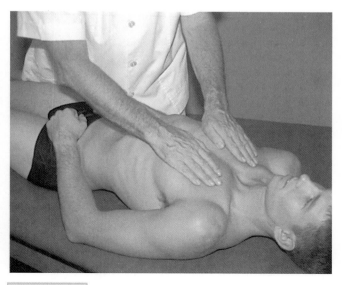

FIGURE 15.21

RIB CAGE

Diagnosis

Supine

Identification of "key rib"

1. Patient is supine with the operator standing at the side with dominant eye over the midline.
2. Operator symmetrically places a finger on the superior aspect of a pair of ribs and follows inhalation and exhalation effort (Fig. 15.22).
3. The rib that stops first during inhalation effort has inhalation restriction.
4. The rib that stops first during exhalation effort has exhalation restriction.

Note: The "key" rib designation denotes the rib that seems to prevent the ribs below (in inhalation restriction) and the ribs above (in exhalation restriction) from moving in their normal fashion.

RIB CAGE

Diagnosis

Prone

Respiratory Movement of the 11th and 12th Ribs

1. Patient is prone on the table with the operator standing at the side and dominant eye over the midline.
2. Operator identifies the tip of the 11th rib usually found in the midaxillary line just superior to the iliac crest.
3. Operator follows the contour of the 11th rib medially and places the thumbs and the thenar eminences over the posterior shaft of the 11th and 12th ribs (Fig. 15.23).
4. Operator follows inhalation and exhalation effort of the patient.
5. The 11th and 12th ribs that do not move posteriorly during inhalation have inhalation restriction.
6. The 11th and 12th ribs that do not move anteriorly during exhalation have exhalation restriction.
7. The 12th rib is notoriously asymmetric but always follows the 11th rib.

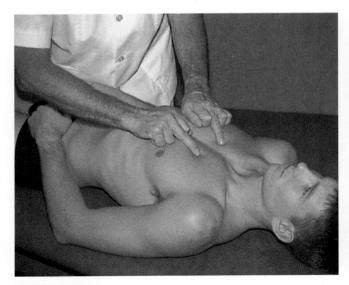

FIGURE 15.22

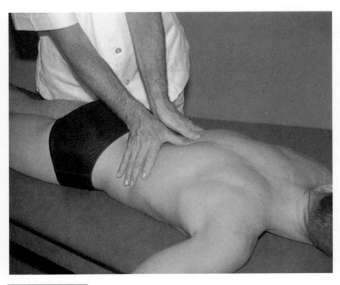

FIGURE 15.23

RIB CAGE SOMATIC DYSFUNCTION

Rib dysfunctions are classified as structural and respiratory. The structural rib dysfunctions include

1. Anterior and posterior subluxation,
2. Superior subluxation of the first rib,
3. Anteroposterior compression,
4. Lateral compression.

The subluxations and compressions follow acute or chronic recurrent trauma which damages the integrity of the costotransverse and/or costovertebral ligamentous articulations. They are frequently related to motor vehicle and sports injuries. In many instances, their presentation suggests that a rib is fractured but imaging studies fail to demonstrate a fracture. They frequently present as intercostal neuralgia. If a patient presents with intercostal neuralgia symptoms and no structural rib dysfunctions are identified, the practitioner should consider organic neurologic disease as the cause of the symptoms.

Another rib dysfunction that some classify as structural is *rib torsion*. Usually accompanying a nonneutral dysfunction of the thoracic spine, particularly of the extended, rotated, and side-bent (ERS) variety, rib torsional dysfunctions frequently resolve when the nonneutral thoracic spine dysfunction has been successfully treated. In other instances, particularly if the torsion has been present for a long time, the rib undergoes torsional deformity that persists and is a leading cause of recurrence of the thoracic spine dysfunction. This chronic torsion alters the bony architecture and that is why some call it a structural rib dysfunction.

Another rib dysfunction classified by some as structural is observed at rib 2 and is described as being "laterally flexed." Another term used is "bucket-bail." In this dysfunction, the rib behaves as though the anterior and posterior ends of the first rib were fixed in a true bucket-handle fashion and the traumatic episode results in the rib being laterally flexed. This usually occurs in a superior direction. Some authors describe this as a major bucket-handle exhalation restriction and it does not respond to the usual respiratory rib techniques. Other authors suggest that there is a subluxation of the rib shaft on top of the transverse process of the associated vertebra. While radiographs have demonstrated this phenomenon in the superior subluxation of rib 1, it has not been demonstrated in the laterally flexed rib. They usually result from acute side-bending injuries to the cervical thoracic junction. Shortening and hypertonicity of the posterior scalene muscles is an important associated finding.

The diagnostic criteria for structural rib dysfunctions are as follows:

1. Anterior Subluxation:
   - Rib angle less prominent in posterior rib cage contour.
   - Rib angle tender with tension of iliocostalis muscle.
   - Prominence of anterior extremity of the rib in the anterior rib cage contour.
   - Marked motion restriction of inhalation and exhalation.
   - Frequently present with complaint of "intercostal neuralgia" in adjacent interspace.

2. Posterior Subluxation:
   - Rib angle more prominent in posterior rib cage contour.
   - Rib angle tender with tension of iliocostalis muscle.
   - Anterior extremity of the rib less prominent in anterior rib cage contour.
   - Marked restriction of rib in inhalation and exhalation movement.
   - Frequent complaint of "intercostal neuralgia" in adjacent interspace.

3. Superior First Rib Subluxation:
   - Palpation of the superior aspect of the first rib anterior to the upper trapezius muscle shows dysfunctional rib to be 5 to 6 mm cephalic in relation to the contralateral side.
   - Marked tenderness of the superior aspect of the first rib.
   - Restriction of respiratory motion primarily exhalation.
   - Hypertonicity of scalene muscles on ipsilateral side.

4. Anteroposterior Rib Compression:
   - Less prominence of the rib shaft in the anterior and posterior convexities of the thoracic cage.
   - Prominence of the rib shaft in the midaxillary line.
   - Tenderness and tension of the intercostal space above and below the dysfunctional rib.
   - Frequent complaint of chest wall pain of the "intercostal neuralgia" type.
   - Motion restriction of respiratory activity.

5. Lateral Rib Compression:
   - Prominence of the rib shaft in the anterior and posterior convexities of the rib cage.
   - Dysfunctional rib shaft less prominent in the midaxillary line.
   - Tenderness and tension of the intercostal space above and below the dysfunctional rib.
   - Complaint of chest wall pain consistent with "intercostal neuralgia."
   - Respiratory motion restriction.

Note: Both anteroposterior and lateral rib compressions simulate rib fracture and typically are associated with trauma.

6. External Rib Torsion:
   - Superior border of the dysfunctional rib more prominent posteriorly.
   - Inferior border of the dysfunctional rib less prominent posteriorly.
   - Tension and tenderness at iliocostalis muscle attachment at the rib angle.
   - Widened intercostal space above and narrowed intercostal space below the dysfunctional rib with tension of the intercostal muscles on the inferior interspace.
   - Respiratory motion restriction primarily of exhalation.
   - These dysfunctions are frequently the key rib in exhalation group rib restrictions.

Note: External torsional dysfunctions are commonly associated with ERS dysfunction to the ipsilateral side. Internal torsional dysfunction has the reverse findings and is usually found on the contralateral side. Rib torsion dysfunctions are seldom found associated with flexed, rotated, and side-bent (FRS) dysfunctions.

7. Lateral Flexed Rib:
- Prominence of the rib shaft in the midaxillary line.
- Marked respiratory rib restriction usually exhalation.
- Asymmetry of interspace above and below the dysfunctional rib with the superior usually narrow and the inferior wider.
- Marked tenderness of the interspace usually the one above.
- Most commonly seen in rib 2, being dysfunctional in a superior position (laterally flexed superiorly).
- Marked tenderness of the superior intercostal space of rib 2 at its lateral aspect just beneath the lateral extremity of the clavicle.
- Frequently associated with brachalgia-type symptoms in the upper extremity.

RESPIRATORY RIB DYSFUNCTIONS

A single rib, or a group of ribs, can demonstrate restriction of either inhalation or exhalation movement. When a group of ribs has restriction of inhalation or exhalation function, we look for the "key rib." The key rib is the major restrictor of the group's ability to move into either inhalation or exhalation. The key rib is found at the upper or lower end of the group. In exhalation group rib restriction, the key rib is at the bottom of the group. In inhalation group rib restriction, the key rib is at the upper end of the group. *The key rib is frequently one of the structural rib dysfunctions. If a structural rib dysfunction is identified, it should be appropriately treated before dealing with the respiratory rib restrictions.* In treating group respiratory rib restrictions of the inhalation and exhalation type, the key rib is the rib usually addressed in the treatment procedure. Caution must be advised for the beginning student when assessing for respiratory restrictions. *The diagnostic criterion is based on the rib group that stops first during inhalation or exhalation. It is not the rib group that has the alteration in the excursion of range.*

Exhalation Restriction

1. A rib or group of ribs that ceases movement first during exhalation effort.

2. The key rib is at the bottom of the group.
3. Assessment is made as to which of the pump-handle or bucket-handle component is the most restricted.

Inhalation Restriction

1. A rib or group of ribs that ceases movement first during inhalation effort.
2. The key rib is at the top of the group.
3. Assessment is made as to whether the pump-handle or bucket-handle component is most restricted.

In group rib respiratory restrictions, there may be more than one key rib. Each rib must be assessed for its compliance in the overall inhalation and exhalation effort of that group of ribs.

TREATMENT OF RIB CAGE DYSFUNCTION

There are general principles of treatment sequence that should be followed for the successful treatment of rib cage dysfunction. As a general rule, treatment of the thoracic spine should precede treatment of the ribs, either individual or in groups. Torsional rib dysfunction frequently responds simultaneously with the treatment of the associated nonneutral thoracic dysfunction. The unique anatomy at the thoracic inlet requires that T1 be adequately evaluated and treated before addressing dysfunction of ribs 1 and 2. The unifacet for the first rib on the lateral side of T1 allows a great deal of variable motion of the first rib.[2–4]

The second principle of treating rib dysfunctions is to *address the structural rib dysfunctions prior to treatment of respiratory rib restriction.*[5,6] The key rib of a group of respiratory rib restriction is usually a structural rib dysfunction at the top or bottom of the group. Appropriate treatment to the structural rib dysfunction frequently restores normal movement to the group of ribs and their respiratory capacity. Following treatment of structural rib dysfunction, the respiratory rib restrictions are addressed with the goal of restoration of maximal, symmetric, inhalation/exhalation movement.

Technique of rib cage dysfunction and restriction is usually direct action with combined activating forces of muscle energy, respiratory effort, and operator guiding.

RIB CAGE

Structural Rib Dysfunction

Diagnosis

Superior Subluxation First Rib (Example: left side)

1. Patient sits with the operator standing behind.

2. Patient's right arm is draped over the operator's right thigh with foot on the table.

3. Operator's right hand and forearm control the patient's head and neck with the fingers of the left hand overlying the upper trapezius muscle that is pulled posteriorly (Fig. 15.24).

4. Operator's left thumb contacts the posterior shaft of the first rib through the trapezius muscle (Fig. 15.25).

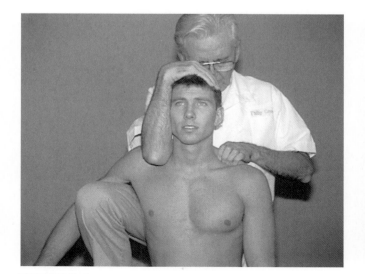

FIGURE 15.24

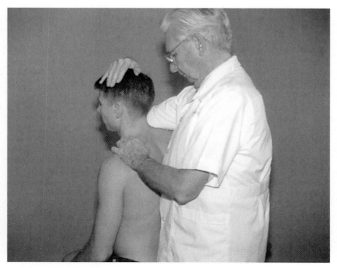

FIGURE 15.25

5. Operator's right hand introduces left-side bending and rotation of the patient's neck to unload T1 and the left scalene muscles. With the tips of the forefingers continuing to maintain the trapezius posteriorly, a caudal force is placed upon the shaft of the first rib (Fig. 15.26).

6. Simultaneously, the operator's left thumb maintains an anterior force on the posterior aspect of the shaft of the first rib to slide it anterior and medial in relation to the left transverse process of T1 (Fig. 15.27).

7. Patient performs a right-side bending effort of the head and neck against operator's resistance through the right hand activating the right scalene muscles and resulting in inhibition of the left scalenes.

8. Two to three efforts may be necessary before release is felt of the superior subluxation restoring symmetry with the opposite side.

9. Retest.

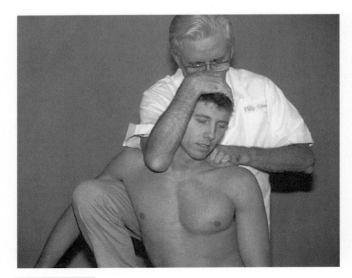

FIGURE 15.26

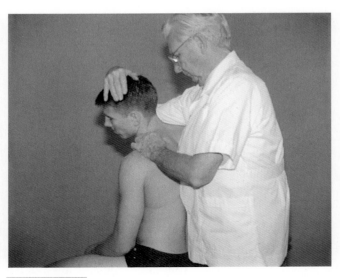

FIGURE 15.27

RIB CAGE

Structural Rib Dysfunction

Diagnosis

Anterior Subluxation (Example: right fifth rib)

1. Patient sits on the table with the right hand holding the left shoulder.

2. Operator stands behind the patient with the right thumb on the shaft of the fifth rib medial to the rib angle (Fig. 15.28) and with the left hand controlling the patient's right elbow (Fig. 15.29).

3. Operator lifts the elbow to localize forces to the dysfunctional rib.

4. Operator applies and maintains a posterolateral "pull" force on the rib shaft (Fig. 15.30).

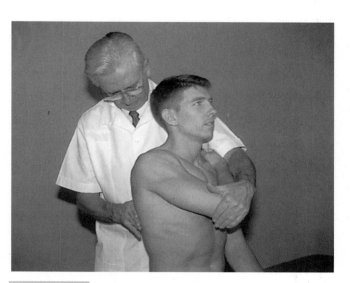

FIGURE 15.29

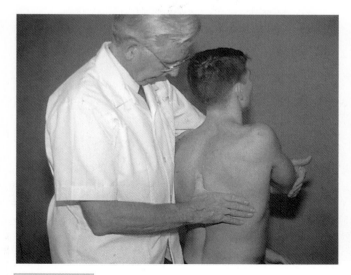

FIGURE 15.28

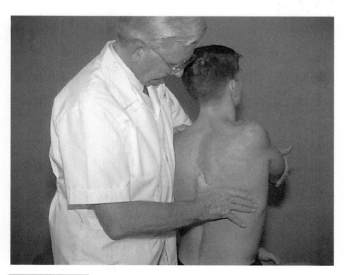

FIGURE 15.30

5. Patient is instructed to "pull" the right elbow laterally or caudally (Fig. 15.31). Three to five repetitions are made of a 3- to 5-second muscle contraction of the patient with operator monitoring rib motion.

6. Patient's left fist can be applied to the anterior extremity of the dysfunctional rib so that when the caudad pulling motion is performed there is anterior-to-posterior force directed at the dysfunctional rib (Fig. 15.32).

7. Retest.

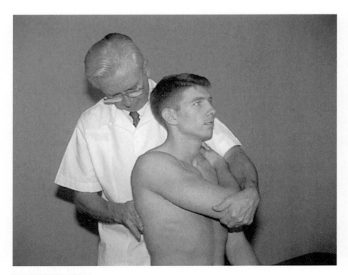

FIGURE 15.31

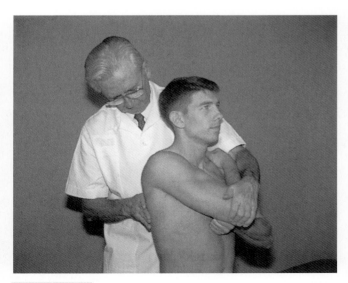

FIGURE 15.32

RIB CAGE

Structural Rib Dysfunction

Diagnosis

Posterior Subluxation (Example: right fifth rib)

1. Patient sits on the table with the right hand grasping the left shoulder.

2. Operator stands behind the patient with the thumb placed on the shaft of the right fifth rib lateral to the angle (Fig. 15.33) and with the left hand holding the patient's right elbow (Fig. 15.34).

3. Operator lifts the elbow to localize forces to the appropriate rib.

4. Operator maintains an anteromedial "push" force on the rib shaft and resists the patient's instructed "push" of the elbow to the left (Fig. 15.35) or a "push" of the right elbow toward the ceiling (Fig. 15.36).

5. Three to five repetitions of a 3- to 5-second muscle effort are usually necessary to restore symmetry.

6. Retest.

Note: Rib subluxations are frequently hypermobile, and following treatment stabilization of the rib cage by strapping or a rib belt is frequently useful.

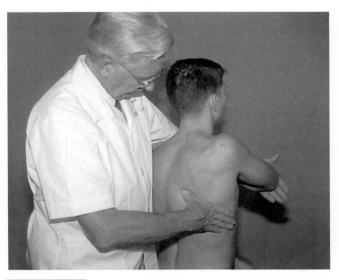

FIGURE 15.33

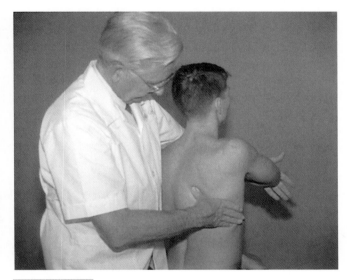

FIGURE 15.35

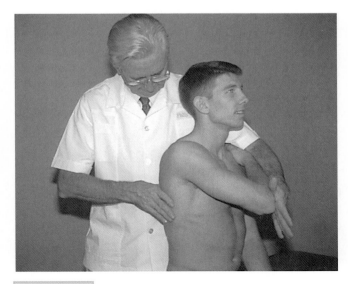

FIGURE 15.34

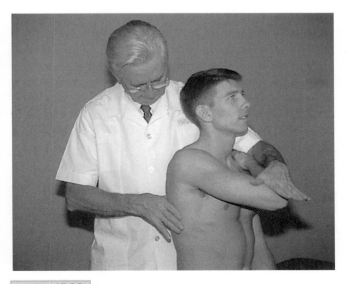

FIGURE 15.36

RIB CAGE

Structural Rib Dysfunction

Diagnosis

Rib Torsion (Example: right fifth rib)

1. Patient sits on the table with the right hand holding the left shoulder.
2. Operator stands behind with the thumb contacting the rib angle of the right fifth rib in a vertical fashion (Fig. 15.37).
3. Operator lifts the elbow to localize forces to the appropriate rib.
4. With external torsional restriction, the thumb applies an anterior force on the superior border of the dysfunctional rib.

5. For internal torsional restriction, the operator's thumb applies an anterior force on the inferior margin of the dysfunctional rib.
6. Patient is instructed to alternately pull the elbow to the lap (Fig. 15.38) and push toward the ceiling (Fig. 15.39) with the operator maintaining the appropriate compressive force on the superior or inferior aspect of the rib shaft.
7. Pulling toward the lap introduces internal torsional movement, and pushing toward the ceiling introduces external torsional movement. Operator resists the rib motion during the appropriate muscle effort and takes up the slack to the new barrier during each relaxation.
8. Three to five repetitions of 3- to 5-second contractions are made.
9. Retest.

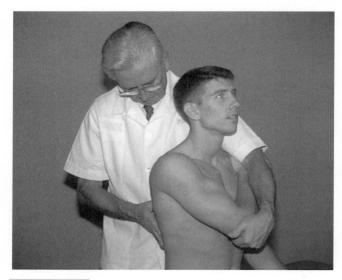

FIGURE 15.38

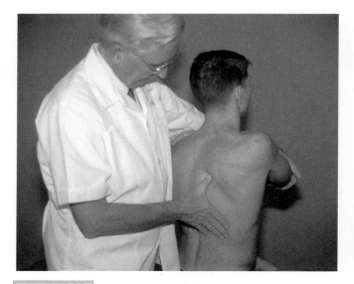

FIGURE 15.37

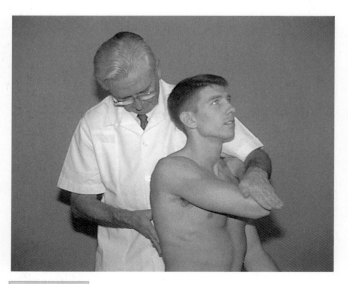

FIGURE 15.39

RIB CAGE

Structural Rib Dysfunction

Diagnosis

External Torsion (Example: right fifth rib)

1. Patient sits on the table with the right hand grasping the left shoulder.

2. Operator stands behind with the left arm controlling the patient's trunk with the left axilla over the patient's left shoulder and the left hand grasping the right shoulder. Operator's right hand identifies the dysfunctional rib angle and the shaft (Fig. 15.40).

3. Operator introduces small amount of flexion, left-side bending, and left rotation of the trunk and right hand follows the right fifth rib anteriorly (Fig. 15.41).

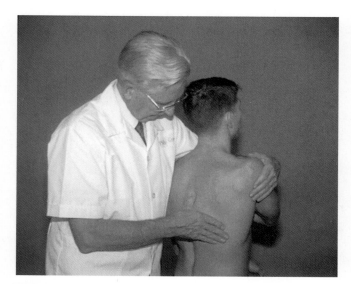

FIGURE 15.40

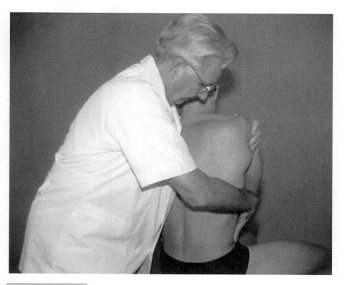

FIGURE 15.41

4. Operator's thumb and thenar eminence contact the anterior shaft of the right fifth rib exerting an internal rotary force over the prominent inferior margin of the shaft (Fig. 15.42).

5. Operator increases the forward bending, left-side bending, and left rotation of the trunk (Fig. 15.43).

6. Operator resists a right rotation, right-side bending, and extension effort of the patient while maintaining a compressive force on the inferior margin of the anterior shaft of the fifth rib (Fig. 15.44).

7. Three to five repetitions of a 3- to 5-second effort are made with the operator engaging a new barrier after each effort.

8. Retest.

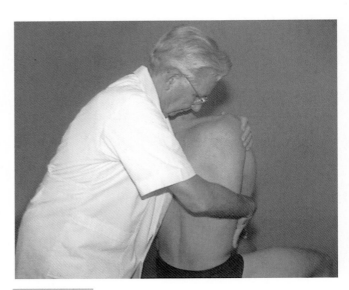

FIGURE 15.43

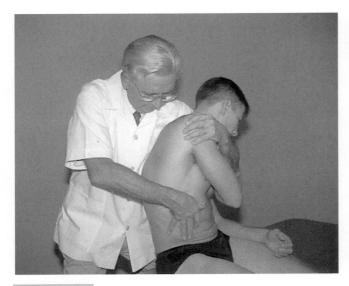

FIGURE 15.42

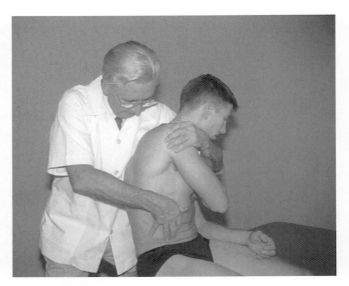

FIGURE 15.44

RIB CAGE

Structural Rib Dysfunction

Diagnosis

Anteroposterior Compression (Example: right sixth rib)

1. Patient sits on the end of the table with the operator standing on the side opposite to the dysfunction and the patient's arm is draped over the operator's shoulder (Fig. 15.45).

2. Operator's middle fingers of both hands contact the prominent rib shaft in the midaxillary line (Fig. 15.46).

3. Operator side bends patient to the right while applying a medial compressive force on the shaft of the dysfunctional rib (Fig. 15.47).

4. Patient is instructed to deeply inhale, hold the breath, and perform a left-side bending effort of the trunk against operator resistance while the operator maintains a medial compressive force on the dysfunctional rib (Fig. 15.48).

5. Three to five repetitions are made.

6. Retest.

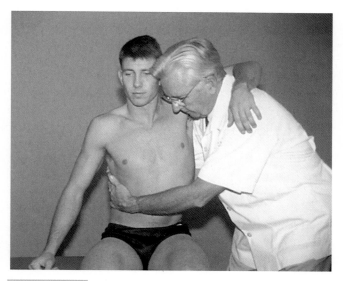

FIGURE 15.45

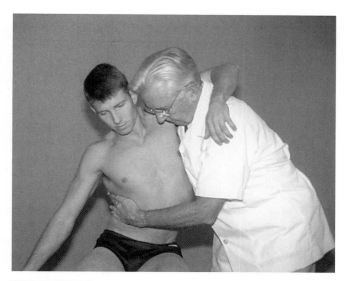

FIGURE 15.47

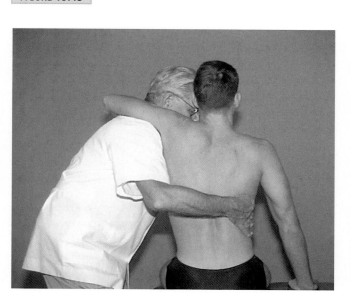

FIGURE 15.46

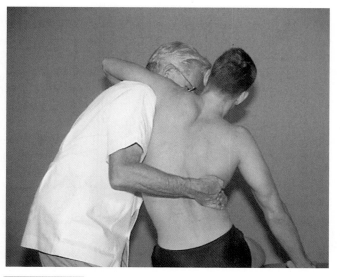

FIGURE 15.48

RIB CAGE

Structural Rib Dysfunction

Diagnosis

Lateral Compression (Example: left fifth rib)

1. Patient sits on the end of the table with the operator standing on the side of the dysfunction with the patient's left arm draped over the operator's right shoulder (Fig. 15.49).

2. Operator places the thenar eminence of each hand over the prominent posterior and anterior shaft of the dysfunctional fifth rib (Fig. 15.50).

3. Operator side bends the patient to the right while maintaining anteroposterior compression on the dysfunctional rib (Fig. 15.51).

4. Patient takes a deep breath, holds the breath, and performs a left-side bending effort against the resistance to the operator's shoulder (Fig. 15.52).

5. Three to five repetitions of a 3- to 5-second effort are performed with the operator engaging a new barrier after each effort.

6. Retest.

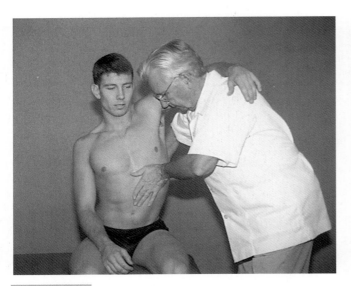

FIGURE 15.49

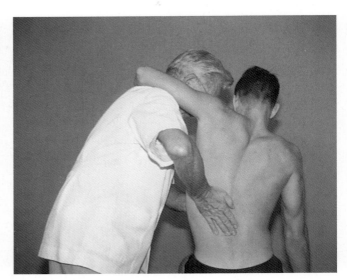

FIGURE 15.51

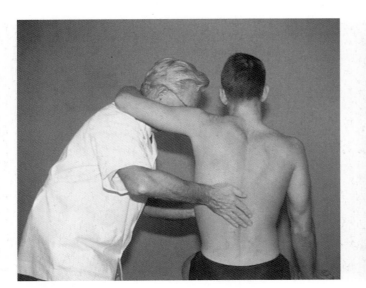

FIGURE 15.50

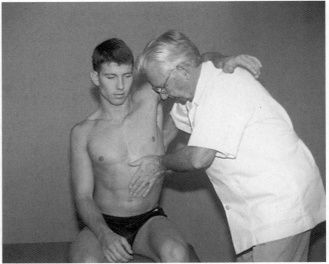

FIGURE 15.52

RIB CAGE

Structural Rib Dysfunction

Diagnosis

Laterally Flexed Superior (Example: left second rib)

1. Patient is supine on the table with the operator standing on the side of the dysfunction facing cephalad with the right hand against the midaxillary line of the patient's thorax (Fig. 15.53).

2. Operator slides the right hand cephalically along the lateral rib shaft with the left hand holding the patient's left arm inferiorly (Fig. 15.54).

3. Operator's left hand introduces left-side bending of the head and neck and the patient is instructed to fully exhale and reach toward the left knee to increase left-side bending (Fig. 15.55).

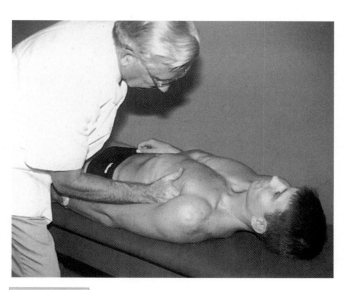

FIGURE 15.54

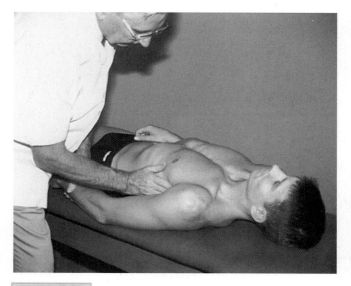

FIGURE 15.53

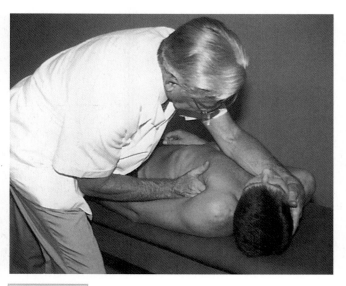

FIGURE 15.55

4. After several respiratory efforts with increased left-side bending, the operator's right hand grasps the superior aspect of the shaft of the second rib and the left hand is switched to the opposite side of the patient's head (Fig. 15.56).

5. While holding the superior aspect of the dysfunctional rib, the operator's left hand introduces acute right-side bending of the head and neck, stretching the left scalene muscles (Fig. 15.57).

6. Retest.

Note: This dysfunction is exquisitely tender to the patient and the treatment procedure is significantly painful. The patient should be appropriately informed.

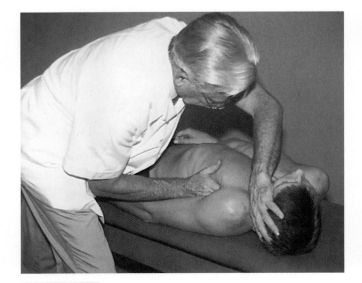

FIGURE 15.56

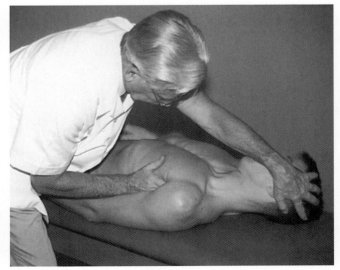

FIGURE 15.57

RIB CAGE

Structural Rib Dysfunction

Laterally Flexed Rib (Example: left second rib)

1. Patient is supine on the table with the operator sitting at the head.

2. Operator's right hand contacts the superior aspect of the left second rib as far laterally as possible and maintains a caudad pressure (Fig. 15.58).

3. Operator's left hand stabilizes the thoracic inlet and the lower cervical spine.

4. Patient abducts, externally rotates the left arm, dorsiflexes the left hand, and provides an on-and-off dural mobilization of the left upper extremity with a median nerve bias (Fig. 15.59). The operator frequently feels a release of the restricted rib during the mobilization by the patient.

5. Retest.

Note: This technique uses operator guiding and dural mobilization as the activating forces. It is much more comfortable for the patient than the previous technique. If ineffective, the previous direct action technique can be used.

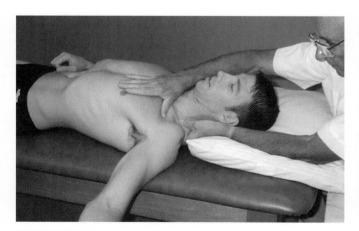

FIGURE 15.58

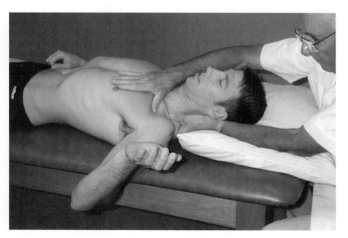

FIGURE 15.59

RESPIRATORY RIB RESTRICTIONS

Following the treatment of structural rib dysfunctions, respiratory rib restrictions are addressed. The respiratory rib restrictions are more myofascial problems than the bone and joint restrictions of the structural rib dysfunctions.

PRINCIPLES OF TREATMENT OF INHALATION RESTRICTION

The goal here is to use a "concentric isotonic" muscle energy technique which will allow the origin and insertion of the specific muscle to approximate.

1. Operator distracts the rib angle laterally and caudad to disengage the rib head at the costovertebral articulation and to allow the anterior rib cage to elevate.
2. Operator abducts and externally rotates the ipsilateral upper extremity to allow the thoracic spine to extend, again allowing the anterior rib cage to elevate.
3. Patient applies the respiratory activating force by deep inhalation.
4. Patient's muscle activating force uses scalenes to lift ribs 1 and 2, pectoralis minor to lift ribs 3 through 5, and serratus anterior to lift ribs 6 through 9.

PRINCIPLES OF TREATMENT OF EXHALATION RESTRICTION

Shortening of the intercostal muscles and their associated fascias hold the key rib in an exhalation restriction up or in an inhalation position. The fascial restriction of the soft tissues above the key rib is where to focus treatment of the exhalation restrictions.

1. Operator positions the patient in combined side bending and flexion to localize forces to the rib dysfunction.
2. Operator contacts the superior shaft and the costochondral junction of the dysfunctional rib.
3. Patient provides a maximum exhalation effort while operator follows and holds the dysfunctional rib in an exhalation position.
3. Patient provides a series of deep respirations; inhalation lifts the upper group of ribs amongst the operator held dysfunctional rib, allowing for focused intercostal soft tissue mobilization above the dysfunctional rib. Exhalation is followed and held.
4. Following a series of patient respirations, the operator returns the patient to a neutral trunk position while holding the rib in an exhalation position and slowly releases pressure on the rib shaft.

RIB CAGE

Respiratory Restriction

Ribs 1 and 2

Diagnosis

Inhalation Restriction (Example: right side)

1. Patient is supine with the operator standing on the left side of the table.

2. The fingers of the operator's left hand contact the medial aspect of the first and second ribs as close to the transverse process as possible (Fig. 15.60).

3. Patient's trunk is returned to the table with the operator's elbow on the table and the operator's hand providing a lateral and inferior pull on the first and second ribs.

4. Operator's right hand introduces left-side bending and rotation of the head and neck putting the right scalenes on tension (Fig. 15.61).

5. Patient is instructed to deeply inhale and lift the head off the table for pump-handle restriction or to side bend the head to the right for bucket-handle restriction against the resistance of the operator's right hand (Fig. 15.62).

6. Three to five repetitions are made of a 3- to 5-second effort.

7. This can be done in the presence of pathology of the right shoulder. If the right shoulder is healthy, an alternate hand position has the patient's forearm resting against the head (Fig. 15.63) reducing the caudad traction on the first and second ribs by the fascia of the right upper extremity.

8. Retest.

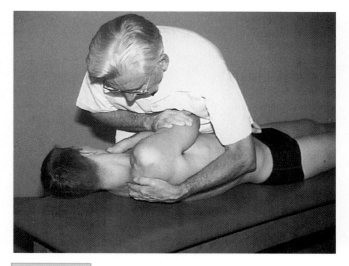

FIGURE 15.60

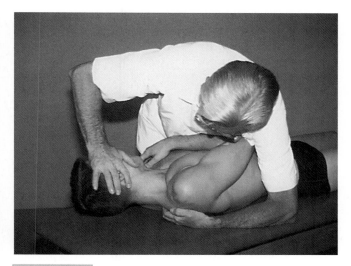

FIGURE 15.62

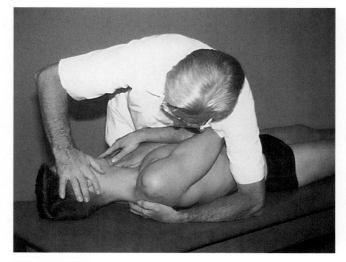

FIGURE 15.61

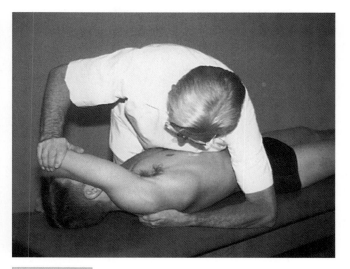

FIGURE 15.63

RIB CAGE

Respiratory Restriction

Ribs 3 to 5

Diagnosis

Inhalation Restriction (Example: right side)

1. Patient is supine on the table with the operator standing on the left side and with the left hand grasping the shafts of ribs 3, 4, and 5 medial to the angle (Fig. 15.64).

2. Operator returns the patient to neutral on the table and with the left forearm on the table applies a lateral and caudad distraction on the dysfunctional ribs.

3. Patient's right arm is elevated and abducted, lifting the anterior ribs and putting the pectoralis minor muscle on stretch.

4. Patient is instructed to take and hold a deep breath.

5. Patient performs a muscle effort of adduction against the operator's resistance for bucket-handle restriction (Fig. 15.65) or a flexion effort against operator resistance for a pump-handle restriction (Fig. 15.66).

6. Patient performs three to five repetitions of a 3- to 5-second contraction.

7. In the presence of the right shoulder pathology, the alternative procedure finds the operator's thumb medial to the right coracoid process to resist an anterior motion of the right shoulder girdle (Fig. 15.67).

8. Retest.

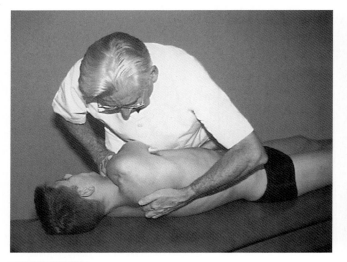

FIGURE 15.64

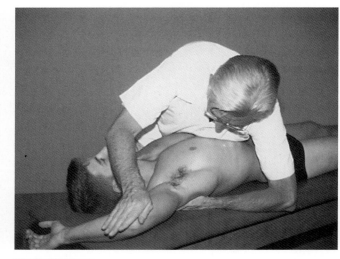

FIGURE 15.66

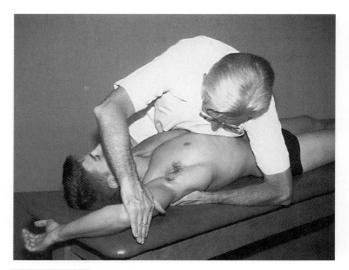

FIGURE 15.65

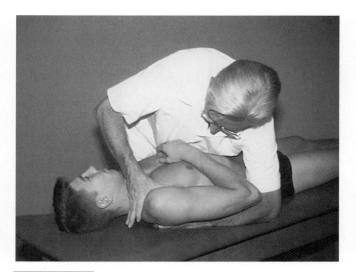

FIGURE 15.67

RIB CAGE

Respiratory Restriction

Ribs 6 to 9

Diagnosis

Inhalation Restriction (Example: right side)

1. Patient is supine on the table with the operator standing on the left side.

2. The fingers of the operator's left hand contact the sixth, seventh, eighth, and ninth ribs medial to the angle (Fig. 15.68).

3. Operator returns the patient to neutral position and with the left elbow on the table puts a lateral and caudad distractive force on the four ribs.

4. Operator's right hand controls the patient's abducted and elevated right upper extremity.

5. Patient is instructed to take and hold a deep breath, and for a pump-handle restriction, the patient flexes the upper extremity against the operator's resistance (Fig. 15.69), or in a lateral direction for bucket-handle restriction (Fig. 15.70).

6. Patient performs three to five repetitions of a 3- to 5-second muscle effort.

7. In the presence of shoulder dysfunction, the operator resists a protraction action of the right scapula at the inferior scapular angle (Fig. 15.71).

8. Retest.

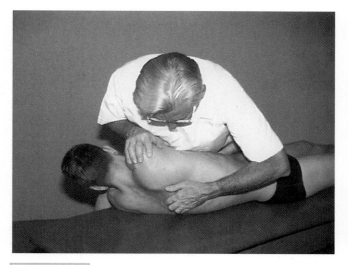

FIGURE 15.68

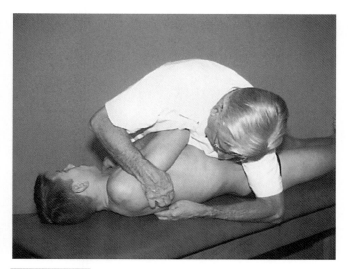

FIGURE 15.70

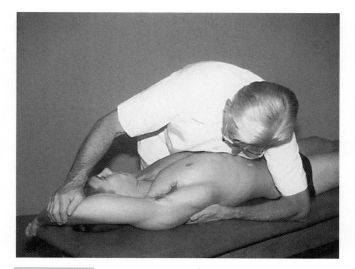

FIGURE 15.69

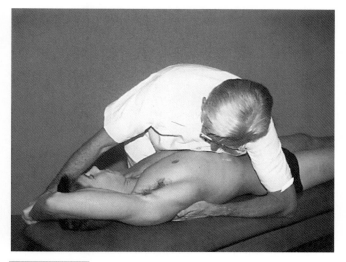

FIGURE 15.71

RIB CAGE

Respiratory Restriction

Lower ribs

Diagnosis

Exhalation Restriction (Example: left side)

1. Patient is supine on the table with the operator standing at the left side of the head of the table.

2. Operator's left thumb and thenar eminence contact the superior aspect of the dysfunctional key rib, including the costochondral junction (Fig. 15.72).

3. Operator's right hand supports the head, neck, and upper thorax to control patient body position (Fig. 15.73).

4. Operator introduces left-side bending and flexion of the trunk down to the key rib (Fig. 15.74).

5. Patient is instructed to exhale completely.

6. Operator follows exhalation movement of the rib and holds it in that position.

7. Operator resists the patient's inhalation respiratory effort. During the patient's next exhalation, a new barrier is engaged by trunk flexion and side bending (Fig. 15.75).

8. After three to five repetitions of maximum exhalation, the patient's head, neck, and upper trunk are returned to neutral while the operator holds the key rib in an exhalation position.

9. Operator slowly releases the left thumb from the key rib.

10. Retest.

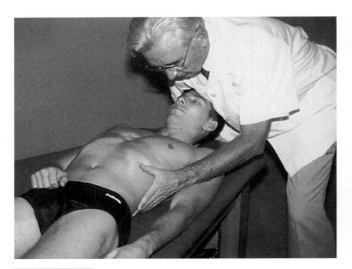

FIGURE 15.72

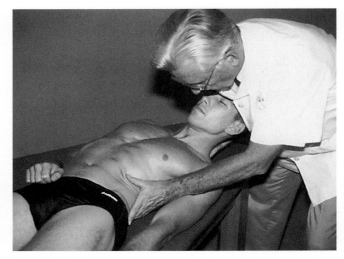

FIGURE 15.74

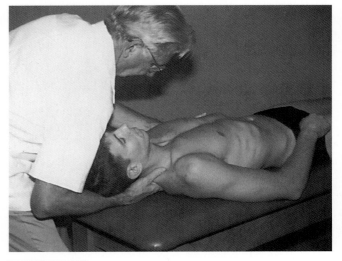

FIGURE 15.73

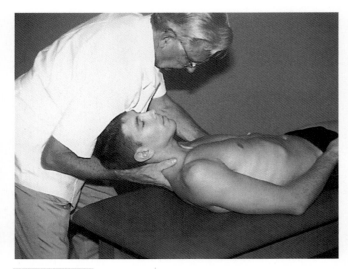

FIGURE 15.75

RIB CAGE

Respiratory Restriction

Upper Ribs

Diagnosis

Exhalation Restriction (Example: left side)

1. Patient is supine on the table with the operator standing at the left side of the head of the table.

2. Operator's left thumb and thenar eminence contact the superior aspect of the shaft of the dysfunctional rib spanning the costochondral junction. Note that the more cephalic the rib, the more medial the costochondral junction (Fig. 15.76).

3. Operator's right hand controls the patient's head, neck, and upper thorax and introduces flexion and side bending to focus forces at the key rib (Fig. 15.77).

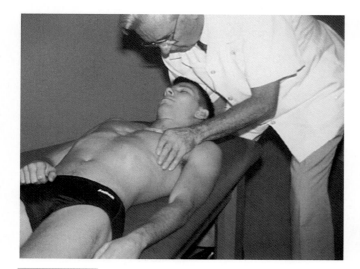

FIGURE 15.76

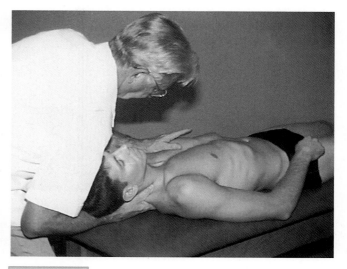

FIGURE 15.77

4. Operator introduces more flexion for pump-handle component and side bending for the bucket-handle component (Fig. 15.78).

5. Patient is instructed to exhale completely, while the operator follows the rib in exhalation with increasing flexion and side bending (Fig. 15.79).

6. Three to five repetitions are performed. When maximum exhalation movement has been achieved, the patient's head and neck are returned to neutral, while the operator holds the dysfunctional rib in exhalation position (Fig. 15.80).

7. Operator slowly releases the compressive left thumb.

8. Retest.

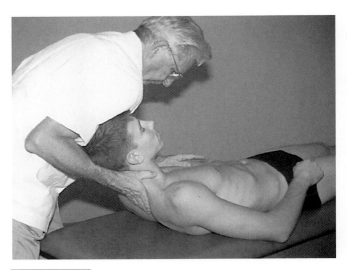

FIGURE 15.79

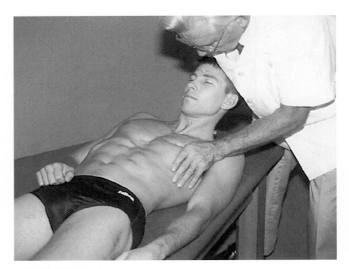

FIGURE 15.78

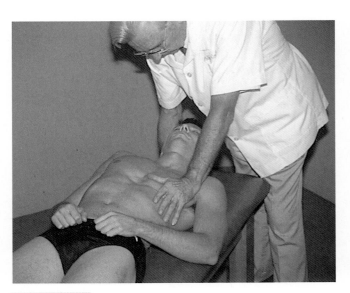

FIGURE 15.80

RIB CAGE

Respiratory Restriction

Upper Ribs

Diagnosis

Exhalation Restriction (Example: left side)

1. Patient is supine with the operator standing at the head of the table.

2. Operator's left hand controls the patient's head and neck, while the right thumb and thenar eminence contact the shaft and costochondral articulation of the dysfunction rib (Fig. 15.81).

3. Operator introduces flexion and side bending down to the key rib.

4. Patient is instructed to fully exhale and the operator follows the dysfunctional rib into an exhalation position and holds it there (Fig. 15.82).

5. Following several respiratory efforts with increasing flexion and side bending, the operator returns the head to neutral and slowly releases the compressive force on the dysfunctional rib.

6. Retest.

Note: This alternative position avoids compressive force on breast tissue particularly in females. It is also particularly valuable for the pump-handle component of upper rib restrictions.

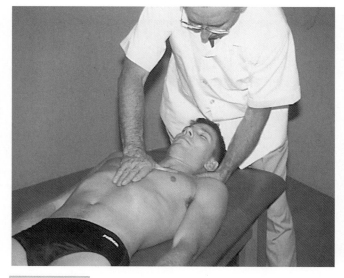

FIGURE 15.81

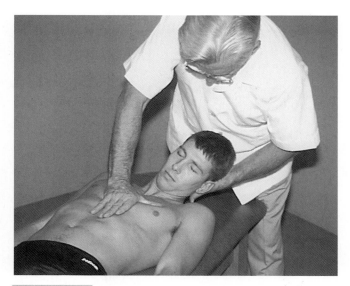

FIGURE 15.82

RIB CAGE

Respiratory Restriction

First Rib

Diagnosis

Exhalation Restriction: pump-handle component (Example: left side)

1. Patient is supine on the table with the operator sitting at the head.

2. Operator's right hand controls the patient's head, while the left thumb contacts the superior aspect of the anterior extremity of the first rib, either lateral to or between the heads of the sternocleidomastoid muscle (Fig. 15.83).

3. Operator introduces head and neck flexion with some left-side bending to unload or loose pack T1 (Fig. 15.84).

4. Patient fully exhales while the operator increases flexion and left-side bending following the left first rib into exhalation (Fig. 15.85).

5. Operator resists inhalation movement of the first rib and during the patient's next exhalation follows the first rib into the exhalation position.

6. Three to five efforts are performed and when maximum exhalation has been achieved, the operator returns the head to neutral and slowly releases the contact on the first rib.

7. Retest.

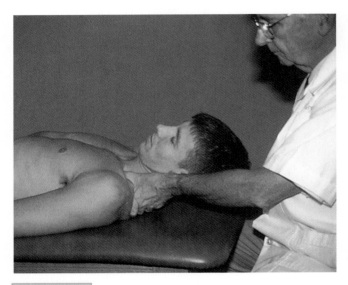

FIGURE 15.84

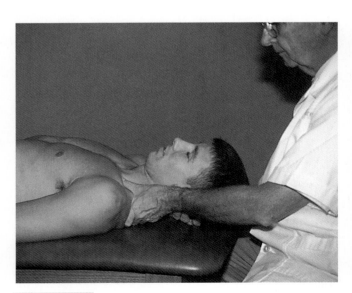

FIGURE 15.83

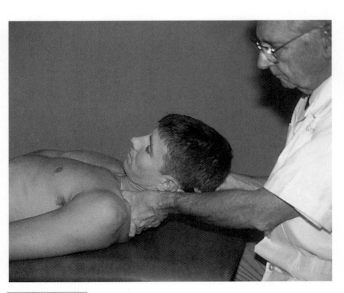

FIGURE 15.85

RIB CAGE

Respiratory Restriction

First Rib

Diagnosis

Exhalation Restriction: bucket-handle component (Example: left side)

1. Patient is supine with the operator sitting at the head of the table.

2. Operator's right hand grasps the patient's head and neck, while the left thumb contacts the superior aspect of the lateral shaft of the first rib just anterior to the trapezius and posterior to the clavicle (Fig. 15.86).

3. Patient performs a forced exhalation while the operator side bends the head and neck to the left with a small amount of flexion and follows the lateral shaft of the rib into exhalation (Fig. 15.87).

4. Operator continues holding the first rib in exhalation and the patient repeats the maximal exhalation effort with increasing left-side bending of the head and neck by the operator's right hand (Fig. 15.88).

5. When maximal exhalation effort has been achieved, the operator holds the first rib in exhalation position and returns the head to neutral.

6. Operator's left thumb is released slowly.

7. Retest.

Note: The goal of head and neck flexion and side bending is to loose pack and maintain freedom of motion of the articular surface of the first rib with T1.

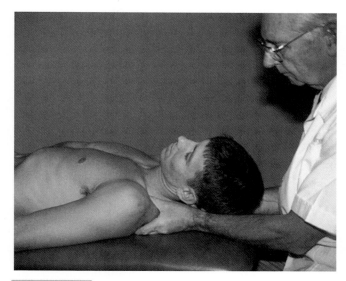

FIGURE 15.87

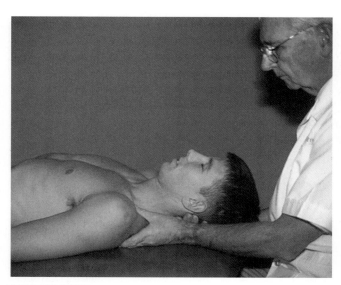

FIGURE 15.86

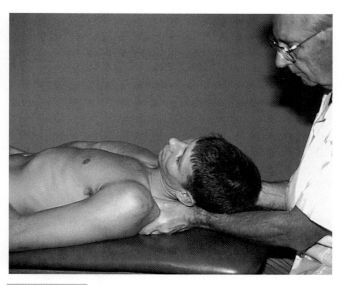

FIGURE 15.88

RIB CAGE

Respiratory Restriction

Ribs 11 and 12

Diagnosis

Exhalation Restriction (Example: right side)

1. Patient is prone on the table with the operator standing on the left side of the patient.

2. Operator's heel of the left hand contacts the medial side of the shafts of the 11th and 12th ribs (Fig. 15.89).

3. Patient's right arm is placed on the table and reaches toward the feet with the trunk side bending toward the right.

4. Operator's right hand grasps the patient's right anterior superior iliac spine (Fig. 15.90).

5. Patient is instructed to maximally exhale.

6. Operator's left hand carries the 11th and 12th ribs in a lateral and caudad direction.

7. At the end of full exhalation, the patient pulls the right anterior superior iliac spine toward the table for 3 to 5 seconds (Fig. 15.91).

8. After each effort, the operator engages a new barrier. Three to five repetitions are made.

9. Retest.

Note: In this situation, the patients' quadratus lumborum muscle is used to pull down the 11th and 12th ribs and mobilize the intercostal soft tissues above the key rib.

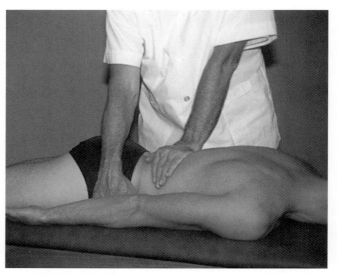

FIGURE 15.90

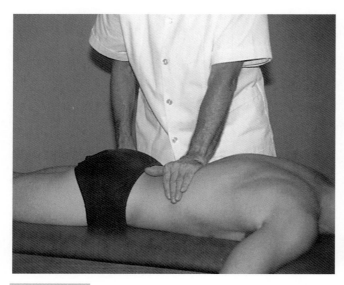

FIGURE 15.89

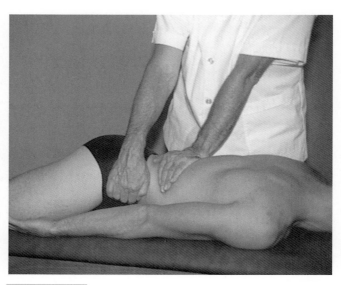

FIGURE 15.91

RIB CAGE

Respiratory Restriction

Ribs 11 and 12

Diagnosis

Inhalation Restriction (Example: right side)

1. Patient is prone on the table with the operator standing on the left side.

2. Operator's heel of the left hand contacts the medial aspect of the patient's 11th and 12th ribs (Fig 15.92) and exerts a lateral and cephalic force.

3. Patient's right hand is placed over the head and the feet to the left introducing left-side bending (Fig. 15.93).

4. Operator's right hand grasps the right anterior superior iliac spine.

5. Patient is instructed to take and hold a maximal inhalation effort.

6. Operator lifts the patient's right pelvis off the table and resists the patient's effort to pull the right anterior superior iliac spine down to the table (Fig. 15.94).

7. Three to five repetitions are made with a new barrier being engaged after each effort.

8. Retest.

Note: This treatment stretches the hypertonic ipsilateral quadratus lumborum muscle which holds the 11th and/or 12th rib down into the inhalation restriction.

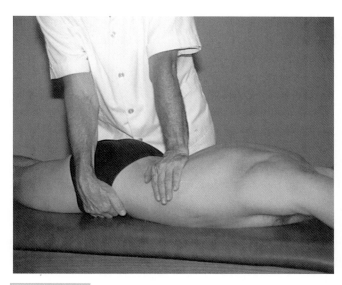

FIGURE 15.93

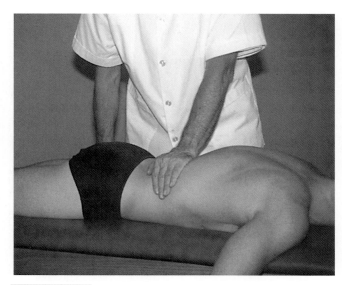

FIGURE 15.92

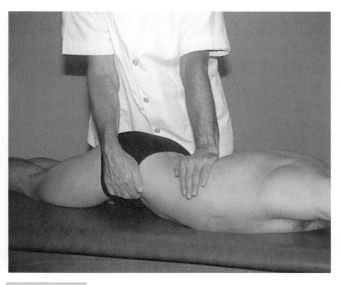

FIGURE 15.94

MOBILIZATION WITH IMPULSE (HIGH-VELOCITY THRUST) DIRECT ACTION TECHNIQUE FOR RIB DYSFUNCTION

The major restrictors of rib cage dysfunction are primarily myofascial. Occasionally, a rib will become dysfunctional with palpable characteristics of deep articular and periarticular tissue reaction. Mobilization with impulse technique would then be of assistance in the management of the rib cage. Mobilization with impulse technique can be used to treat single rib and group rib dysfunctions of both the structural and respiratory type. Mobilizations with impulse techniques are contraindicated in the presence of rib subluxations, which are typically due to articular trauma with hypermobility. The treatment sequence is the same as previously described.

The structural rib dysfunction most frequently treated with mobilization with impulse technique is external rib torsional dysfunction associated with a nonneutral ERS dysfunction of the thoracic spine.

RIB CAGE

Respiratory Restriction

Mobilization with Impulse Technique

Supine

Diagnosis

External Torsion Dysfunction (Example: left fifth rib)

1. Patient and operator positions are the same as for the thoracic spine, mobilization with impulse technique for an ERS left dysfunction at T4 to T5 (Figs. 14.68 and 14.69).

2. Operator establishes lever arm.

3. Operator's right hand establishes a fulcrum to stabilize both transverse processes of T5 with the thenar eminence on the inferior aspect of the left fifth rib.

4. Following the return of the patient to neutral position and the establishment of the lever arm to the fulcrum, the operator's left hand introduces flexion, right-side bending, and right rotation of the neck and upper thoracic spine down to the left fifth rib.

5. The force through the lever arm to the fulcrum is somewhat more to the left side than midline as for the thoracic dysfunction, and a high-velocity, low-amplitude thrust is made by the body weight of the operator on the lever arm to the fulcrum resulting in flexion, right-side bending, right rotation of T4 on T5, the opening of the left zygapophysial joint, and the mobilization of the left fifth rib. The thenar eminence of the operator's right hand maintains a cephalic pressure on the inferior aspect of the fifth rib at the time of the thrust.

6. Commonly, two cavitation pop sounds occur in rapid sequence when the thrust is applied.

7. Retest.

RIB CAGE

Respiratory Restriction

Mobilization with Impulse Technique

Rib 1

Diagnosis

Inhalation or Exhalation Restriction (Example: left first rib)

1. Patient is supine on the table with the operator standing on the right side and sliding an arm under the patient with fingers of the right hand grasping the superior aspect of the left first rib (Fig. 15.95).

2. With exhalation restriction, the operator depresses the anterior aspect of the rib shaft. With inhalation restriction, the operator depresses the posterior aspect of first rib.

3. Operator's left hand side bends patient's head and neck to the left and rotates to the right, localizing to T1 (Fig. 15.96).

4. A mobilization with impulse thrust is performed by the operator with either an acute exaggeration of the head and neck position into left-side bending or stabilizing the head and neck with the left hand and performing an acute caudad thrust through the right hand along an axis of the right forearm.

5. Retest.

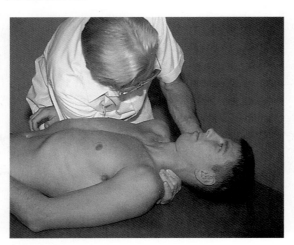

FIGURE 15.95

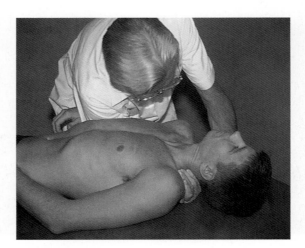

FIGURE 15.96

RIB CAGE

Respiratory Restriction

Mobilization with Impulse Technique

Rib 1

Diagnosis

Exhalation Restriction (Example: left first rib)

1. Patient sits on the table with the operator standing behind.

2. Operator's right foot is placed on the table and the patient's right upper extremity is draped over the operator's right thigh.

3. Operator's right hand contacts the right side of the head and neck of the patient, while the left hand contacts the left first rib over its anterior and posterior extremity (Fig. 15.97).

4. Operator's left forearm is angled from above downward against the hand contact on the first rib (Fig. 15.98).

5. Operator introduces left-side bending and right rotation of the patient's head and neck localized at T1 (Fig. 15.99).

6. A mobilization with impulse thrust is performed through the operator's left forearm in a caudad and medial direction (Fig. 15.100).

7. Retest.

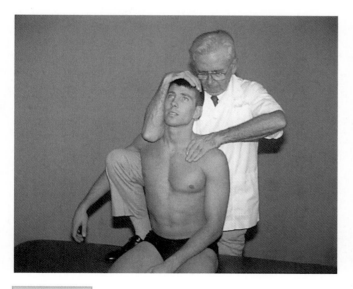

FIGURE 15.97

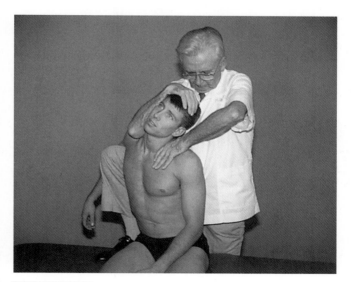

FIGURE 15.99

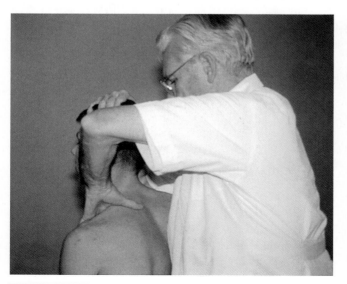

FIGURE 15.98

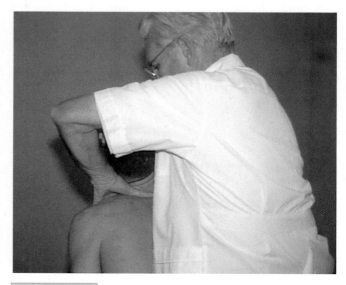

FIGURE 15.100

RIB CAGE

Respiratory Restriction

Mobilization with Impulse Technique

Rib 2

Diagnosis

Exhalation Restriction (Example: left second rib)

1. Patient sits on the table with the operator standing behind with the right foot on the table and the patient's right arm draped over the operator's right thigh.

2. Operator's right hand controls the right side of the patient's head and neck and the left hand is over the patient's left shoulder (Fig. 15.101).

3. Operator's left thumb is on the posterior shaft of the rib 2 (Fig. 15.102).

4. Operator introduces left-side bending and right rotation of the head and neck, with translation of the trunk from left to right localizing to T1 to T2 and the left second rib (Fig. 15.103).

5. When the barrier is engaged, a mobilization with impulse technique is performed through the left forearm with an anterior and medial thrust against the resistance of the stabilizing right arm (Fig. 15.104).

6. Retest.

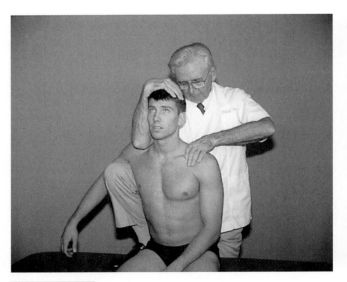

FIGURE 15.101

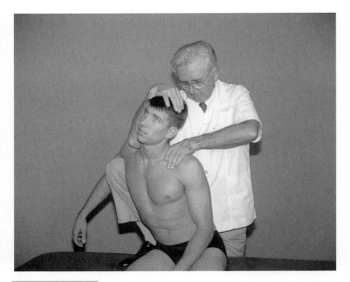

FIGURE 15.103

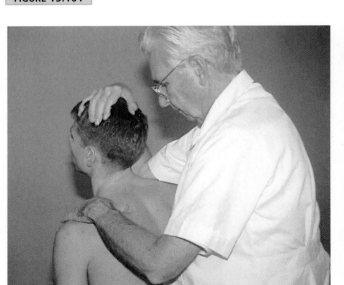

FIGURE 15.102

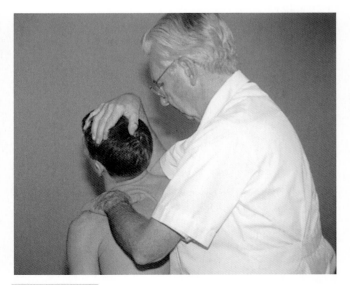

FIGURE 15.104

RIB CAGE

Respiratory Restriction

Mobilization with Impulse Technique

Typical Ribs (3 to 10)

Diagnosis

Inhalation or Exhalation Restriction (Example: left ribs)

1. Operator's thumb and thenar eminence function as the fulcrum. The thumb contacts either the superior or the inferior aspect of the dysfunctional rib (Fig. 15.105).

2. For inhalation restriction, the thumb and thenar contact is on the superior aspect of the rib shaft with the rib being carried caudad (Fig. 15.106).

3. For exhalation restriction, the thumb is placed below the rib shaft and exerts a superior force (Fig. 15.107).

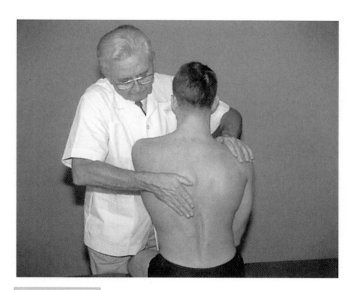

FIGURE 15.106

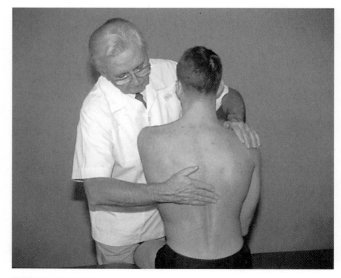

FIGURE 15.105

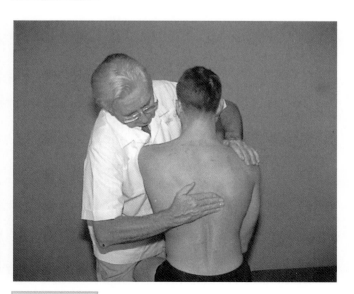

FIGURE 15.107

4. Patient's left hand grasps the right shoulder establishing the lever arm (Fig. 15.108).

5. Operator places the fulcrum on the dysfunctional rib as appropriate for the respiratory restriction (Fig. 15.109).

6. Patient's trunk is returned to midline and the operator's body (either chest wall or abdomen) localizes to fulcrum through the lever arm (Fig. 15.110).

7. A mobilization with impulse thrust is made by the operator's body dropped through the lever arm to the fulcrum with the right thumb and thenar eminence exerting a cephalic-directed force for exhalation restriction and a caudad-directed force for inhalation restriction.

8. A respiratory assist of inhalation or exhalation can be made, but usually exhalation for relaxation of the patient is more helpful.

9. Retest.

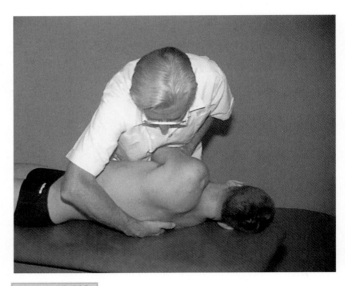

FIGURE 15.109

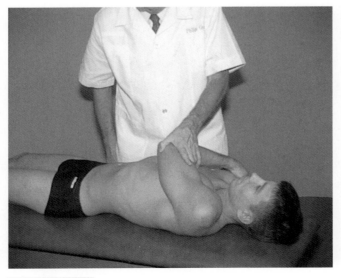

FIGURE 15.108

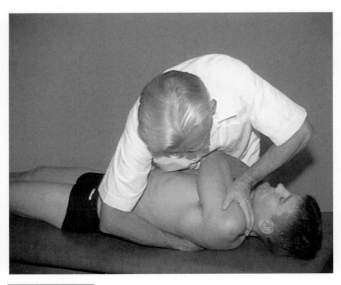

FIGURE 15.110

RIB CAGE

Respiratory Restriction

Mobilization with Impulse Technique

Lower Typical Ribs and Ribs 11 and 12

Diagnosis

Inhalation or Exhalation Restriction (Example: left side)

1. Patient is in lateral recumbent position with the dysfunctional side up.

2. Operator stands in front of the patient with the pisiform of the right hand in contact with the posterior aspect of the dysfunctional rib (Fig. 15.111).

3. Operator's left hand contacts the anterior aspect of the patient's left shoulder.

4. For exhalation restriction, the pisiform contact is on the inferior aspect of the rib shaft and the operator's right forearm directs the rib in an anterior and superior direction (Fig. 15.112).

5. For inhalation restriction, the pisiform contact is on the superior aspect of the rib shaft and the operator's right arm carries it caudally (Fig. 15.113).

6. A mobilization with impulse thrust is performed by a body drop of the operator directing force through the right forearm in the appropriate direction for inhalation or exhalation restriction.

7. Retest.

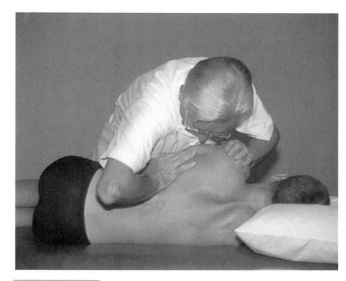

FIGURE 15.112

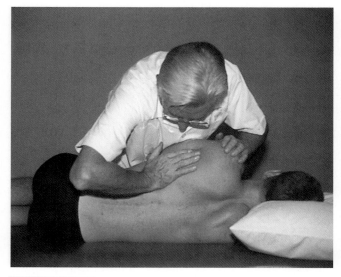

FIGURE 15.111

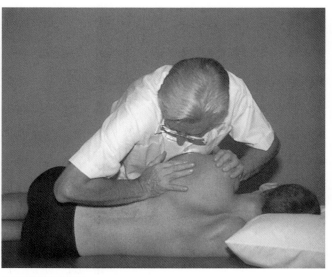

FIGURE 15.113

RIB CAGE

Respiratory Restriction

Mobilization with Impulse Technique

Diagnosis

Ribs 11 and 12 (Example: right side)

1. Patient is prone on the table with the operator standing on the left side with the left hand medial to the shafts of ribs 11 and 12 and the right hand grasping the patient's right anterior superior iliac spine.

2. For exhalation restriction, the patient is side bent to the right with the right arm reaching toward the right knee (Fig. 15.114).

3. For inhalation restriction, the patient is left-side bent with the right hand over the head (Fig. 15.115).

4. The barrier is engaged by lifting the anterior superior iliac spine from the table.

5. A mobilization with impulse thrust is performed through the operator's left hand in a lateral and inferior direction for exhalation restriction and in a lateral and superior direction for inhalation restriction.

6. Retest.

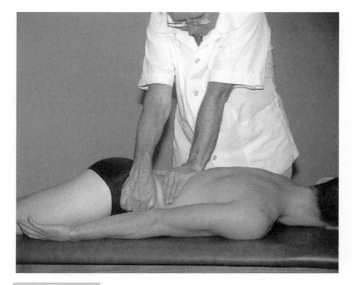

FIGURE 15.114

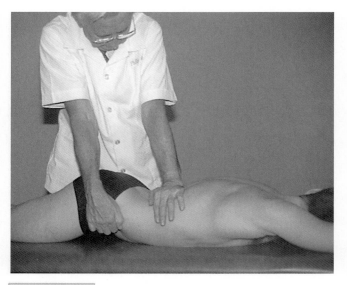

FIGURE 15.115

CONCLUSION

Dysfunction of the rib cage is highly significant in many problems of the musculoskeletal system. The structural rib dysfunctions can be major pain generators. Respiratory rib restriction compromises the patient's capacity for respiration and efficient circulation of the low-pressure venous and lymphatic systems. There are extensive muscle attachments to the rib cage that can serve as restrictors of the cervical spine, the upper extremities, the lumbar spine, and even the pelvis and lower extremities. Restoration of symmetric thoracic cage function for respiration and circulation is as important as restoring symmetric mobility of the lumbar spine, pelvis, and lower extremities in the walking cycle.

REFERENCES

1. Andriacchi T, Schultz A Belytschko T, et al. A model for studies of mechanical interactions between the human spine and rib cage. *J Biomech* 1974;7: 497–507.
2. Lee R, Farquharson T, Domelo S. Subluxation and locking of the first rib: A cause of thoracic outlet syndrome. *Aust Assoc Man Med Bull* 1988;6:50–51.
3. Lindgren KA, Leino E. Subluxation of the first rib: A possible thoracic outlet syndrome mechanism. *Arch Phys Med Rehabil* 1988;68:692–695.
4. Lindgren KA, Mannimen H, Rytkonen H. Thoracic outlet syndrome: A functional disturbance of the upper thoracic aperture? *Muscle Nerve* 1995;5:526–530.
5. Bourdillon J. Treatment of respiratory rib dysfunctions. *J Orthop Med* 1990; 12:63–68.
6. Bourdillon J. Treatment of structural rib dysfunctions. *J Orthop Med* 1991; 13:20–22.

The lumbar spine and pelvic girdle (see Chapter 17) contain many of the structures incriminated in the complaint of "low back pain." The classic report of Mixter and Barr[1] in 1934 brought the lumbar intervertebral disk to the attention of physicians in many disciplines. The differential diagnosis of low back pain continues to be a dilemma for the examining physician. About 60% to 80% of cases of low back pain are still classified as idiopathic.[2] After the exclusion of organic and pathologic conditions by orthodox orthopedic and neurologic testing, the examiner is left with the difficulty of determining if any other treatable source for the back pain can be identified. It is in these patients that the ability to identify and treat functional abnormalities of the musculoskeletal system has been found to be clinically effective. It is strongly recommended that the structural diagnostic procedures identified here, and in Chapter 17, be used concurrently with orthopedic and neurologic testing of the lower trunk and the lower extremities. Including functional diagnosis in these patients greatly reduces the number that needs to be classified as idiopathic. More clinical research is needed into the origin of pain in dysfunctions of the lumbar spine and pelvis, the efficacy, and the mechanisms of manual medicine therapeutic applications.

FUNCTIONAL ANATOMY

The five lumbar vertebrae are the most massive in the vertebral column. The vertebral bodies are kidney shaped and are solidly constructed to participate in weight bearing of the superincumbent vertebral column. The posterior arches are strongly developed with large spinous processes projecting directly posterior from the vertebral bodies. The transverse processes are quite large and those at L3 are usually the broadest. The lumbar lordosis has an anterior convexity with L3, usually the most anterior segment. L4 and L5 have limited motion because of the strong attachments of the iliolumbar ligaments to the osseous pelvis; therefore, L3 becomes the first lumbar segment that is freely movable.[3]

The articular pillar has a superior zygapophysial joint that faces posteriorly and medially and an inferior zygapophysial joint that faces laterally and anteriorly. The superior facet is somewhat concave and the inferior facet somewhat convex.[4] The facing of the lumbar zygapophysial joint is variable and asymmetry is quite common. Because of the shape of the zygapophysial joints, only a small amount of axial rotation movement is present. When the plane of the zygapophysial joints is more sagittal, there appears to be increased stability of the lumbar spine. The more coronal facing the lumbar zygapophysial joints are, the more mobility and potential hypermobility appear to be present. The presence of asymmetry, with one zygapophysial joint being sagittal and the other being coronal, appears to increase the risk of disc degeneration and herniation,

with a tendency toward herniation on the side of the coronal facing facet.[5] Asymmetric zygapophysial joints also appear to influence the motion characteristics of the segment and are frequently found in patients with recurrent and refractory dysfunctional problems in the lumbar spine. Between the superior and inferior zygapophysial joints lies a structure called the pars interarticularis. Disruption through the pars without separation is called spondylolysis. With separation at this level, the body, pedicle, and superior articular pillar slide anteriorly while the spinous process, laminae, and inferior articular pillar are held posteriorly, resulting in spondylolisthesis.

The lower lumbar region is frequently the site of developmental variations. In addition to asymmetric development of the zygapophysial joints, other variations in the posterior arch occur resulting in unilateral and bilateral changes in size and shape of the transverse process, culminating in a transitional lumbosacral vertebra that may have lumbar or sacral characteristics, (previously referred to as lumbarization and sacralization). Failure of closure of the posterior arch is not infrequently seen and occasionally, the spinous process of L5 is missing. Absence of these structures must result in alteration of the usual ligamentous and muscular attachments in the region.

LUMBAR MOTION

The motions available in the lumbar spine are primarily flexion and extension. There is a small amount of right- and left-side bending and a minimal amount of rotation. The coupled movements of side bending and rotation available in the lumbar spine are both neutral (type I) and nonneutral (type II). In the absence of dysfunction, when in the neutral and the backward-bent positions, side bending and rotation are coupled to opposite sides. In the forward-bent position, side bending and rotation couple to the same side (nonneutral mechanics). Neutral coupling is the lumbar motion that occurs during normal gait. The lumbar lordosis is present and the lumbar spine side bends and rotates to opposite sides with each step. The nonneutral behavior of the lumbar spine, when it is forward bent, places the lumbar spine at risk for injury of the zygapophysial joints for dysfunction, the paravertebral muscles for strain, the posterior ligaments for sprain, and the intervertebral disk for torsional injury and potentially herniation.[6] The L4 and L5 segments have less mobility than the upper three due to the attachment of the iliolumbar ligaments with the osseous pelvis.

MOTION AT THE LUMBOSACRAL JUNCTION

During neutral vertebral mechanics, and in the absence of dysfunction, the lumbar spine and the sacrum move in opposite directions. As the sacrum moves into anterior nutation (sacral flexion), the lumbar spine moves into backward bending (extension) in relation to the sacrum. With the sacrum moving into posterior nutation (sacral extension), the lumbar moves into forward bending (flexion) in relation to the sacrum. With side bending right and rotation left of the sacrum between the hip bones, the lumbar spine adapts by side bending left and rotating right in the three-dimensional space. Sometimes, this lumbar to sacral coupling occurs at the lumbosacral junction (L5 on S1) and occasionally, it occurs at L4-L5. The reason for the difference may be in the location of the lower lumbar segments in relation to the hip bones. Previous studies have shown that if L5 is located deep within the pelvis, the L4-L5 disc is more likely to herniate. If L5 is high and above the level of the hip bones, the L5-S1 disc is more likely to herniate. This may be due to the different orientation of the iliolumbar ligaments. The obvious conclusion is that the torsional load on the disc is different. This anatomy may also explain the different coupling seen at the lumbosacral junction. Suffice it to say, the lumbar spine and the sacrum, as units, should move in opposite directions during neutral mechanics.

In the absence of dysfunction, all lumbar segments should follow the segment below during the forward-bending/backward-bending arc. The paired transverse processes of each segment should remain in the same relevant plane as the segment below. Loss of the normal, neutral, relationship of the lumbar spine to the sacrum is of great clinical significance and is termed "nonadaptive lumbar response" to sacral function. Restoration of this normal relationship at the lumbosacral junction (whether at L4-L5 or L5-S1) is one of the major reasons for diagnosing and treating lumbar spine dysfunctions before addressing the two sacroiliac joints. Many of the techniques to be described in Chapter 17 require the normal, neutral, relationship of L5 to the sacrum.

STRUCTURAL DIAGNOSIS OF LUMBAR SPINE DYSFUNCTION

The lumbar spine has the capacity for three dysfunctions. There can be the two nonneutral (type II) dysfunctions of either the extended, rotated, and side-bent (ERS) type or the flexed, rotated, and side-bent (FRS) type or a neutral (group) dysfunction. Group dysfunctions frequently occur in the upper lumbar spine and carry over into the lower thoracic spine segments. In the presence of flattening of the lumbar lordosis, the probability of FRS dysfunction with extension restriction is high. If the lumbar lordosis is increased, the probability of ERS dysfunction with flexion restriction is high. The diagnosis of lumbar segmental dysfunction combines tissue texture changes of the deeper layers of paravertebral muscles, particularly hypertonicity of the multifidi, rotatores, and intertransversarii, and alteration in motion characteristics. Evaluation of lumbar segmental motion can be done in a variety of ways. For the reasons described in Chapter 6, the recommended process is to evaluate the location of the posterior aspect of the transverse processes in three positions. This process requires the assessment of the superior segment in relation to the inferior. In the lumbar spine, this requires that L5 be assessed in relation to the sacrum. Therefore, assessment of the lumbar spine begins by identifying the sacral base, the posterior aspect of the transverse processes of S1. Because of the anatomy of the

lumbosacral junction, it is not possible to palpate the transverse processes of L5. Instead, the examiner identifies the symmetric portions of the posterior arch of L5, as far laterally as possible, to assess rotation of L5 in relation to S1.

The diagnostic procedure requires the assessment of the paired transverse processes in neutral, forward-bent, and backward positions. A sequence that is the easiest for a beginning student is to first assess in the prone (neutral) position on the table (Fig. 16.1). Beginning at the sacral base, each lumbar vertebra is assessed for its relationship to the one below up to the thoracolumbar junction. Assessment is now made in the backward-bent (extended) prone prop position on the table (sphinx position) (Fig. 16.2). Despite the mass size of the lumbar musculature, the transverse processes are quite easily palpated in this position. Assessment is then made in the fully forward-bent

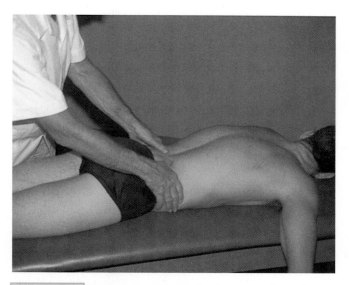

FIGURE 16.1 Transverse process palpation, neutral position.

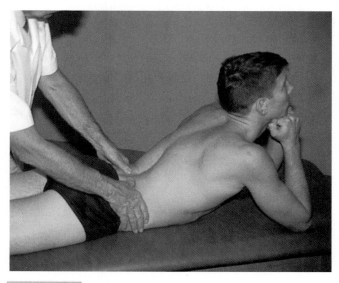

FIGURE 16.2 Transverse process palpation, backward-bent (extended) position (prone prop).

position with the patient seated with the feet on the floor or a stool. Assessment is made from below upward in a similar fashion. It is more difficult to palpate transverse processes in this position because of the tension through the lumbar muscles and the lumbodorsal fascia (Fig. 16.3). If one transverse process is more posterior in the fully forward-bent position and becomes symmetric in the prone prop (sphinx position), a nonneutral (type II) ERS dysfunction is present at this level. If one transverse process is more prominent in the prone prop (sphinx position) and becomes symmetric in the forward-bent position, a nonneutral (type II) FRS restriction is present. If three or more transverse processes remain prominent throughout all three positions, a neutral (type I) dysfunction is present. It is difficult to evaluate the functional capacity of the upper lumbar segments until those identified as dysfunctional in the lower region are successfully treated. Nonneutral dysfunctions are common at L4 and L5, as well as at the thoracolumbar junction. Nonneutral

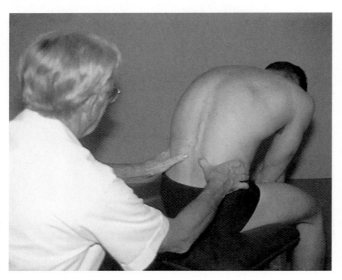

FIGURE 16.3 Transverse process palpation, forward-bent position.

dysfunctions at L4 and L5 are frequently seen in association with dysfunction of the sacroiliac joints.

The lumbar spine also has the capacity for bilateral dysfunction at the same vertebral motion segment. The most common is bilateral flexed or bilateral extended dysfunction. These are seen more frequently at the lumbosacral and the thoracolumbar junctions. These dysfunctions are more difficult to diagnose since there is no rotational asymmetry. The major clue to their existence is bilateral tissue texture abnormality at a given segment and some overall motion loss. The diagnosis is made by finding no change in the interspinous space between the two segments during the forward-bending–backward-bending arc. The segment is either bilaterally flexed or bilaterally extended. These dysfunctions are classified as "sagittal plane dysfunctions."

In the presence of unleveling of the sacrum and in the absence of dysfunction of the lumbar spine, there will be a side bending and rotation to opposite sides of the lumbar vertebra in order to compensate and maintain the trunk erect. This adaptive response is only found in neutral positions. The longer this is present, the more likely it is to develop a neutral (group) dysfunction.

MANUAL MEDICINE PROCEDURES FOR DYSFUNCTIONS OF LUMBAR SPINE

The treating clinician needs to have manual medicine techniques to treat group (type I) dysfunctions and the nonneutral (type II) ERS and FRS dysfunctions. In the treatment sequence, it is recommended that nonneutral dysfunctions be treated first and group dysfunctions last. Usually, one begins by treating the lower segments first and sequentially from below upward. Exceptions to this below upward rule are those cases in which the major restrictor is higher in the lumbar spine or in which the lowest segment is so acute that it is difficult to directly address it. One should be able to treat a patient in the erect sitting posture or recumbent on the table. It is frequently valuable to treat a large patient in the sitting position so that gravity can be used as an assisting activating force.

LUMBAR SPINE

Muscle Energy Technique

Sitting

Nonneutral Dysfunction (Example: L4 ERS$_{left}$)

Position: Backward bent (extended), rotated left, and side bent left (ER$_{left}$S$_{left}$)

Motion Restriction: Forward bending (flexion), right-side bending, and right rotation

1. Patient sits on the stool with the left hand holding the right shoulder and the right arm dropped at the side.

2. Operator stands at the left side of the patient straddling the patient's left knee with the left hand grasping the patient's right shoulder and controlling the left shoulder with the left axilla (Fig. 16.4). The operator's right middle finger monitors the L4-L5 interspinous space and the right index finger monitors the left transverse process of L4.

3. The forward-bending (flexion) barrier is engaged by an anterior-to-posterior translatory movement at L4-L5 (Fig. 16.5).

4. Right-side bending and right rotation are introduced at L4-L5 by the operator's left arm and by asking the patient to reach to the floor with the right hand (Fig. 16.6).

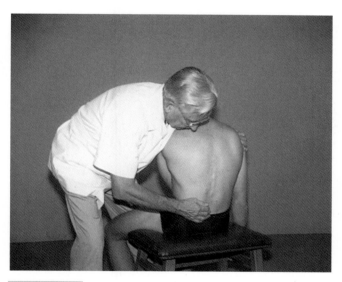

FIGURE 16.5

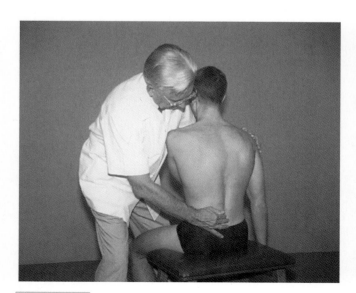

FIGURE 16.4

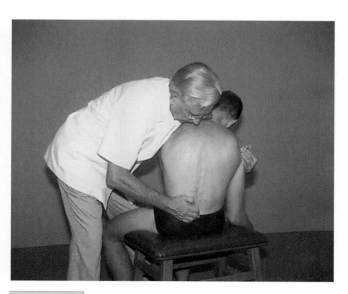

FIGURE 16.6

5. Patient is instructed to side bend to the left against equal resistance for 3 to 5 seconds using an isometric contraction. Following relaxation, a new forward-bending, right-side bending, and right-rotational barrier is engaged and three to five repetitions are made of the left-side bending isometric effort.

6. When all right rotation and right-side bending restrictions are removed, the operator forward bends the patient while maintaining right rotation (Fig. 16.7).

7. Operator's left hand resists a patient trunk extension effort, fully forward bending the segment and opening both zygapophysial joints at L4-L5 (Fig. 16.8).

8. Retest.

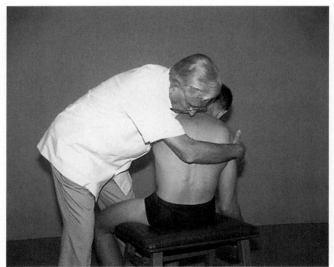

FIGURE 16.7

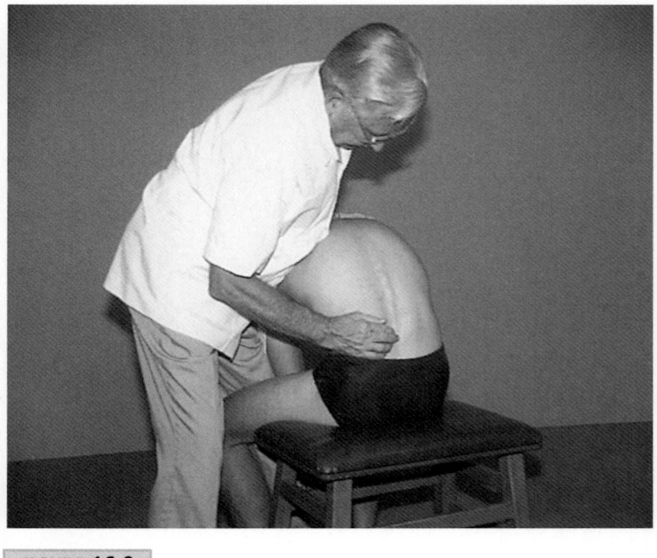

FIGURE 16.8

LUMBAR SPINE

Muscle Energy Technique

Sitting

Nonneutral Dysfunction (Example: L3 FRS$_{left}$)

Position: Forward bent (F), rotated (left), and side bent (left)

Motion Restriction: Backward bending (extension), side bending right, and rotation right

1. Patient sits on the stool with the operator sitting behind controlling the patient's trunk with the right hand and monitoring the interspinous space of L3-L4 with the left index finger and the left transverse process of L3 with the left middle finger.

2. Operator introduces side bending left and rotation right in neutral mechanics by the patient dropping the left shoulder and shifting the weight to the right buttock.

3. Three to four repetitions of an isometric left rotation effort by the patient pushing the right shoulder into the operator's right hand introduces right rotation at L3 on L4 (Fig. 16.9).

4. Operator introduces extension and right-side bending while maintaining this right rotation by pressing inferiorly on the right shoulder allowing the patient to shift his weight to the left buttock and project the abdomen over the left knee (Fig. 16.10).

5. Operator resists a series of three to five isometric contractions of 3 to 5 seconds with the patient either pulling the right shoulder forward against resistance or lifting the right shoulder toward the ceiling against resistance (Fig. 16.11). After each repetition, a new barrier is engaged.

6. When all right-side bending and right rotation restriction is removed, the operator maintains extension and straightens the patient's shoulders, while blocking the L4 segment bilaterally with the left hand (Fig. 16.12). The operator's right hand resists flexion effort by the patient's trunk to fully extend L3 on L4, closing both zygapophysial joints.

7. Retest.

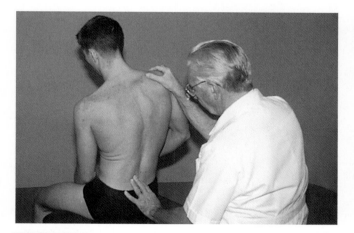

FIGURE 16.9

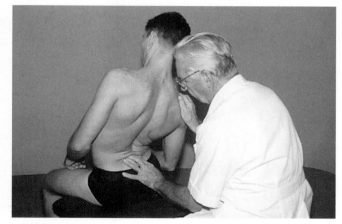

FIGURE 16.11

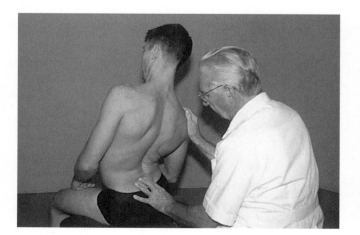

FIGURE 16.10 Observation of gait from the left side.

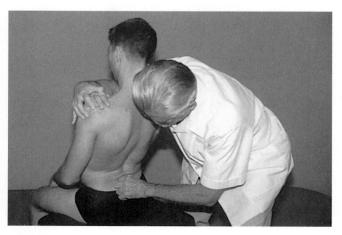

FIGURE 16.12

LUMBAR SPINE

Muscle Energy Technique

Sitting

Neutral (Group Dysfunction)

Variation 1

Position: Neutral, side bent right, and rotated left ($NS_{right}R_{left}$ or EN_{left})

Motion Restriction: Side bending left and rotation right

1. Patient sits on the table with the right hand grasping the left shoulder. The operator stands behind with the right arm under the patient's right axilla and grasping the patient's left shoulder to control the upper trunk (Fig. 16.13).

2. Operator's left thumb is placed at the apex of the left lumbar convexity for localization (Fig. 16.14).

3. Operator introduces left-side bending and right rotation by left-to-right translation localized by the left thumb contact at the apex of the left lumbar convexity (Fig. 16.15).

4. Operator resists a series of 3- to 5-second right-side bending efforts against the operator's resistance through the right hand (Fig. 16.16). The localizing thumb maintains a force anteromedially against the left lumbar curve.

5. Retest.

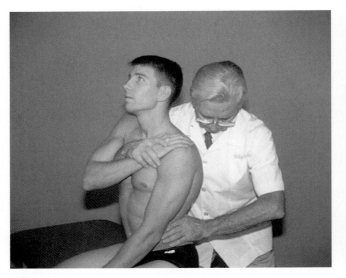

FIGURE 16.13

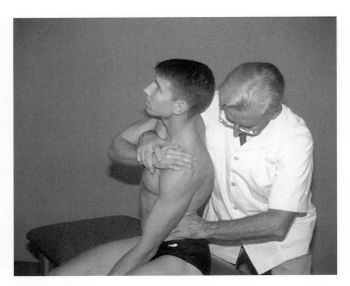

FIGURE 16.15

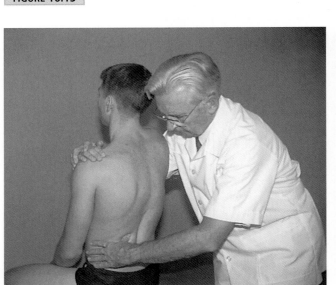

FIGURE 16.14

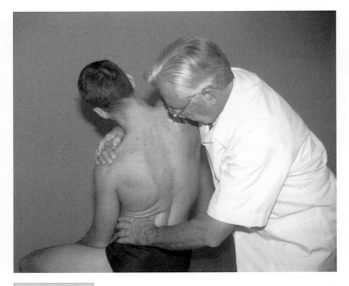

FIGURE 16.16

LUMBAR SPINE

Muscle Energy Technique

Sitting

Neutral (Group Dysfunction)

Variation 2

Position: Neutral, side bent right, and rotated left ($NS_{right}R_{left}$ or EN_{left})

Motion Restriction: Side bending left and rotation right

1. Patient sits on the table with the left hand holding the right shoulder. The operator stands behind with the left hand grasping the patient's right shoulder and with the left axilla over the patient's left shoulder. The operator's right thumb is at the apex of the left lumbar convexity pressing anteromedially (Fig. 16.17).

2. Operator introduces left-side bending and right rotation through the left arm contact with translation from left to right at the apex of the curve localized by the right thumb (Fig. 16.18).

3. Operator resists patient's right-side bending effort of 3 to 5 seconds repeated three to five times (Fig. 16.19).

4. Following each effort, the operator engages the new left-side bending and right-rotational barrier with left-to-right translation localized at the apex.

5. Retest.

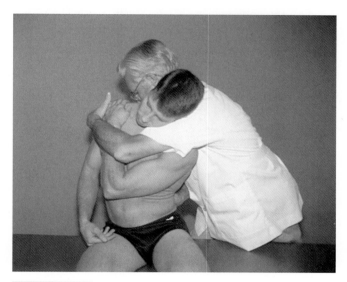

FIGURE 16.18

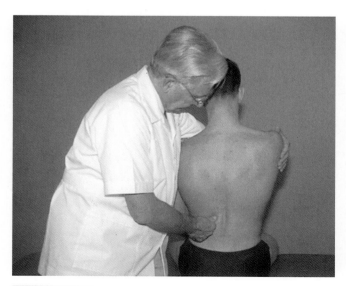

FIGURE 16.17

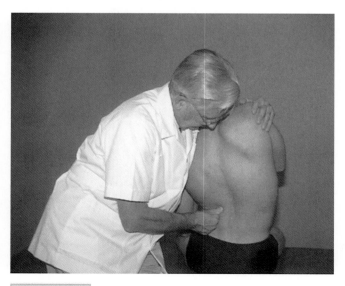

FIGURE 16.19

LUMBAR SPINE

Muscle Energy Technique

Sitting

Bilateral Extension Restriction (Example: L1-L2)

    Position: Bilaterally flexed

    Motion Restriction: Bilateral extension

1. Patient sits on the table with the hands holding the opposite shoulder. The operator stands behind with the left hand holding both the elbows to control the patient's trunk (Fig. 16.20).

2. The heel of the operator's hand blocks the L2 segment in the midline (Fig. 16.21).

3. Operator engages extension barrier by backward bending the trunk while translating from posterior to anterior through the right hand (Fig. 16.22). Note the blocking of the right elbow against the operator's trunk.

4. Operator's left arm resists a forward bending effort by the patient with a 3- to 5-second contraction repeated three to five times (Fig. 16.23).

5. The extension barrier is engaged after each patient effort.

6. Retest.

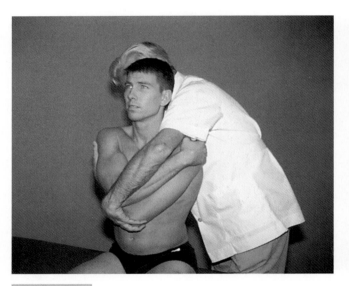

FIGURE 16.20

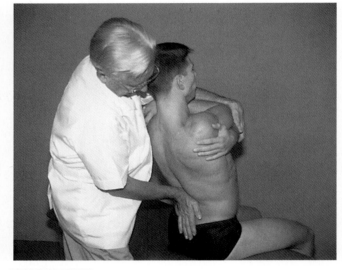

FIGURE 16.22

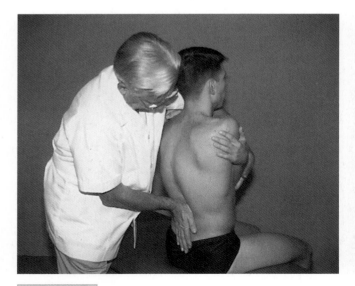

FIGURE 16.21

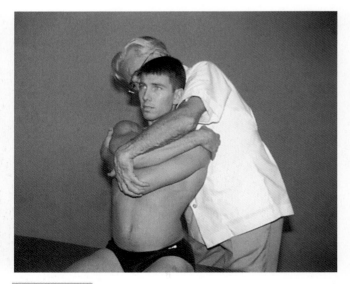

FIGURE 16.23

LUMBAR SPINE

Muscle Energy Technique

Sitting

Lateral Recumbent (Sims Position)

Nonneutral Dysfunction (Example: L4 ERS$_{right}$)

Position: Backward bent, extended and side bent right (ERS$_{right}$)

Motion Restriction: Forward bending (flexion), rotation left, and side bending left

1. Patient is prone on the table with the operator standing at the right side. The operator flexes the patient's knees and rolls the lower extremity onto the left hip into the Sims position (Fig. 16.24).

2. Operator's left middle finger palpates the L4-L5 interspace with the index finger over the right transverse process of L4. The operator's right hand introduces left rotation of the trunk down to L4. The patient assists by reaching toward the floor (Fig. 16.25).

3. Operator switches hands with the right hand monitoring the L4-L5 level and simultaneously uses his left arm and left thigh to flex the patient's knees up to L5, engaging the flexion barrier (Fig. 16.26).

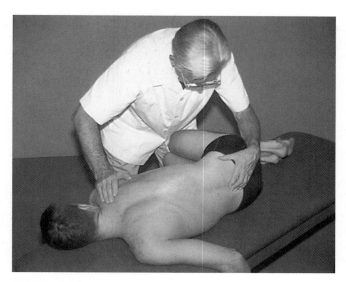

FIGURE 16.25

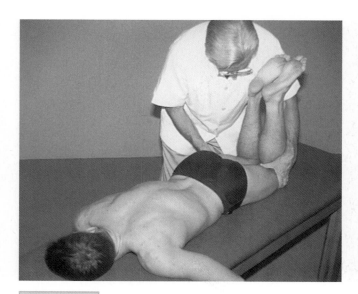

FIGURE 16.24

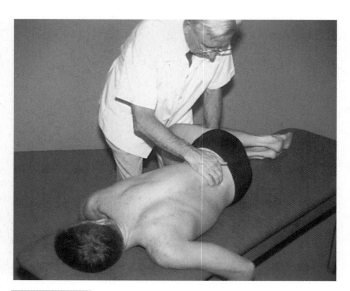

FIGURE 16.26

4. While continuing to monitor the L4-L5 level, the operator drops both of the patient's feet to the floor introducing left-side bending to the barrier (Fig. 16.27). Note that the patient's knees are resting on the operator's left thigh.

5. Operator resists a muscle effort by the patient to lift the feet to the ceiling attempting to introduce a right-side bending effort against resistance (Fig. 16.28). The operator's right hand monitors over the L4-L5 level ensuring localization of muscle contraction at that level.

6. Three to five repetitions of a 3- to 5-second muscle contraction are performed by the patient with the operator engaging a new flexion, left rotation, and left-side bending barrier after each effort.

7. Retest.

Note: Caution must be used to protect the lateral aspect of the patient's left thigh against the edge of the table. If the operator is unable to stabilize the patient's legs against the left thigh, a rolled towel or a small pillow can be placed between the patient's thighs and the edge of the table. Another option is for the operator to sit on the end of the table with the left hand monitoring the L4-L5 level, controlling the lower extremities with the right hand, with the patient's left knee over the operator's left thigh.

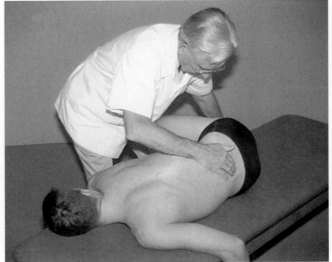

FIGURE 16.27

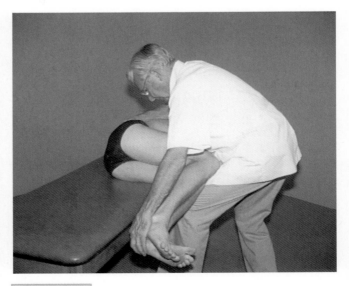

FIGURE 16.28

LUMBAR SPINE

Muscle Energy Technique

Lateral Recumbent

Nonneutral Dysfunction (Example: L4 ERS$_{left}$)

　Position: Backward bent, rotated and side bent left (ERS$_{left}$)

　Motion Restriction: Forward bending (flexion), rotation right, and side bending right

1. Patient is in the left lateral recumbent position with the neck supported by a pillow, the feet and knees together, and the shoulders and hips perpendicular to the table. The operator stands in front of the patient and with the right hand flexes the patient's trunk down to L4 from above maintaining the shoulders perpendicular to the table for right-side bending (Fig. 16.29).

2. Operator flexes the lower extremities up to L5 while monitoring the interspinous space at the L4-L5 level with the right hand (Fig. 16.30).

3. Operator introduces right rotation through the right forearm rotating the patient's right shoulder posteriorly while monitoring at the L4-L5 level with the right hand.

4. Operator introduces right-side bending by lifting both of the patient's feet toward the ceiling (Fig. 16.31), engaging the combined right rotation, right-side bending barrier.

5. Operator resists patient effort to pull the feet back toward the table (a left-side bending effort) while monitoring for contraction of the erector spinae muscles at the L4-L5 level.

6. Patient performs three to five repetitions of a 3- to 5-second contraction. During each relaxation phase, the operator reengages the forward bending, right rotation, right-side bending barrier.

7. Retest.

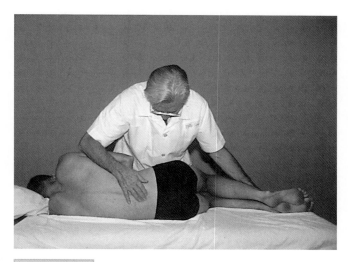

FIGURE 16.30

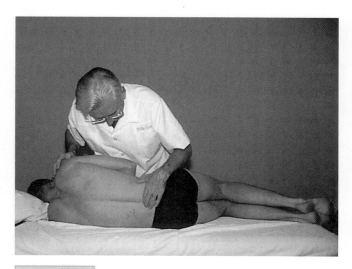

FIGURE 16.29

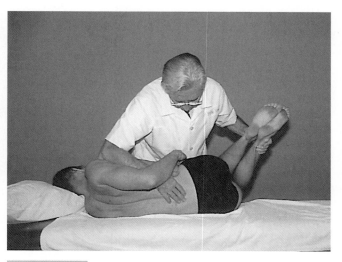

FIGURE 16.31

LUMBAR SPINE

Muscle Energy Technique

Lateral Recumbent

Nonneutral Dysfunction (Example: L4 FRS$_{left}$)

Position: Forward bent, rotated and side bent left (L4 FRS$_{left}$)

Motion Restriction: Backward bending (extension), right rotation, and right-side bending

1. Patient is in the left lateral recumbent position with the knees and feet together and with the shoulders and pelvic perpendicular to the table (begins right-side bending by position).

2. Operator stands in front of the patient and with hands contacting the L4-L5 level (Fig. 16.32).

3. Operator first engages the initial backward-bending (extension) barrier by translating the L4-L5 level from posterior to anterior (Fig. 16.33).

Note: Patient is lying on a sheet or a towel to facilitate sliding on the table.

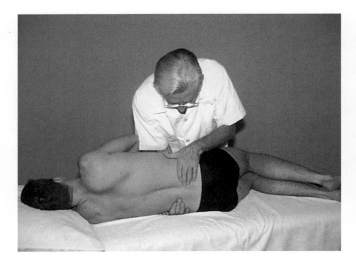

FIGURE 16.32

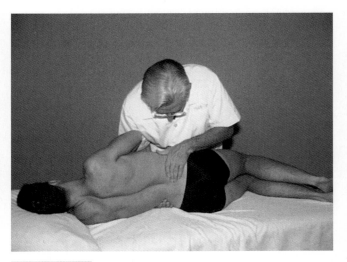

FIGURE 16.33

4. While monitoring the interspinous space at the L4-L5 level, the operator fine-tunes backward-bending (extension) barrier from above by translating the left shoulder posteriorly, maintaining both the shoulders perpendicular to the table, and monitoring with the left hand for motion down to L4 (Fig. 16.34).

5. Operator fine-tunes backward-bending (extension) barrier from below by extending the lower extremities and monitoring with the right hand for movement up to L5 (Fig. 16.35).

6. Operator engages right-rotation barrier by rotating the right shoulder posteriorly with the right hand monitoring for rotation to L4 with the left hand (Fig. 16.36). The patient grasps the edge of the table to maintain right rotation and to introduce more extension.

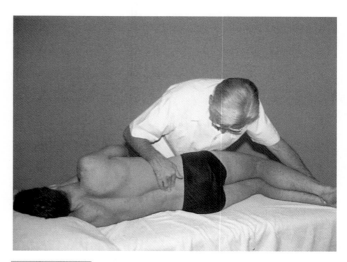

FIGURE 16.35

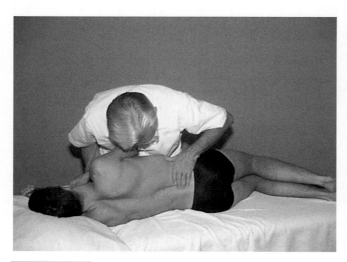

FIGURE 16.34

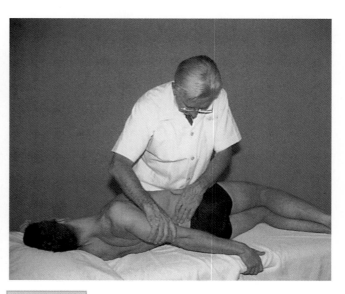

FIGURE 16.36

7. Operator's left hand lifts the right leg to engage the right-side bending barrier while monitoring with the right hand at the L4-L5 level (Fig. 16.37).

8. Patient pulls the right knee down toward the left knee for three to five repetitions of a 3- to 5-second muscle contraction against resistance provided by the operator's left hand. After each effort, the operator engages a new right-side bending barrier by lifting the knee toward the ceiling and a new backward bending barrier by translating L4-L5 anteriorly by the right hand.

9. Operator returns the patient's right knee to the table and places the right forearm against the patient's right shoulder maintaining right rotation. Operator's right hand monitors at the interspinous space at the L4-L5 level. Operator's left hand on patient's right buttock engages right-side bending barrier by cephalic translation (Fig. 16.38). Operator resists with the right forearm a left rotation effort of the patient's trunk by pushing the right shoulder into the operator's right forearm or a left-side bending effort by pushing the right buttock caudad. Again, three to five repetitions are performed.

10. Retest.

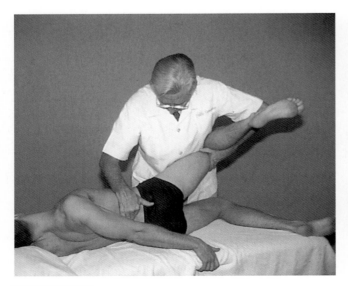

FIGURE 16.37

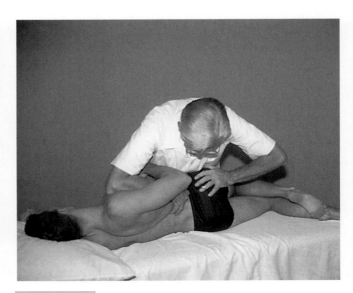

FIGURE 16.38

LUMBAR SPINE

Muscle Energy Technique

Lateral Recumbent Position

Neutral (Group Dysfunction) (Example: L1-L4 convex left)

Position: Neutral, side bent right, and rotated left ($NS_{right}R_{left}$ or EN_{left})

Motion Restriction: Left-side bending and right rotation

1. Patient is in right lateral recumbent position with the shoulders and pelvis perpendicular to the table and with the knees and feet together. Operator stands in front of the patient.

2. Operator flexes and extends the lower extremities to ensure the point of maximum ease of the forward-bending/backward-bending movement of the L1-L4 lumbar neutral curve. Operator monitors with the left hand (Fig. 16.39).

3. Operator lifts both feet toward the ceiling, introducing a left-side bending and a right-rotational movement to the lumbar spine (Fig. 16.40).

4. Operator's right hand resists patient's effort of pulling the feet back to the table for 3 to 5 seconds and three to five repetitions (a right-side bending effort).

5. Operator's left hand monitors the muscle contraction and postcontraction stretch of the right paravertebral muscles (the concavity).

6. Retest.

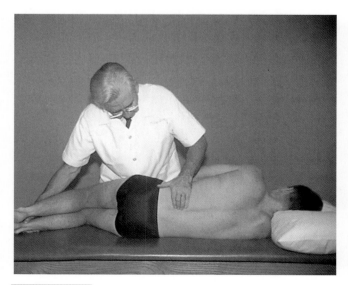

FIGURE 16.39

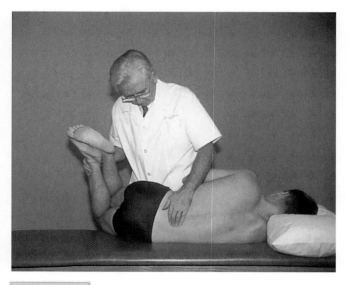

FIGURE 16.40

LUMBAR SPINE

Mobilization with Impulse Technique

Lateral Recumbent Position

Neutral (Group) Dysfunction (Example: L1-L4 convex left)

  Position: Neutral, side bent right, and rotated left ($NS_{right}R_{left}$ or EN_{left})

  Motion Restriction: Side bending left and rotation right

1. Patient is in the left lateral recumbent position (most posterior transverse processes toward the table) with the operator standing in front.

2. Patient's lower extremities are flexed and extended to the point of maximum ease of the forward-bending/backward-bending range of the lumbar lordosis.

3. Operator monitors the dysfunctional lumbar segments with the left hand and grasps the patient's left elbow (Fig. 16.41).

4. Operator pulls the patient's left elbow forward and caudad (Fig. 16.42), introducing left-side bending and right rotation from above (Fig. 16.43).

5. Operator's right forearm in contact with the patient's right axilla and pectoral region maintains right rotation from above, while the operator's left forearm pulls the patient's pelvis into left rotation (Fig. 16.44). The transverse processes of the apex of the dysfunctional group are perpendicular to the table.

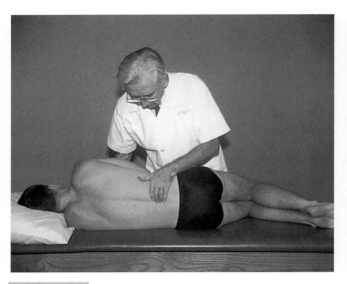

FIGURE 16.41

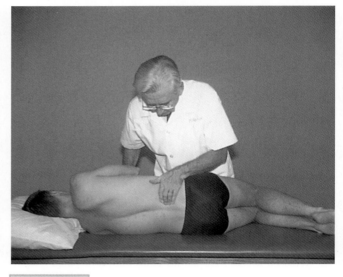

FIGURE 16.43

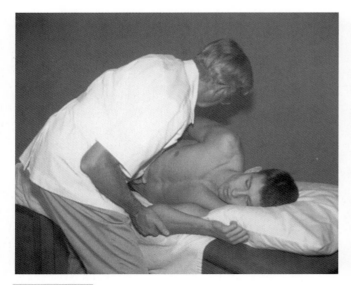

FIGURE 16.42

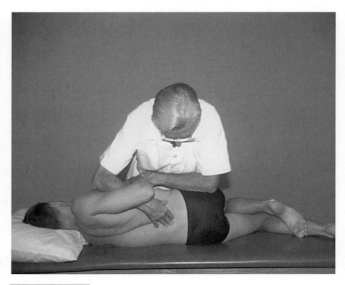

FIGURE 16.44

6. A mobilization with impulse thrust is made through the left forearm by the operator's body drop rotating the pelvis anteriorly into left rotation.

7. An alternate arm position finds the operator's right forearm stabilizing the patient's right shoulder and pectoral region and both hands monitoring at the dysfunctional lumbar segments. Again, an anterior rotary thrust is applied through the left forearm by an operator body drop (Fig. 16.45).

8. An alternate arm position has the operator's right hand stabilizing the anterior aspect of the pectoral region (not grasping the humerus) and the left forearm incorporated as part of the operator's body provides the anterior rotational thrust. Note the operator's left hand monitoring the dysfunctional segments (Fig. 16.46).

9. Retest.

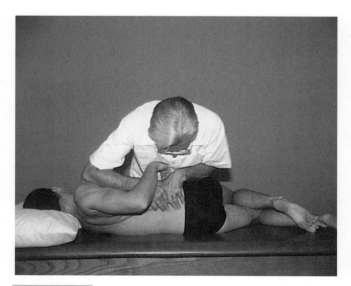

FIGURE 16.45

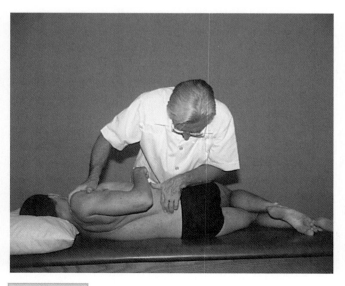

FIGURE 16.46

LUMBAR SPINE

Mobilization with Impulse Technique

Lateral Recumbent Position

Nonneutral Dysfunction (Example: L4 ERS$_{left}$)

    Position: Backward bent, rotated and side bent left (ERS$_{left}$)

    Motion Restriction: Forward bending (flexion), right rotation, and right-side bending

1. Patient is in the left lateral recumbent position (most posterior transverse process toward the table) with a pillow supporting the cervical spine, knees and feet together, and the shoulders and pelvis perpendicular to the table (initiating beginning right-side bending). Operator stands in front monitoring the L4-L5 interspinous space with the left hand (Fig. 16.47).

2. While maintaining the patient's shoulders perpendicular to the table, the operator introduces forward bending down to L4 from above by curling the patient's trunk forward (Fig. 16.48).

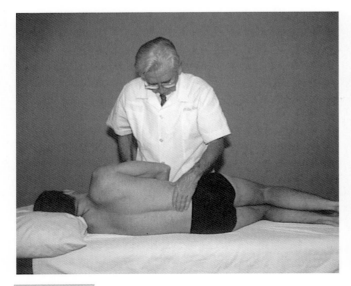

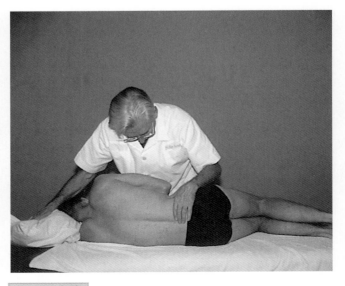

3. Operator now monitors the L4-L5 interspinous space with the right hand and flexes the lower extremities up to L5 (Fig. 16.49).

4. Operator brings the patient's right knee forward and places the right foot in the left popliteal space. The operator's right forearm introduces right rotation down to L4 (Fig. 16.50).

5. Operator's left forearm in contact with the patient's right buttock rotates the pelvis anteriorly and superiorly (Fig. 16.51).

6. Operator fine-tunes forward bending, right rotation, and right-side bending to the elastic barrier and provides an anterior and cephalad thrust through the left forearm by a body drop. The localization attempts to maintain the transverse processes of L4 perpendicular to the table.

7. Retest.

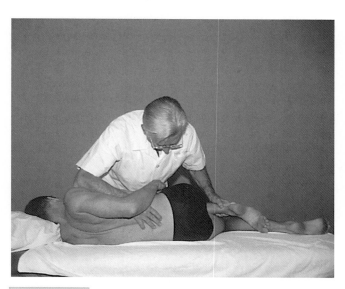

FIGURE 16.50

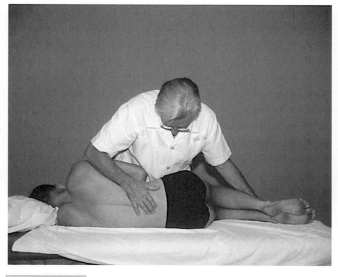

FIGURE 16.49

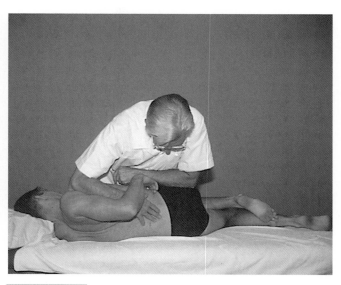

FIGURE 16.51

LUMBAR SPINE

Mobilization with Impulse Technique

Lateral Recumbent Position

Nonneutral Dysfunction (Example: L4 FRS$_{left}$)

    Position: Forward bent rotated left, side bent left (FRS$_{left}$)

    Motion Restriction: Backward bending (extension), rotation right, side bending right

1. Patient lies in the left lateral recumbent position (most posterior transverse process toward the table) with a pillow under the cervical spine, knees and feet together, and the shoulders and pelvis perpendicular to the table.

2. Operator stands in front and grasps the L4-L5 segment level between the hands (Fig. 16.52).

3. Operator's hands localize to the initial backward-bending barrier by translating the patient's trunk from posterior to anterior (Fig. 16.53).

4. Operator fine-tunes extension barrier from above by translating the patient posteriorly through the operator's right forearm (Fig. 16.54) while monitoring with the left hand at the L4-L5 interspinous space (Fig. 16.55).

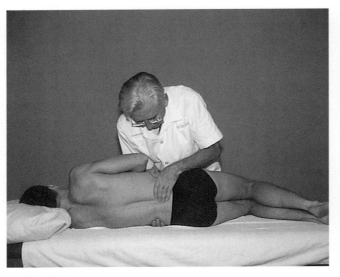

FIGURE 16.52

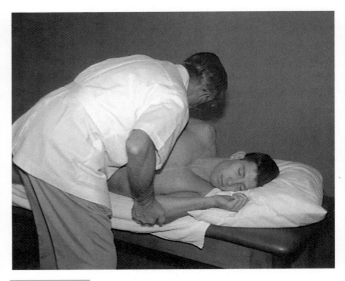

FIGURE 16.54

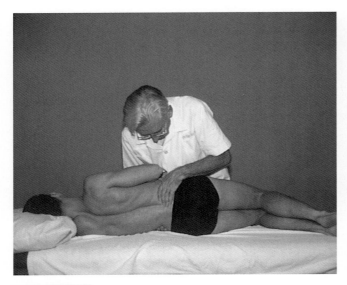

FIGURE 16.53

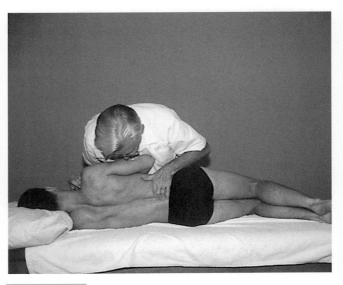

FIGURE 16.55

5. Operator fine-tunes extension barrier from below by extending the lower extremities with the left arm for movement up to L5 being monitored by the right hand (Fig. 16.56).

6. Operator's left hand brings the patient's right knee forward and places the right foot in the left popliteal space. The right forearm, in contact with the patient's right pectoral region, introduces right rotation from above monitoring with the fingers of the right hand over the L4-L5 level (Fig. 16.57).

7. Operator's left forearm contacts the patient's right buttock and introduces anterior and cephalad rotation of the pelvis engaging the barrier at the L4-L5 level (Fig. 16.58).

8. Operator introduces mobilizing thrust through the left forearm by a body drop in an anterior and cephalad direction.

9. Retest.

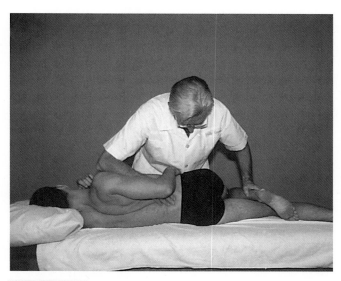

FIGURE 16.57

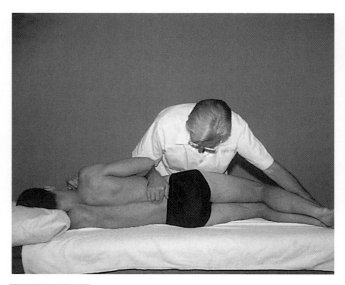

FIGURE 16.56

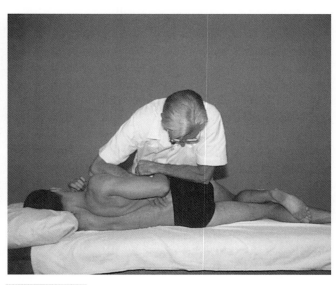

FIGURE 16.58

LUMBAR SPINE

Mobilization with Impulse Technique

Sitting

Sagittal Plane Restriction (Example: L1 bilaterally flexed)

> Position: Bilaterally forward bent (flexed)

> Motion Restriction: Bilateral backward bending (extension)

1. Patient sits on the table with arms crossed holding the opposite shoulder. The operator stands behind grasping the patient's elbows for trunk control (Fig. 16.59).

2. The heel of the operator's right hand is placed in the midline over the spinous process of L2 with localization to the inferior segment (Fig. 16.60).

3. Operator applies a backward-bending (extension) thrust by lifting the patient's trunk through the elbows over the fulcrum applied by the right hand on L2 (Fig. 16.61).

4. An alternate thrust is a body drop of the operator's body through a lever arm of the right forearm in an anterior direction against the right hand contact on L2 (Fig. 16.62).

5. When using either of the thrust options, the operator tries to thrust only with one hand while the other maintains stabilization. However, both options require two-handed coordination.

6. Retest.

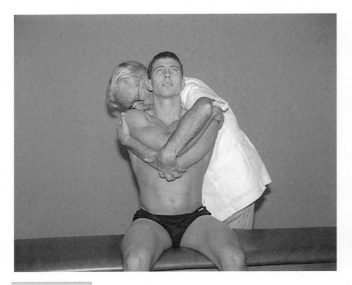

FIGURE 16.59

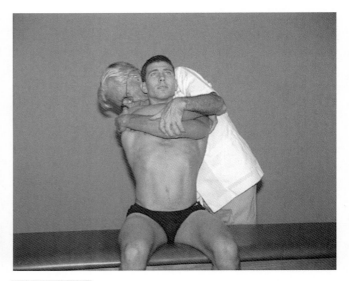

FIGURE 16.61

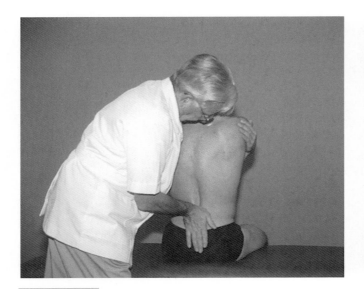

FIGURE 16.60

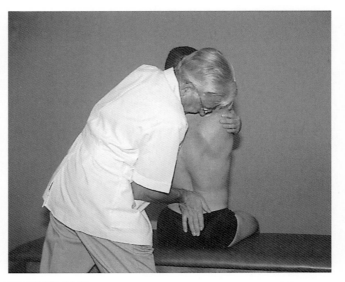

FIGURE 16.62

LUMBAR SPINE

Mobilization with Impulse Technique

Sitting

Nonneutral Dysfunction (Example: L3 ERS$_{left}$)

Position: Backward bent, rotated and side bent right (ERS$_{left}$)

Motion Restriction: Forward bending (flexion), rotation right, and side bending right.

1. Patient sits astride the table with arms crossed holding each shoulder.

2. Operator stands at the right side of the patient with the right hand grasping the patient's left shoulder and right axilla over the patient's right shoulder. Operator's reinforced left thumb is in contact with the right side of the spinous process of L3 (Fig. 16.63).

3. Operator engages the forward bending, right-side bending, and right-rotational barrier through movement of the patient's trunk by the right arm and with right-to-left pressure of the left thumb on the spinous process of L3 (Fig. 16.64).

4. The mobilizing thrust is applied by exaggerating the patient's body position by dropping the operator's weight toward the floor while simultaneously thrusting from right to left with the left thumb on the spinous process of L3.

5. An alternative localizing hand position is the use of the left pisiform through the operator's hypothenar eminence on the right side of the spinous process of L3 (Fig. 16.65). Note the blocking of the operator's left forearm against the left hip.

6. Retest.

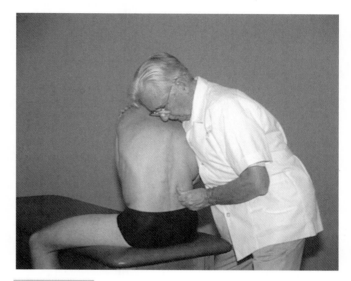

FIGURE 16.64

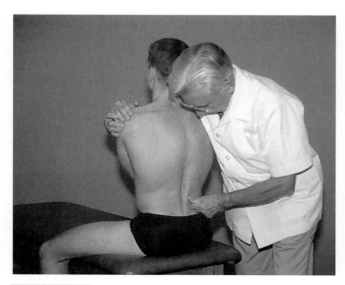

FIGURE 16.63

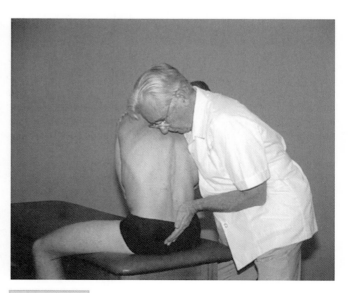

FIGURE 16.65

LUMBAR SPINE

Mobilization with Impulse Technique

Sitting

Nonneutral Dysfunction (Example: L3 FRS$_{left}$)

> Position: Forward bent (flexed), rotated left, and side bent left
>
> Motion Restriction: Backward bending (extension), rotation right, and side bending right

1. Patient sits astride the table with the right hand holding the left shoulder.

2. Operator stands at the right side with the right hand holding the patient's left shoulder and the right axilla on top of the patient's right shoulder. Operator's reinforced left thumb is on the right side of the spinous process of L3 (Fig. 16.66).

3. Operator introduces backward bending, right-side bending, and right rotation through the right arm contact with the patient's trunk, while localizing by translation from right to left on the spinous process of L3 (Fig. 16.67).

4. The mobilizing thrust is introduced by the inferior body drop of the operator on the patient's right shoulder and a right-to-left force through the left thumb.

5. An alternative hand contact is the operator's pisiform through the left hypothenar eminence on the right side of the spinous process of L3 (Fig. 16.68). Note that operator's left elbow is in contact with the left hip, providing a lever arm to the contact on L3.

6. Retest.

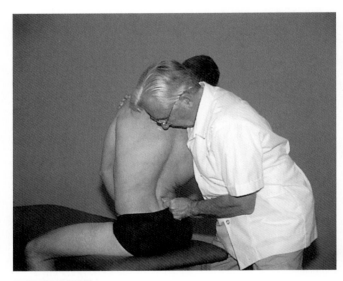

FIGURE 16.67

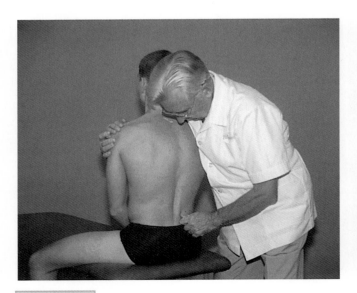

FIGURE 16.66

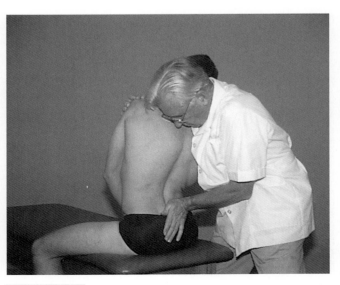

FIGURE 16.68

LUMBAR SPINE

Mobilization with Impulse Technique

Sitting

Neutral (Group Dysfunction) (Example: L1-L4 convex left)

Position: Neutral, side bent right, rotated left ($NS_{right}R_{left}$ or EN_{left})

Motion Restriction: Side bending left and rotation right

1. Patient sits astride the table with the left hand on the right shoulder.

2. Operator stands at the left side of the patient with the left hand holding the right shoulder, the left axilla on top of the patient's left shoulder, and the reinforced thumb in the inter-transverse space between L2-L3 (Fig. 16.69).

3. Operator engages the left-side bending and right-rotation barrier through the control of the patient's trunk with the left arm while maintaining an anteromedial-localizing fulcrum with the right thumb (Fig. 16.70).

4. The mobilizing thrust is a body drop of the operator toward the floor enhancing the left-side bending and right rotation with localization at the apex of the curve.

5. An alternate hand position is the use of the right pisiform and right hypothenar eminence at the apex of the lumbar curve (Fig. 16.71).

6. Retest.

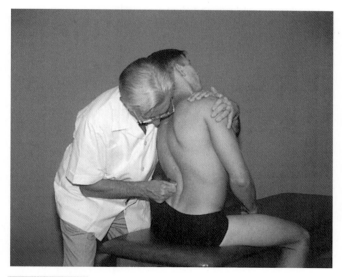

FIGURE 16.70

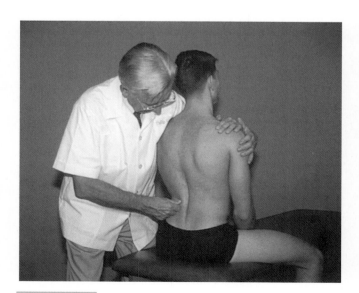

FIGURE 16.69

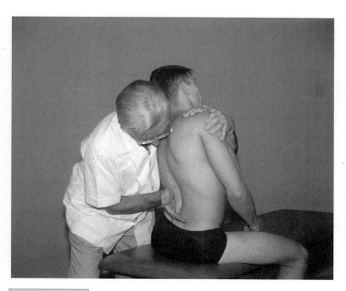

FIGURE 16.71

LUMBAR SPINE

Mobilization without Impulse (Articulatory) Technique

Activating Force Variations

1. All previous mobilization with impulse techniques can be modified using a mobilization without impulse activating force.

2. Patient and operator positions remain the same.

3. Follow the principles found in Chapter 7.

4. Use repetitive oscillatory operator efforts in the direction of the restrictive barrier, gradually increasing the range of movement.

5. This technique is frequently applied before the use of final mobilizing with impulse thrust.

6. Retest.

LUMBAR SPINE

Muscle Energy Activating Force

1. Any of the mobilizing with impulse techniques can be modified to use a muscle intrinsic activating force.

2. Patient's activating force is in the direction opposite to the operator-localized position.

3. Three to five repetitions of a 3- to 5-second muscle contraction are used with the operator reengaging the new barrier after each patient contraction.

4. Frequently, two or three muscle energy efforts are used before the application of a mobilization with impulse thrust.

5. Retest.

CONCLUSION

The lumbar spine is a frequent site of dysfunction, particularly nonneutral dysfunctions of the FRS type. These dysfunctions are frequently associated with a herniated intervertebral disk at the same level. Restoration of more normal mobility at the segment is frequently most helpful in managing the discogenic radiculopathy, if present (See Chapter 20).

The lumbar spine should be examined, and treated if dysfunctional, before addressing the pelvis, as many of the techniques for sacral dysfunction use the lumbar spine as a lever.

REFERENCES

1. Mixter WJ, Barr SS. Rupture of the intervertebral disk with involvement of the spinal canal. *N Eng J Med* 1934;211:210–215.
2. Bogduk N. The innervation of the lumbar spine. *Spine* 1983;8:286–293.
3. Cossette JW, Farfan HF, Robertson GH, et al. The instantaneous center of rotation of the third lumbar intervertebral joint. *J Biomech* 1971;4:149–153.
4. Bogduk N, Towmey L. *Clinical Anatomy of the Lumbar Spine*. London: Churchill Livingstone, 1987.
5. Farfan HF, Sullivan JD. The relation of facet orientation to intervertebral disk failure. *Can J Surg* 1967;10:179–185.
6. Farfan HF. The effects of torsion on the intervertebral joints. *J Bone Joint Surg Am* 1970;52:468–497.

PELVIC GIRDLE DYSFUNCTION

The growth in research activities in the past 10 to 15 years has diminished the controversy surrounding the role of the sacroiliac joint in causing lower back pain. Several world congresses in the past decade addressed the role of the sacroiliac joint in back pain. Sacroiliac joint motion has been reported in the medical literature since mid-19th century.[1] Some of the orthopedic literature in the first half of the 20th century included descriptions of pain syndromes related to the joint and various therapeutic methods for its control. Despite these publications, many authorities held the view that there was no movement at the sacroiliac joints and therefore it was not clinically significant. Based on the recent contributions from basic and clinical science, there has been a change in perception of the role of the sacroiliac joint in clinical pain syndromes.[2,3] Movement within the sacroiliac joint, although small, is now generally recognized.[4,5] Controversy continues as to the type of motion available and the axes of motion. Sacroiliac arthrography has demonstrated that some sacroiliac joints are painful on injection and pain relief occurs following instillation of local anesthetic.[6] Normal sacroiliac joints do not appear to be painful on injection.[7] Controversy continues as to the ability of a clinician to use physical assessment to identify a significant sacroiliac dysfunction.[8,9] Additional basic research and clinical research are clearly needed.

It is beyond the scope of this volume to review all of the research on sacroiliac motion. The generally accepted pelvic girdle motions will be discussed and a diagnostic and therapeutic system for pelvic girdle dysfunction will be described. The system described will allow the clinician to diagnose and treat all of the physical findings of pelvic girdle dysfunctions. It builds on the current knowledge of pelvic girdle movement and dysfunction and adds a theoretic construct and terminology to describe the various physical findings encountered during examination of the pelvic girdle.

MODELS OF PELVIC GIRDLE DYSFUNCTION

The postural–structural, or biomechanical, model is the one most commonly used by the manual medicine practitioner in dealing with the pelvis because it is the key to the gait cycle on which all activities of daily living are based. The pelvis links the mobile extremities with the trunk in the highly complex mechanism of ambulation. Manual medicine management of the pelvic girdle restores functional symmetry to the three bones and joints of the pelvic girdle during the walking cycle. The superior surface of the body of the sacrum supports the vertebral column. Alteration in the sacrum has a significant effect on the vertebral function above. We owe a large debt of gratitude to Mitchell,[10] for his seminal work in defining the role of the pelvis in musculoskeletal function. He is acknowledged as the father of the muscle energy system of manual medicine, but his insight into the pelvic girdle could be viewed as a more significant contribution to the field. Instead of referring to his work as the muscle energy system, we could describe it as the *Mitchell pelvic biomechanical model*.

The pelvic girdle is also important in the respiratory–circulatory model because of its relationship to the pelvic diaphragm.[11] Dysfunction of the osseous pelvis alters the functional capacity of the muscles of the pelvic diaphragm in a manner similar to those of thoracic spine and rib dysfunctions on the thoracoabdominal diaphragm. Many patients with pelvic girdle dysfunction have vague and persistent symptoms of the lower urinary tract, the genital system, and the rectum that resolve when pelvic girdle function is restored.

The sacral component of the pelvis is of importance within the craniosacral system. The sacrum has inherent mobility between the two hip bones (innominates) as part of craniosacral rhythm and is linked with the motion of the occiput. Altered mechanical function of the pelvic girdle can negatively influence the craniosacral mechanism and, alternatively, altered craniosacral mechanics can influence the biomechanical function of the osseous pelvis. The osseous pelvis has a significant contribution to the functional capacity of the musculoskeletal system and warrants appropriate investigation and management in all patients.

FUNCTIONAL ANATOMY

The pelvic girdle consists of three bones and three joints (Fig. 17.1). The sacrum is formed by the fused elements of the sacral vertebrae and articulates superiorly with the last lumbar vertebra and caudally with the coccyx. The sacrum should be viewed as a component part of the vertebral axis. In many ways, the sacrum functions as an atypical lumbar vertebra between the two hip bones, with the sacroiliac joints as atypical zygapophysial joints.[12] The right and left hip bones consist of the fused elements of the ilium, ischium, and pubis. The two hip bones are joined anteriorly by the symphysis pubis joint. Each hip bone articulates cephalically with the sacrum at the ipsilateral sacroiliac joint and caudally with the femur at the hip joint. Functionally, the hip bone should be viewed as a lower extremity bone and the two sacroiliac joints as the junction of the trunk and the lower extremity.

The joints of the pelvic girdle consist of the symphysis pubis and the two sacroiliac joints. The symphysis pubis is an amphiarthrosis with strong superior and inferior ligaments and a thinner posterior ligament. The opposing surfaces can range from being symmetrically flat to quite asymmetric and interlocking. The minimal amount of

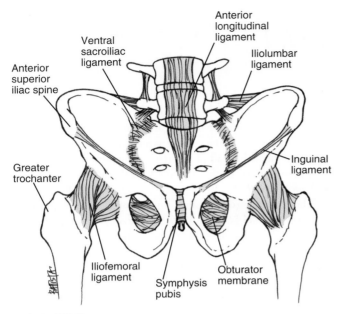

FIGURE 17.1   Anterior sacroiliac ligaments

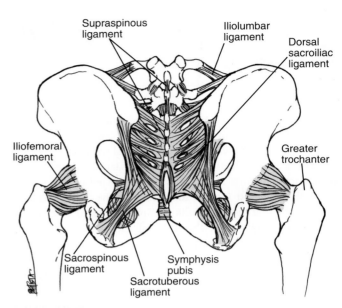

FIGURE 17.2   Sacroiliac joint. Note long arm and short arm.

motion available at this joint is strongly influenced by the shape of the joint, the ligamentous integrity of the joint (particularly under the influence of hormonal changes), and the actions of the abdominal muscles from above and the adductor muscles of the lower extremity below.[13,14]

The sacroiliac joints are true arthrodial joints with a joint space, synovial capsule, and articular cartilage. They are unique in that the cartilage on the sacral side is hyaline cartilage and the cartilage on the ilial side is fibrocartilage.[15] The articular cartilage on the sacral side is much thicker than that on the ilial side. The joints are L-shaped in contour with a shorter upper arm and a longer lower arm (Fig. 17.2). The joint contour usually has a depression on the sacral side at approximately S2 and a corresponding prominence on the ilial side. The shape of the sacroiliac joint varies markedly from individual to individual and from side to side in the same individual. During the aging process, there is an increase in the grooves on the opposing surfaces of the sacrum and ilium that appear to reduce available motion and enhance stability.[9] It is of interest to note that the age at which the incidence of disabling back pain is highest (range: 25 to 45 years) is the same age when the greatest amount of motion is available in the sacroiliac joints. Asymmetric dysfunction of this movement may contribute to disabling back pain. The sacroiliac joint usually has a change in the anteroposterior beveling at approximately the junction of the upper and lower arms. The plane of the upper portion is convergent from behind forward whereas the lower portion is divergent from behind forward, resulting in an interlocking mechanism centering at approximately S2. This interlocking mechanism of joint beveling and the concave–convex relationship at S2 provides some stability of the joint and is described as *form closure*.[16] Occasionally, the opposing joint surfaces are quite flat and do not have the

interlocking joint bevel change at S2 or the ilial prominence within the sacral depression. This type of sacroiliac joint is much less stable and the possibility of superior and inferior translatory movement, or shearing, exists. Occasionally, the sacral concavity is replaced by a convexity with the ilial side being more concave. This joint structure provides increased mobility, primarily in rotation medially and laterally, around a vertical axis.[17]

Much of the integrity of the sacroiliac joint depends on ligamentous structures (Figs. 17.1 and 17.3). The *iliolumbar ligaments* attach to the transverse processes of L4 and L5 and to the anterior surface of the iliac crest. The lower fibers extend inferiorly and blend with the anterior sacroiliac ligaments. The *anterior sacroiliac ligaments* are two relatively flat and thin bands. They can be viewed as providing a sling from the two hip bones for the anterior surface of the sacrum. They are the anterior aspect of the synovial portion of the joint.[18] The *posterior sacroiliac ligaments* have three layers. The deepest layer consists of short interosseous ligaments running from the sacrum to the ilium. The intermediate layer runs from the posterior arches of the sacrum to the medial side of the ilium, occupying most of the space overlying the posterior aspect of the sacroiliac joint. The *long posterior sacroiliac ligaments* blend together and course vertically from the sacral crest to the ilium. Inferiorly, these posterior sacroiliac ligaments blend with the accessory sacroiliac ligaments, the *sacrotuberous and the sacrospinous*.[14] Of particular interest is the *long dorsal sacroiliac ligament* that courses from the posterior superior iliac spine (PSIS) inferiorly and inserts into S4. The role of this ligament is to prevent posterior sacral nutation.[19,20] In sacral dysfunctions with a posterior sacral base this ligament is under tension stress and may become painful to palpation. Tenderness in the region of this ligament is one of the more reliable physical findings in

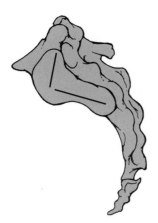

FIGURE 17.3 **Posterior sacroiliac ligaments.**

symptomatic sacroiliac combined with nonadaptive lumbar dysfunction.[21] The sacrotuberous ligament runs from the inferior lateral angle (ILA) of the sacrum to the ischial tuberosity and has a crescent-shaped medial border. It is continuous with the fascia of the hamstring muscles and forms an important link between the lower extremity and the trunk. The sacrotuberous ligament restricts anterior nutation of the sacrum and is under tension stress in sacral dysfunctions with an anterior base and can become tender at its sacral or ischial end.[19] The sacrospinous ligament lies under the sacrotuberous and runs from the ILA of the sacrum to the ischial spine. These two accessory ligaments contribute to the formation of the greater and lesser sciatic notches that are divided by the sacrospinous ligament.

Muscular attachment to the pelvic girdle is extensive but there are few muscles that directly influence sacroiliac motion. Movement of the sacroiliac mechanism appears to be mainly passive, in response to muscle action in the surrounding areas above and below. The abdominal muscles, including the transversus, the two obliques, and the rectus abdominus, insert in the superior aspect of the pelvic girdle and are joined posteriorly by the quadratus lumborum, the lumbodorsal fascia, and the erector spinae mass. Six groups of hip and thigh muscles attach to the pelvic girdle and lower extremities. These hip muscles strongly influence the movement of the two hip bones within the pelvic girdle. Anterior to the sacroiliac joints are two highly significant muscles, the psoas and piriformis. The psoas crosses over the anterior aspect of the sacroiliac joints in its travel from the lumbar region to insert into the lesser trochanter of the femur. The right and left piriformis muscles originate from the anterior surface of the sacrum, travel through the sciatic notch, and insert into the greater trochanter of the femur. Asymmetry of length and tone of the piriformis is frequently observed in recurrent dysfunction of the sacroiliac joints.

Two other muscles have recently been shown to be highly significant in sacroiliac motion and dysfunction. They are the gluteus maximus and the latissimus dorsi muscles. The gluteus maximus attaches to the posterolateral aspect of the sacrum,

and the latissimus dorsi attaches to the base of the sacrum through the lumbodorsal fascia. Contraction of these muscles provides a force that helps the joint to be stable during the stance phase of gait and mobile during the swing phase. The fiber directions of these four muscles form an "X" on the dorsal aspect of the back. Gluteal function coupled with the contralateral latissimus dorsi is important in what is currently called "force closure of the sacroiliac joint." *The form closure of the joints beveling, the force closure of the gluteal–latissimus mechanism, and the strength of the posterior sacroiliac ligaments provide for sacroiliac stability.*[22]

Muscle imbalance in any of these groups affects pelvic girdle function. Gluteus maximus contraction is known to become inhibited in the presence of sacroiliac joint and lower extremity joint dysfunctions.[23,24] Imbalance in piriformis length and strength strongly influences movement of the sacrum between the hip bones. Imbalance of the pelvic diaphragm is significant in patients with rectal, gynecologic, and urologic problems. The reader is encouraged to review the anatomy of all these muscles in a standard anatomic text.

MOTION IN THE PELVIC GIRDLE

The pelvic girdle functions as an integrated unit with all three bones moving at all three joints, influenced by the lower extremities below and the vertebral column and trunk above. This integration results in torsional movement of the pelvis, both left and right, around a vertical (*y*) axis. In torsional movement to the left, the symphysis turns left of the midline, the right hip bone is carried forward, the left hip bone is carried backward, and the sacrum faces somewhat to the left (counterclockwise pelvic rotation). Torsion to the right (clockwise rotation) is just the reverse.

CLINICAL PEARL

A simple screening test for global pelvic torsional movement involves the patient in the supine position with the operator placing the palm of the hands over each anterior superior iliac spine (ASIS). Alternate rocking of the osseous pelvis by pushing posteriorly on each ASIS results in a sensation of symmetry or asymmetry. If movement seems to be more restricted when pushing posteriorly on the right ASIS than with the left, one can presume that the pelvic girdle is torsioned to the left and that there is some restrictor in the mechanism that needs further evaluation.

The amount of movement present at the symphysis pubis and at both sacroiliac joints is certainly not great and more biomechanical research is needed to identify the specific motions available and to determine their axes. The descriptions that follow are based on current biomechanical information and clinical observations. Many of the clinical observations cannot be adequately explained by current biomechanical information. A theoretic construct is offered to explain some of the clinical observations and to establish a vocabulary to describe both available normal motions and dysfunctions.

MOVEMENT AT THE SYMPHYSIS PUBIS

Movement at the symphysis pubis is quite small. It occurs in one-legged standing and during the walking cycle. Strong ligaments maintain the normal integrity of the joint, primarily superiorly and inferiorly. The ligaments become more lax as a result of hormonal change in females, particularly during pregnancy and delivery, and separation occurs to widen the internal pelvic diameter during delivery. There is a normal superior shearing movement if one-legged standing is maintained for several minutes.[13] If one-legged standing on one side is habitual, chronic recurrent pubis dysfunction appears. Muscle imbalance between the abdominal muscles above and the thigh adductors from below is secondary to prolonged one-legged standing. After standing on the opposite leg, or with prolonged standing on both legs, the shearing movement should return to normal. During normal walking, the symphysis pubis serves as the anterior axis for alternating hip bone rotation.[25] Symphysis pubis dysfunction, either superior or inferior, alters the anterior and posterior hip bone rotation during walking.

SACROILIAC MOTION

Sacroiliac motion is the movement of the sacrum between the two hip bones and requires the participation of both sacroiliac joints. Nutation and counternutation (anterior nutation–posterior nutation) is the sacral motion about which the most is known from biomechanical and radiographic research. "Nutation" and "counternutation" are the terms used in the anatomic literature, but this author prefers the use of anterior nutation for nutation and posterior nutation for counternutation, because this terminology allows one to describe a neutral point between anterior and posterior nutation. Nutation (anterior nutation) is a forward nodding movement of the sacrum between the hip bones with the sacral base moving anteriorly and inferiorly and the sacral apex moving posteriorly and superiorly (Fig. 17.4). Counternutation (posterior nutation) occurs when the sacral base moves posteriorly and superiorly and the sacral apex moves anteriorly and inferiorly (Fig. 17.5).

This is the sacroiliac movement that occurs in a two-legged stance with trunk forward and backward bending. Many other structures participate in the trunk forward and backward bending, but the sacroiliac motion is described as nutation and counternutation.

The horizontal axis around which this anteroposterior nutation occurs has been described differently by various investigators but appears to be related to the upper and lower limbs of the sacroiliac joint and their junction somewhere around S2. This axis is the *middle transverse axis* in Mitchell terminology. A superior-to-inferior translatory movement accompanies the overturning of anterior and posterior nutation. During anterior nutation (nutation), there is an inferior translatory movement of the sacrum. During posterior nutation (counternutation), there is a superior translatory movement. This superior-to-inferior translatory movement accompanying the overturning of anterior and posterior nutation has some authors describing it as "shear" and using the "shear" term as part of the description of unilateral dysfunction. "Shear" is not an appropriate term as it is not a true shearing motion but rather the normal translation component of the nutational movement. Bilateral symmetry of anteroposterior nutation depends on the symmetry of the two sacroiliac joints. With asymmetry of a patient's two sacroiliac joints being so common, asymmetry of this anteroposterior nutation is also quite common. This explains why it is possible for unilateral restriction to occur.

There is a craniosacral component to anterior and posterior nutational movement of the sacrum that follows the cranial rhythmic impulse. The axis for this motion is called the *superior transverse axis* in Mitchell terminology. Anterior nutation is called sacral flexion in the biomechanical model and sacral extension in the craniosacral model. Posterior nutation is called sacral extension in the biomechanical model and sacral flexion in the craniosacral model (see Table 12.1).

Movement of the sacrum between the two hip bones during walking is more complex and less well understood. If one palpates the right side of the sacral base with the right thumb, the right ILA with the right index finger, the left

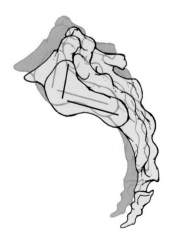

FIGURE 17.4 Sacral nutation.

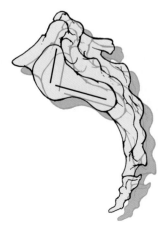

FIGURE 17.5 Sacral counternutation.

sacral base and left ILA with the left thumb and index finger, and follows movement of the sacrum during walking, the sacrum appears to have an oscillatory movement: first left, then right. The right base appears to move anteriorly while the left ILA moves posteriorly, and then the reverse occurs, with the left sacral base moving anteriorly and the right ILA moving posteriorly. This sacral motion has been described as torsion to describe the coupling of side bending and rotation to opposite sides.

Most of the studies of sacral side bending and rotational coupling have them always couple to opposite sides. In only one cadaveric study, using a unilateral preparation, the coupling of sacral side bending and rotation appeared to depend on whether side bending or rotation was introduced first. Clinical observation of the walking cycle demonstrates that sacral side bending and rotation couple to opposite sides. In left torsional movement, the anterior surface of the sacrum rotates to face left (left rotation), while the superior surface of S1 (sacral base plane) declines to the right (right-side bending). Right torsion is the exact opposite. For descriptive purposes, this complex, polyaxial, torsional movement is considered to occur around an oblique axis. By convention, and from the Mitchell terminology, the left oblique axis runs from the upper extremity of the left sacroiliac joint to the lower end of the right sacroiliac joint, and the right oblique axis runs from the upper end of the right sacroiliac joint to the lower extremity of the left sacroiliac joint[10] (Fig. 17.6). Although the biomechanics of the torsional movements of the sacrum are unknown, the hypothetic left and right oblique axes are useful for descriptive purposes.

In the normal walking cycle, the sacrum appears to move anterior in oscillating fashion around alternating oblique axes. For example, during right midstance (midleft swing phase), the sacral base on the left begins to move into anterior nutation as it is carried forward by the advancing left ilia. As it begins to rotate to the right, it side bends to the left. The oblique hypothetical torsional axis that is produced from this polyaxial movement is right. So, during right midstance gait, the sacrum begins to move into right rotation about a right oblique axis. The lumbar spine will concurrently rotate to the left and side bend to the right (Fig. 17.7). During left midstance gait the sacral base on the right begins to move into anterior nutation as it is carried forward by the advancing right ilium. As it begins to rotate to the left, it side bends to the right. The oblique hypothetical torsional axis that is produced from this polyaxial movement is left. So, during left midstance gait, the sacrum begins to move into left rotation about a left oblique axis. The lumbar spine will concurrently rotate to the right and side bend to the left.[26]

To summarize the normal walking cycle, the sacrum appears to move with left torsion on the left oblique axis, return to neutral, rotate in right torsion on the right oblique axis, and then return to neutral. Because the nutational component of this normal walking movement is anterior in direction, left torsion on the left oblique axis and right torsion on the right oblique axis are described as *anterior torsional movements*. The nutational movement in normal walking is anterior on one side, returns to neutral, anterior to the opposite side, and returns to neutral. Posterior nutational movement does not appear past neutral in the normal walking cycle.

Since much of the activity of the musculoskeletal system involves the walking cycle, maintenance of normal left-on-left and right-on-right sacral movements is an important therapeutic objective. Since walking occurs with the vertebral column in the erect, neutral (neither flexed nor extended) position, the anterior torsional sacral movements are called neutral mechanics. During walking, the thoracolumbar spine side bends left and

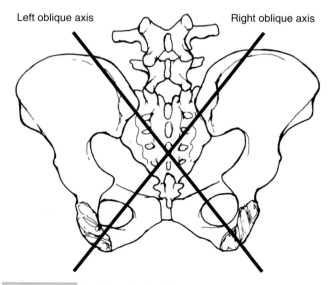

FIGURE 17.6 Right and left oblique axes.

Left oblique axis   Right oblique axis

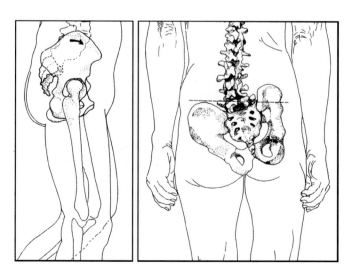

FIGURE 17.7 Anterior motion of the sacrum during right midstance.

rotates right, then side bends right and rotates left with each step. This neutral movement of the vertebral column requires normal segmental mobility, and starts with the response of the lumbar spine, usually L5, at the lumbosacral junction. (See Chapter 16 for description of lumbar linkage to the sacrum.) As the sacrum side bends right and rotates left, L5 side bends left and rotates right. Each vertebra above L5 should appropriately respond as part of the adaptive neutral curve. A vertebra, particularly in the lower lumbar spine, with nonneutral dysfunction results in a "nonadaptive" vertebral response to the sacrum. Treatment of lumbar spine dysfunction should always precede treatment of sacroiliac dysfunction because many sacroiliac treatments require the use of the lumbar spine as a lever.

A third sacral movement occurs when the trunk is forward bent and side bent or rotated to one side. This maneuver results in the nonneutral behavior of the lumbar spine with side bending and rotation coupled to the same side. The sacrum between the hip bones participates in this maneuver by backward or posterior torsional movement. Posterior torsional movement occurs on the left or right oblique axes, and the coupling of side bending and rotation occurs to opposite sides. In posterior torsional movement, one side of the sacral base moves beyond neutral into posterior nutation. In posterior or backward torsion to the right on the left oblique axis, the sacrum rotates right, side bends left, and the right base moves into posterior nutation. In backward or posterior torsion to the left on the right oblique axis, the sacrum rotates left, side bends right, and the left base goes into posterior nutation. These posterior torsional movements are nonneutral sacroiliac mechanics and are not part of the normal walking cycle.

The sacroiliac joint is at risk for injury, as is the lumbar spine, when the trunk is forward bent and side bending/rotation is introduced. In this posture, the lumbar spine is at risk for annular tear of the disc, strain of deep lumbar muscles, and sprain of the zygapophysial joints. The posterior torsional movement of the sacrum appears to sprain the posterior sacroiliac ligaments. Nonneutral dysfunction of the lower lumbar spine and backward torsional dysfunction of the sacroiliac joint occur in the well-known syndrome of "the well man bent over and the cripple stood up."

ILIOSACRAL MOVEMENT

The sacroiliac mechanism can be viewed from the perspective of each hip bone articulating with the sacrum. The motion can be described as one hip bone moving on one side of the sacrum (iliosacral movement). Each hip bone in the walking cycle rotates anteriorly and posteriorly around the anterior axis at the symphysis pubis, and anteriorly and posteriorly with each side of the sacrum on a posterior axis (the inferior transverse axis in Mitchell terminology). In anterior hip bone rotation, the hip bone rotates forward in relation to the sacrum with the ASIS being carried anterior, inferior, and a little laterally; the PSIS is carried anterior and superior; and the ischial tuberosity is carried posterior and superior. In posterior hip bone rotation, the ASIS is carried superior, posterior, and a little medially; the PSIS is carried posterior and inferior; and the

ischial tuberosity is carried anterior and superior. Anterior and posterior hip bone rotations occur in the presence of normal sacroiliac joint contour. If the opposing surfaces of the sacrum and ilium at the sacroiliac joint are altered, atypical movements appear clinically. In approximately 10% to 15% of the population, the sacroiliac joint does not have the form closure of the bevel change and convex-to-concave relationship at S2. The opposing joint surfaces are more flat and parallel. This configuration makes the joint susceptible to a superior-to-inferior translatory movement that can become dysfunctional. This is a true "shear" motion of one joint surface on the other.[27] In those sacra in which the sacral side is convex and the ilial side concave, internal and external rotation around a vertical axis appears possible. These very rare movements can occasionally become dysfunctional and are termed "in-flare" and "out-flare," describing the medial and lateral rotation around a vertical axis observed clinically.

Somatic dysfunction can occur with any of these motions within the pelvic girdle. Each of these motions is quite small, but when lost, each has a significant clinical effect. In dysfunctions within the pelvic girdle, it is common to find restriction of several movements within the mechanism.

STRUCTURAL DIAGNOSIS OF PELVIC GIRDLE SOMATIC DYSFUNCTION

In the structural diagnosis of the pelvic girdle, the examiner looks for the diagnostic triad of asymmetry, range of motion alteration, and tissue texture abnormality. Evaluation is made of asymmetry of paired anatomic landmarks within the pelvic girdle and lower extremity; altered range of motion (by the standing and seated flexion tests, the stork test, and various springing movement tests of the sacroiliac joints); and tissue texture abnormality in the deep fascia and ligaments over the sacroiliac joints, the sacrotuberous ligament, and the gluteal and perineal muscles. A combination of findings within the asymmetry, range of motion, tissue texture abnormality (ART) diagnostic triad leads to the diagnosis of pelvic girdle dysfunction. The diagnostic process identifies dysfunction at the symphysis pubis (dysfunction between the two pubic bones), the sacroiliac joints (sacrum between the two hip bones), and the iliosacral joints (each hip bone as it articulates with its respective side of the sacrum). The diagnostic sequence is standing, sitting with feet on floor or supported on a stool, supine, prone, and supine again.

The motion tests of the standing and seated flexion test have been classically used to assess sacroiliac restriction on one side. Recent research has shown that even in a symptomatic sacroiliac dysfunction, the joint still moves, albeit somewhat less than normal. *What is important is that these tests show relative asymmetry of pelvic motion and are useful in lateralizing the relative restriction to one side.* The two flexion tests are very sensitive but not very specific for joint restriction. The standing flexion test is highly sensitive to restrictors influencing the pelvis from the lower extremity, and the seated flexion test takes out the influence of the lower extremities and is more sensitive to restrictors from the sacroiliac joints and the trunk.

PELVIC GIRDLE

Diagnosis: Standing

1. Patient stands with his weight equally distributed on both feet acetabular distance apart.

2. Operator stands or sits behind the patient with the dominant eye in the midline and on the horizontal plane where the hands are placed.

3. Operator palpates the superior aspect of each iliac crest, evaluating the relative height (Fig. 17.8).

4. Operator palpates superior aspect of the greater trochanter of each femur evaluating the relative height (Fig. 17.9).

5. If one crest and greater trochanter are higher than the other, there is presumptive evidence of anatomic shortening of lower extremity.

6. Level crest height but unlevel trochanters or unlevel crests and equal trochanters are presumptive evidence of bony asymmetry of the pelvic girdle.

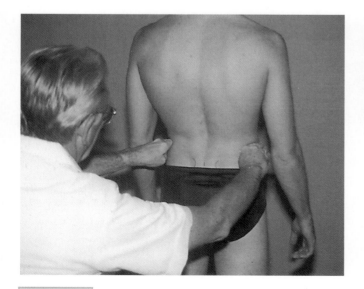

FIGURE 17.8

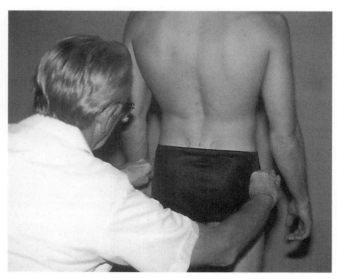

FIGURE 17.9

PELVIC GIRDLE

Diagnosis: Standing Flexion Test

1. Patient stands with his weight equally distributed on both feet acetabular distance apart.

2. Operator stands or sits behind the patient.

3. Operator's hands grasp along the posterior aspect of each ilia with the pads of the thumbs placed just under the inferior slope of the PSIS (Fig. 17.10).

4. Patient is instructed to smoothly bend forward as far as possible without bending the knees (Fig. 17.11).

5. Operator's hands follow the motion of the ilia with a visual focus on the excursion of each PSIS. The test is deemed positive on the side that the PSIS appears to move more cephalad and/or ventral.

6. The standing flexion test is used to identify the side of restricted pelvic motion for pubic and iliosacral dysfunction. False positives are found with asymmetric tightness of the contralateral hamstring and of the ipsilateral quadratus lumborum. The test is sensitive to the role of the long fasciae of the lower extremity on pelvic mobility.

7. Operator observes the response of the vertebral column for dysrhythmia and the presence of altered lateral curvatures.

Note: If both thumbs move symmetrically, the interpretation is that the test is negative; however, it might also be a bilaterally positive test.

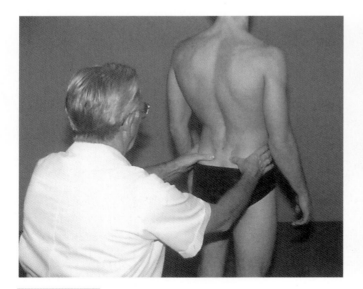

FIGURE 17.10

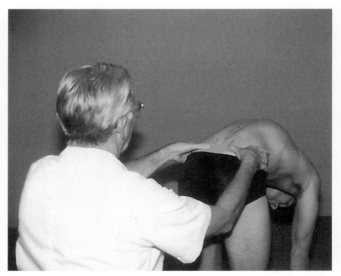

FIGURE 17.11

PELVIC GIRDLE

Diagnosis: One-legged Stork Test (Gillet)

1. Operator stands or sits behind the standing patient.

2. The operator's right hand grasps along the posterior aspect of the right ilia, with the pad of the thumb placed just under the inferior slope of the PSIS and the left thumb on the midline of the sacral promontory at the same level (Fig. 17.12).

3. Patient raises the right knee toward the ceiling.

4. Motion of the right ilia is followed with a focus on the thumb. A normal response finds the thumb on the PSIS moving caudad in relation to the thumb on the sacrum (Fig. 17.13).

5. A positive response finds the thumb on the PSIS not moving or moving cephalically (Fig. 17.14).

6. Comparison is made with the opposite side by reversing the procedure.

7. Lower pole movement is tested by placing the left thumb on the sacral hiatus and the right thumb at the same level on the posterior inferior aspect of the iliac bone (Fig. 17.15).

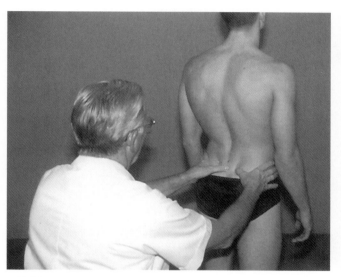

FIGURE 17.12

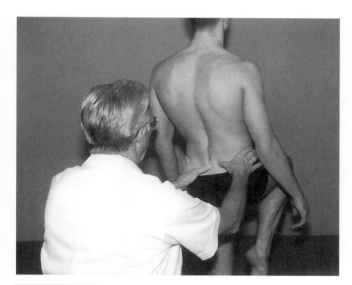

FIGURE 17.14

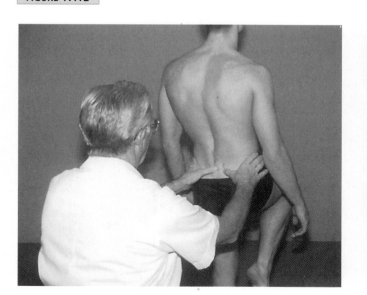

FIGURE 17.13

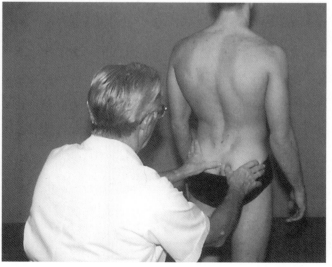

FIGURE 17.15

8. Patient lifts the right knee toward the ceiling.

9. A normal response finds the right thumb moving laterally, caudally, and ventrally (Fig. 17.16).

10. A positive response finds the right thumb moving cephalad in relation to the left thumb on the sacrum (Fig. 17.17).

11. If the patient is unable to do the one-legged standing required for this test, suspect sensory motor balance dysfunction and assess accordingly (see Chapter 20).

Note: Although the upper and lower pole "stork tests" findings are sensitive for sacroiliac joint restrictions, the upper pole test is more specific for upper pole sacroiliac joint dysfunctions such as posterior torsions[8] whereas the lower pole test is more specific for lower pole sacroiliac joint dysfunctions, such as anterior torsions or unilateral sacral dysfunctions.

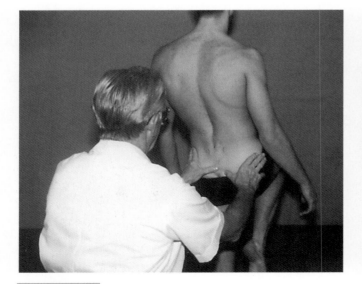

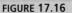
FIGURE 17.16

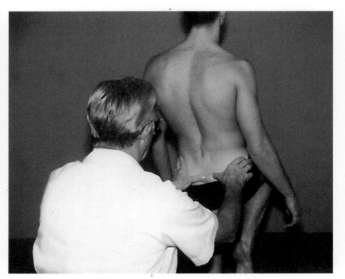
FIGURE 17.17

PELVIC GIRDLE

Diagnosis: Standing

Trunk Side Bending

1. Operator stands or sits behind the patient standing with feet acetabular distance apart.

2. Operator palpates each PSIS with the thumbs (Fig. 17.18).

3. Patient side bends trunk to the left (Fig. 17.19) without forward bending, while operator observes behavior of the induced lumbar curve and the pelvic motion.

4. Patient performs side bending trunk to the right (Fig. 17.20).

5. Operator observes symmetry of induced side-bending curve. A normal response is a smooth C-curve of the spine with fullness of the side of the convexity. A positive finding is a straightening of the lumbar curve and/or fullness of the side of concavity which suggests nonneutral behavior of the lumbar spine.

6. Operator observes behavior of the pelvis during trunk side bending. The normal response is pelvic rotation opposite to the induced lumbar rotation above. A positive response is any other pelvic motion.

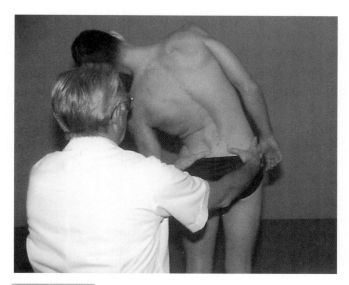

FIGURE 17.19

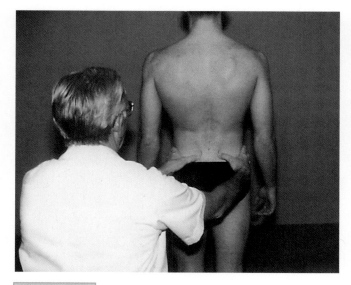

FIGURE 17.18

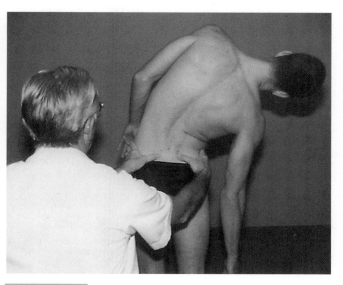

FIGURE 17.20

PELVIC GIRDLE

Diagnosis: Sitting

Sitting Flexion Test

1. Patient sits on examining stool with feet on the floor or on the table with feet supported.

2. Operator sits or kneels behind the patient, the hands grasp along the posterior aspect of each iliac crest with the pads of the thumbs placed just under the inferior slope of the PSIS (Fig. 17.21).

3. Unleveling of the crest in the seated position is strong evidence of bony asymmetry in the bony pelvis.

4. Patient is asked to smoothly forward bend as far as possible with the arms between the knees (Fig. 17.22). Operator's hands follow the excursion of the ilia with a visual focus on the thumbs.

5. A positive finding has the PSIS on one side moving more cephalad and/or more ventral than the other. A false-positive response is found in the presence of ipsilateral quadratus lumborum tightness.

6. Operator observes the behavior of the lumbar and lower thoracic spines for dysrhythmia and abnormal lateral curves. Comparison is made with that observed while standing.

7. With the patient in the fully forward-bent position, operator palpates the posterior aspect of the ILA of the sacrum, searching if they are symmetrically in the coronal plane or if one is more posterior than the other (Fig. 17.23). This finding will be used in sacroiliac diagnosis.

Note: The seated flexion test is sensitive to sacroiliac joint dysfunctions and will correlate to the same side of the lower and upper pole stork test. If altered vertebral mechanics are more severe during the standing flexion test than when seated, major restriction in the lower extremities is suggested. If vertebral dysrhythmia is worse during the seated flexion test, major restriction above the pelvic girdle is suggested.

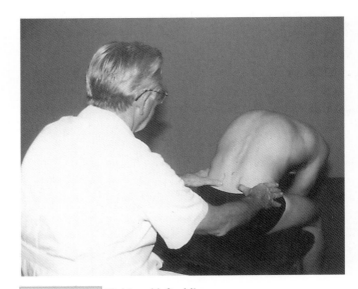

FIGURE 17.22 Right and left oblique axes.

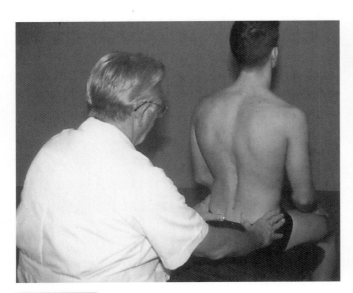

FIGURE 17.21

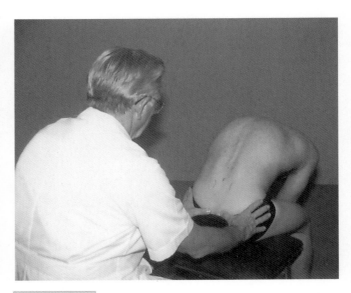

FIGURE 17.23

PELVIC GIRDLE

Diagnosis: Supine

Pubic Symphysis Height

1. Patient is supine on the table.
2. Operator stands at the side of the table with dominant eye over the midline.
3. Operator places the palm of the hand on the abdomen and moves caudally until the heel of the hand strikes the superior aspect of the symphysis pubis (Fig. 17.24).
4. Operator places the pads of the index fingers on the superior aspect of the symphysis pubis (Fig. 17.25).

5. Operator moves the index finger pads laterally approximately 2 cm, palpating the superior aspect of the pubic tubercles (Fig. 17.26).
6. A positive finding is one pubic tubercle being more superior or inferior to the other and tension and tenderness of the medial attachment of the inguinal ligament.

Note: If a positive finding for dysfunction of the pubic symphysis is found, it should be appropriately treated before proceeding with the diagnostic process of the rest of the pelvis.

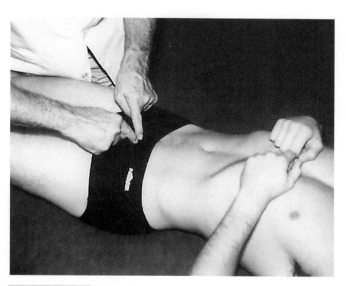

FIGURE 17.25

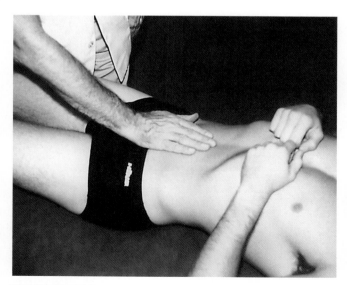

FIGURE 17.24

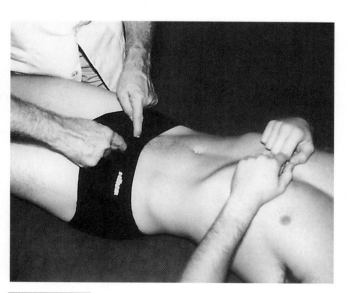

FIGURE 17.26

PELVIC GIRDLE

Diagnosis: Supine and Prone

Iliac Crest Height

1. Patient is supine on the table with the operator standing at the side with dominant eye over the midline.

2. Operator palpates the superior aspect of each iliac crest in relation to the horizontal plane by symmetric placement of the index fingers (Fig. 17.27).

3. Patient is prone on the table with the operator standing at the side with dominant eye over the midline.

4. Operator palpates the superior aspect of each iliac crest in relation to the horizontal plane with the index fingers (Fig.17.28).

5. If one crest is higher than the other, operator is highly suspicious of the presence of a hip bone shear dysfunction. If subsequently verified, it should be treated before proceeding with the remaining examination of the pelvic girdle.

PELVIC GIRDLE

Diagnosis: Prone

Leg Length at Medial Malleolus

1. Patient is prone on the table with the dorsum of the foot free and the distal tibia and fibula at the edge of the table.

2. Operator stands at the end of the table and palpates the most inferior aspect of each medial malleolus, determining if one is longer or shorter than the other (Fig. 17.29).

3. A confirmatory test is to dorsiflex the feet and sight down perpendicularly on the pads of each heel to determine which is longer or shorter.

4. Inequality may be a function of asymmetric leg length.

5. In the presence of symmetric leg length, inequality in the medial malleolus is usually a function of the adaptation of the lumbar spine to sacral base unleveling in sacroiliac dysfunction.

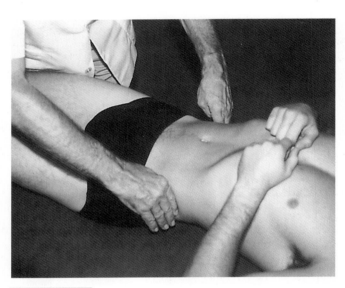

FIGURE 17.27

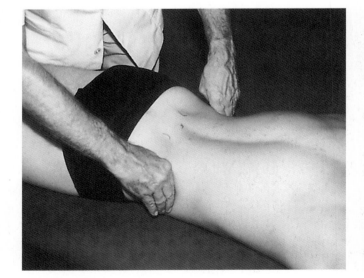

FIGURE 17.28

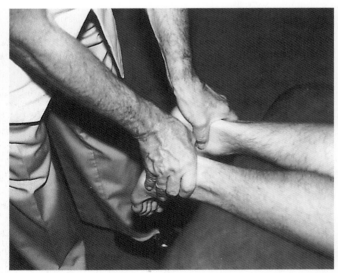

FIGURE 17.29

PELVIC GIRDLE

Diagnosis: Prone

Ischial Tuberosity Level

1. Patient is prone on the table with the operator standing at the side and dominant eye over the midline.

2. Operator places the sides of the thumbs in gluteal fold and presses ventrally into the posterior aspect of the hamstring fascia (Fig. 17.30).

3. Operator's thumbs move superiorly until the pads strike the inferior aspect of the ischial tuberosities (Fig. 17.31).

4. Evaluation is made of the level of the ischial tuberosities against the horizontal plane.

5. Unleveling of the ischial tuberosity the width of the thumb (6 mm) is considered positive.

Note: Care must be exercised to palpate the inferior aspect of the ischial tuberosity, as the structure is quite round.

PELVIC GIRDLE

Diagnosis: Prone

Sacrotuberous Ligament Tension

1. Patient is prone with the operator standing at the side with dominant eye over the midline.

2. Operator's thumbs are placed on the inferior aspect of the ischial tuberosities (Fig. 17.31).

3. Operator's thumbs stay on the bone and move medially, curl cephalad, and hook out posterolaterally on each side under each sacrotuberous ligament (Fig. 17.32).

4. Operator assesses the symmetry of tone of the sacrotuberous ligament. Laxity or increased tension with associated tenderness is a positive finding.

5. Unleveling of the ischial tuberosity and asymmetric tension of the sacrotuberous ligaments are positive findings for hip bone shear dysfunction.

Note: Tenderness of the sacrotuberous ligament is common in association with sacroiliac dysfunction.

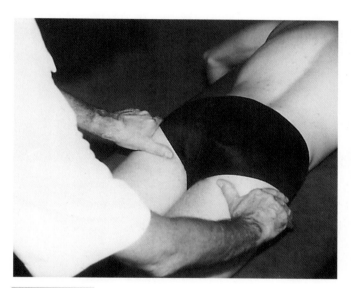

FIGURE 17.30

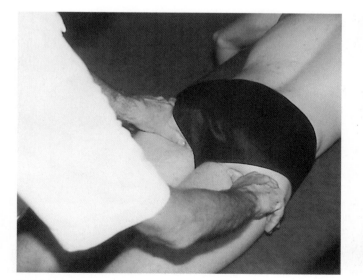

FIGURE 17.31

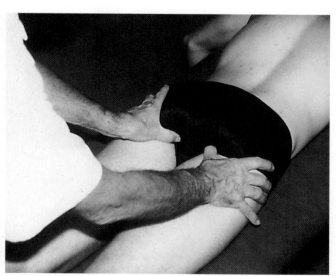

FIGURE 17.32

PELVIC GIRDLE

Diagnosis: Prone

Inferior Lateral Angle (ILA)

1. Patient is prone on the table with the operator standing at the side with dominant eye over the midline.

2. Operator palpates the sacral hiatus at the caudal end of the sacral crest (Fig. 17.33).

3. Operator identifies the posterior aspect of the ILA 1.5 to 2 cm lateral to the sacral hiatus (Fig. 17.34).

4. Operator places the pad of each thumb over the posterior aspect of the ILA evaluating the level against the coronal

plane. A small depression of bone makes this landmark easily palpable (Fig. 17.35).

5. Operator's thumbs are turned under the inferior aspect of the ILA (without lifting thumbs off the bony contact) for evaluation of the level against the horizontal plane (Fig. 17.36).

6. In the presence of a symmetrically shaped sacrum, a posterior ILA is always inferior, and an inferior ILA is always posterior. Occasionally, the finding is more posterior than inferior or more inferior than posterior.

7. While palpating the inferior aspect of the ILA, tension and tenderness of the superior attachment of the sacrotuberous ligament are assessed. Sacrotuberous ligament is palpably tense and usually tender in the presence of many sacroiliac dysfunctions.

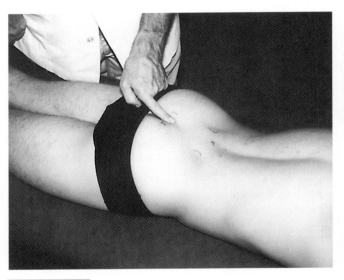

FIGURE 17.33

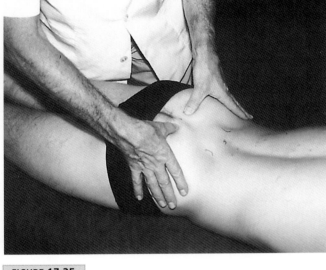

FIGURE 17.35

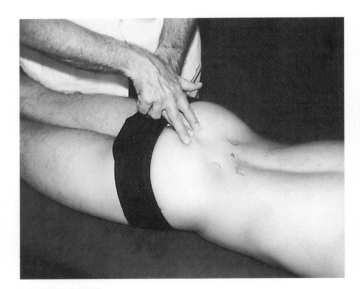

FIGURE 17.34

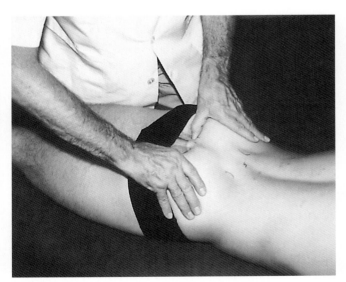

FIGURE 17.36

PELVIC GIRDLE

Diagnosis: Prone

Posterior Superior Iliac Spine, Sacral Base, and L5

1. Patient is prone on the table with the operator standing at the side with dominant eye over the midline.

2. Operator places thumb pads on the inferior slope of the PSIS to assess the level against the horizontal plane (Fig. 17.37).

3. Operator places the pads of the thumbs on the most posterior aspect of the PSIS and curls thumbs medially and caudally approximately 30 degrees. The tip of the thumb strikes the sacral base. Assessment is made of the level of the sacral base against the coronal plane (Fig. 17.38).

4. Operator's thumbs begin at the same most posterior aspect of the PSIS and curl medially and cephalad approximately 30 degrees to strike the posterior arch of L5 (Fig. 17.39). Assessment is made of the level of L5 against the coronal plane.

5. The level of the sacral base is frequently referred to as "depth of the sacral sulcus." If one sacral base is more anterior than the other, the sacral sulcus is said to be "deep" on that side. The term "depth of the sacral sulcus" should be reserved for a finding of depth difference from the PSIS to a sacral base that is level in the coronal plane.

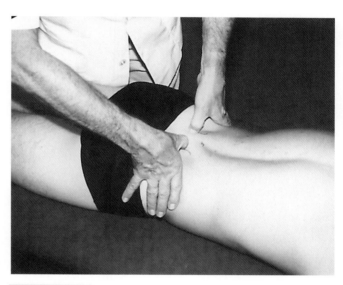

FIGURE 17.38

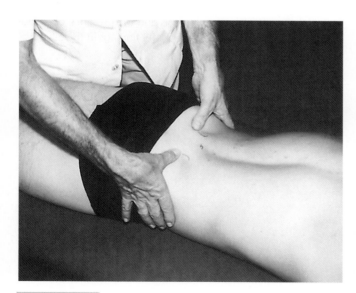

FIGURE 17.37

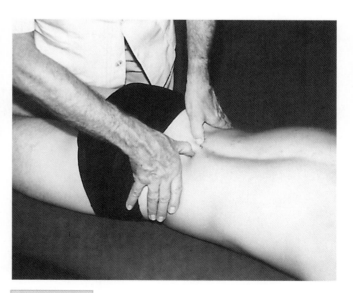

FIGURE 17.39

PELVIC GIRDLE

Diagnosis: Prone

Four-Point Sacral Motion

1. Patient is prone on the table with the operator standing at the side and the dominant eye over the midline.

2. Operator's thumbs are on the posterior aspect of each ILA and the index fingers are over each side of the sacral base (Fig. 17.40). Assessment is made of the level of the ILA and the sacral base against the coronal plane.

3. Operator monitors the movement of the four-point contact on the sacrum while the patient deeply inhales and exhales several times. Normal function finds the sacral base to move

dorsally and the sacral ILA to move ventrally during deep inhalation and the reverse during exhalation.

4. Patient is asked to assume trunk extension through the prone prop position with the chin in the hands (Fig. 17.41). Assessment is made as to the level of the ILA and sacral base against the coronal plane in comparison with the prone neutral position.

5. The level of the ILA during trunk forward bending has previously been assessed (Fig. 17.23).

6. The behavior of the ILA and sacral base during the three positions of neutral, backward bent (prone prop position), and forward bent (during seated flexion) is the most reliable sign of sacroiliac dysfunction.

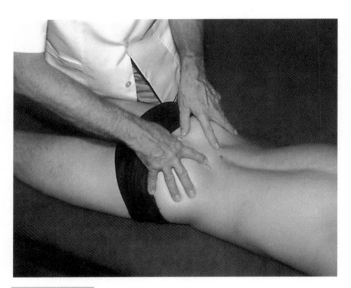

FIGURE 17.40

PELVIC GIRDLE

Diagnosis: Prone

Spring Test

1. Patient is prone on the table with the operator standing at the side with dominant eye over the midline.

2. Operator places the palm of the hand over the midline of the lumbar region with the heel of the hand over the lumbosacral junction and the middle finger over the lumbar spinous processes (Fig. 17.42).

3. Operator evaluates the lumbar lordosis for normal, increase, or flattening.

4. Operator provides a short quick push with the heel of the hand toward the table evaluating for yielding of the lumbar spine. This maneuver should cause lumbar spine extension and sacral nutation (anterior nutation).

5. If the operator feels no resistance, and there is yielding of the lumbar lordosis, the test is recorded as negative.

6. A lumbar spine resisting this maneuver is recorded as positive.

7. The status of the lumbar lordosis and the presence of a positive or negative spring test are useful findings in the diagnosis of sacroiliac dysfunction.

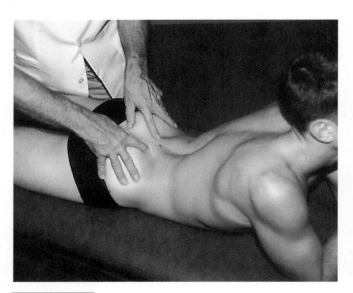

FIGURE 17.41

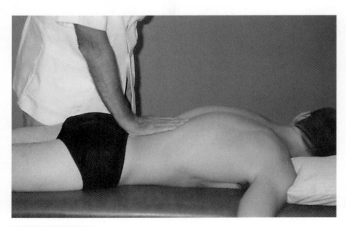

FIGURE 17.42

PELVIC GIRDLE

Diagnosis: Prone

Sacroiliac Rocking Test

1. Patient is prone on the table with the operator standing at the side.

2. Operator places the right thumb over the left ILA and the left thumb over the left sacral base (Fig. 17.43).

3. Alternate ventral pressure of each thumb tests the capacity of the left sacroiliac joint to nutate anteriorly and posteriorly across the transverse axis.

4. Operator's thumbs are placed over the right ILA and sacral base (Fig. 17.44), and the right sacroiliac joint is similarly tested for nutation anteriorly and posteriorly across the transverse axis.

5. Operator's right thumb is over the posterior aspect of the left ILA and the left thumb over the right sacral base (Fig. 17.45).

6. Alternate ventral pressure by the thumbs tests the capacity of the sacrum's torsional movement around the left oblique axis.

7. Operator's right thumb is over the right ILA and the left thumb over the left sacral base (Fig. 17.46). A similar ventral pressure motion tests the capacity of the sacrum to move around the right oblique axis.

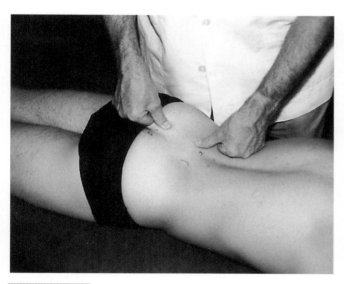

FIGURE 17.43

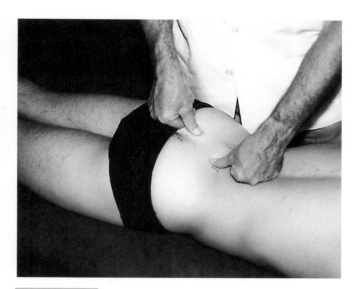

FIGURE 17.45

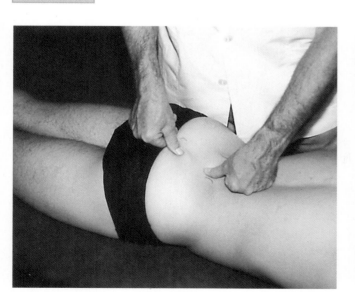

FIGURE 17.44

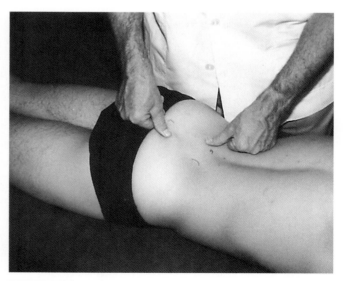

FIGURE 17.46

PELVIC GIRDLE

Diagnosis: Prone

Sacroiliac Motion Spring Test

1. Patient is prone on the table with the operator standing at the side.

2. Operator's right thenar eminence is over the left ILA and the index and middle fingers of the left hand are over the left sacral base (Fig. 17.47).

3. Ventral pressure through the right hand while monitoring movement at the left fingers tests for posterior nutation capacity of the left sacroiliac joint.

4. Operator places the right thenar eminence over the right ILA and the left fingers over the right sacral base and springs ventrally, testing posterior nutation capacity of the right sacroiliac joint.

5. Operator places right thenar eminence over the left ILA and the monitoring left fingers are over the right sacral base (Fig. 17.48).

6. Ventral springing through the right thenar eminence with monitoring of motion of the right sacral base identifies coupled side bending and rotational torsional movements around the left oblique axis.

7. Operator places right thenar eminence over the right ILA and the left fingers monitor the left sacral base (Fig. 17.49). Ventral pressure through the right hand monitored at the left base identifies torsional movement around the right oblique axis.

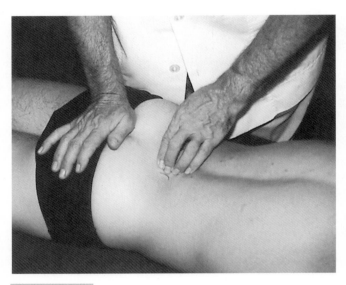

FIGURE 17.48

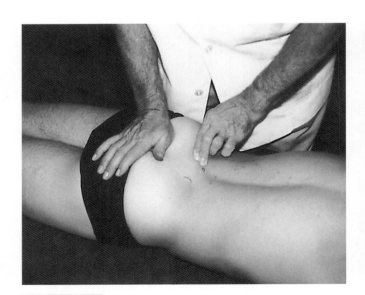

FIGURE 17.47

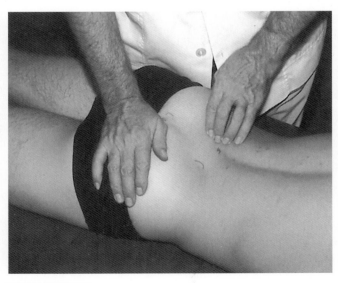

FIGURE 17.49

PELVIC GIRDLE

Diagnosis: Prone

Sacroiliac Motion Test by Gapping

1. Patient is prone on the table with the operator standing at the side.

2. Operator's fingers of the left hand overlie the posterior aspect of the left sacroiliac joint while the right hand controls the left lower extremity, knee flexed, with contact at the ankle (Fig. 17.50).

3. With patient's knee below 90 degrees of flexion, operator introduces internal rotation of the lower extremity through the femur, hip joint, and hip bone while monitoring movement of the left sacroiliac joint.

4. The normal motion is gapping of the joint posteriorly.

5. Internal rotation of the leg with the knee below 90 degrees primarily tests the lower pole of the left sacroiliac joint.

6. Operator repeats the maneuver with the knee flexed above 90 degrees (Fig. 17.51), which primarily tests movement of the upper pole.

PELVIC GIRDLE

Diagnosis: Supine

Leg Length

1. Patient is supine with the operator standing at the end of the table.

2. Operator grasps patient's feet and ankles with the thumbs under the inferior aspect of each medial malleolus (Fig. 17.52).

3. Operator sights down perpendicular to each thumb, identifying which leg appears longer or shorter.

4. In the absence of anatomic difference in leg length, inequality of leg length in the supine position is a function of hip bone rotation due to iliosacral dysfunction.

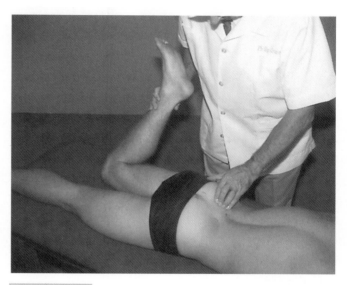

FIGURE 17.51

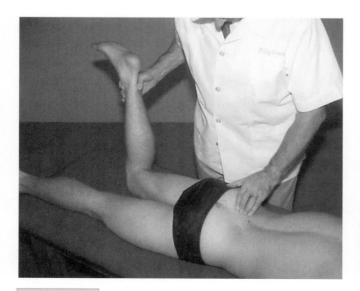

FIGURE 17.50

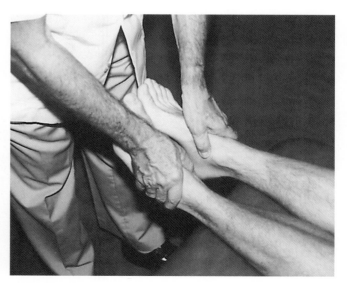

FIGURE 17.52

PELVIC GIRDLE

Diagnosis: Supine

Anterior Superior Iliac Spine

1. Patient is supine with the operator standing at the side with dominant eye over the midline.

2. Operator places the palms of the hands over each ASIS for precise localization (Fig. 17.53).

3. Operator places both thumbs on the inferior aspect of the ASIS testing against the horizontal plane for hip bone rotation (Fig. 17.54).

4. Operator places each thumb on the anterior aspect of the ASIS testing against the coronal plane to determine if one hip bone is more anterior or posterior than the other (Fig. 17.55).

5. Operator's thumbs are placed on the medial side of the ASISs, testing their relationship to the midsagittal plane to see if one is more medial or lateral than the other (Fig. 17.56).

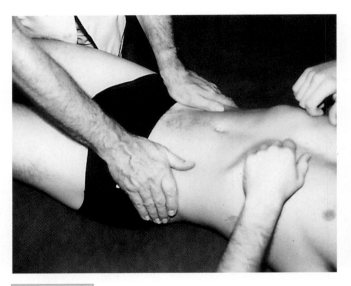

FIGURE 17.53

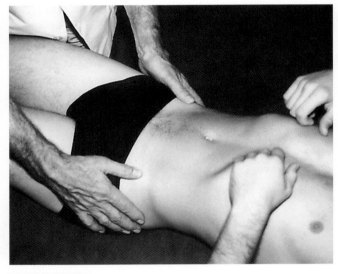

FIGURE 17.55

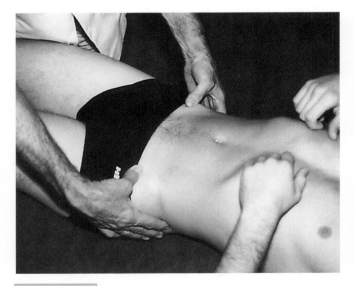

FIGURE 17.54

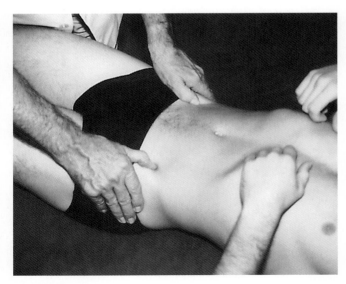

FIGURE 17.56

PELVIC GIRDLE DYSFUNCTIONS

There are 14 different dysfunctions possible within the pelvic girdle (Table 17.1). It is seldom that one finds a single dysfunction within the pelvis. Combinations of dysfunctions of the pubis, sacroiliac, and iliosacral mechanisms are quite common.

Diagnosis of these dysfunctions is made from a combination of physical findings of asymmetry of osseous parts, asymmetric range of motion of the right and left side of the pelvis, and tissue texture abnormalities, primarily of ligamentous tension and tenderness.

Pubic Symphysis Dysfunction

Dysfunctions of the symphysis pubis are very common and frequently overlooked. The main reason they are overlooked is that they seldom have associated local pain. The unleveling of the pubic symphysis could also be called a subluxation. It is always either superior or inferior. A unilateral anterior or posterior symphysis does not occur except in association with pelvic ring fracture. Muscle imbalances between the abdominals above and the adductors below are major contributors to the presence and persistence of this dysfunction. They frequently result from the chronic posture of one-legged standing. Pubic dysfunction restricts symmetric motion of the hip bones during the walking cycle and interferes with all other motions in the pelvis. The diagnostic criteria for pubic dysfunction are based on three diagnostic findings. The determination of the side of restriction is based on the standing flexion test as the motion test. The asymmetry finding is that one pubic tubercle is either high or low on one side against the horizontal plane. The third finding is tension and tenderness on the insertion of the inguinal ligament. The most common dysfunctions are of the right inferior pubic symphysis and left superior pubic symphysis.

TABLE 17.1   *Pelvic Girdle Dysfunctions*

Pubis
1. Superior
2. Inferior

Sacroiliac
1. Bilaterally nutated anteriorly
2. Bilaterally nutated posteriorly
3. Unilaterally nutated anteriorly (sacrum flexed)
4. Unilaterally nutated posteriorly (sacrum extended)
5. Torsioned anteriorly (left on left or right on right)
6. Torsioned posteriorly (left on right or right on left)

Iliosacral
1. Rotated anteriorly
2. Rotated posteriorly
3. Superior (cephalic) shear
4. Inferior (caudad) shear
5. Rotated medially (in-flare)
6. Rotated laterally (out-flare)

Right Inferior Pubic Symphysis

- Positive right standing flexion test
- Right pubis inferior
- Tension and tenderness of right inguinal ligament

Left Superior Pubic Symphysis

- Positive left standing flexion test
- Left pubis superior
- Tension and tenderness of the left inguinal ligament

The less common right superior and left inferior dysfunctions differ only on the level of the pubis against the horizontal plane. If these less common dysfunctions are present, suspect a more complex musculoskeletal problem.

Sacroiliac Dysfunctions

The sacrum becomes dysfunctional between the two iliac bones either unilaterally or bilaterally (Table 17.2). The bilaterally anteriorly and bilaterally posteriorly nutated dysfunctions are rare, probably because symmetry of both sides of a sacrum is so rare. They are frequently missed because of the findings of the bilateral positive standing flexion test initially appearing negative. The one-legged stork test then becomes most valuable, as it will be bilaterally positive indicating bilateral restriction. Another reason they are missed is that the sacral base and ILAs are level against the coronal plane. They also are frequently related to bilateral dysfunction of L5 with a bilaterally extended L5 associated with a bilaterally anteriorly nutated sacrum and a bilaterally flexed L5 with the bilaterally posteriorly nutated sacrum. The rocking, springing, and gapping sacroiliac motion tests are valuable in diagnosing the bilateral sacral dysfunctions.

A difficult concept to grasp is the unilateral anteriorly or posteriorly nutated sacrum. One wonders how rigid bones can anteriorly nutate (flex) or posteriorly nutate (extend) on one side. In fact, the bone does not twist or change its shape; the findings are the result of the unilateral restriction of both the overturning and translatory movement on one side relative to its ilia. One-sided dysfunction is easily explained by the common asymmetry of the two sacroiliac joints. One appears to continue to function normally and the other becomes restricted, either anteriorly or posteriorly nutated. The unilaterally nutated dysfunctions have also been described as "sacral shear," either superior or inferior. The "shear" term comes from the observation of the ILA being more inferior than posterior in its asymmetry. It is as though the sacrum "sheared" either down or up. "Shear" is a misnomer because the joint surfaces do not actually shear against each other; rather the translatory component of the nutational motion causes the inferiority or superiority of the ILA. The incidence of the anteriorly nutated (flexed) sacrum is high and it is usually found on the left, although it does occur on the right. The incidence of posteriorly nutated sacrum is rare, but when it does occur it is usually found on the right side. Since the asymmetry of the sacral base and the ILA is the same in both dysfunctions, the differences in the motion tests and the spring test are needed for an accurate diagnosis.

TABLE 17.2	*Sacroiliac Dysfunctions*							
Diagnosis	Seated Flexion Test Positive	Base of Sacrum	ILA Position	ILA Motion	Lumbar Scoliosis	Lumbar Lordosis[a]	Medial Malleolus Prone
Unilateral nutated anteriorly (flexed)	Right	Anterior right	Inferior right	—	Convex right	Normal to increased	Long right
	Left	Anterior left	Inferior left	—	Convex left	Normal to increased	Long left
Unilateral nutated posteriorly (extended)	Right	Posterior right	Superior right	—	Convex left	Reduced	Short right
	Left	Posterior left	Superior left	—	Convex right	Reduced	Short left
Anterior torsion	Left on left	Right	Anterior right	Posterior left	Left, increased on forward bending	Convex right	Increased	Short left
	Right on right	Left	Anterior left	Posterior right	Right, increased on forwardbending	Convex left	Increased	Short right
Backward torsion	Right on left	Right	Posterior right	Posterior right	Right, increased on forward bending	Convex left	Reduced	Short right
	Left on right	Left	Posterior left	Posterior left	Left, increased on backward bending	Convex right	Reduced	Short left
Bilateral nutated anteriorly (flexed)	—	Bilateral	Anterior	Posterior	—	—	Increased	Even
Bilateral nutated posteriorly (extended)	—	Bilateral	Posterior	Anterior	—	—	Reduced	Even

[a]Reduced is also a positive spring test.

The bilateral anterior and posterior nutated dysfunctions and the unilateral anteriorly and posteriorly nutated dysfunctions are all related to the transverse axis. The bilateral dysfunctions involve both joints, whereas the unilateral dysfunctions only involve restriction on one side. The torsional restrictions include both joints and involve the oblique axes. Remember, the oblique axis is a descriptive one and the coupled side bending and rotation to the opposite side result from a complex polyaxial system.

The diagnostic finding that identifies the torsional dysfunctions is the sacral base and ILA being posterior on the same side. *A posterior base and an ILA on the same side is always a torsion.* The differentiation between an anterior and posterior torsional dysfunction is primarily made by the behavior of the sacral base and ILA in the forward bending and backward bending of the trunk. *Forward torsions become asymmetric in forward bending and become symmetric in backward bending. The posterior torsions are the reverse. They get more asymmetric in backward bending and symmetric in forward bending.* With the torsional dysfunctions the ILA become symmetric in one position, trunk either forward or backward bent. This is not true of the unilaterally nutated sacrum, either anterior or posterior, as the ILA in these dysfunctions is never symmetric,

either forward bent or backward bent. The unilaterally anteriorly nutated sacrum may seem to get a little more asymmetric in forward bending, and the unilaterally posteriorly nutated sacrum a little more asymmetric in backward bending, but they never become symmetric.

The behavior of the ILA in the forward-bent position then becomes a very valuable clue to sacroiliac dysfunction. If the ILA is symmetric in the forward-bent position while doing the seated flexion test, the examiner has ruled out four of the possible sacroiliac dysfunctions, the two unilaterally nutated restrictions and the forward torsions. If the seated flexion test is positive on one side, the examiner has ruled out the bilaterally anteriorly or posteriorly nutated sacral dysfunctions as well. The only possibility left is one of the posterior torsion dysfunctions.

Iliosacral Dysfunctions

The diagnosis of iliosacral dysfunction follows the diagnosis and treatment of the pubic and sacroiliac dysfunctions (Table 17.3). The iliosacral dysfunctions are unilateral dysfunctions, although there may be one on each side of the pelvis. Remember that there are two different axes for motion of the ilium: the symphysis pubis is in front, with the sacrum posteriorly. The examiner primarily

TABLE 17.3		*Iliosacral Dysfunctions*						
Diagnosis		**Standing Flexion Test Positive**	**ASIS Supine**	**Medical Malleolus Supine**	**Posterior Superior Iliac Spine Prone**	**Sacral Sulcus Prone**	**Ischial Tuberosity Prone**	**Sacrotuberous Ligament Prone**
Anterior rotated	Right	Right	Inferior right	Long right	Superior right	Shallow right	—	—
	Left	Left	Inferior left	Long left	Superior left	Shallow left	—	—
Posterior rotated	Right	Right	Superior right	Short right	Inferior right	Deep right	—	—
	Left	Left	Superior left	Short left	Inferior left	Deep left	—	—
Rotated lateral (out-flare)	Right	Right	Lateral right	—	Medial right	Narrow right	—	—
	Left	Left	Medial left	—	Lateral left	Narrow left	—	—
Rotated medial (in-flare)	Right	Right	Medial right	—	Lateral right	Wide right	—	—
	Left	Left	Medial left	—	Lateral left	Wide left	—	—
Superior shear (upslip)	Right	Right	Superior right	Short right	Superior right	—	Superior right	Lax right
	Left	Left	Superior left	Short left	Superior left	—	Superior left	Lax left
Inferior shear (downslip)	Right	Right	Inferior right	Long right	Inferior right	—	Inferior right	Tight right
	Left	Left	Inferior left	Long left	Inferior left	—	Inferior left	Tight left

assesses the hip bones with the patient in the supine position. Therefore, the pelvis must be balanced and symmetrically placed on the sacrum if possible. The bony asymmetries most important for the iliosacral dysfunctions are the level of the ischial tuberosities; the anterior or posterior, inferior or superior, medial or lateral placement of the anterior iliac spines; and the level of the medial malleolus in the supine position.

The superior and inferior hip bone shear dysfunctions are true "shears" as the joint apposition is altered. They can also be classified as true subluxations. They occur in those patients who do not have good form closure of the sacroiliac joint. They are the result of a shearing force, either superior or inferior, on one sacroiliac joint. The inferior shears will frequently self-correct on loading of the involved leg, whereas the superior shears persist unless appropriately treated. The superior shear results from some trauma such as a slip and fall of the buttocks or during a motor vehicle collision when the patient has one foot firmly placed on the brake pedal when the impact occurs. Another characteristic of the shear dysfunctions is symptom severity that appears to be greater than expected from the injury described. They are common in the patient with chronic lower back pain syndrome and, when present, interfere with all other motions within the pelvis. The hip bone shears also have a characteristic tissue texture finding in the sacrotuberous ligament. The ligament is lax in the superior shear and under great tension

in the inferior shear. It is usually tender on the side of dysfunction.

The more common iliosacral dysfunctions are the anterior- and posterior-rotated hip bones. They both have asymmetries of the ASIS and the medial malleolus. The assessment of the ASIS is made to see if one is more anterior or posterior, more superior or inferior, and more medial or lateral than its fellow on the other side. An assessment is made of the length of the medial malleolus in the supine position. The findings are correlated with the positive motion tests of the standing flexion test and the one-legged stork test. The most common are a right anterior hip bone dysfunction and a left posterior hip bone dysfunction. The asymmetry findings are the same and the differentiating finding is the positive motion test, right or left.

The medially or laterally rotated hip bone dysfunctions (in-flare and out-flare) are quite rare and are only found in those sacroiliac joints that have altered convex-to-concave relationships at S2 with convexity on the sacral side and concavity on the ilial side. They can only be diagnosed after the correction of any hip bone rotational dysfunction that is present. There is a little lateral component to the anterior hip bone and a little medial component to the posterior hip bone dysfunction. If one only looks at the medial and lateral aspects of the ASISs and overlooks the superior-to-inferior and anterior-to-posterior aspects, one can erroneously make a diagnosis of a medial or lateral rotated hip bone.

Symmetry of hip bone rotation, alternately anterior and posterior on each side, is an essential component of the gait cycle. Altered hip bone rotation is frequently associated with altered muscle balance in the trunk and lower extremity. For example, a short, tight quadratus femoris muscle is frequently associated with an anterior hip bone on that side, and a short, tight hamstring muscle is frequently associated with a posterior hip bone on that side. Treating the joint restriction without also dealing with the muscle imbalance is one reason for chronicity.

MANAGEMENT OF PELVIC GIRDLE DYSFUNCTION

The goal of manual medicine treatment to pelvic girdle dysfunction is to restore the mechanics of the normal walking cycle. In the overall treatment of the patient, one should treat the lumbar spine prior to the treatment of the pelvis because many sacroiliac techniques require the use of the lumbar spine as a lever arm. The pelvis is the bony attachment of many muscles of the trunk above and of the extremities below. Treatment of the pelvic girdle should always be accompanied by the diagnosis and treatment of muscle imbalance both above and below the pelvis to prevent recurrence of dysfunction and to enhance the therapeutic outcome.

Treatment Sequence

The recommended treatment sequence is symphysis pubis, hip bone shear dysfunction, sacroiliac dysfunction, and iliosacral dysfunction. In the diagnostic sequence, one assesses for pubic dysfunctions early. If dysfunction is found, it should be treated before proceeding with the diagnostic sequence. Recall that the major criterion for sacroiliac dysfunction is identified with the patient in the prone position. If there is residual dysfunction of the symphysis pubis in front, the patient is not symmetric in the prone position on the tripod of the two ASISs and the symphysis pubis.

Following the diagnosis and treatment of the pubic dysfunction, the next major assessment is for the presence of hip bone shear dysfunction. The major index of suspicion occurs with unleveling of the iliac crests in the unloaded position. When a hip bone shear dysfunction is present, it appears to restrict all other motions within that sacroiliac joint. Therefore, it deserves attention early in the diagnostic and treatment process. A second reason for treating the hip bone shear early is the need to have two symmetric hip bones available to assess the sacrum's position in between the bones. Sacroiliac dysfunction is then addressed in order to restore its symmetry to the coronal plane when the patient is supine on the examining table to allow for assessment of each hip bone in relation to the fixed sacrum on the table.

PELVIC GIRDLE

Symphysis Pubis

Muscle Energy Technique

Supine

Position: Symphysis either superior or inferior ("shotgun" technique)

1. Patient is supine with the hips and knees flexed and the feet together.

2. Operator stands at the side of the table, holding the patient's knees together.

3. Operator resists two to three patient efforts of knee abduction for 3 to 5 seconds (Fig. 17.57).

4. Operator places the forearm between the patient's knees (Fig. 17.58).

5. A series of adduction efforts of both knees attempts to distract the symphysis pubis.

6. Retest.

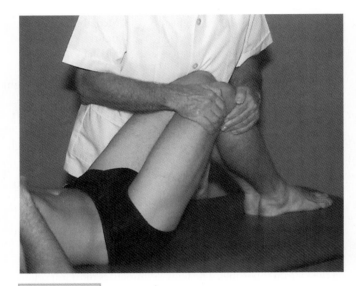

FIGURE 17.57

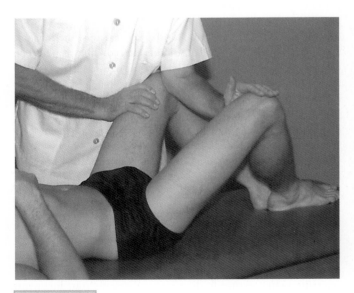

FIGURE 17.58

PELVIC GIRDLE

Symphysis Pubis

Muscle Energy Technique

Supine

Position: Left superior symphysis

1. Patient is supine on the table with the operator standing on the left side (Fig. 17.59).

2. Operator slides patient's pelvis to the left side of the table, maintaining the left hip bone on the edge. Patient's left arm holds the right shoulder for trunk stability (Fig. 17.60).

3. Operator's legs support the patient's freely hanging left leg.

4. Operator's left hand stabilizes the right side of the patient's pelvis and right hand is placed above the patella over the patient's distal left femur.

5. Patient performs a series of three to five repetitions of 3- to 5-second muscle contractions of hip flexion against the operator's right hand (Fig. 17.61).

6. After each patient effort, the operator engages a new barrier by additional left leg extension.

7. Retest.

Note: With the patient's leg in an abducted and extended position, hip flexion activates left adductor muscle group, pulling left symphysis inferiorly by concentric isotonic muscle contraction.

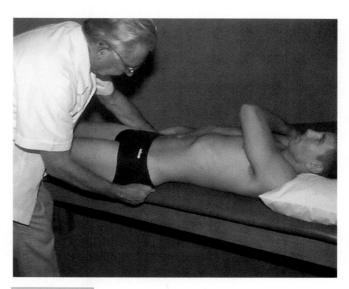

FIGURE 17.60

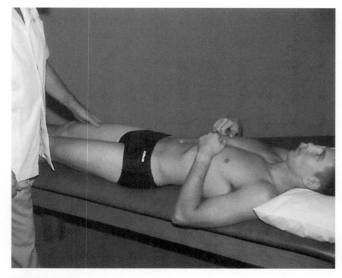

FIGURE 17.59

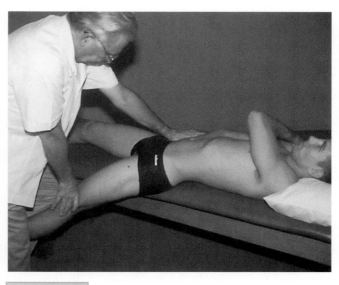

FIGURE 17.61

PELVIC GIRDLE

Symphysis Pubis

Muscle Energy Technique

Supine

Diagnosis

Position: Right symphysis inferior

1. Patient is supine on the table with the right knee and hip flexed, adducted, and slightly internally rotated to close pack the ipsilateral sacroiliac joint.

2. Operator stands on the left side and rolls the patient's pelvis to the left to place operator's left hand to control the patient's right hip bone (Fig. 17.62).

3. Operator places patient's right PSIS between the operator's left middle and ring fingers with heel of hand in contact with the ischial tuberosity (Fig. 17.63).

4. Operator returns the patient's pelvis to the table with the right hip bone in contact with the left hand and a superior and medial compressive force of the heel of the left hand applied against the ischial tuberosity (Fig. 17.64).

5. Operator resists three to five efforts of a 3- to 5-second muscle contraction by the patient to straighten the right leg in the caudad direction.

6. After each effort, the operator engages new barriers by more hip flexion and compression against the right ischial tuberosity.

7. Alternative operator position is with the patient's right knee in the operator's right axilla with right hand holding the edge of the table (Fig. 17.65).

8. Retest.

Note: Flexion, internal rotation, and adduction of the right hip close pack the right sacroiliac joint so that the hip extension effort transmits operator force against the ischial tuberosity in a cephalad and medial direction toward the symphysis pubis.

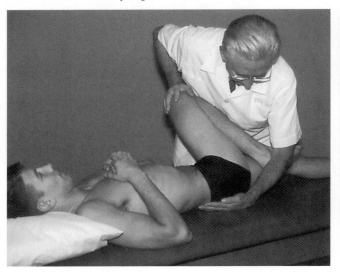

FIGURE 17.62

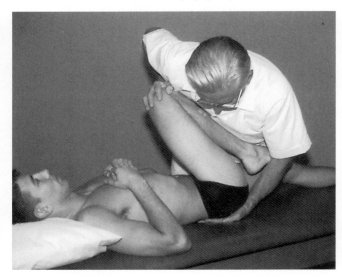

FIGURE 17.64

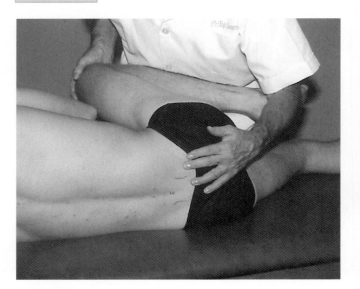

FIGURE 17.63

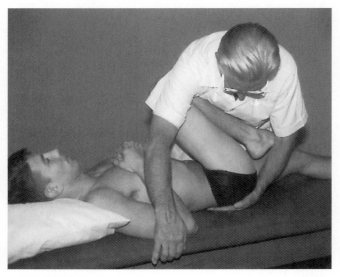

FIGURE 17.65

PELVIC GIRDLE

Iliosacral

Muscle Energy Technique

Supine

Diagnosis

Position: Left superior hip bone shear dysfunction

1. Patient is supine with the feet off end of table.

2. Operator stands at the end of the table with the left thigh against the patient's right foot and both hands grasping the patient's left leg just proximal to the ankle (Fig. 17.66). An assistant may be used to stabilize the patient's right leg.

3. Operator abducts the extended left leg 10 to 15 degrees to loose pack the left sacroiliac joint (Fig. 17.67).

4. Operator internally rotates the extended, abducted left leg to close pack the left hip joint (Fig. 17.68).

5. Operator puts long-axis extension on the left leg while the patient performs a series of inhalation and exhalation efforts (Fig. 17.69).

6. Three to four respiratory cycles are performed and during the last exhalation effort the patient is instructed to cough while, simultaneously, the operator tugs the left leg in a caudad direction.

7. Retest.

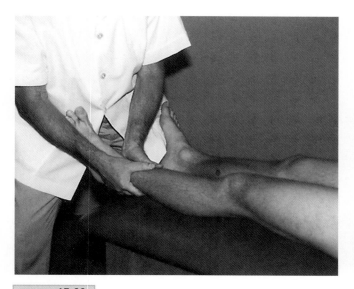

FIGURE 17.66

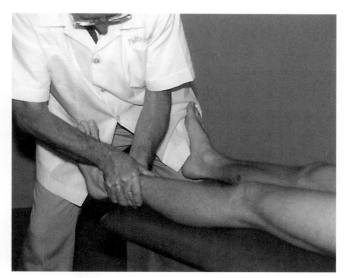

FIGURE 17.68

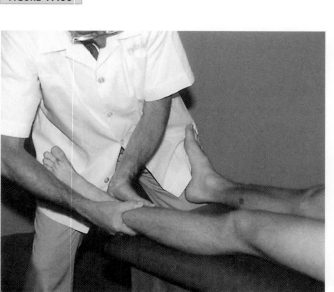

FIGURE 17.67

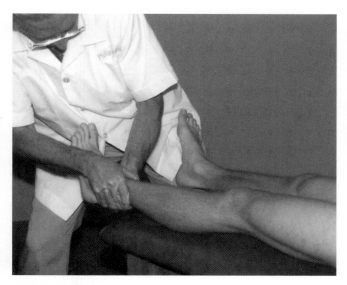

FIGURE 17.69

PELVIC GIRDLE

Iliosacral

Muscle Energy Technique

Lateral Recumbent

Diagnosis

Position: Right inferior hip bone shear

1. Patient lies in the left lateral recumbent position.

2. Operator stands in front (or back) of the patient with the right arm and shoulder supporting the weight of the right lower extremity. An assistant may help by holding the weight of the right leg.

3. Operator's left hand grasps the posterior aspect of the right hip bone from the ischial tuberosity to the PSIS (Fig. 17.70).

4. Operator's right hand grasps the right hip bone from the ischial tuberosity to the inferior pubic ramus (Fig. 17.71).

5. Operator's two hands distract the right hip bone laterally (toward the ceiling) and exert a cephalic directional force on the right hip bone.

6. Patient performs a series of deep inhalation and exhalation efforts while operator maintains distraction of the right hip bone in a cephalic direction.

7. Retest.

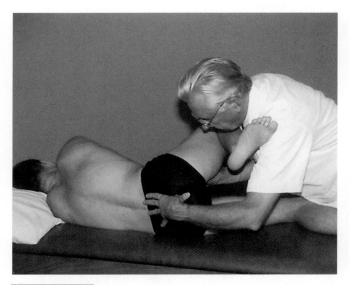

FIGURE 17.70

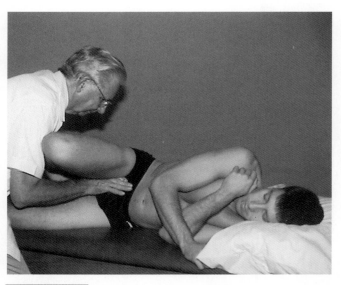

FIGURE 17.71

PELVIC GIRDLE

Iliosacral

Muscle Energy Technique

Prone

Diagnosis

Position: Right inferior hip bone shear

1. Patient is prone on the table with the operator standing on the right side.

2. Operator places the patient's right foot between the knees and the extended right arm and hand control the right knee to loose pack the right sacroiliac joint (Fig. 17.72).

3. Operator's left hand contacts the right ischial tuberosity and maintains a force in the cephalic direction.

4. Patient performs a series of deep inhalation and exhalation efforts.

5. Patient attempts to straighten the right arm against a hand contact on the table leg resulting in a caudad force through the trunk.

6. A combination of the operator's force on ischial tuberosity, patient's right arm muscle effort against trunk, and respiratory effort provides superior shearing movement of the right hip bone against the sacrum.

7. Retest.

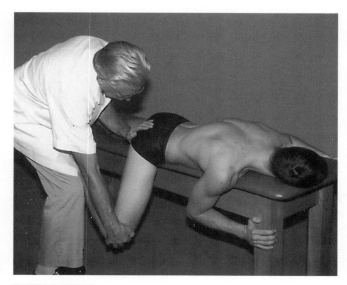

FIGURE 17.72

PELVIC GIRDLE

Sacroiliac

Muscle Energy Technique

Prone

Diagnosis

Position: Left unilateral anterior nutated sacrum (left sacrum flexed)

Motion Restriction: Left unilateral posterior nutation

1. Patient is prone with the operator standing on the left side.

2. Operator's fingers of the left hand monitor the left sacral base while operator's right arm introduces abduction of patient's left leg to approximately 15 degrees (Fig. 17.73).

3. Operator internally rotates left leg gapping the posterior aspect of the left sacroiliac joint. Patient holds the leg in that position (Fig. 17.74).

4. With right arm straight, operator places the heel of the hand on the left ILA and springs sacrum from above and below and from side to side until a point of maximum motion is identified at the left sacral base (Fig. 17.75).

5. Patient takes a maximum inhalation and holds breath as operator maintains a ventral and cephalic compressive force on the left ILA.

6. As patient exhales, operator maintains pressure.

7. Patient performs a series of forced inhalation efforts while the operator maintains force on ILA.

8. Retest.

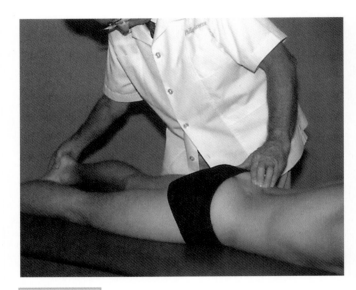

FIGURE 17.74

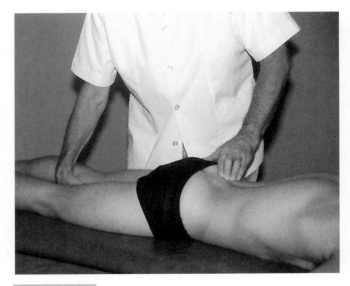

FIGURE 17.73

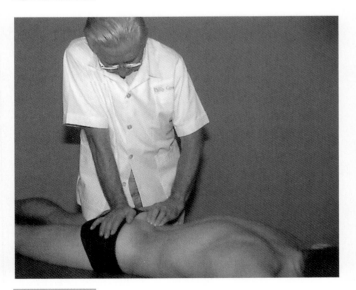

FIGURE 17.75

PELVIC GIRDLE

Sacroiliac

Muscle Energy Technique

Prone

Diagnosis

Position: Right posterior nutated sacrum (right extended sacrum)

Motion Restriction: Anterior nutation of right sacrum

1. Patient is prone on the table with the operator standing on the right side.

2. Operator's right hand monitors the right sacroiliac joint as the left hand abducts right leg to approximately 15 degrees, loose packing the right sacroiliac joint (Fig. 17.76).

3. Operator externally rotates the right abducted leg gapping the anterior aspect of the right sacroiliac joint. Patient is instructed to hold right leg in that position (Fig. 17.77).

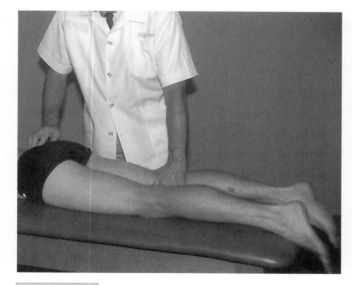

FIGURE 17.76

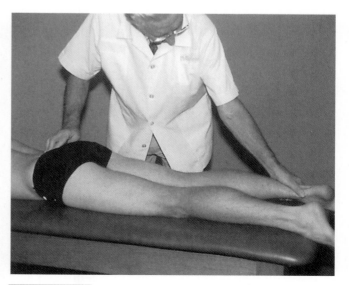

FIGURE 17.77

4. Patient's trunk is extended by prone prop position while operator's right pisiform is in contact with the right sacral base, maintaining a ventral and caudad directional force (Fig. 17.78).

5. Operator's left hand on the right ASIS provides a counterforce against the compression through the right hand (Fig. 17.79).

6. Patient performs a series of forced exhalation efforts while the operator maintains ventral and caudad compressive forces against the right sacral base.

7. At the end of each exhalation effort, the patient is instructed to pull the right ASIS toward the table as a muscle activating force.

8. After three to five repetitions, the operator maintains the sacral compression against the counterforce on the ASIS and the patient is instructed to return to the neutral position (Fig. 17.80).

9. Retest.

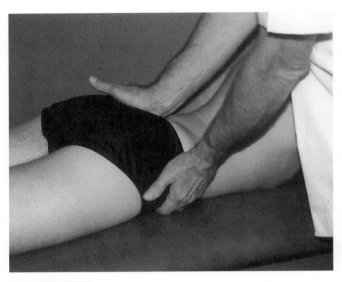

FIGURE 17.79

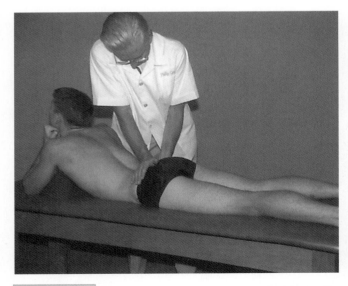

FIGURE 17.78

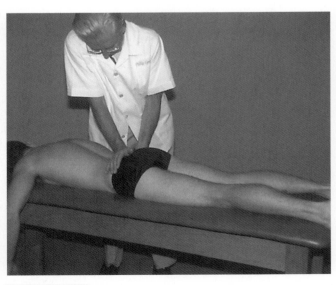

FIGURE 17.80

PELVIC GIRDLE

Sacroiliac

Muscle Energy Technique

Sims position

Diagnosis: Left-on-left forward (anterior) sacral torsion

Position: Sacrum left rotated, right-side bent, and anteriorly nutated at right base

Motion Restriction: Right rotation, left-side bending, and posterior nutation of right base

1. Patient is prone on the table.

2. Operator stands on the right side and flexes patient's knees to 90 degrees (Fig. 17.81).

3. Operator rolls the patient onto the left hip introducing the Sims position (Fig. 17.82).

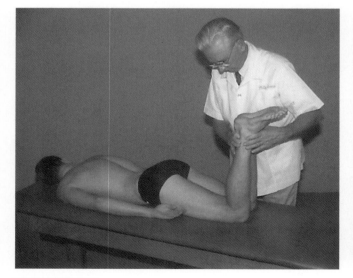

FIGURE 17.81

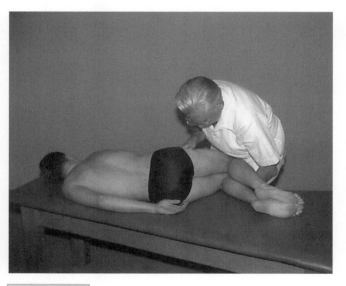

FIGURE 17.82

4. Operator controls patient's knees on operator's left thigh, monitors lumbosacral junction with left hand, and introduces trunk rotation to the left through the right hand until L5 begins to rotate left (Fig. 17.83).

5. Operator's right hand now monitors the lumbosacral junction and right sacral base while left hand introduces left-side bending (Fig. 17.84).

6. Operator flexes the lower extremities until right sacral base begins to move posteriorly, then resists an effort by the patient of lifting both feet toward the ceiling against resistance offered by the left hand (Fig. 17.85).

7. Patient performs three to five muscle contractions of lifting the feet to the ceiling for 3 to 5 seconds against resistance offered by the operator with an engagement of the flexion and side-bending barrier between each effort.

8. Retest.

Note: Lumbar rotation to the left from the top down and stopping at L5 carries the sacrum into relative right rotation against its initial barrier. This critical step requires that lumbar treatment precedes sacral treatment.

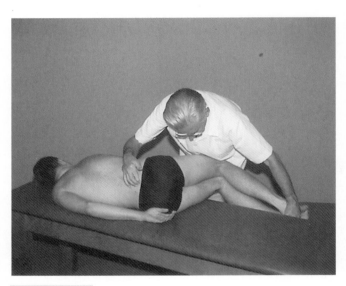

FIGURE 17.84

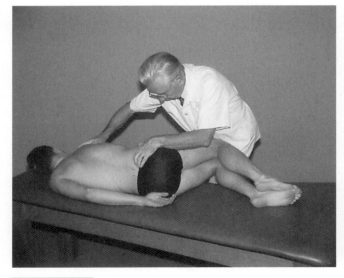

FIGURE 17.83

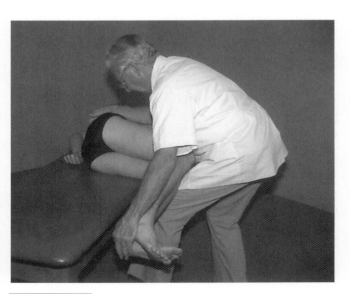

FIGURE 17.85

PELVIC GIRDLE

Sacroiliac

Muscle Energy Technique

Lateral Recumbent

Diagnosis: Left-on-left forward (anterior) sacral torsion

Position: Left rotated, right-side bent, and anteriorly nutated right sacral base

Motion Restriction: Right rotation, left-side bending, and posterior nutation of right sacral base

1. Patient lies in the right lateral recumbent position with the operator standing in front, monitoring the lumbosacral junction (Fig. 17.86).
2. Operator introduces neutral side bending right, rotation left, through the lumbar spine until L5 first begins to rotate left (Fig. 17.87).

Note: Lumbar rotation to the left from the top down, stopping at L5 carries the sacrum into relative right rotation against its initial barrier.

3. Operator flexes the thighs and pelvis until first posterior movement of the right sacral base.
4. Operator introduces left-side bending by lifting the feet toward the ceiling (Fig. 17.88).
5. Patient performs three to five muscle contractions for 3 to 5 seconds by pulling the feet down toward the table.
6. Operator engages new barriers by increasing hip flexion and side bending by lifting knees to the ceiling between each muscle effort.
7. Retest.

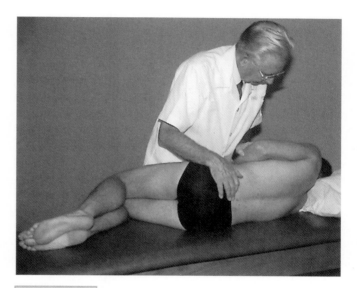

FIGURE 17.87

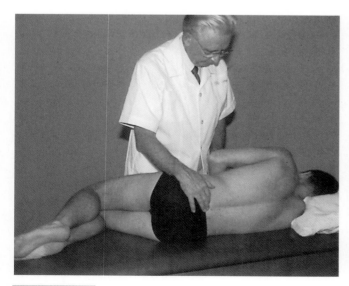

FIGURE 17.86

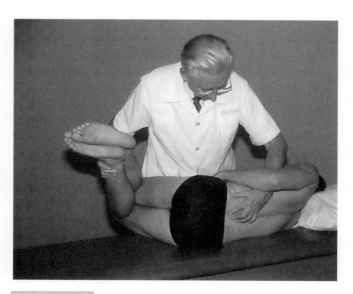

FIGURE 17.88

PELVIC GIRDLE

Sacroiliac

Muscle Energy Technique

Lateral Recumbent

Diagnosis: Right-on-left backward (posterior) sacral torsion

Position: Right rotated, left-side bent, posteriorly nutated right sacral base

Motion Restriction: Left rotation, right-side bending, and anterior nutation of right sacral base

1. Patient lies in the left lateral recumbent position with the operator standing in front, monitoring the lumbosacral junction with the left hand (Fig. 17.89).

2. Operator pulls the patient's left arm anterior and caudad introducing neutral left-side bending and right rotation of the lumbar spine until L5 first rotates to the right (Fig. 17.90).

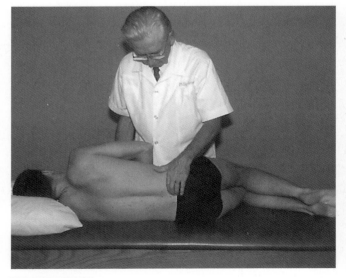

FIGURE 17.89

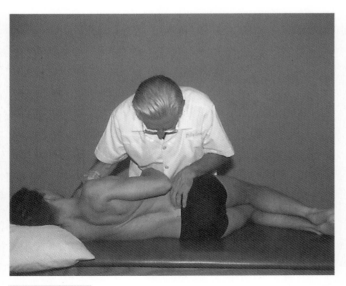

FIGURE 17.90

Note: Lumbar rotation to the right from the top down, stopping at L5 carries the sacrum into relative left rotation against its initial barrier.

3. Operator introduces extension of both legs through the left hand while the right hand monitors the right sacral base until the base first moves anteriorly (Fig. 17.91).

4. Operator drops the right leg in front of the left knee and places the left hand against the patient's distal right femur (Fig. 17.92).

5. Operator's right forearm maintains L5 rotation to the right while the left hand resists the patient's effort of lifting the right knee toward the ceiling (Fig. 17.93).

6. Patient performs three to five muscle contractions for 3 to 5 seconds with the operator engaging the new barriers between each effort by further extending the bottom leg and dropping the right leg more toward the floor.

7. Retest.

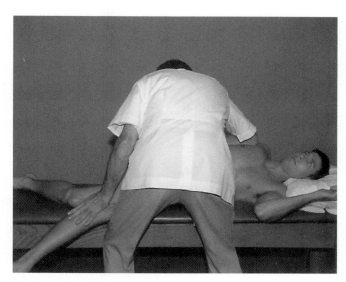

FIGURE 17.92

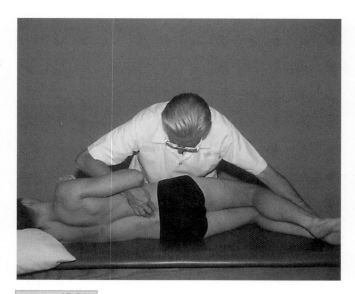

FIGURE 17.91

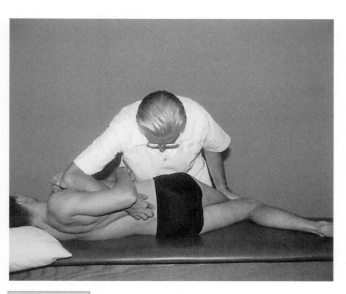

FIGURE 17.93

PELVIC GIRDLE

Sacroiliac

Muscle Energy Technique

Sitting

Diagnosis: Bilateral anterior nutated (flexed) sacrum

   Position: Bilateral anterior nutated

   Motion Restriction: Bilateral posterior nutation

1. Patient sits on a stool with the feet apart and the legs internally rotated (Fig. 17.94).

2. Patient flexes the trunk forward.

3. Operator places the heel of the right hand over the apex of the sacrum and the left hand over the patient's thoracic spine (Fig. 17.95).

4. Operator maintains the ventral pressure on the sacral apex and resists the patient's instruction to lift shoulders toward the ceiling with the patient's breath at full inhalation.

5. Patient performs three to five efforts of 3 to 5 seconds of muscle contraction to restore posterior nutational movement of the sacral base.

6. The full inhalation helps move the sacral base posteriorly.

7. Retest.

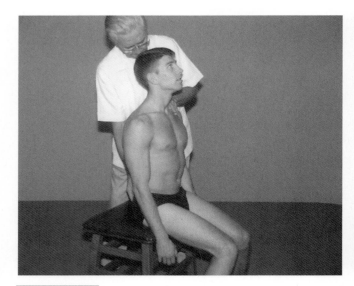

FIGURE 17.94

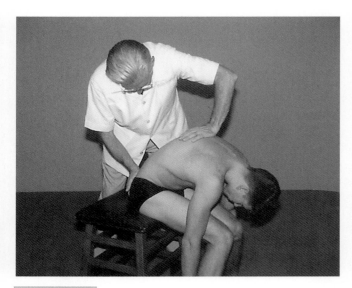

FIGURE 17.95

PELVIC GIRDLE

Sacroiliac

Muscle Energy Technique

Sitting

Diagnosis: Bilateral posterior nutated (extended) sacrum

    Position: Bilaterally posterior nutated

    Motion Restriction: Bilateral anterior nutation

1. Patient sits on a stool with the feet together and the knees apart, externally rotating the legs; arms crossed.

2. Operator stands at the side with the right hand on the sacral base and the left hand controlling the patient's trunk (Fig. 17.96).

3. Patient is instructed to arch the back by pushing the abdomen toward the knees with full exhalation while the operator maintains a ventral compressive force with the right hand on the sacral base (Fig. 17.97).

4. Operator's left hand resists three to five repetitions of 3- to 5-second muscle contraction of trunk flexion.

5. The exhalation effort assists in moving the sacral base anteriorly.

6. Retest.

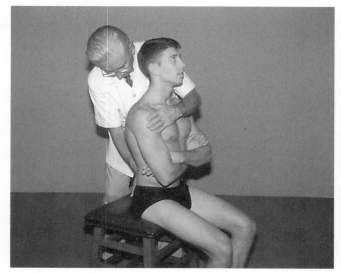

FIGURE 17.96

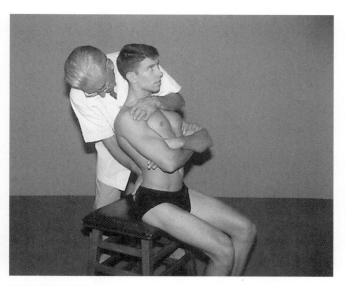

FIGURE 17.97

PELVIC GIRDLE

Iliosacral

Muscle Energy Technique

Supine

Diagnosis: Left posterior hip bone

Position: Hip bone rotated posteriorly

Motion Restriction: Anterior rotation of hip bone

1. Patient is supine on the table with the operator standing on the left side.

2. Operator slides the patient's pelvis until the sacrum is at the edge of the table (Fig. 17.98).

3. Operator controls the left lower extremity between the knees.

4. Operator stabilizes the right side of pelvis at the right ASIS (Fig. 17.99).

5. Operator's right hand contacts distal femur above the patella.

6. Operator resists the patient's hip flexion effort for 3 to 5 seconds.

7. Operator engages a new barrier by dropping the patient's left leg toward the floor and repeats the resistance to hip flexion effort three to five times.

8. Retest.

Note: This procedure is similar to that for a superior pubic symphysis dysfunction; the difference is that the sacrum and the posterior aspect of the hip bone are the fixed point on the edge of the table.

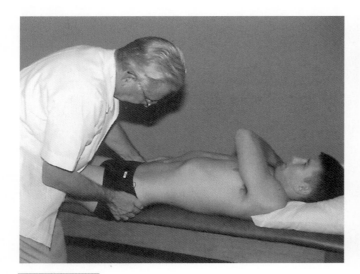

FIGURE 17.98

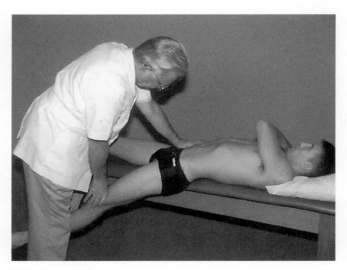

FIGURE 17.99

PELVIC GIRDLE

Iliosacral

Muscle Energy Technique

Prone

Diagnosis: Left posterior hip bone

    Position: Left hip bone rotated posteriorly

    Motion Restriction: Anterior rotation of left hip bone

1. Patient is prone on the table with the operator standing on the right side.

2. Operator controls the patient's left leg by grasping the flexed knee in the left hand. Left leg is abducted to loose pack the left sacroiliac joint.

3. Operator's right hand is on the left iliac crest, 5 to 6 cm anterior to the PSIS (Fig. 17.100).

4. Operator extends the patient's leg to barrier while exerting pressure with the right hand in the direction of the iliac crest (Fig. 17.101).

5. Patient's muscle effort is a series of three to five contractions for 3 to 5 seconds of hip flexion (pull leg to table) against operator resistance.

6. After each muscle effort, the operator engages a new extension barrier.

7. Retest.

Note: This dysfunction frequently accompanies a left sacrum anteriorly nutated (flexed). A combination technique can be performed as the last step of the muscle energy procedure for the left sacrum flexed. While holding the sacrum in the posteriorly nutated position with the right hand, the operator's left hand extends the left hip, rotating the left hip bone anteriorly, and resists the muscle effort of pulling the knee to the table (Fig. 17.102).

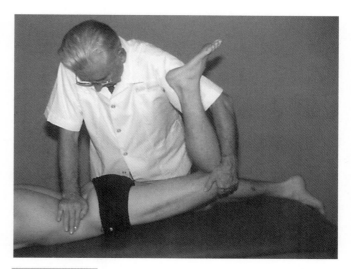

FIGURE 17.101

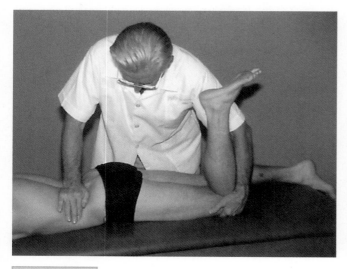

FIGURE 17.100

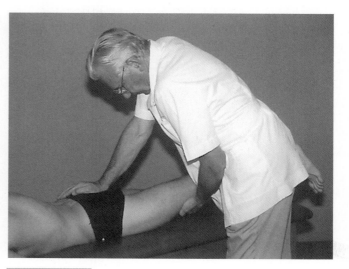

FIGURE 17.102

PELVIC GIRDLE

Iliosacral

Muscle Energy Technique

Lateral Recumbent

Diagnosis: Left posterior hip bone

    Position: Left hip bone rotated posteriorly

    Motion Restriction: Left hip bone anterior rotation

1. Patient lies in the right lateral recumbent position with the operator standing behind.

2. Operator's right hand is placed on the iliac crest 5 to 6 cm anterior to the PSIS (Fig. 17.103).

3. Operator grasps patient's flexed left knee in the left hand and, supporting the left lower extremity, loose packs the left sacroiliac joint (Fig. 17.104).

4. Operator extends the patient's leg to barrier while exerting anterior pressure along the iliac crest with the right hand (Fig. 17.105).

5. Patient provides muscle contraction to pull the leg anteriorly against the operator's resistance for three to five repetitions of 3 to 5 seconds.

6. Operator engages a new extension barrier after each muscle effort.

7. Retest.

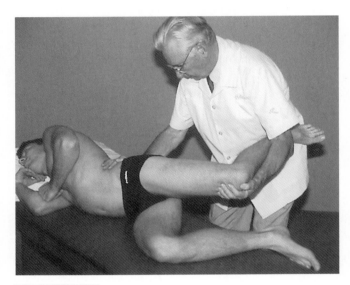

FIGURE 17.104

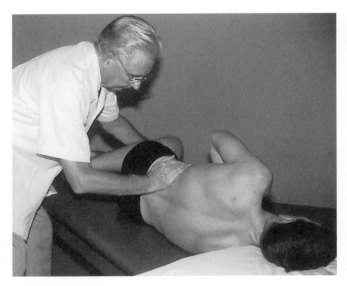

FIGURE 17.103

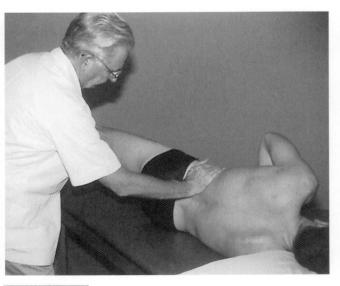

FIGURE 17.105

PELVIC GIRDLE

Iliosacral

Muscle Energy Technique

Prone

Diagnosis: Right anterior hip bone

    Position: Right hip bone anteriorly rotated

    Motion Restriction: Posterior rotation of right hip bone

1. Patient is in the prone position with the operator standing at the right side.

2. Operator grasps the pelvis and slides the patient's lower trunk to the right edge of the table (Fig. 17.106).

3. Operator controls the patient's right leg by placing the foot between the operator's knees and grasping the right knee with the right hand.

4. Operator's left hand stabilizes the sacrum in the midline with the left index finger monitoring the right sacroiliac joint (Fig. 17.107).

5. Operator controls patient's right leg with abduction, external rotation, and flexion to engage barrier to posterior rotational movement (Fig. 17.108).

6. Patient performs muscle effort for 3 to 5 seconds with three to five repetitions of extending the right leg by pushing the right foot against the operator's thigh.

7. Operator engages a new barrier of posterior rotation between each patient contraction.

8. Retest.

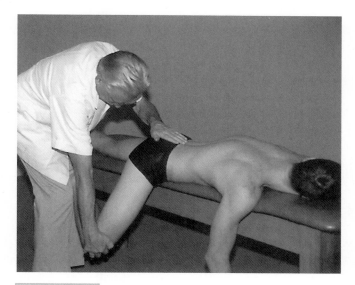

FIGURE 17.107

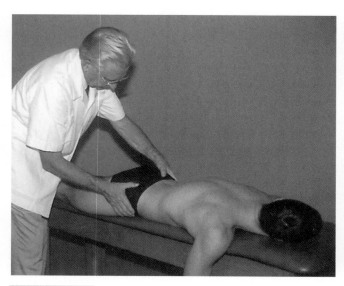

FIGURE 17.106

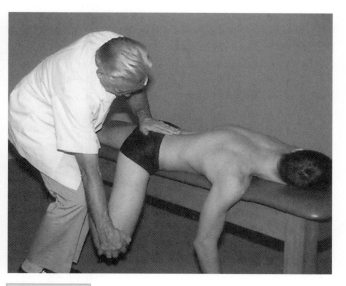

FIGURE 17.108

PELVIC GIRDLE

Iliosacral

Muscle Energy Technique

Supine

Diagnosis: Right anterior hip bone

   Position: Right hip bone anteriorly rotated

   Motion Restriction: Posterior rotation of right hip bone

1. Patient is in the supine position with the right hip and knee flexed.

2. Operator stands on the patient's left side with the heel of the left hand contacting the right ischial tuberosity and the fingers of the left hand monitoring motion of the sacroiliac joint (Fig. 17.109).

3. Operator flexes, externally rotates, and abducts patient's right leg, loose packing the right sacroiliac joint.

4. Operator exerts a cephalad and lateral force against the right ischial tuberosity.

5. Patient performs three to five muscle contractions for 3 to 5 seconds to extend the right leg against resistance offered by the operator's right hand and trunk (Fig. 17.110).

6. Between each patient effort, the operator increases posterior rotation of the right hip bone while monitoring loose-packed position of the right sacroiliac joint with the left hand.

7. Retest.

Note: This procedure is similar to that of an inferior symphysis pubis dysfunction. The differences are loose packing the right sacroiliac joint and the cephalad and lateral force of the left hand on the ischial tuberosity that directs hip bone rotation rather than force toward the symphysis pubis.

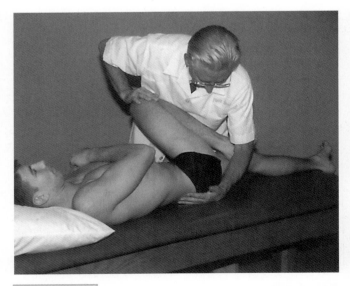

FIGURE 17.109

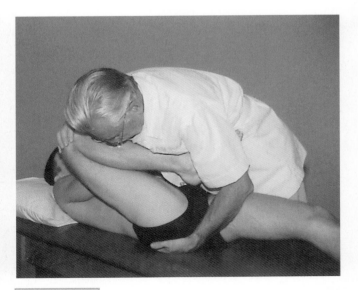

FIGURE 17.110

PELVIC GIRDLE

Iliosacral

Muscle Energy Technique

Lateral Recumbent

Diagnosis: Right anterior hip bone

    Position: Right hip bone anteriorly rotated

    Motion Restriction: Posterior rotation of right hip bone

1. Patient is in the left lateral recumbent position with the operator facing the patient.

2. Patient's right leg is flexed at the hip and the knee with the foot placed against the operator's hip.

3. Operator's left hand is placed on the right hip bone with the fingers monitoring motion at the right sacroiliac joint and the heel of the hand against the ischial tuberosity (Fig. 17.111).

4. Operator engages barrier by introducing abduction, external rotation, and flexion of the right leg (Fig. 17.112).

5. Patient performs three to five muscle contractions of 3 to 5 seconds attempting to straighten the right leg against operator resistance.

6. Operator engages a new barrier after each patient relaxation.

7. Retest.

Note: Muscle efforts other than hip extension can be adduction or abduction of the right knee against operator resistance.

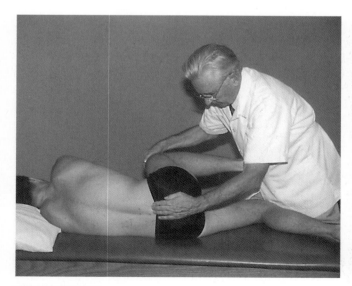

FIGURE 17.111

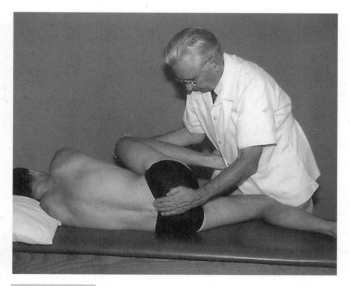

FIGURE 17.112

PELVIC GIRDLE

Iliosacral

Muscle Energy Technique

Supine

Diagnosis: Right hip bone internally rotated (in-flare)

   Position: Right hip bone internally rotated

     Motion Restriction: External rotation of right hip bone

1. Patient is supine on the table with the operator standing on the right side.

2. Operator flexes the patient's right hip and knee placing the right foot on the left knee (Fig. 17.113).

3. Operator's left hand stabilizes the left pelvis at the left ASIS.

4. Operator's right hand on the medial side of the patient's right knee externally rotates the hip until barrier is engaged (Fig. 17.114).

5. Patient performs three to five muscle contractions for 3 to 5 seconds attempting to internally rotate the right leg against resistance by operator.

6. Operator engages a new external rotation barrier after each patient contraction.

7. Retest.

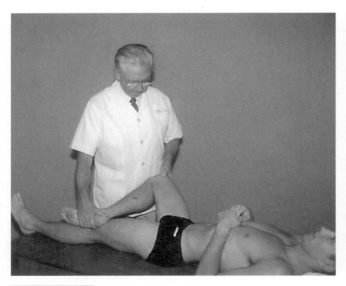

FIGURE 17.113

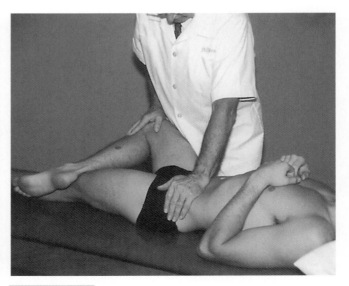

FIGURE 17.114

PELVIC GIRDLE

Iliosacral

Muscle Energy Technique

Supine

Diagnosis: Left hip bone externally rotated (out-flare)

>   Position: Left hip bone externally rotated

>   Motion Restriction: Internal rotation of left hip bone

1. Patient is supine on the table with the operator standing on the left side.

2. Operator flexes the patient's left hip and knee rolling the patient's pelvis to the right. Operator's fingers of the right hand grasp the medial side of the left PSIS (Fig. 17.115).

3. Patient's pelvis returned to neutral with the left hip bone resting on the operator's hand.

4. Operator's left hand adducts the left femur to the internal rotational barrier of the left hip bone while maintaining lateral traction on the left PSIS by the right hand.

5. Patient performs three to five muscle efforts for 3 to 5 seconds attempting to abduct and externally rotate the left leg against resistance of the operator's left hand (Fig. 17.116).

6. Operator engages new internal rotational barrier after each patient relaxation.

7. Retest.

Note: Operator's left hand also maintains pressure through the left thigh toward the table to prevent the pelvis from rotating to the right during muscle contraction.

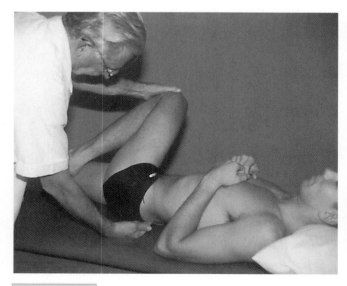

FIGURE 17.115

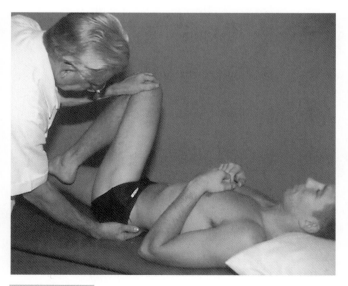

FIGURE 17.116

PELVIC GIRDLE

Symphysis Pubis

Mobilization With Impulse Technique

Supine

Diagnosis: Pubic dysfunction either superior or inferior ("shotgun" technique)

1. Patient is supine on the table with the operator standing at the side.

2. Operator's knees and hip are flexed with the feet on the table.

3. Operator's two hands are between the patient's knees (Fig. 17.117).

4. Patient is instructed to hold the knees together.

5. Operator provides mobilization with impulse thrust by separating both knees with both hands against patient resistance (Fig. 17.118).

6. Retest.

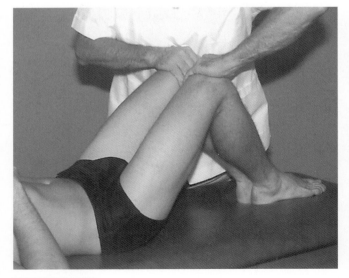

FIGURE 17.117

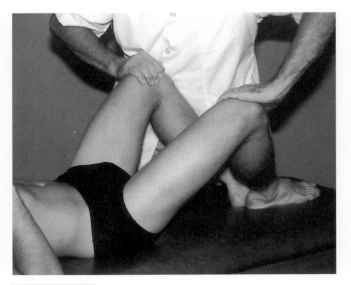

FIGURE 17.118

PELVIC GIRDLE

Sacroiliac

Mobilization With Impulse Technique

Lateral Recumbent

Diagnosis: Left unilateral anterior nutated sacrum (left sacrum flexed)

    Position: Left sacrum anteriorly nutated

    Motion Restriction: Posterior nutation of left sacral base

1. Patient is in the left lateral recumbent position with the knees and feet together.

2. Operator stands in front and monitors the lumbosacral junction with the left hand (Fig. 17.119).

3. Operator's right hand pulls the patient's left shoulder anterior and caudad, introducing neutral left-side bending right rotation of the lumbar spine until L5 begins to rotate to the right.

4. Operator's left hand contacts the sacrum with the pisiform on the left ILA and with left forearm parallel to the table.

5. Operator's right hand and forearm stabilize the trunk and monitor at the lumbosacral junction.

6. Operator performs mobilizing thrust through the left arm in a cephalic direction parallel to the table (Fig. 17.120).

7. An alternate right hand position stabilizes the right shoulder for the thrust through the left forearm (Fig. 17.121). This position may offer better leverage for the cephalic thrust through the left arm.

8. Retest.

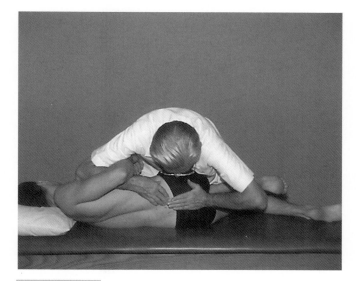

FIGURE 17.120

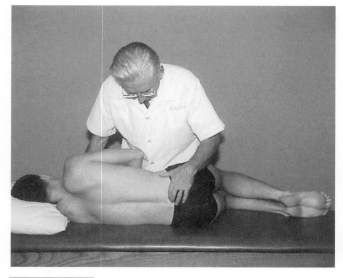

FIGURE 17.119

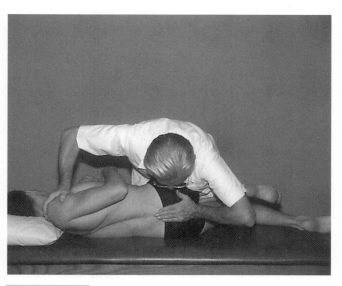

FIGURE 17.121

PELVIC GIRDLE

Sacroiliac

Mobilization With Impulse Technique

Prone

Diagnosis: Left unilateral anterior nutated sacrum (left sacrum flexed)

    Position: Left sacrum anteriorly nutated

    Motion Restriction: Posterior nutation of left sacral base

1. Patient is prone on the table with the operator standing on the left side.

2. Operator's left hand monitors the left sacroiliac joint while the right hand abducts the left leg to the loose-packed position (approximately 15 to 20 degrees). Left leg is internally rotated and held by the patient (Fig. 17.122).

3. Operator's right thenar eminence contacts the left ILA.

4. Operator engages posterior nutational barrier by springing the sacrum.

5. Patient deeply inhales and operator delivers a mobilization with impulse thrust in an anterior and superior direction through the right hand (Fig. 17.123).

6. Retest.

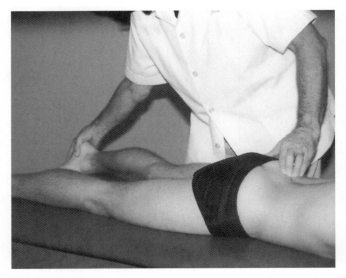

FIGURE 17.122

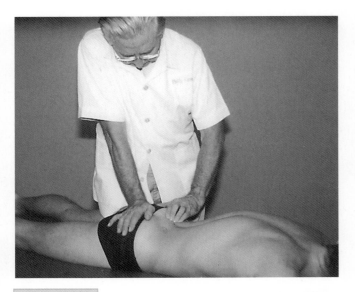

FIGURE 17.123

PELVIC GIRDLE

Sacroiliac

Mobilization With Impulse Technique

Left Lateral Recumbent

Diagnosis: Left-on-left anterior (forward) sacral torsion

> Position: Sacrum left rotated, right-side bent, and anteriorly nutated right base

> Motion Restriction: Sacral right rotation, left-side bending, and posterior nutation right base

1. Patient is in the left lateral recumbent position with the knees and feet together and shoulders perpendicular to the table.

2. Operator stands in front and flexes and extends the lower extremities, maintaining neutral mechanics in the lumbar spine and engaging the first posterior nutational barrier of the sacrum (Fig. 17.124).

3. Operator's right hand on the right shoulder introduces side bending right and rotation left of the lumbar spine by pushing the shoulder caudally until L5 rotates left.

4. Operator's left hand contacts the sacrum with the left pisiform against the left ILA (Fig. 17.125).

5. The barrier is engaged through the operator's right forearm and left hand contacting the sacrum with the left pisiform in the direction of the right shoulder.

6. A mobilization with impulse thrust is provided in a scooping fashion of the left hand on the left ILA in the direction of the resistant right hand on the right shoulder.

7. Retest.

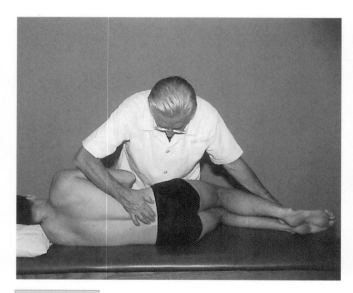

FIGURE 17.124

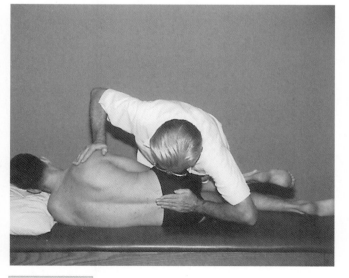

FIGURE 17.125

PELVIC GIRDLE

Sacroiliac

Mobilization With Impulse Technique

Supine

Diagnosis: Right-on-left backward (posterior) sacral torsion

Position: Sacrum right rotated, left-side bent, and posteriorly nutated right base

Motion Restriction: Left rotation, right-side bending, and anterior nutation of the right sacral base

1. Patient is supine with the operator standing on the left side of the table.

2. Operator translates the pelvis from right to left introducing right-side bending of the trunk (Fig. 17.126). Patient clasps the hands behind the neck.

3. Operator side bends the trunk to the right through the lumbar spine, including the sacrum (Fig. 17.127).

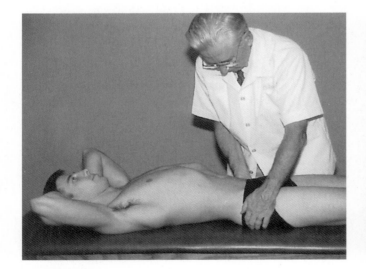

FIGURE 17.126

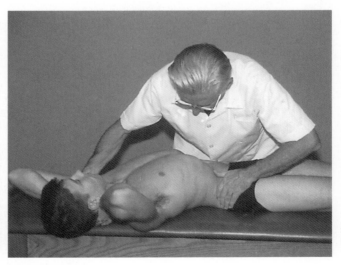

FIGURE 17.127

4. Operator threads the right forearm through the patient's right arm. The back of the operator's right hand is against the sternum (Fig. 17.128).

5. Operator stabilizes the right hip bone through the left-hand contact on the right ASIS.

6. Operator engages the barrier by left rotation of the trunk into and including the sacrum, being careful not to lose the right-side bending (Fig. 17.129).

7. Operator performs mobilization with impulse thrust by enhanced trunk rotation to the left against the stabilized right hip bone resulting in left rotation, right-side bending, and anterior nutation of the right sacral base.

8. Retest.

Note: This technique is also effective for a unilateral right posterior nutated sacrum (extended).

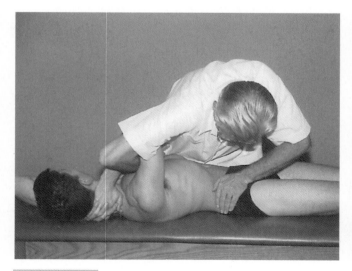

FIGURE 17.128

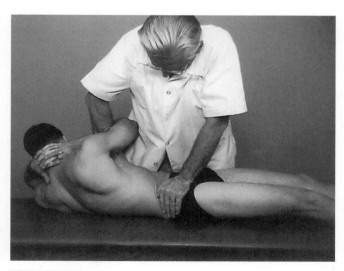

FIGURE 17.129

PELVIC GIRDLE

Sacroiliac

Mobilization With Impulse Technique

Sitting

Diagnosis: Left-on-left forward (anterior) sacral torsion

Position: Sacrum left rotated, right-side bent, and anteriorly nutated right sacral base

Muscle Restriction: Right rotation, left-side bending, and posteriorly nutated right sacral base

1. Patient sits astride the table with the left hand grasping the right shoulder.

2. Operator stands at the right side with the right hand grasping the patient's left shoulder and the right axilla controlling the right shoulder.

3. Operator's left pisiform contact is on the left sacral base (Fig. 17.130).

4. Operator's right arm introduces lumbar forward bending, right-side bending, and right rotation (nonneutral mechanics) while left hand prevents left rotation of the left sacral base (Fig. 17.131).

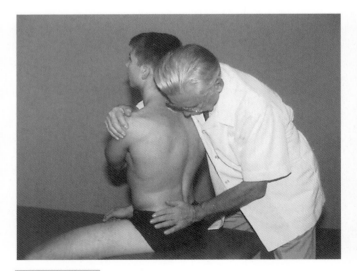

FIGURE 17.130

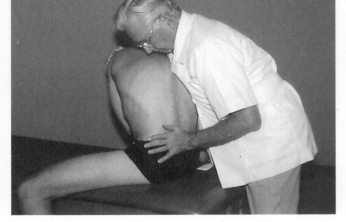

FIGURE 17.131

5. Operator's right arm maintains trunk right-side bending as nonneutral mechanics, flexion, and right rotation are released into neutral lumbar spine (Fig. 17.132).

6. While maintaining the right-side bending, left rotation is introduced through the trunk as an anterior thrust is delivered by the left forearm through the contact of the left pisiform on the left sacral base (Fig. 17.133).

7. Retest.

Note: Initially nonneutral lumbar mechanics are used, then released into neutral mechanics so that L5 rotates left and the sacrum rotates to the right, bringing the right sacral base posteriorly.

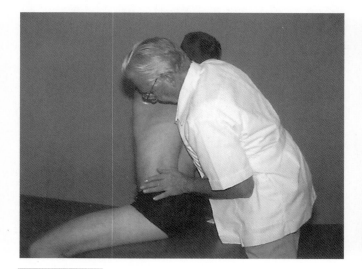

FIGURE 17.132

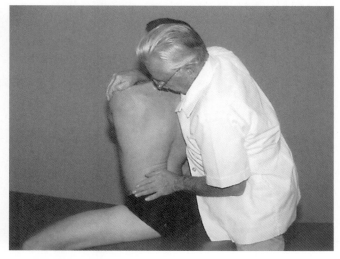

FIGURE 17.133

PELVIC GIRDLE

Sacroiliac

Mobilization With Impulse Technique

Sitting

Diagnosis: Right-on-left backward (posterior) sacral torsion

Position: Sacrum right rotated, left-side bent, posteriorly nutated right sacral base

Motion Restriction: Left rotation, right-side bending, and anterior nutation of right sacral base

1. Patient sits astride the table with the left hand grasping the right shoulder.

2. Operator stands at the left side with the left hand grasping the patient's right shoulder and the left axilla controlling the patient's left shoulder. Operator's right pisiform contacts the right sacral base (Fig. 17.134).

3. Operator introduces left-side bending and right rotation of the trunk down to L5, rotating the sacrum to the left. Operator puts anterior compression on the right sacral base (Fig. 17.135).

4. Operator reverses trunk mechanics into right-side bending and left rotation down to and including the sacrum (Fig. 17.136).

5. Operator performs mobilizing with impulse thrust through the right forearm to pisiform contact on right sacral base while exaggerating trunk extension while side bent right and rotated left.

6. Retest

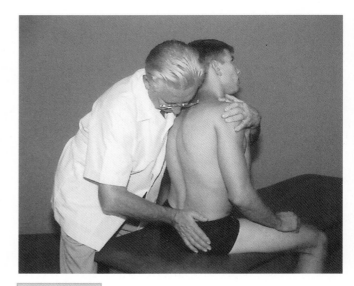

FIGURE 17.135

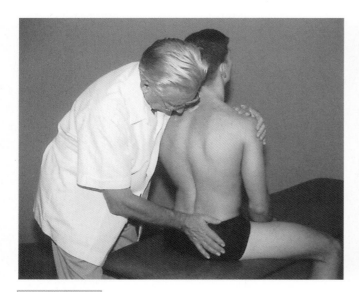

FIGURE 17.134

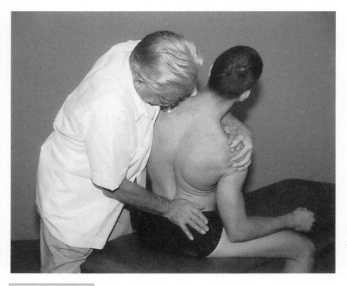

FIGURE 17.136

PELVIC GIRDLE

Iliosacral

Mobilization With Impulse Technique

Supine

Diagnosis: Left superior hip bone shear

1. Patient is supine with the operator standing at the end of the table.
2. Operator grasps the distal tibia and fibula above the ankle (Fig. 17.137).

3. Patient flexes the knee and the hip with slight abduction of the left lower extremity but without rotation (Fig. 17.138).
4. When the left leg is controlled with left sacroiliac joint plane loose packed, operator provides mobilization with impulse thrust by long-axis extension, carrying knee extension and hip extension to the left sacroiliac joint (Fig. 17.139).
5. Retest.

Note: This procedure is not indicated in the presence of knee or hip joint pathology.

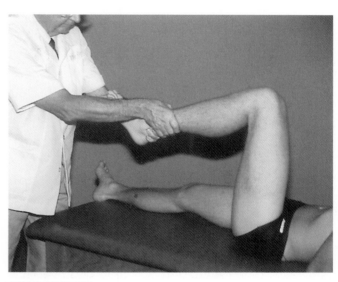

FIGURE 17.138

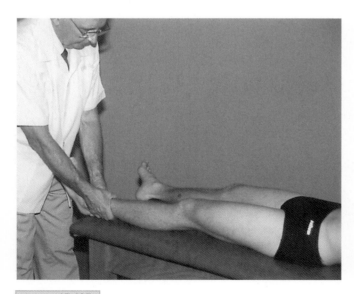

FIGURE 17.137

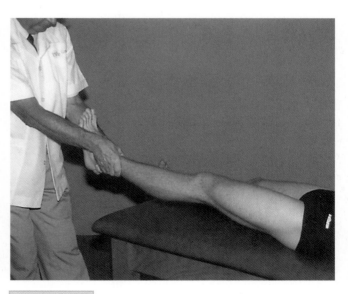

FIGURE 17.139

PELVIC GIRDLE

Iliosacral

Mobilization With Impulse Technique

Lateral Recumbent

Diagnosis: Right inferior hip bone shear dysfunction

1. Patient is in the left lateral recumbent position with the operator standing in front, monitoring the lumbosacral junction (Fig. 17.140).

2. Operator introduces neutral left-side bending right rotation of the lumbar spine down to and including the lumbosacral junction (Fig. 17.141).

3. Operator places the patient's right foot in the left popliteal space (Fig. 17.142).

4. Operator stabilizes the trunk with the right forearm and right hand monitoring at the right sacroiliac joint.

5. Operator's left forearm contacts the inferior aspect of the patient's right ischial tuberosity (Fig. 17.143).

6. Operator provides mobilization with impulse thrust in a cephalic direction against the right ischial tuberosity with the plane of the right sacroiliac joint parallel to the table resulting in superior translatory movement of the right hip bone.

7. Retest.

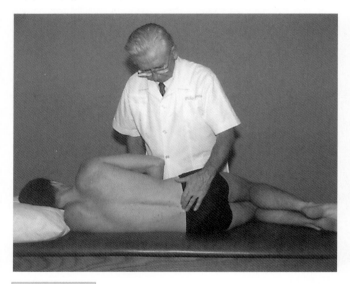

FIGURE 17.140

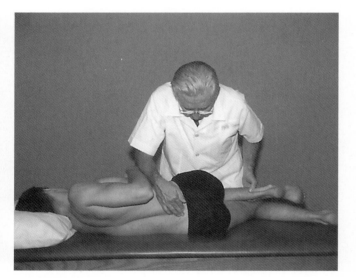

FIGURE 17.142

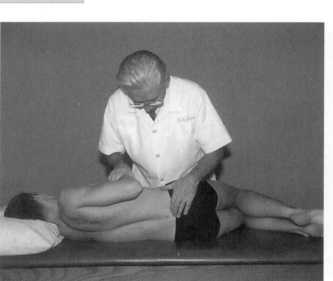

FIGURE 17.141

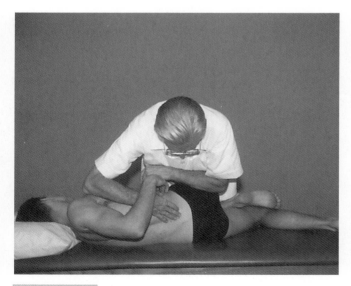

FIGURE 17.143

PELVIC GIRDLE

Iliosacral

Mobilization With Impulse Technique

Diagnosis: Right anterior hip bone

    Position: Right hip bone anteriorly rotated

    Motion Restriction: Posterior rotation right hip bone

1–4. These steps are identical to the technique for right inferior hip bone shear (Figs. 17.140–17.142).

5. Operator's right hand grasps the right ASIS and the left hand grasps the right ischial tuberosity (Fig. 17.143).

6. With the plane of the right sacroiliac joint parallel to the table, operator rotates hip bone posteriorly to the barrier and provides a mobilization with impulse thrust with both hands in a counterclockwise direction (Fig. 17.144).

7. An alternate hand position finds the operator's left forearm on the right ischial tuberosity. The right hand stabilizes the trunk with the right sacroiliac joint plane parallel to the table. A mobilization thrust is made by the left forearm in an anterior and superior direction rotating the left hip bone posteriorly (Fig. 17.145).

8. Retest.

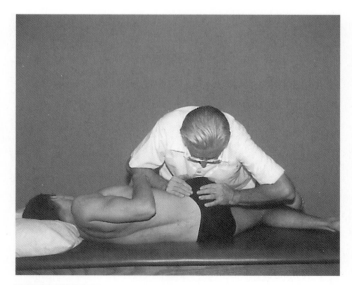

FIGURE 17.144

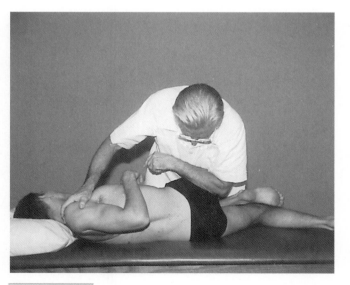

FIGURE 17.145

PELVIC GIRDLE

Iliosacral

Mobilization With Impulse Technique

Lateral Recumbent

Diagnosis: Left posterior hip bone

  Position: Left hip bone posteriorly rotated

  Motion Restriction: Anterior rotation of left hip bone

1. Patient is in the right lateral recumbent position with the operator standing in front, monitoring the lumbosacral junction (Fig. 17.146).

2. Operator introduces neutral side bending right and rotation left lumbar curve to include the lumbosacral junction.

3. Operator extends the lower extremities until the sacral base first starts to move forward (Fig. 17.147). Patient's left knee is placed in the right popliteal space.

4. With the left arm stabilizing the trunk and maintaining the plane of the left sacroiliac joint parallel to the table, operator's right pisiform contacts the left PSIS (Fig. 17.148).

5. Operator's body drop provides a mobilization with impulse technique through the right forearm, turning the left hip bone anteriorly.

6. An alternate contact is the operator's right forearm along the posterior aspect of the patient's left iliac crest (Fig. 17.149).

7. Operator's body drop provides a mobilization with impulse thrust through the left forearm contact rotating the left hip bone anteriorly.

8. Retest.

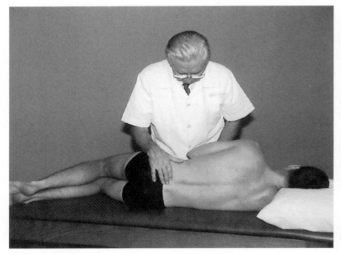

FIGURE 17.146

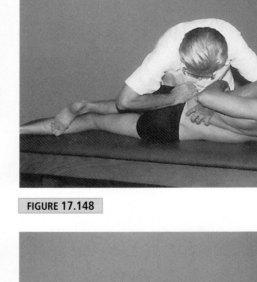

FIGURE 17.148

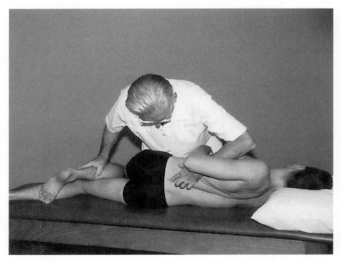

FIGURE 17.147

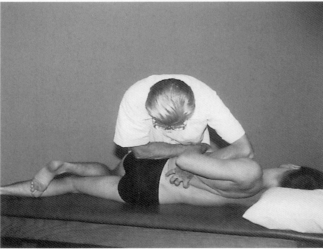

FIGURE 17.149

MUSCLE DYSFUNCTIONS OF THE PELVIC GIRDLE

Dysfunctions of the pelvic girdle always involve the many muscles to which it is related. Frequently seen is alteration in the pelvic diaphragm. This is particularly common in dysfunctions of the symphysis pubis and the hip bone shear dysfunctions. Widespread symptoms of the lower urinary tract, genitalia, and rectum are frequently present. Restoration of the function of the pelvic diaphragm is described in Chapter 7. Dysfunction of the muscles of the lower extremity and trunk need to be assessed and treated appropriately. These are described in Chapter 20.

CONCLUSION

Dysfunction of the pelvic girdle is complex and not easily understood. It is common to find several dysfunctions within the same pelvic girdle. Each needs to be individually diagnosed and appropriately treated. The diagnostic and therapeutic system described allows the operator to deal with any combination of physical findings that are found within the pelvic girdle. Restoration of pelvic girdle function within the walking cycle is a major therapeutic goal, particularly from the biomechanical postural–structural model.

REFERENCES

1. Weisel H. Movement of the sacroiliac joint. *Acta Anat* 1955;23:80–91.
2. Bernard TN, Kirkaldy-Willis WH. Recognizing specific characteristics of non specific low back pain. *Clin Orthop* 1987;217:266–280.
3. Greenman PE, Tate B. Structural diagnosis in chronic low back pain. *Man Med* 1998;3:114–117.
4. Sturesson B, Selvik G, Udén A. Movements of the sacroiliac joints. A roentgen stereophotogrammetric analysis. *Spine* 1989;14:162–165.
5. Vleeming A, van Wingerden JP, Dijkstra PF, et al. Mobility in the SI-joints in old people: A kinematic and radiologic study. *Clin Biomech* 1992;7:170–176.
6. Fortin JD, April CN Ponthieux B, Pier J. Sacroiliac joint: Pain referral maps upon applying a new injection/arthrography technique. 1: Asymptomatic volunteers. *Spine* 1994;19:1475–1482.
7. Fortin JD, Dwyer AP, West S, et al. Sacroiliac joint: Pain referral maps upon applying a new injection/ arthrography technique. 2: Clinical evaluation. *Spine* 1994;19:1483–1489.
8. DonTigny RL. Dysfunction of the sacroiliac joint and its treatment. *J Orthop Sports Phys Ther* 1979;1:23–35.
9. Bernard TN, Cassidy JD. The sacroiliac syndrome: Pathophysiology, diagnosis, and management. In: Frymoyer JW, ed. *The Adult Spine, Principles and Practice.* 2nd Ed. New York: Raven Press, 1991:2343–2366.
10. Mitchell FL Sr. *Structural Pelvic Function.* Carmel, CA: Yearbook of the American Academy of Osteopathy, 1958:71–90.
11. Beal MC. The sacroiliac problem: Review of anatomy, mechanics, and diagnosis. *J Am Osteopath Assoc* 1982;81:667–679.
12. Alderink GJ. The sacroiliac joint: Review of anatomy, mechanics, and function. *J Ortho Sports Phys Ther* 1991;13:71–84.
13. Chamberlain WE. The symphysis pubis in the roentgen examination of the sacroiliac joint. *Am J Roentgenol* 1930;24:621–625.
14. Lee D. *The Pelvic Girdle.* 3rd Ed. Edinburgh: Churchill Livingstone, 2004.
15. Bowen V, Cassidy JD. Macroscopic and microscopic anatomy of the sacroiliac joint until the eighth decade. *Spine* 1981;6:620–628.
16. Vleeming A, Stoeckart R, Volkers ACW, et al. Relation between form and function in the sacroiliac joint. 2: Biomechanical aspects. *Spine* 1990;15:130–132.
17. Stevens A: Side-bending and axial rotation of the sacrum inside the pelvic girdle. In: Vleeming A, Mooney V, Snijders CJ, et al., eds. *First Interdisciplinary World Congress on Low Back Pain and Its Relation to the Sacroiliac Joint.* San Diego, CA, 5–6 November 1992:209–230.
18. Bogduk NLT. *Clinical Anatomy of the Lumbar Spine and Sacrum.* 3rd Ed. New York: Churchill Livingstone, 1997.
19. Vleeming A, Pool-Goudzwaard AL, Hammudoghlu D, et al. The function of the long dorsal sacroiliac ligament: Its implication for understanding low back pain. *Spine* 1996;21(5):556.
20. Pool-Goudzwaard AL, Kleinrensink GJ, Snijders CJ, et al. The sacroiliac part of the iliolumbar ligament. *J Anat* 2001;199(Pt 4):457–463.
21. Fortin JD, Falco FJ. The Fortin finger test: An indicator of sacroiliac pain. *Am J Orthop* 1997;26(7):477–480.
22. Vleeming A, Pool-Goudzwaard AL, Stoeckart R, et al. The posterior layer of the thoracolumbar fascia: Its function in load transfer from spine to legs. *Spine* 1995;20(7):753–758.
23. Bullock-Saxton JE, Janda V, Bullock MI. The influence of ankle sprain injury on muscle activation during hip extension. *Int J Sports Med* 1994;15(6):330–334.
24. Bullock-Saxton JE, Janda V, Bullock MI. Reflex activation of gluteal muscles in walking. An approach to restoration of muscle function for patients with low-back pain. *Spine* 1993;18(6):704–708.
25. Pitkin HC, Pheasant HC. Sacroarthrogenic telalgia. *J Bone Joint Surg* 1936;18:111–133.
26. Greenman PE. Clinical aspects of sacroiliac function in walking. *J Man Med* 1990;5:125–130.
27. Greenman PE. Innominate shear dysfunction in the sacroiliac syndrome. *Man Med* 1986;2:114–121.

Highly developed hand dexterity is one of the distinguishing characteristics of humans. Upper extremity function places the hand in positions that allow it to perform its unique, intricate movements. The upper extremity is attached to the trunk primarily through muscular attachments. The only articulation of the upper extremity with the trunk is the sternoclavicular joint. The arrangements of the muscular attachments allow the extremity a wide range of movement in relation to the trunk. The upper extremity has a strong interrelationship with the cervical spine, thoracic spine, and thoracic cage through the multiple muscle relationships.

In approaching dysfunctions within the upper extremity, the operator should first examine and treat any dysfunctions within the cervical spine, thoracic spine, and thoracic cage. The cervicothoracic junction is one of the major transitional regions of the body. The relationship of T1 with the first rib and the sternoclavicular joint is of major significance in upper extremity problems. T1 dysfunctions influence the first rib and lead to dysfunctions there. Dysfunctions of the first rib influence the manubrium of the sternum and the sternoclavicular joint. *Evaluation of symptoms in the upper extremity should proceed from proximal to distal because of the influence of the cervical spine and thoracic inlet on circulatory and neural functions.* Whether the practitioner is using a circulatory or a neurologic model, evaluation of the cervical and thoracic spine is appropriate before moving distally to the upper extremity.

BRACHALGIA

One of the common mistakes the operator makes in evaluating upper extremity complaints is to evaluate only at the joint where the symptom is present and proximal thereto. From the structural diagnostic perspective, a patient with pain in the upper extremity under the general rubric of "brachalgia" has five potential entrapment sites for elements of the brachial plexus.

1. The cervical roots are at risk at the intervertebral foramen as they exit from the vertebral canal. Productive change of the uncovertebral joint of Luschka and posterolateral protrusion of intervertebral disk material may narrow the intervertebral canal anteriorly, reducing the space available for the roots. Dysfunction or disease of the zygapophysial joints may negatively affect the foraminal size and shape from the posterior direction, reducing space for the nerve roots. In addition to significant osseous change, swelling and congestion from acute or chronic inflammation can also cause entrapment.

2. The roots are transported through the intertransversarii muscles between the transverse processes of the cervical vertebrae. Hypertonicity of these short, fourth-layer spinal muscles, with accompanying chronic passive congestion, may also be a site of potential entrapment. Hypertonicity of these muscles is common with segmental dysfunction at the same level.

3. The roots forming the brachial plexus pass through the scalene muscles. Hypertonicity and passive congestion of these muscles, commonly found in cervical and upper rib cage dysfunction, negatively influence the brachial plexus.

4. As the plexus traverses laterally, it passes through the costoclavicular canal. The lateral portion of the second rib and the posterior aspect of the clavicle bind this triangular-shaped region. Dysfunctions of the second rib, particularly where it is held in an inhalation position in the lateral bucket-handle range, and of the sternoclavicular and acromioclavicular articulations can result in potential entrapment at the costoclavicular canal. A large amount of soft tissue occupies space within this region and if congested, the costoclavicular canal can narrow.

5. More laterally, the neurovascular bundle passes under the insertion of the pectoralis minor tendon to the coracoid process of the scapula. Hypertonicity, shortening, and thickening of the pectoralis muscle and its tendon can compress the nerves as they pass distally.

In addition to the neural structures, the vascular and lymphatic channels are at risk as they pass in close proximity to the scalenes, first rib, costoclavicular canal, and underlying the pectoralis minor tendon. The examiner must thoroughly evaluate the cervical, upper thoracic, and upper rib cage areas before proceeding with the evaluation and management of the distal region of the upper extremity.

The screening examination (see Chapter 2) for the upper extremities involves the patient actively abducting the upper extremities with the elbows extended and attempting to bring the backs of the hands together over the head. Inability to symmetrically accomplish this maneuver demands further diagnostic evaluation. The upper extremities should be evaluated by traditional orthopedic and neurologic testing. A recent addition to testing of the neural structures is the neural dynamic testing of the nervous system for neural and "dural" restrictions.

There are many systems for the structural diagnosis and manual medicine treatment of the extremities. This author has found many of the procedures found in Mennell's *Joint Pain*[1] to be of considerable therapeutic value. Only a few of these procedures will be repeated here and the reader is encouraged to study Mennell's text.

The shoulder, elbow, and wrist are not single joints; each of the regions contains several articulations. For that reason, we will approach the upper extremity on a regional basis and evaluate the specific articulations individually.

SHOULDER REGION

The shoulder region consists of the sternoclavicular, acromio-clavicular, and glenohumeral articulations. The scapulocostal junction is not a true articulation. The ability of the concave costal surface of the scapula to smoothly move over the thoracic cage is of major importance in upper extremity function, particularly the shoulder region. The direct restrictors of scapulo-costal motion are the muscles and fasciae that hold the scapula to the trunk. These myofascial elements are best approached by soft-tissue and myofascial release techniques. Particular attention must be given to the trapezius, sternocleidomastoid, levator scapulae, rhomboids, serratus anterior, and latissimus dorsi muscles and their fasciae. Evaluation and treatment of these muscles should precede the articulations in the shoulder region.

Sternoclavicular Joint

The medial end of the clavicle articulates with the manubrium of the sternum. Within this joint is a meniscus. The medial end of the clavicle is intimately related to the anterior aspect of the first rib. The joint is polyaxial in its movement with abduction, horizontal flexion, and rotation as the primary motions. As the clavicle is abducted, it externally (posteriorly) rotates, and as it returns to neutral, it internally (anteriorly) rotates. Rotation then becomes a coupled movement with abduction.

UPPER EXTREMITY

Sternoclavicular Joint

Diagnosis

Test for Restricted Abduction

1. Patient is supine on the table with arms resting easily at the side.

2. Operator stands at the side or at the head of the table with paired fingers over the superior aspect of the medial end of the clavicle (Fig. 18.1).

3. Patient is asked to actively "shrug the shoulders" by bringing the shoulder tip to the ear bilaterally (Fig. 18.2).

4. Operator's palpating fingers follow the movement at the medial end of the clavicle.

5. The normal finding is the equal movement of the medial end of both clavicles in a caudad direction.

6. A positive finding is the failure of one clavicle to move caudad when compared to the opposite. It appears to be held in the original starting position.

Note: This test can also be done with patient sitting.

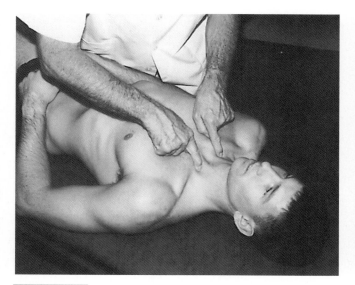

FIGURE 18.1

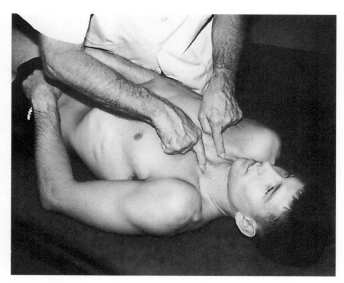

FIGURE 18.2

UPPER EXTREMITY

Sternoclavicular Joint

Mobilization without Impulse (Articulatory Treatment)

Diagnosis: Restricted abduction

1. Patient sits on the examining table or stool.

2. Operator stands behind the patient with the thenar eminence of one hand over the superior aspect of the medial end of the dysfunctional clavicle; the other hand grasps the patient's forearm (Fig. 18.3).

3. Operator abducts the extended upper extremity to the resistant barrier (Fig. 18.4) and sweeps it across the patient's torso in the direction of the opposite knee while constant caudad pressure is maintained by the thenar eminence on the medial end of the clavicle (Fig. 18.5).

4. Several repetitions are done, increasing the abduction movement of the patient's extended arm. (A high-velocity thrust by the thenar eminence may be used.)

5. Retest.

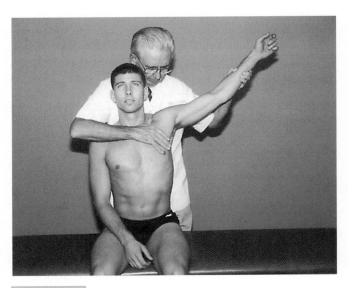

FIGURE 18.4

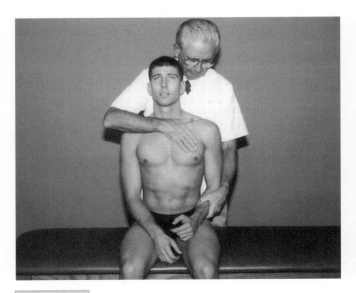

FIGURE 18.3

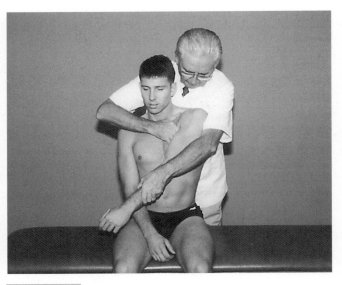

FIGURE 18.5

UPPER EXTREMITY

Sternoclavicular Joint

Muscle Energy Technique

Supine

Diagnosis: Restricted abduction

1. Patient is supine on the table with the dysfunctional upper extremity at the edge of the table.
2. Operator stands on the side of the dysfunction facing cephalad.
3. Operator places one hand over the medial end of the dysfunctional clavicle while the other grasps the patient's forearm just above the wrist (Fig. 18.6).

4. Operator internally rotates the dysfunctional upper extremity and carries it into extension off the edge of the table to the resistant barrier while monitoring with the opposite hand at the sternoclavicular region (Fig. 18.7).
5. Patient performs a 3- to 5-second muscle contraction to lift the arm toward the ceiling against the operator's resistance for three to five repetitions.
6. Following each relaxation, the operator increases the extension of the upper extremity to a new resistant barrier and patient again repeats the effort of lifting the arm toward the ceiling.
7. Retest.

Note: This procedure also increases internal (anterior) rotation at the sternoclavicular joint.

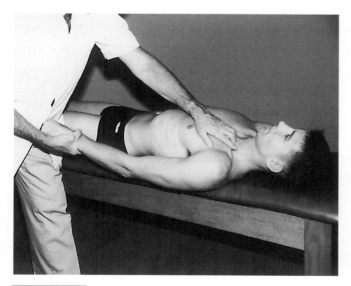

FIGURE 18.6

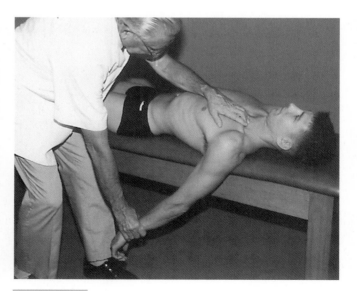

FIGURE 18.7

UPPER EXTREMITY

Sternoclavicular Joint

Muscle Energy Technique

Sitting

Diagnosis: Restricted abduction

1. Patient sits on the table or stool.

2. Operator stands behind the patient with the thenar eminence of one hand in contact with the superior aspect of the medial end of the dysfunctional clavicle and the other hand controlling the dysfunctional upper extremity at the elbow (Fig. 18.8).

3. With the elbow at 90 degrees, the upper extremity is externally rotated and abducted to approximately 90 degrees with additional abduction until the resistant barrier is engaged (Fig. 18.9).

4. Patient performs muscle contraction to adduct the upper extremity three to five times for 3 to 5 seconds against resistance offered at the elbow by the operator.

5. After relaxation, the operator engages a new barrier.

6. Retest.

Note: This procedure also enhances the external (posterior) rotation at the sternoclavicular joint.

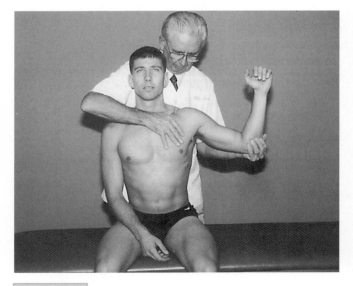

FIGURE 18.8

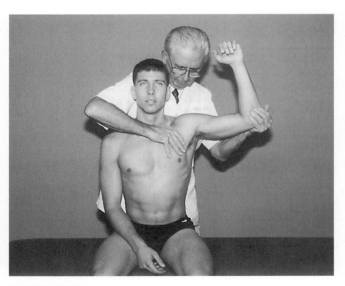

FIGURE 18.9

UPPER EXTREMITY

Sternoclavicular Joint

Diagnosis

Test for Restricted Horizontal Flexion

1. Patient is supine on the table.

2. Operator stands at the side or the head of the table with fingers symmetrically placed on the anterior aspect of the medial end of each clavicle (Fig. 18.10).

3. Patient extends the upper extremities in front of the body and then reaches toward the ceiling.

4. Operator evaluates movement of the medial end of each clavicle (Fig. 18.11).

5. The normal finding is for each clavicle to move symmetrically in a posterior direction as the lateral end of the clavicle moves anteriorly.

6. A positive finding is for one clavicle not to move in a posterior direction during the reaching effort.

Note: This test can also be done with the patient sitting.

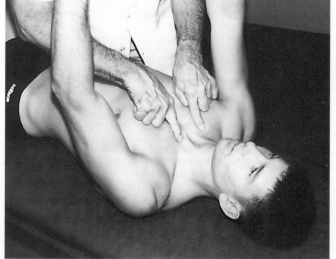

FIGURE 18.10

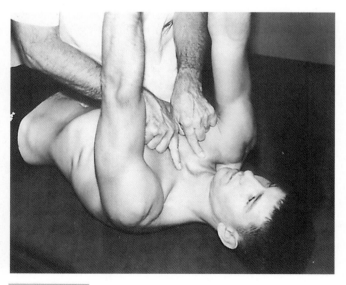

FIGURE 18.11

UPPER EXTREMITY

Sternoclavicular Joint

Mobilization without Impulse (Articulatory) Treatment

Diagnosis: Restricted horizontal flexion

1. Patient sits on the table.

2. Operator stands behind with one hand on the anterior aspect of the medial end of the dysfunctional clavicle and the lateral hand grasping the forearm (Fig. 18.12).

3. Operator takes the upper extremity into horizontal extension (Fig. 18.13) and sweeps it forward in horizontal flexion (Fig. 18.14) with increasing arcs of movement, while the thenar eminence of the opposite hand maintains a posterior compressive force on the medial end of the dysfunctional clavicle. (A high-velocity thrust by the thenar eminence may be substituted.)

4. Retest.

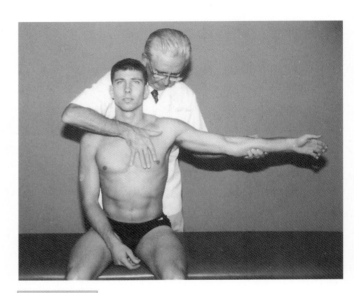

FIGURE 18.13

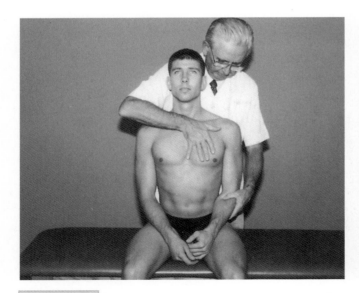

FIGURE 18.12

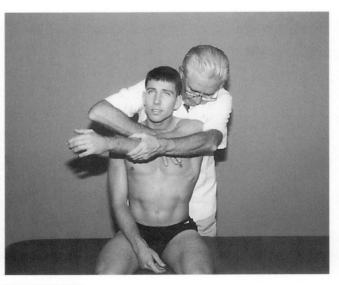

FIGURE 18.14

UPPER EXTREMITY

Sternoclavicular Joint

Muscle Energy Technique

Supine

Diagnosis: Restricted horizontal flexion

1. Patient is supine on the table.

2. Operator stands on the side of the table opposite the dysfunctional sternoclavicular joint.

3. Operator places the cephalic hand over the medial end of the dysfunctional clavicle and the caudad hand grasps the patient's shoulder girdle over the posterior aspect of the scapula (Fig. 18.15).

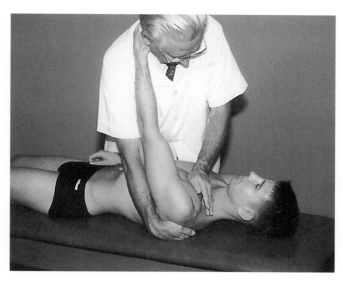

FIGURE 18.15

4. Patient's hand grasps the back of the operator's neck with an extended arm.

5. Operator engages the horizontal flexion barrier by standing more erect and lifting the dysfunctional scapula (Fig. 18.16).

6. Patient pulls down upon the operator's neck with 3- to 5-second muscle effort for three to five repetitions, while the operator maintains posterior compression on the anterior aspect of the medial end of the dysfunctional clavicle.

7. Operator engages a new barrier after each of the patient's muscle contraction.

8. Retest.

UPPER EXTREMITY

Sternoclavicular Joint

Mobilization Without Impulse (Articulatory) Technique
Diagnosis: Restricted horizontal flexion

1. Patient is supine; the operator stands on the opposite side of the dysfunction.

2. Operator webs the caudad forearm between the patients chest and humerus and grasps the side of the table.

3. Patient's opposite hand reaches across the abdomen and grasps the wrist of the dysfunctional extremity.

4. Operator's cephalic hand applies pressure on the medial end of the dysfunctional clavicle (Fig. 18.17).

5. Patient pulls on the wrist distracting the clavicle while the operator springs the medial end of the clavicle posteriorly.

6. Retest.

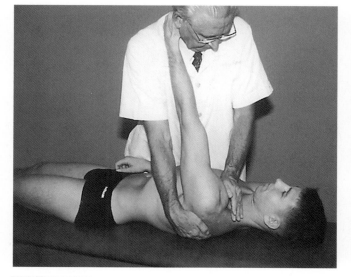

FIGURE 18.16

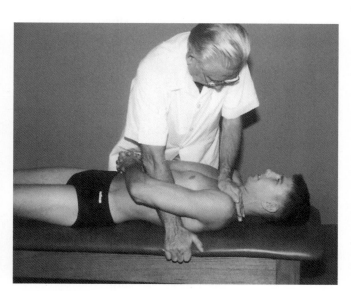

FIGURE 18.17

ACROMIOCLAVICULAR JOINT

The acromioclavicular joint contributes only a small amount of motion to the shoulder region, but its contribution to total upper extremity abduction is critical. The primary movements of this articulation are abduction and internal and external rotations. The joint is angled laterally at approximately 30 degrees from front to back. The joint largely depends on ligaments for its integrity and frequently separates during trauma. Productive change at this joint is common. Clinical experience has shown that loss of acromioclavicular joint function is highly significant, particularly the loss of abduction. This is important to remember during motion testing of the shoulder girdle. Dysfunction of this joint is one of the most frequently overlooked in the upper extremity.

UPPER EXTREMITY

Acromioclavicular Joint

Diagnosis: Test for restricted abduction and adduction

1. Patient sits with the operator standing behind.
2. Operator's medial hand palpates the superior aspect of the acromioclavicular joint and the lateral hand controls the patient's proximal forearm (Fig. 18.18).

3. Operator introduces adduction and external rotation of the forearm monitoring a gapping movement at the acromioclavicular joint (Fig. 18.19).
4. Absence of the gapping movement is evidence of restriction of adduction movement.
5. Comparison is made with the opposite side.
6. Operator introduces abduction movement while monitoring at the joint for movement (Fig. 18.20).
7. Comparison is made with the opposite side.

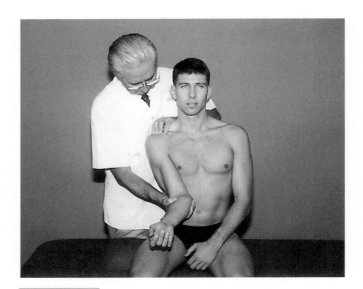

FIGURE 18.19

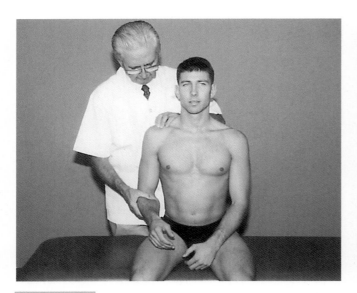

FIGURE 18.18

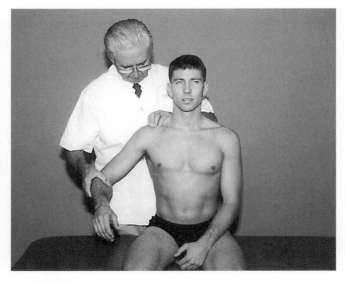

FIGURE 18.20

UPPER EXTREMITY

Acromioclavicular Joint

Muscle Energy Technique

Sitting

Diagnosis: Restricted abduction

1. Patient sits on the table or stool with the operator standing behind.

2. Operator maintains compressive force on the lateral end of the clavicle, medial to the acromioclavicular joint.

3. Operator's lateral hand takes the patient's upper extremity to horizontal flexion of 30 degrees and abducts to the barrier (Fig. 18.21).

4. Patient pulls the elbow to the side against resistance offered by the operator for 3 to 5 seconds and three to five repetitions.

5. Operator engages new abduction barrier after each muscle effort.

6. Retest.

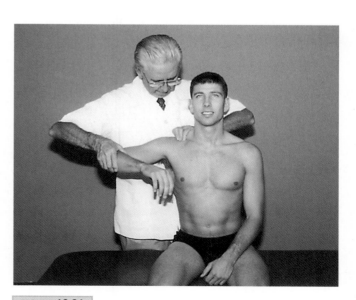

FIGURE 18.21

UPPER EXTREMITY

Acromioclavicular Joint

Diagnosis: Test for restricted internal and external rotation

1. Patient sits on the table or stool with the operator standing behind.

2. Operator's medial hand palpates the superior aspect of the acromioclavicular joint.

3. Operator's lateral hand moves the upper extremity into horizontal flexion to 30 degrees and abduction to the first barrier (Fig. 18.22).

4. Operator introduces internal rotation (Fig. 18.23) and external rotation (Fig. 18.24) while monitoring mobility of the acromioclavicular joint.

5. Comparison is made with the opposite side.

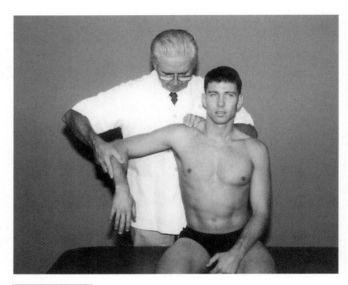

FIGURE 18.23

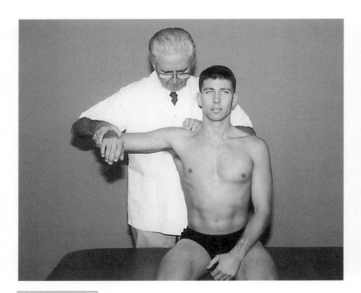

FIGURE 18.22

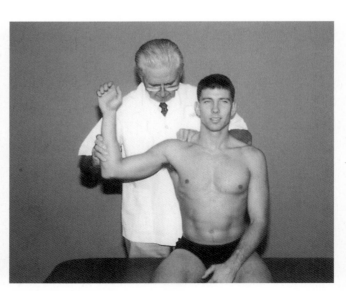

FIGURE 18.24

UPPER EXTREMITY

Acromioclavicular Joint

Muscle Energy Technique

Diagnosis: Restricted internal or external rotation

1. Patient sits on the table or stool with the operator standing behind.

2. Operator's medial hand stabilizes the lateral aspect of the clavicle and monitors the acromioclavicular joint.

3. Operator takes the upper extremity to 30 degrees of horizontal flexion and abduction to 90 degrees.

4. External rotational barrier is engaged with the operator's lateral hand grasping the patient's wrist and places the forearm to patient's forearm (Fig. 18.25).

5. Operator engages internal rotation barrier by threading lateral forearm under the patient's elbow and grasping the distal forearm (Fig. 18.26).

6. Patient provides muscle contraction for 3 to 5 seconds and three to five repetitions against resistance of either internal or external rotation.

7. Operator engages a new barrier after each muscle contraction.

8. Retest.

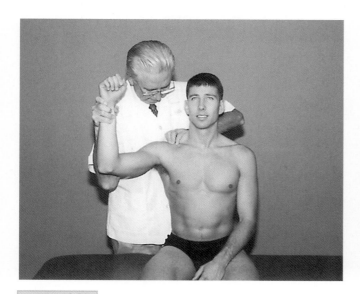

FIGURE 18.25

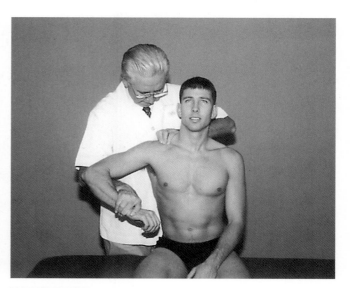

FIGURE 18.26

GLENOHUMERAL JOINT

The glenohumeral joint has one of the widest ranges of movement of any joint within the body. The depth of the glenoid is increased by the cartilaginous glenoidal labrum. For this joint to perform its normal function, it is dependent upon the ability of the scapula to move on the thoracic cage with the glenoid being elevated for upper extremity abduction. For this reason, the muscular attachments to the scapula must perform their normal actions. Tightness and shortening of the levator scapulae and the latissimus dorsi muscles are notoriously found in a dysfunctional upper extremity, particularly the impingement syndrome of the rotator cuff. The articular capsule is normally quite lax and loose, particularly inferiorly, providing for a wide range of movement. Joint integrity is maintained by the intimate attachment of the rotator cuff muscles (supraspinatus, infraspinatus, teres minor, and subscapularis) to the articular capsule.

The extensive movements of this joint are described in relation to the vertical and horizontal planes. In the vertical or neutral plane, the humerus is at the side of the body. Movement then occurs in flexion, extension, internal rotation, and external rotation. In the horizontal plane, with the humerus at 90 degrees to the trunk, it is also possible to have flexion, extension, internal rotation, and external rotation. Adduction moves the humerus toward the body and in front of the chest, and abduction moves the arm away from the body with full range extending so that the elbow can touch the ear. All of these motions should be tested and compared with the opposite side. The primary movement loss in the glenohumeral joint involves the functions of external rotation and abduction. The humeral head must move from cephalad to caudad on the glenoid during abduction; loss of this ability to track from superior to inferior during abduction results in major restriction at the glenohumeral joint.

Because the vast majority of dysfunctions within the glenohumeral joint are muscular in origin, muscle energy diagnostic and therapeutic techniques are most effective.

The principles of diagnosis and treatment are

1. to evaluate range of motion in all of the motion directions described above,
2. to evaluate the strength of each of the muscle groups,
3. to treat restricted range of movement by postisometric relaxation technique at the restrictive barrier, and
4. if weakness is identified, to treat by means of a series of concentric isotonic contractions. Each motion should be compared with that available on the opposite side.

GLENOHUMERAL JOINT

Muscle Energy Procedure

1. Patient sits on the table or stool with the operator standing behind.

2. Range of motion is tested in all directions by engaging the restrictive barrier. Comparison is made with the opposite side.

3. If motion is restricted, the operator engages resistant barrier. Patient performs three to five repetitions of a 3- to 5-second isometric contraction against operator resistance.

4. The operator performs strength testing by having the patient contract the muscle in the direction of operator resistance. Comparison is made with the opposite side. If one muscle group is weak, the patient performs a series of three to five concentric isotonic contractions through the total range of movement against progressively increasing resistance by the operator.

5. Operator's medial hand stabilizes the shoulder girdle with the fingers on the coracoid process, the web of the hand over the acromioclavicular joint, and the thumb posterior and inferior over the spine of the scapula.

6. Operator's lateral hand controls the patient's elbow and forearm.

7. Operator introduces the following motions and treats accordingly:

   - Neutral flexion (Fig. 18.27)
   - Neutral extension (Fig. 18.28)
   - Neutral external rotation (Fig. 18.29)
   - Neutral internal rotation, stage 1 (Fig. 18.30)
   - Neutral internal rotation, stage 2 (Fig. 18.31)
   - Adduction (Fig. 18.32)
   - Abduction (Fig. 18.33)
   - Horizontal flexion (Fig. 18.34)
   - Horizontal extension (Fig. 18.35)
   - Horizontal internal rotation (Fig. 18.36)
   - Horizontal external rotation (Fig. 18.37)

8. Retest.

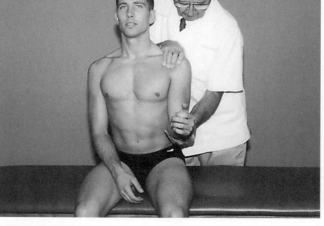

FIGURE 18.27

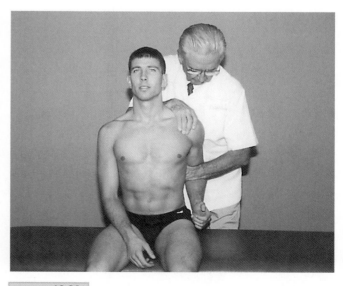

FIGURE 18.28

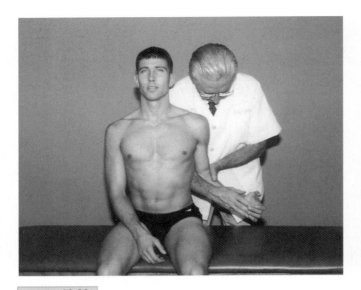

FIGURE 18.29

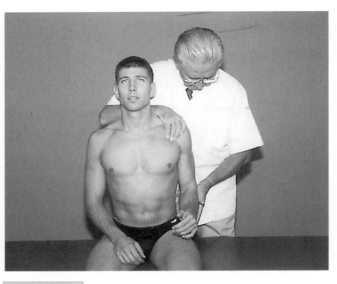

FIGURE 18.32

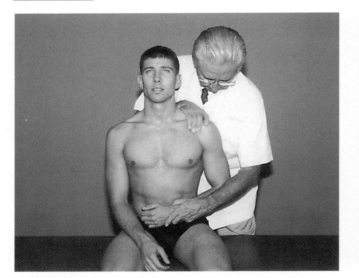

FIGURE 18.30

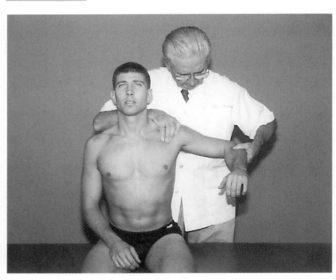

FIGURE 18.33

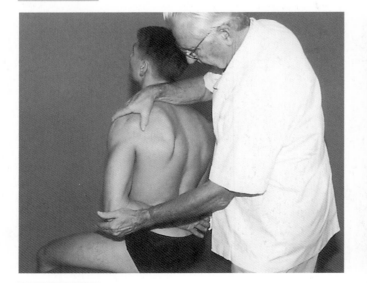

FIGURE 18.31

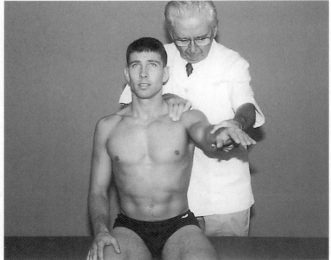

FIGURE 18.34

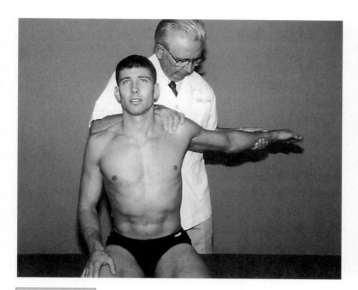

FIGURE 18.35

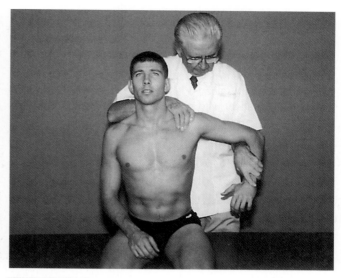

FIGURE 18.36

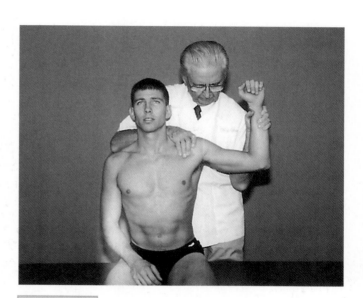

FIGURE 18.37

GLENOHUMERAL JOINT

Glenoidal Labrum (Green's) Technique

This technique enhances movement of the humeral head within the glenoid and the glenoid labrum and is useful as the initial treatment in a patient with *adhesive capsulitis* (*frozen shoulder*).

1. Patient is prone with the involved arm off the edge of the table and the operator sitting at the side facing the dysfunctional shoulder (Fig. 18.38).

2. Operator grasps the distal humerus in both hands and applies caudad and anterior traction with internal and external rotation two to three times (Fig. 18.39).

3. Operator next grasps patient's humeral neck with thumbs on the greater tuberosity, the index and middle fingers on the attachment of the rotator cuff, and the ring and little fingers surrounding the proximal shaft, controlling the humeral shaft against the thenar eminences (Fig. 18.40).

4. Operator applies movement through the humeral head in an anterior–posterior, cephalic–caudal, and medial and lateral traction—distraction directions.

5. Operator induces circular and figure-eight motions, enhancing range in all directions.

6. Operator emphasizes increase in caudal translatory movement of the humeral head on the glenoid.

7. Retest.

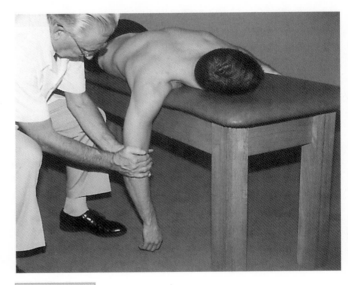

FIGURE 18.39

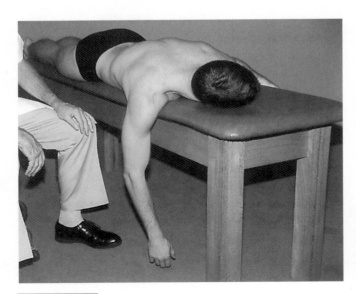

FIGURE 18.38

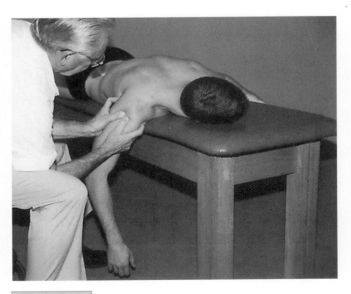

FIGURE 18.40

GLENOHUMERAL JOINT

Spencer Seven-Step Technique

The principle is a sequential, direct action, mobilization without impulse (articulatory) technique against motion resistance.

1. Patient is in lateral recumbent position with the affected shoulder uppermost, head supported, and knees flexed.

2. Operator stands facing the patient.

3. Operator's proximal hand stabilizes the shoulder girdle including the clavicle and the scapula.

4. Step 1: Operator gently flexes (Fig. 18.41) and extends the arm (Fig. 18.42) in the sagittal plane with the elbow flexed. Repetitions are made within the limits of pain provocation.

5. Step 2: Operator flexes patient's arm in the sagittal plane with the elbow extended in a rhythmic swinging movement, increasing range so that the patient's arm covers the ear (Fig. 18.43).

6. Step 3: Operator circumducts the patient's abducted humerus with the elbow flexed. Clockwise and counterclockwise concentric circles with gradual increase in range are made within limits of pain (Fig. 18.44).

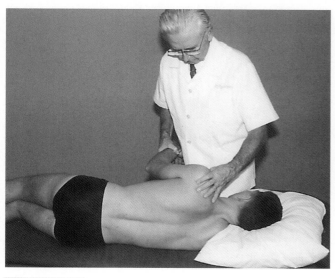

FIGURE 18.41

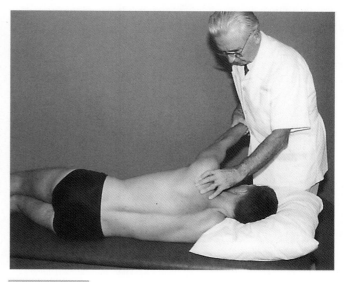

FIGURE 18.43

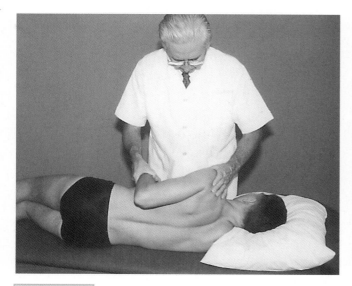

FIGURE 18.42

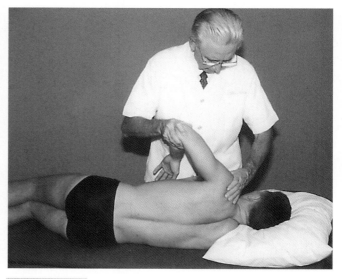

FIGURE 18.44

7. Step 4: Operator circumducts the patient's humerus with the elbow extended in clockwise and counterclockwise circles, increasing range as permitted by pain (Fig. 18.45).

8. Step 5: Operator abducts the patient's arm with the elbow flexed with gradual increases of range of abduction against the stabilized shoulder girdle (Fig. 18.46).

9. Step 6: Operator places the patient's hand behind the rib cage and gently springs the elbow forward and inferior, increasing internal rotation of the humerus (Fig. 18.47).

10. Step 7: Operator grasps the patient's proximal humerus with both hands and applies lateral and caudad traction in a pumping fashion (Fig. 18.48).

11. Retest.

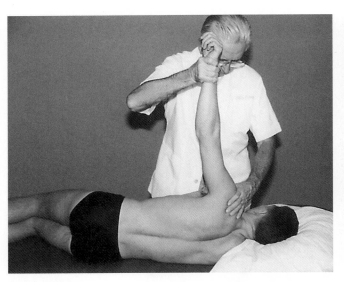

FIGURE 18.45

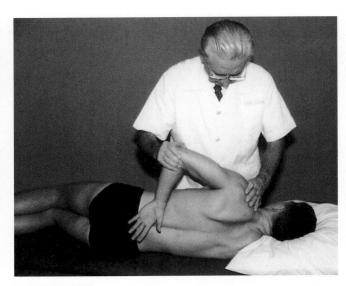

FIGURE 18.47

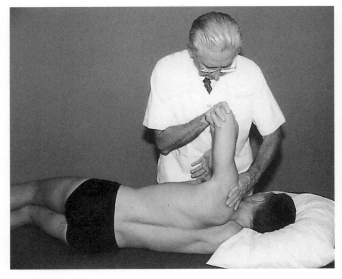

FIGURE 18.46

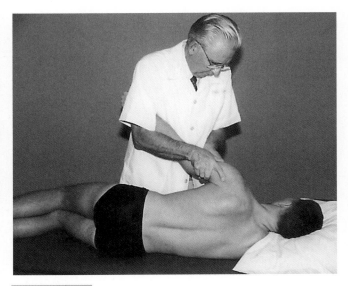

FIGURE 18.48

ELBOW REGION

There are three joints at the elbow region: the humeroulnar joint, the humeroradial joint, and the proximal radioulnar joint. The primary movements are flexion–extension, pronation–supination, and a small amount of abduction–adduction. All joints participate in the elbow function. Flexion–extension is the primary movement at the humeroulnar joint, and pronation–supination is a combined humeroradial and proximal radioulnar joint movement. Abduction–adduction movement is primarily a joint play movement at the humeroulnar joint, and, when dysfunctional, reduces the flexion–extension range. The elbow region has a number of related pain syndromes that are frequently described as "tennis elbow." Many of these patients present with pain on the lateral aspect of the elbow, radiating into the forearm, which is aggravated by activity. Dysfunction of the radial head involving the proximal radioulnar and humeroradial joints is a frequent finding. *Radial head dysfunction is the most common somatic dysfunction within the elbow region.*

ELBOW REGION

Diagnosis: Restricted abduction–adduction (humeroulnar joint)

1. Patient sits on the table with the operator standing in front.
2. Operator's two hands circumferentially grasp the proximal radioulnar region.
3. Operator supports the patient's hand and wrist between the medial side of the elbow and the trunk.

4. Operator's hands introduce translatory movement medially (Fig. 18.49) and laterally (Fig. 18.50) through the arc from flexion to extension testing for resistance.
5. Comparison is made with the opposite side.
6. A direct action mobilization without impulse, progressively carried through to mobilization with impulse, has the operator engage either the adduction or abduction barrier while extended (Fig. 18.51). Mobilization without impulse repetitions are made against the resistant barrier with a final mobilization with impulse performed.
7. Retest.

Note: Adduction restriction is more common than abduction.

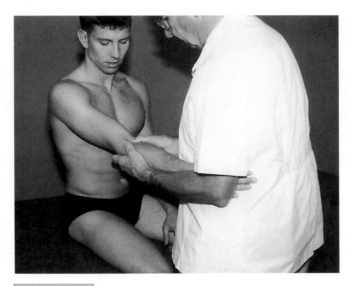

FIGURE 18.50

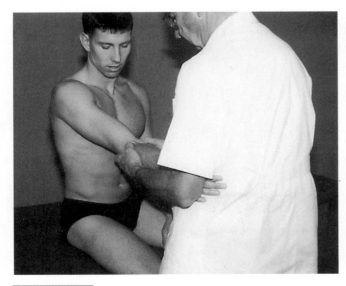

FIGURE 18.49

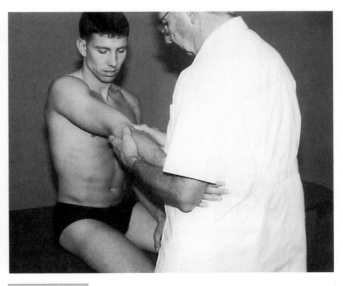

FIGURE 18.51

ELBOW REGION

Muscle Energy Technique

Restricted Elbow Extension

1. Patient sits on the table with the operator standing in front.

2. Operator's medial hand grasps the patient's distal supinated forearm with the lateral hand stabilizing the elbow.

3. Patient's elbow extension barrier is engaged (Fig. 18.52).

4. Patient performs a series of three to five muscle contractions for 3 to 5 seconds against the operator's resistance.

5. Operator progressively engages elbow extension barrier after each muscle contraction (Fig. 18.53).

6. Retest.

7. An alternate technique has the patient perform a series of isotonic contractions of the triceps muscle through full flexion-to-extension arc.

8. Operator fully flexes the elbow, stabilizing the elbow with the lateral hand, grasping the distal forearm to provide resistance to isotonic contraction (Fig. 18.54).

9. Patient performs three to five repetitions with progressively increasing resistance by the operator's medial hand until full elbow extension is achieved (Fig. 18.55).

10. Retest.

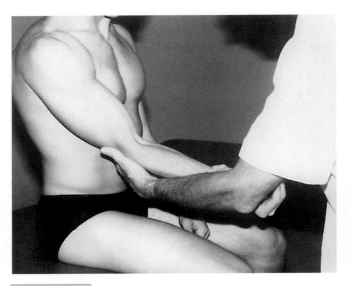

FIGURE 18.52

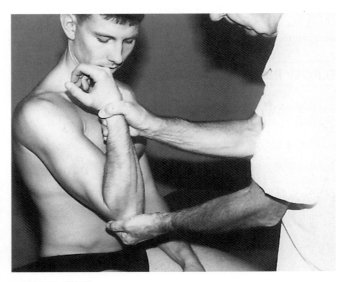

FIGURE 18.54

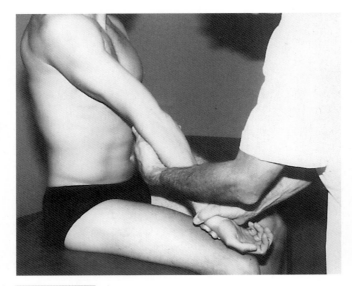

FIGURE 18.53

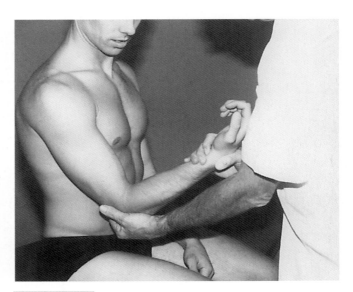

FIGURE 18.55

ELBOW REGION

Muscle Energy Technique

Restricted Pronation and Supination

1. Patient sits on the table with the operator standing in front.

2. Operator's medial hand stabilizes the patient's elbow flexed to 90 degrees. The lateral hand grasps the distal forearm, wrist, and hand with the patient's thumb pointing vertically (Fig. 18.56).

3. Operator introduces supination (Fig. 18.57) and pronation (Fig. 18.58) testing for restriction.

4. Comparison is made with the opposite side.

5. Treatment of restricted supination has the operator's lateral hand stabilizing the flexed elbow and monitoring the radial head while medial hand supinates the forearm to resistant barrier (Fig. 18.59).

6. Patient performs three to five muscle contractions for 3 to 5 seconds against resistance offered by the operator's medial hand.

7. Operator engages a new supination barrier after each patient effort.

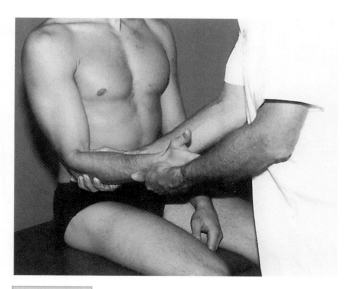

FIGURE 18.56

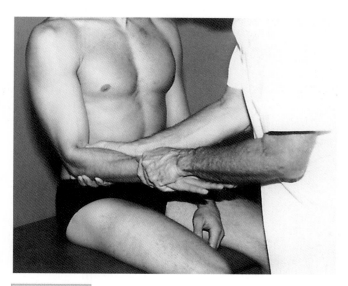

FIGURE 18.58

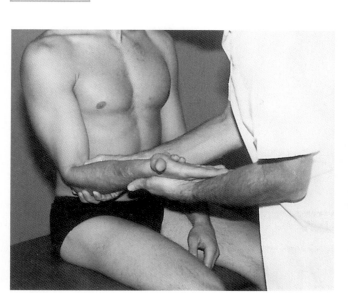

FIGURE 18.57

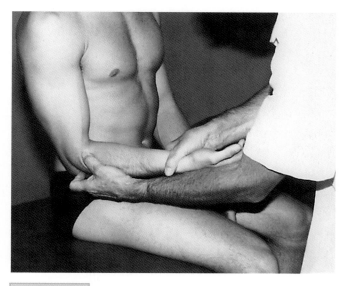

FIGURE 18.59

8. Treatment of restricted pronation has the operator's two hands in the same location but engages the pronation barrier (Fig. 18.60).

9. Patient performs three to five muscle contractions for 3 to 5 seconds against operator resistance.

10. Operator engages a new pronation barrier after each muscle contraction.

11. Retest.

Note: Restricted pronation and supination of the forearm combines the motion of the humeroradial, proximal radioulnar, and distal radioulnar articulations. Supination is the most common restriction.

ELBOW REGION

Diagnosis of Radial Head Dysfunction

Test 1: Palpation for asymmetry

1. Patient sits on the table, elbows flexed to 90 degrees, and the forearm supinated and supported in lap.

2. Operator stands in front and palpates the radial head posteriorly with the index fingers and the soft tissues anteriorly with the thumbs (Fig. 18.61).

3. Operator assesses the symmetric relationship of the radial head to the capitulum of humerus.

4. In addition to asymmetry, the dysfunctional side is usually tender with tension of the periarticular tissues.

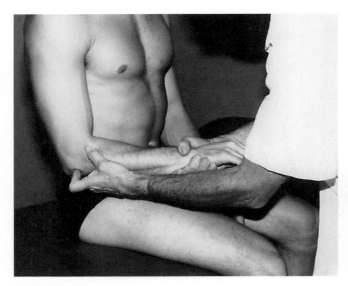

FIGURE 18.60

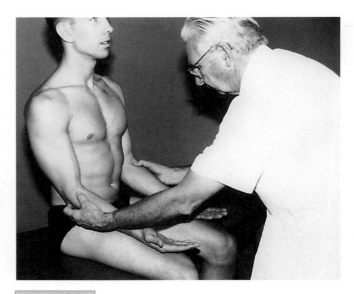

FIGURE 18.61

ELBOW REGION

Diagnosis of Radial Head Dysfunction

Test 2: Motion of the radial head

1. Patient sits on the table with the elbow flexed to 90 degrees.

2. Operator stands in front with the lateral hand palpating the radial head at the humeroradial articulation with the index finger posterior and the thumb anterior.

3. Operator's medial hand grasping the distal radius and ulna introduces supination (Fig. 18.62) and pronation (Fig. 18.63).

4. Comparison is made with the opposite side. In dysfunction, asymmetry is identified in the motion between the radial head and the capitulum.

ELBOW REGION

Diagnosis of Radial Head Dysfunction

Test 3: Motion test

1. Patient sits on the table with the forearms supinated.

2. Patient flexes and brings the elbows to the front of the chest with medial margins of the forearm and the hand approximated (Fig. 18.64).

3. Patient attempts to extend the elbows while maintaining the forearms together (Fig. 18.65).

4. Pronation of the forearm during the elbow extension identifies radial head dysfunction.

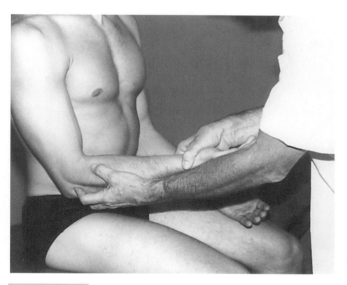

FIGURE 18.62

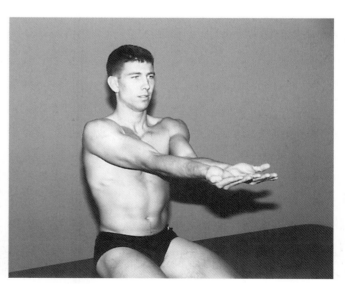

FIGURE 18.64

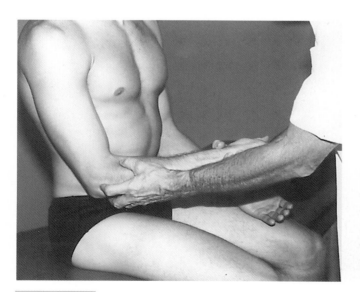

FIGURE 18.63

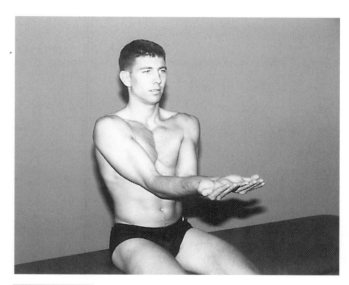

FIGURE 18.65

ELBOW REGION

Muscle Energy Technique

Diagnosis

Position: Radial head posterior

Motion Restriction: Supination

1. Patient sits on the table with the elbow flexed to 90 degrees.

2. Operator stands in front with the lateral hand supporting the proximal forearm and the index finger over the posterior aspect of the radial head.

3. Operator's medial hand grasps the distal forearm and introduces supination to the barrier (Fig. 18.66).

4. Patient pronates the hand against operator resistance for 3 to 5 seconds for three to five repetitions.

5. Operator engages a new supination barrier after each patient effort.

6. With the last patient muscle effort, an attempt is made to flex the elbow against resistance in addition to pronation.

7. Retest.

ELBOW REGION

Mobilization with Impulse Technique

Diagnosis

Position: Radial head posterior

Motion Restriction: Supination

1. Patient sits on the table.

2. Operator stands in front grasping the proximal forearm with the index finger of the lateral hand overlying the posterior aspect of the radial head (Fig. 18.67).

3. Operator controls the patient's distal forearm, hand, and wrist between the elbow and the chest wall.

4. Operator engages a barrier of extension, supination, and slight adduction (Fig. 18.68).

5. Operator performs mobilization with impulse thrust in a medial and anterior direction.

6. Retest.

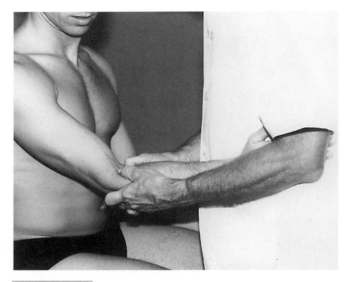

FIGURE 18.67

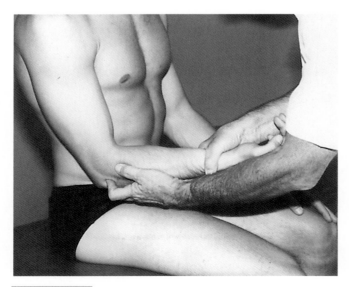

FIGURE 18.66

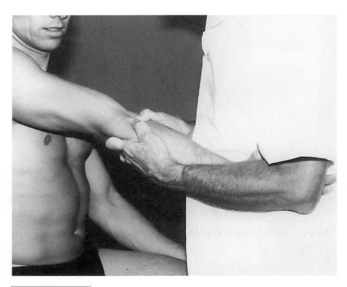

FIGURE 18.68

ELBOW REGION

Mobilization with Impulse Technique

Diagnosis

Position: Radial head anterior

Motion Restriction: Pronation

1. Patient stands or sits on the table.

2. Operator stands in front with the medial hand grasping the proximal forearm and the thumb of the lateral hand over the anterior aspect of the radial head (Fig. 18.69).

3. Operator pronates and flexes the patient's forearm while the thumb holds the radial head posteriorly (Fig. 18.70).

4. When a barrier is engaged, an increasing elbow flexion mobilization with impulse thrust is performed.

5. Retest.

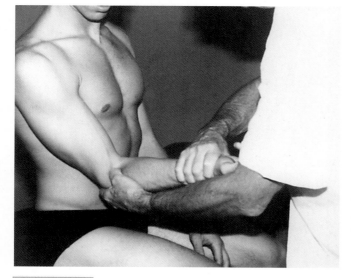

FIGURE 18.69

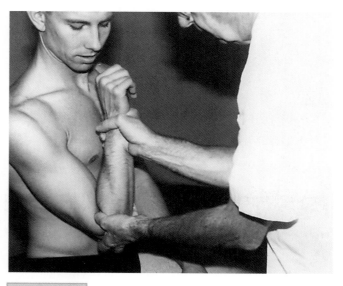

FIGURE 18.70

WRIST AND HAND REGION

Like the elbow, the wrist is not a single articulation but a combination of many. They include the radiocarpal joint with the distal radius articulating with the carpal scaphoid and lunate, the distal radioulnar joint, the ulnar-meniscal-triquetral joint, the intercarpal joint, the carpometacarpal joints, and the proximal and distal interphalangeal joints.[2] Movements at the wrist region include dorsiflexion, palmar flexion, adduction (ulnar deviation), abduction (radial deviation), and pronation and supination. Pronation and supination occur primarily at the distal radioulnar joint and are related to similar pronation–supination movement at the elbow region.

WRIST AND HAND REGION

Diagnosis

1. Patient sits on the table with the operator standing in front.

2. Patient's arms are at the side with elbows flexed to 90 degrees.

3. Operator introduces palmar flexion (Fig. 18.71), dorsiflexion (Fig. 18.72), ulnar deviation pronated (Fig. 18.73), pronated radial deviation (Fig. 18.74), supinated radial deviation (Fig. 18.75), and supinated ulnar deviation (Fig. 18.76), testing for restricted range of movement.

4. Muscle strength testing can be performed in the same directions.

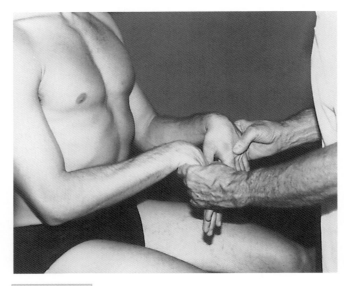

FIGURE 18.71

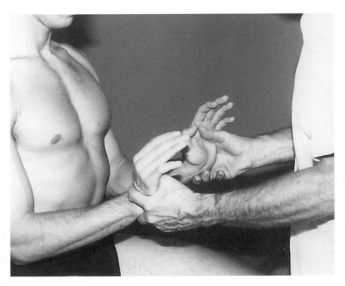

FIGURE 18.72

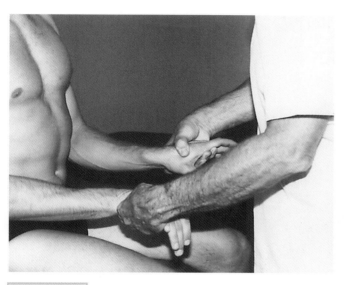

FIGURE 18.73

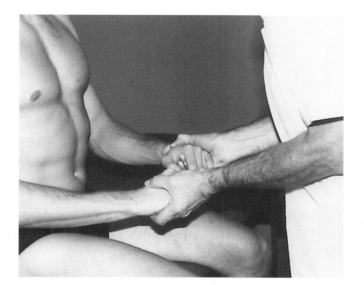

FIGURE 18.74

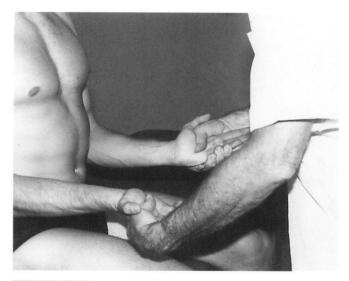

FIGURE 18.75

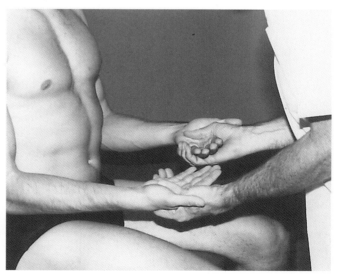

FIGURE 18.76

WRIST AND HAND REGION

Muscle Energy Technique

1. Patient sits on the table with the operator standing in front.

2. Operator's proximal hand stabilizes the patient's distal forearm while the distal hand engages the resistant barrier of the wrist and hand motion.

3. Operator engages resistant barriers in palmar flexion (Fig. 18.77), dorsiflexion (Fig. 18.78), pronated radial deviation (Fig. 18.79), pronated ulnar deviation (Fig. 18.80), supinated radial deviation (Fig. 18.81), and supinated ulnar deviation (Fig. 18.82).

4. Patient performs 3- to 5-second muscle contractions against operator resistance for three to five repetitions.

5. Operator engages a new barrier after each patient effort.

6. Retest.

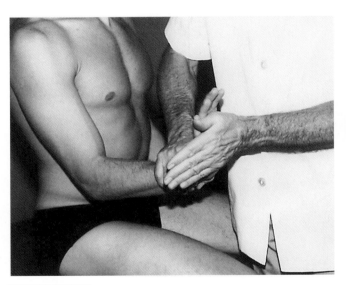

FIGURE 18.78

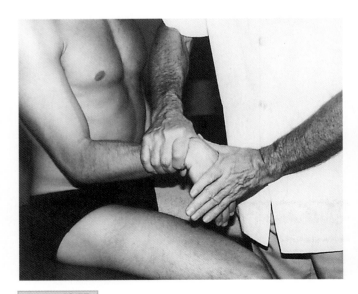

FIGURE 18.77

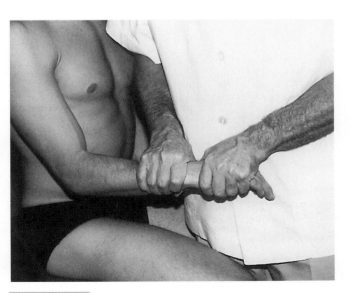

FIGURE 18.79

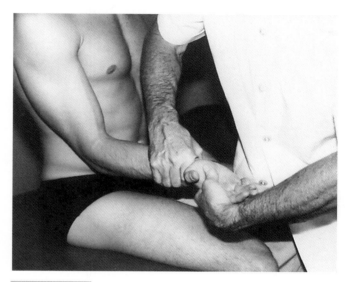

FIGURE 18.81

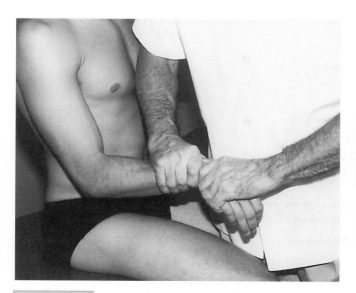

FIGURE 18.80

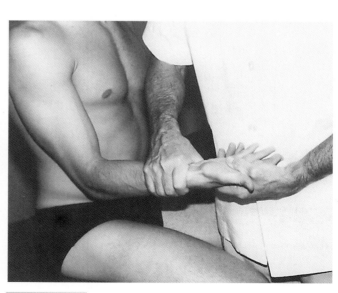

FIGURE 18.82

WRIST AND HAND REGION

Mobilization with Impulse Technique

1. Patient sits on the table with the operator standing in front.

2. Operator's hands grasp the patient's hand and wrist with the operator's thumbs contacting the dorsal aspect of the scaphoid and lunate (Fig. 18.83) and index fingers grasping the volar aspect of the scaphoid and lunate (Fig. 18.84).

3. Operator engages dorsiflexion barrier and applies mobilization with impulse thrust by taking the patient's wrist toward the floor (Fig. 18.85).

4. Operator engages palmar flexion barrier and provides a mobilization with impulse thrust by carrying the wrist toward the ceiling (Fig. 18.86).

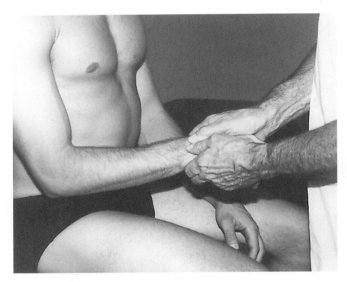

FIGURE 18.83

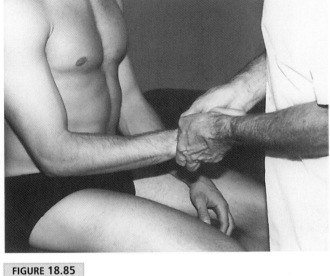

FIGURE 18.85

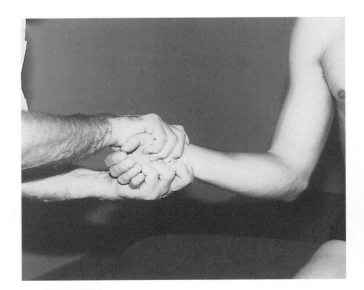

FIGURE 18.84

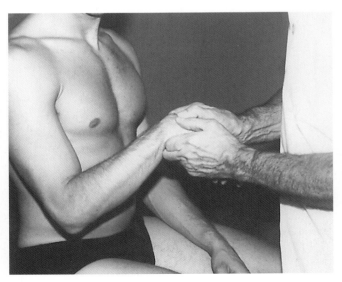

FIGURE 18.86

5. Operator engages radial deviation barrier and performs mobilization with impulse thrust while taking the wrist laterally (Fig. 18.87).

6. Operator engages ulnar deviation barrier and provides mobilization with impulse thrust by taking the wrist medially (Fig. 18.88).

7. Retest.

WRIST AND HAND REGION

Joint Play: Long-axis Extension

Radiocarpal Joint

1. Patient sits or stands on the table with the operator in front.

2. Operator's proximal hand stabilizes the patient's elbow flexed to 90 degrees.

3. Operator's distal hand grasps the radiocarpal joint just distal to the radial and ulnar styloid processes (Fig. 18.89).

4. Operator takes up long-axis extension to the barrier.

5. Operator performs a long-axis extension thrust by the distal hand.

6. Retest.

Note: This technique also performs joint play movement at the proximal radioulnar and humeroradial joints.

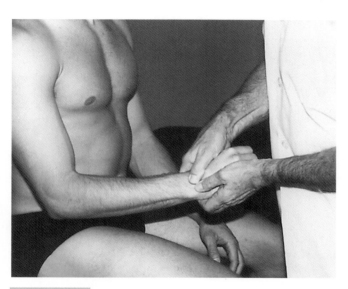

FIGURE 18.87

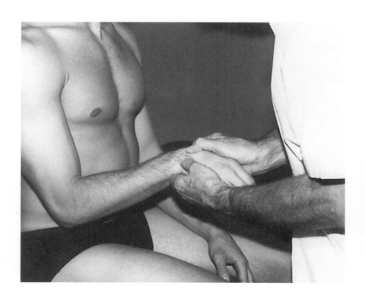

FIGURE 18.88

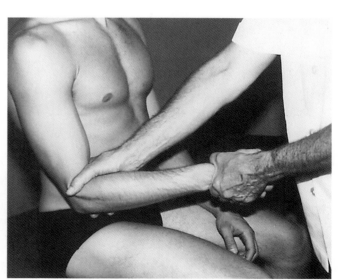

FIGURE 18.89

WRIST AND HAND REGION

Joint Play

Distal Radioulnar and Ulna-Meniscal-Triquetral Articulations

1. Patient stands or sits on the table with the operator in front.

2. Operator stabilizes the patient's hand and radiocarpal region by placing the index finger in the web of the patient's thumb (Fig. 18.90) and the thenar eminences and middle, ring, and little fingers grasping the distal radius and proximal carpals (Fig. 18.91).

3. Operator grasps the distal ulna between the thumb and pads of the fingers (Fig. 18.92).

4. Operator provides anteroposterior glide and medial and lateral rotary joint play movements of the distal ulna (Fig. 18.93).

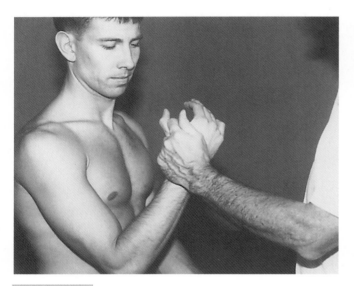

FIGURE 18.90

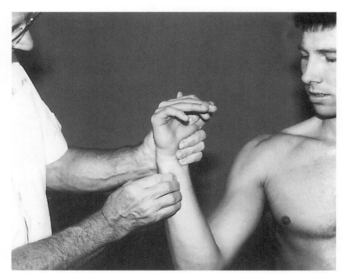

FIGURE 18.92

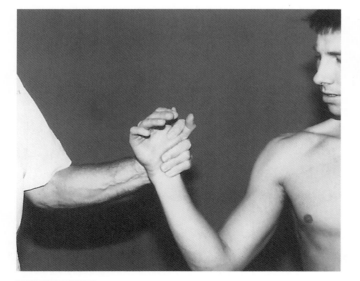

FIGURE 18.91

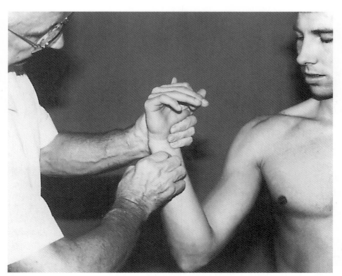

FIGURE 18.93

5. Using the same handhold to stabilize the distal radius and carpals, the operator places the right thumb over the dorsal surface of the distal ulna and the proximal interphalangeal joint of the right index finger over the pisiform bone (Fig. 18.94).

6. Operator squeezes the thumb and the index finger providing an anteroposterior glide joint play movement at the ulnar-meniscal-triquetral joint (Fig. 18.95).

7. The maneuver is a squeeze-and-release process through the operator's right hand.

8. Retest.

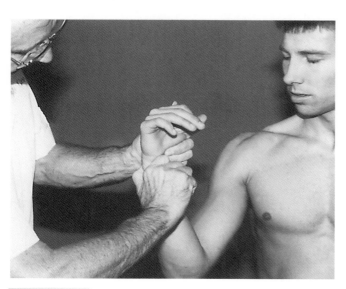

FIGURE 18.94

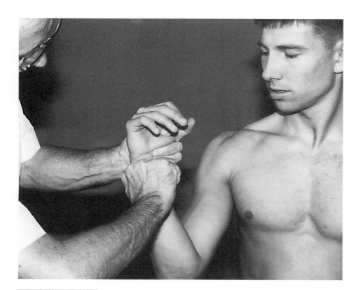

FIGURE 18.95

WRIST AND HAND REGION

Joint Play

Midcarpal Joint

1. Patient stands or sits on the table with the operator at the side.

2. Operator's proximal hand grasps the distal radius and ulna and the fingers contact the proximal row of the carpal bones.

3. Operator's distal hand controls the patient's hand and the distal row of the carpal bones.

4. Operator's knuckles of the index fingers and the thumbs of both hands are together.

5. Operator introduces approximately 15 degrees of palmar flexion to loose pack the midcarpal joint (Fig. 18.96).

6. While maintaining stability with the proximal hand, the distal hand moves toward the ceiling and to the floor providing an anteroposterior glide of the midcarpal joints.

7. Retest.

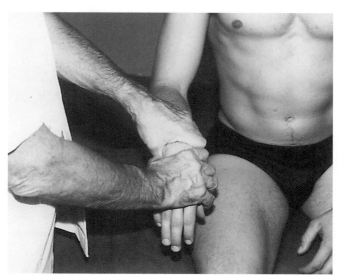

FIGURE 18.96

WRIST AND HAND REGION

Joint Play

Midcarpal Joint Dorsal Tilt

1. Patient stands or sits on the table with the operator standing in front.

2. Operator's right thenar eminence is placed transversely across the proximal crease of the patient's right wrist stabilizing the distal radius, ulna, and proximal row of carpals (Fig. 18.97).

3. Operator identifies the dorsal aspect of the head of the capitate by coursing the left index finger proximally between the shafts of the patient's second and third metacarpal bones (Fig. 18.98).

4. Operator places left pisiform over the head of the patient's capitate with the rest of the hand stabilizing the patient's hand (Fig. 18.99).

5. Operator's two arms are parallel with each other, and by moving both elbows medially, a joint play dorsal tilt of the head of the capitate is performed.

6. Retest.

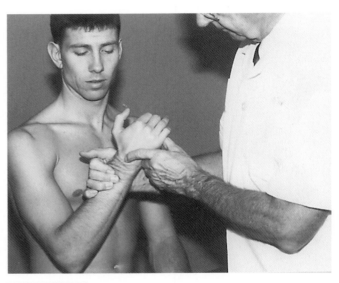

FIGURE 18.98

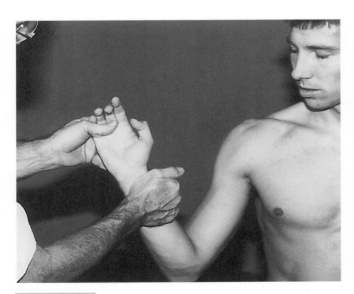

FIGURE 18.97

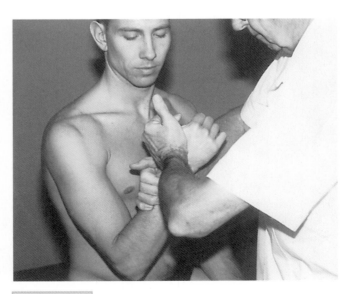

FIGURE 18.99

WRIST AND HAND REGION

Joint Play

First Carpometacarpal Joint

1. Operator's left hand stabilizes the patient's wrist and hand (Fig. 18.100).

2. Operator grasps the patient's thumb and first metacarpal bone, placing the operator's first metacarpals to the patient's (Fig. 18.101).

3. Operator performs joint play mobilizing thrust by tilting the right hand toward the patient (ulnar deviation), resulting in an anteroposterior tilt of the first carpometacarpal joint.

    Note: The operator's combined joint play movement is similar to using a "bottle cap opener."

4. Retest.

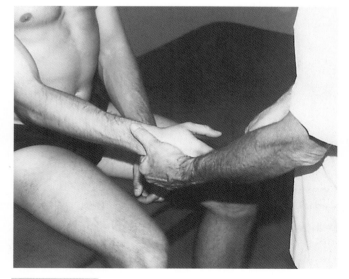

FIGURE 18.100

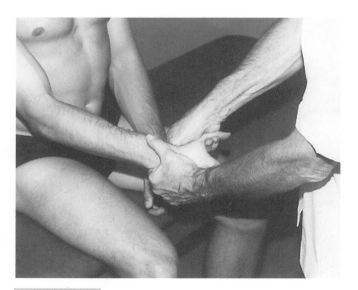

FIGURE 18.101

WRIST AND HAND REGION

Myofascial Release

1. Patient sits on the table with the operator standing in front.

2. Operator's two hands grasp the patient's hand with one hand holding the thumb (Fig. 18.102) and the other holding the ulnar side of the patient's hand (Fig. 18.103).

3. Operator's hand applies abduction and extension load to the thumb while the other hand introduces radioulnar deviation and palmar–dorsiflexion loads in a circular fashion, seeking direct and indirect barriers.

4. Operator localizes to individual carpal bones by contacting the dorsal surface with the tip of the thumb and the volar surfaces with the finger pads (Fig. 18.104).

5. Retest.

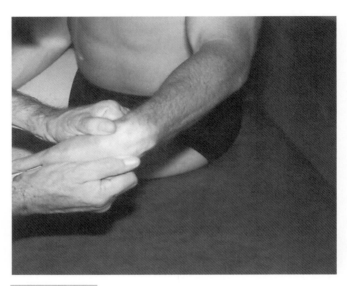

FIGURE 18.103

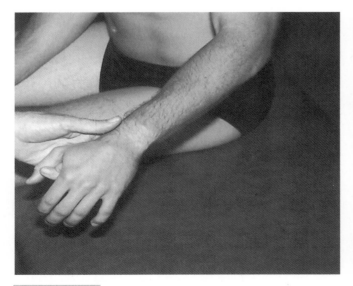

FIGURE 18.102

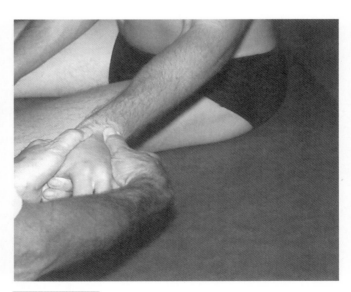

FIGURE 18.104

WRIST AND HAND REGION

Myofascial Release

Wrist Retinaculi (Carpal Tunnel Release)

1. Patient sits on the table with the operator standing in front.

2. Operator's two hands grasp the patient's hand with the thumbs over the lateral attachments of the wrist retinaculum (Fig. 18.105). The fingers overlie the dorsal aspect of the wrist.

3. Operator's hands introduce dorsiflexion of the patient's wrist (Fig. 18.106).

4. Operator applies lateral distraction load until release is achieved (Fig. 18.107).

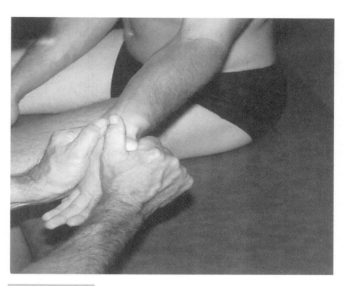

FIGURE 18.106

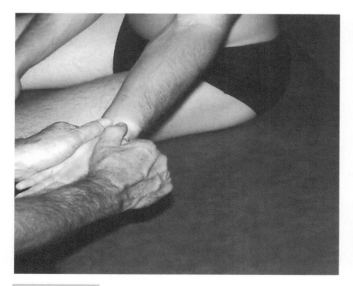

FIGURE 18.105

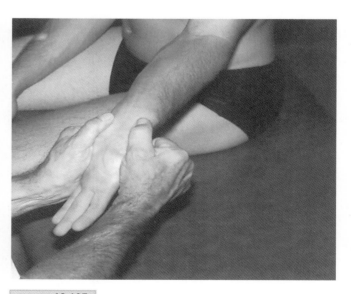

FIGURE 18.107

WRIST AND HAND REGION

Flexor Retinaculi and Flexor Tendons

1. Patient sits on the table with the operator standing in front.

2. Operator interlaces the fingers of both hands applying a thenar eminence contact across the distal radius and ulnar on the dorsal side and the wrist retinaculum on the volar side (Fig. 18.108).

3. Operator maintains anteroposterior compression over the wrist, while the patient actively flexes and extends fingers (Fig. 18.109).

4. Patient repeats flexion and extension efforts several times, mobilizing flexor tendons under the flexor retinaculum while the operator's hands maintain compression resulting in distraction.

5. Retest.

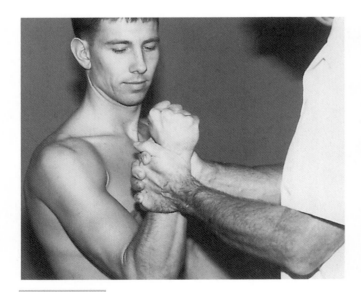

FIGURE 18.108

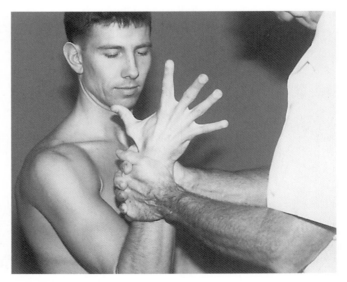

FIGURE 18.109

UPPER LIMB NEURAL TENSION TESTS AND DURAL MOBILIZATION

The work of Elvey[3-4] and Butler[5] has generated an interest in the upper and lower extremities neural tension tests and the use of these diagnostic maneuvers for dural mobilization. The peripheral nervous system has an extensive connective tissue interface that can be subjected to restriction, altered tension, and mobility. The diagnostic tests add another dimension to the neurologic tests of reflex testing, sensory examination, and muscular weakness (strength) testing. Restriction of the peripheral nervous system and its dura is frequently seen in association with somatic dysfunction of the vertebral complex from which the nerve roots emerge and course through the extremities. These maneuvers can be used as an additional activating force in mobilizing areas of somatic dysfunction. Although Butler does not describe the relationship of the peripheral tests and mobilizing procedures with the cranial dura, others knowledgeable about the craniosacral system have found that there is clearly an association, and the use of peripheral dural mobilizing procedures can profoundly influence the dural component of the craniosacral system.

In the upper extremity, there are three upper limb tension tests that are biased toward the median, radial, and ulnar distributions. When using the maneuvers therapeutically in the presence of restricted neural and dural mobility, a gentle on and off of the tension is applied. One does not attempt to "stretch" the nerve but enhance its mobility within its connective tissue.

UPPER LIMB TENSION TEST 1: MEDIAN NERVE BIAS

1. Patient is supine on the table with the operator standing at the side.

2. Operator's left hand depresses the patient's left shoulder to prevent elevation during abduction of the upper extremity by the operator's left thigh (Fig. 18.110).

3. Operator's right hand introduces external rotation of the humerus (Fig. 18.111) and supination of the forearm and wrist with extension of the fingers (Fig. 18.112).

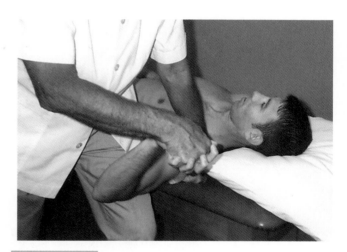

FIGURE 18.111

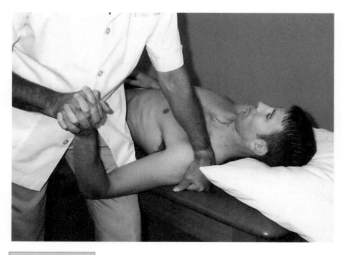

FIGURE 18.110

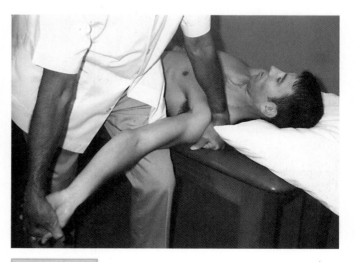

FIGURE 18.112

4. Operator extends the elbow (Fig. 18.113) sensing for restriction in tension and the initiation of painful discomfort in the arm.

5. Patient side bends the head to the left and assessment is again made to see if there is change in the arm symptom (Fig.18.114). Usually, the tension and discomfort are lessened.

6. Patient side bends the head to the right (Fig. 18.115) and assessment is made again. This maneuver usually enhances the sensation of tension and patient symptoms.

7. If used as a therapeutic maneuver, the on and off of elbow extension is done within the limits of the tension.

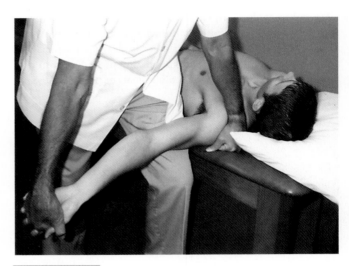

FIGURE 18.114

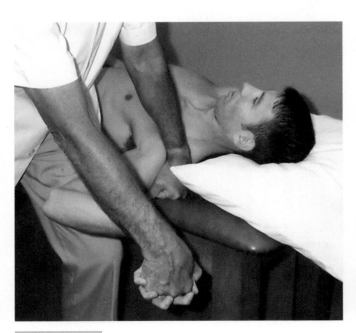

FIGURE 18.113

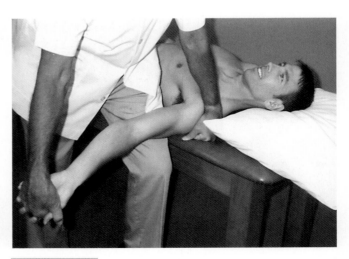

FIGURE 18.115

UPPER LIMB TENSION TEST 2: RADIAL NERVE BIAS

1. Patient is supine with the operator standing at the head of the table.

2. Patient's left arm is off the side of the table with the operator's right thigh stabilizing the patient's left shoulder to prevent elevation.

3. Operator's right hand holds the patient's arm and the left hand controls the left wrist (Fig. 18.116).

4. Operator's left hand flexes the patient's wrist and thumb and applies ulnar deviation (Fig. 18.117).

5. Operator abducts the arm with the elbow straight, sensitizing to the radial nerve distribution.

UPPER LIMB TENSION TEST 3: ULNAR NERVE BIAS

1. Patient is supine on the table with the operator standing at the side.

2. Operator stabilizes the shoulder and the arm at 90 degrees as in upper limb tension test 1 (Fig. 18.110).

3. Patient's wrist is extended, the forearm pronated, and the elbow flexed (Fig. 18.118).

4. Patient's shoulder is abducted directing the patient's left hand toward the left ear (Fig. 18.119).

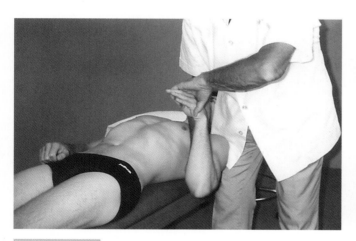

FIGURE 18.116

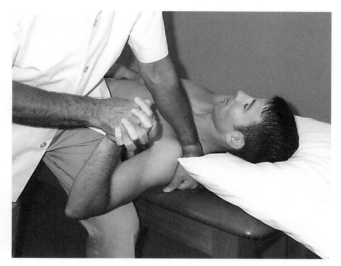

FIGURE 18.118

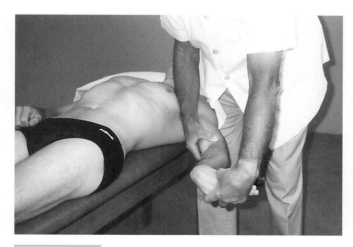

FIGURE 18.117

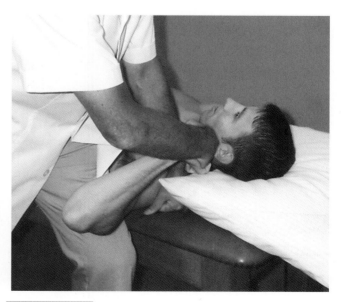

FIGURE 18.119

SUMMARY

Frequent complaints in the upper extremity include bursitis, tendonitis, epicondylitis, tennis elbow, golfer's elbow, carpal tunnel syndrome, and many others. Dysfunction in the symptomatic joint regions is commonly found as are proximal and distal dysfunctions. The examiner should always assess, and appropriately treat, any dysfunction in the trunk proximal to the extremity before addressing the extremity. The identification and appropriate treatment of dysfunctions within the entire upper extremity is helpful in the management of these patients.

REFERENCES

1. Mennell J McM. *Joint Pain*. Boston: Little, Brown and Company, 1964.
2. Mennell J McM. *The Musculoskeletal System: Differential Diagnosis from Symptoms and Physical Signs*. Gaithersburg, MD: Aspen Publishers, 1992.
3. Elvey RL. Brachial plexus tension tests and the pathoanatomical origin of arm pain. In: Glasgow EF, Twomey LT, Scull ER, Kleynhans AM, Idczak RM (Eds) *Aspects of Manipulative Therapy*, 2nd ed. Melbourne: Churchill Livingstone, 1985, pp. 116–122.
4. Elvey RL. Treatment of arm pain associated with abnormal branchial plexus tension. *Aust J Physiother* 1986;32:225–230.
5. Butler DS. *Mobilization of the Nervous System*. Melbourne: Churchill Livingstone, 1991.

The primary function of the lower extremity is ambulation. The complex interactions of the foot, ankle, knee, and hip regions provide a stable base for the trunk in standing and a mobile base for walking and running. Dysfunction in the lower extremities alters the functional capacity of the rest of the body, particularly the pelvic girdle. The screening examination (see Chapter 2) evaluated the lower extremities while standing and during walking, performing the squat test, the straight leg-raising test (for hamstring length), the standing flexion test, and the one-legged stork test. A positive finding of any of these screening tests requires that the examiner proceeds to further evaluation of the hip, knee, foot, and ankle. This chapter deals with the lower extremity from the hip to the distal regions. From the functional perspective, the lower extremity begins at the sacroiliac joint rather than the hip joint. The hip bone functions as a lower extremity bone during the walking cycle. Assessment of lower extremity function must include the pelvic girdle.

As with the upper extremities, evaluation should proceed from proximal to distal for several reasons. First, when considering the respiratory–circulatory model, it is appropriate to proceed from proximal to distal to enhance venous and lymphatic return. If edema and inflammation are part of the restrictive process, this sequence assists fluid movement. Second, proceeding from proximal to distal provides the examiner a point of reference for evaluating one bone in relation to another at an articulation. Structural examination of the lower extremities should be combined with standard orthopedic and neurologic tests and, particularly, some of the newer neural and dural tension signs found within the system of mobilization of the nervous system.[1] *The ultimate goal of evaluation and treatment of the lower extremities is to return the most symmetric walking cycle that is possible*. Anatomic variation in the bones of the lower extremity can result in the "short leg" and pelvic tilt syndromes that have clinical significance in somatic dysfunction of the vertebral column and pelvic girdle. Alteration in the mechanics of the foot with flattening of the medial, transverse, and lateral arches of the knee region, including the tibiofemoral and proximal tibiofibular articulations, and the hip may alter the function within the vertebral axis and pelvic girdle.

As with the upper extremity, several of Mennell's diagnostic and therapeutic joint play techniques are presented. A thorough study of that system is highly recommended and can be found in the publications by Mennell, including *Joint Pain, Foot Pain, and The Musculoskeletal System: Differential Diagnosis from Symptoms and Physical Signs*.[2–4]

HIP JOINT

The hip joint is a ball and socket articulation that has polyaxial movement. There is a cartilaginous lip surrounding the acetabulum, and the hip capsule is intimately related to the extensive musculature surrounding the hip joint. The hip joint movement includes flexion–extension, abduction–adduction, and internal rotation–external rotation. The musculature surrounding the hip joint can be divided into six groups, each responsible for one of the movement directions. In addition to dysfunction of muscle, there are joint play dysfunctions and capsular restrictions that need to be assessed and treated in order to achieve muscle balance surrounding the hip joint.

The balancing of the hip musculature is an important part of the treatment of the patient's musculoskeletal system, particularly those patients with lower back and lower extremity pain syndromes. Many experts debate the exact treatment sequence, but this author has found it most effective to treat shortness and tightness before treating weakness. Clinical observation finds that the short, tight group of muscles reflexly inhibits the antagonist, resulting in apparent weakness of the antagonist muscle. Once the shortness and tightness of the agonist are removed, the apparent weakness of the antagonist is no longer present frequently. If a muscle still appears to be functionally weak after treating the shortness and tightness of its antagonist, it should be treated for weakness using the techniques described. Muscle imbalance patterns are frequently seen in the six muscle groups. It is common to find the right adductors tight with apparent weakness of the left adductors and weakness of the right abductors. The psoas and rectus femoris muscles are frequently tight and need to be stretched so that appropriate hip extension can occur during the walking cycle. The imbalance of tightness and weakness between agonist and antagonist is consistent with the tight–loose concept found when using the myofascial release system of diagnosis and treatment.

HIP JOINT

Supine

Assessment of Hip Capsular Pattern

1. Patient is supine with the operator standing at the side of the table.

2. Operator's distal hand grasps the ankle region while the proximal hand controls the flexed hip and flexed knee.

3. Operator introduces circumduction in clockwise (Fig. 19.1) and counterclockwise directions (Fig. 19.2).

4. Operator increases the circumduction arc to see if the capsular pattern is smooth in all directions.

5. A positive finding is to have a hitch or delay in movement during the circumduction arc that is frequently reported by the patient as being pinching and painful.

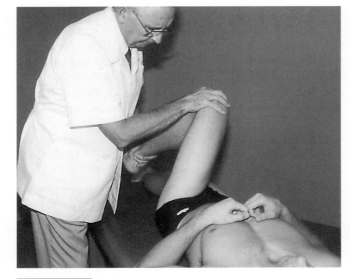

FIGURE 19.1

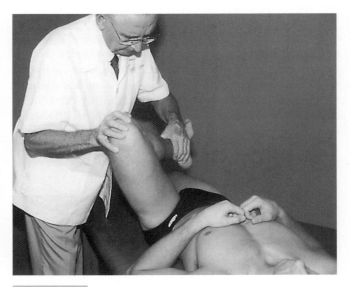

FIGURE 19.2

HIP JOINT

Supine

Joint Play

1. Patient is supine with the operator standing at the side of the table.

2. Operator flexes the patient's hip and knee to 90 degrees.

3. Operator drapes the flexed knee over the shoulder and grasps the anterior aspect of the proximal femur with interlaced hands.

4. When all slack is taken up, a mobilizing joint play distraction thrust is applied in a caudad direction by the two hands (Fig. 19.3).

5. Operator drapes the knee over the neck and with interlaced fingers grasping medial side of proximal femur.

6. When slack is taken out in a medial-to-lateral direction, a joint play thrust is applied in lateral distraction by the two hands (Fig. 19.4).

7. Reassess.

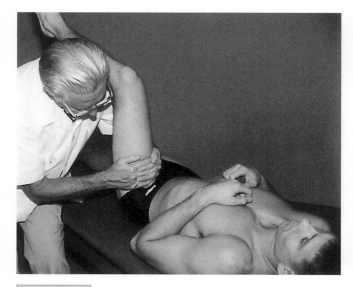

FIGURE 19.3

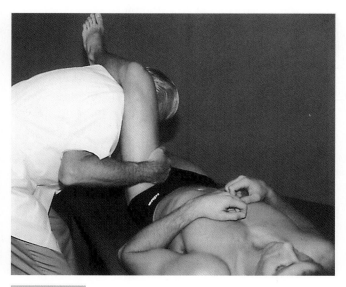

FIGURE 19.4

HIP JOINT

Supine

Acetabular Labrum Technique (Example: left hip)

1. Patient is supine with the operator standing at the side of the table.

2. Operator flexes the knee and hip and controls the left lower extremity with the left arm, axilla, and trunk.

3. Operator places the heel of the right hand against the lateral aspect of the patient's left greater trochanter (Fig. 19.5).

4. Operator applies a series of impaction compressive forces through the right arm in the direction of the femoral head and hip joint, while alternately providing an anteroposterior compressive force through the left arm contact, with some cephalic-to-caudad distraction as well.

5. Various degrees of adduction–abduction and internal–external rotation are used to fine-tune against the resistant barrier.

6. The activating force is mobilization without impulse.

7. Retest.

HIP JOINT

Prone

Mobilization of Anterior Capsule (Example: right hip)

1. Patient is prone with the operator standing at the side of the table.

2. Operator flexes the right knee and grasps the anterior aspect of the distal right femur with the right hand and arm.

3. Operator's left hand contacts the posterior aspect of the proximal right femur with the left arm fully extended (Fig. 19.6).

4. Operator gently lifts the right knee off the table and applies a series of mobilizing without impulse forces in an anterior direction against the proximal femur.

5. Operator fine-tunes against resistant barrier by internally and externally rotating the right femur and by applying medial and lateral directional forces through the left hand.

6. Retest.

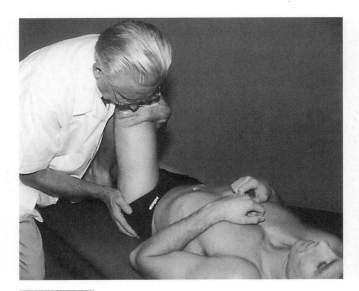

FIGURE 19.5

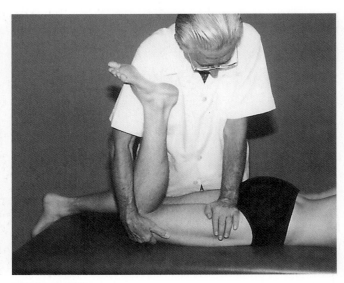

FIGURE 19.6

HIP JOINT

Supine

Mobilization of Posterior Hip Capsule (Example: right hip)

1. Patient is supine with the operator standing on the right side.

2. Operator's right hand is placed over the ischial tuberosity with the left hand controlling the flexed hip and knee (Fig. 19.7).

3. Operator abducts and adducts and internally and externally rotates the right hip against the restrictive barrier.

4. Operator's activating force is repetitive mobilization without impulse in a posterior direction through the shaft of the femur.

5. An alternate position has the operator on the left side of the patient and the patient's left hip bone on the edge of the table.

6. Operator's two hands on the patient's flexed left knee fine-tunes adduction–abduction and internal–external rotation against the barrier and then provides repetitive posterior mobilization without impulse through the shaft of the left femur (Fig. 19.8).

7. Reassess.

The primary dysfunctions of the hip joint are imbalances of length and strength of the six muscle groups. Structural diagnosis and muscle energy techniques for these muscle imbalances are as follows:

1. Operator passively takes the hip joint through a range of motion, evaluating quantity of range, quality of movement during the range, and quality of the end feel.

2. Comparison is made on the opposite side.

3. Asymmetry may be due to shortening of the muscle group on the restricted side or weakness of the contralateral muscle group with increased range.

4. Strength testing is performed by asking the patient to maximally contract the muscle against equal and opposite resistance, comparing one side to the other.

5. Treatment of short and tight muscle groups is achieved by a series of 3- to 5-second isometric contractions against the operator's equal and opposite resistance. After each patient effort, the operator engages the next resistant barrier with gradual lengthening of the shortened muscle by the principle of postisometric relaxation.

6. Treatment of functional weakness of a muscle group is accomplished by asking the patient to perform a series of 3- to 5-concentric isotonic contractions made through the total range of movement against an operator counterforce that is yielding in nature but with progressive increase in resistance with each effort.

7. Retest for length and strength of comparable muscle groups.

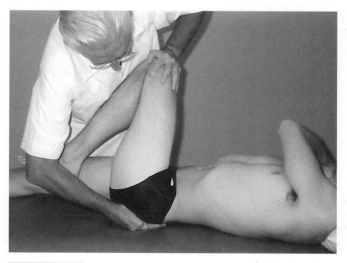

FIGURE 19.7

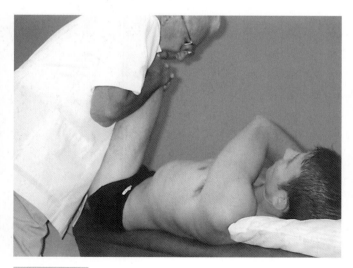

FIGURE 19.8

HIP JOINT

Muscle Energy Technique

Motion Tested: Abduction

Muscles Tested: Adductors (adductor magnus, adductor brevis, and adductor longus)

1. Patient is supine on the table with the operator standing at the end grasping the lower extremity at the ankle.

2. Operator abducts the extended lower extremity to the end point, evaluating total range and quality of movement during the range (Fig. 19.9). During motion testing, the operator prevents the extended leg from moving into external rotation.

3. Operator tests for adductor strength by offering resistance against the patient's extended leg with the knee fully extended. Operator's resistance is above the knee joint to protect the medial collateral ligament (Fig. 19.10).

4. Treat shortness or weakness as appropriate.

5. Retest.

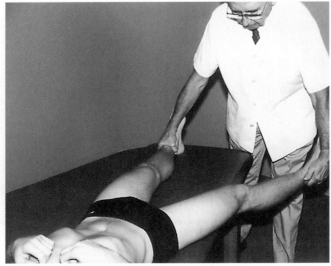

FIGURE 19.9

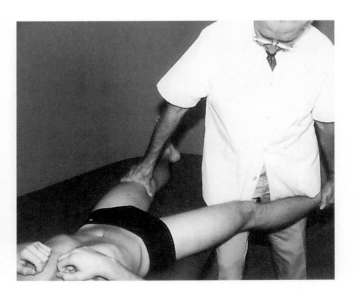

FIGURE 19.10

HIP JOINT

Muscle Energy Technique

Motion Tested: Adduction

Muscles Tested: Abductors (gluteus medius and gluteus minimus)

1. Patient is supine on the table with the operator standing at the end.
2. Operator adducts the extended leg across the front of the opposite leg, testing for range and quality of movement (Fig. 19.11).

3. Operator tests for strength by asking the patient to maximally abduct the leg against resistance offered by the operator holding the leg in the adducted position (Fig. 19.12).
4. Comparison is made with the opposite leg.
5. Treatment for shortness or tightness is accomplished as appropriate.
6. Retest.

Note: An alternate method is to lift the leg not being tested (Fig. 19.13) and adduct the extended leg being tested beneath it (Fig. 19.14). Testing in this position also evaluates the tensor fascia lata muscle.

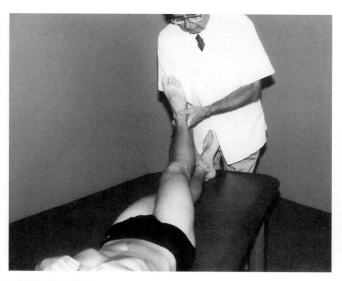

FIGURE 19.11

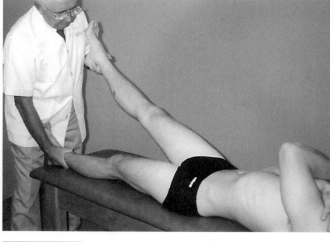

FIGURE 19.13

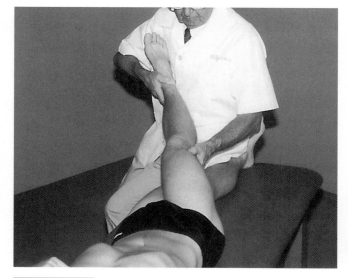

FIGURE 19.12

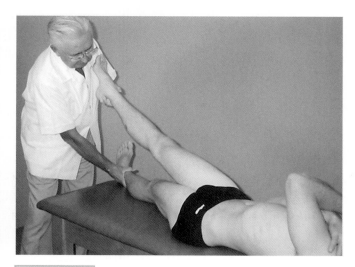

FIGURE 19.14

HIP JOINT

Muscle Energy Technique

Motion Tested: External rotation with hip flexed to 90 degrees

Muscles Tested: Internal rotators (gluteus medius and gluteus minimus)

1. Patient is supine on the table with the operator standing at the side next to the extremity being tested.

2. Operator holds the lower extremity with 90-degree flexion at both the hip and the knee (Fig. 19.15).

3. Operator externally rotates the femur by carrying the foot and ankle medially, evaluating range and quality of movement (Fig. 19.16).

4. Operator performs strength testing by having the patient internally rotate the femur against equal and opposite resistance (Fig. 19.17).

5. Comparison is made with the opposite side.

6. Shortness or weakness is treated as appropriate.

7. Retest.

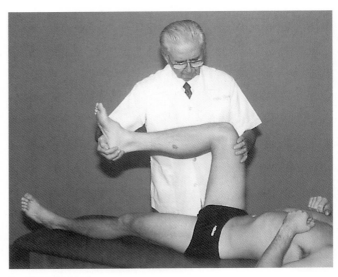

FIGURE 19.16

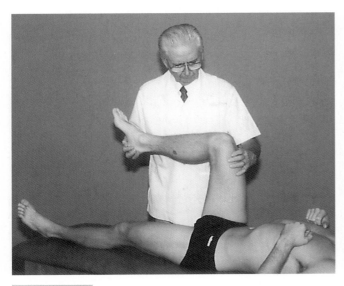

FIGURE 19.15

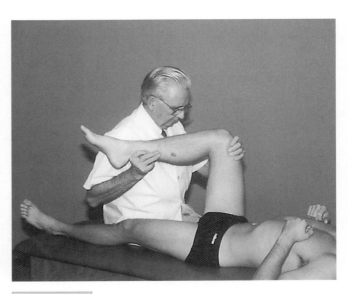

FIGURE 19.17

HIP JOINT

Muscle Energy Technique

Motion Tested: Internal rotation with hip flexed to 90 degrees

Muscles Tested: External rotators (primarily piriformis)

1. Patient is supine on the table with the operator standing at the side next to the extremity being tested.

2. Operator holds the lower extremity with 90-degree flexion at both the hip and the knee (Fig. 19.15).

3. Operator introduces internal rotation testing for range and quality of movement (Fig. 19.18).

4. Operator performs strength testing by asking the patient to externally rotate against the resistance offered by the operator (Fig. 19.19).

5. Comparison is made with the opposite side.

6. Shortness or tightness is treated as appropriate.

7. Retest.

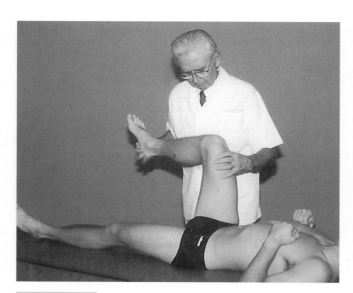

FIGURE 19.18

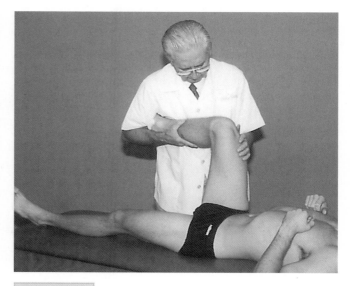

FIGURE 19.19

HIP JOINT

Muscle Energy Technique

Motion Tested: Partial hip flexion (straight leg raising)

Muscles Tested: Hip extensors, primarily hamstring muscles (semitendinosus, semimembranosus, and biceps femoris)

Note: Gluteus maximus and adductor magnus become hip extensors when thigh is flexed.

1. Patient is supine on the table with the operator standing at the side of the table.

2. Operator monitors anterior superior iliac spine on the side opposite the leg being tested.

3. Operator lifts the extended leg introducing hip flexion, testing for range and quality of movement with the end point being the first movement of the opposite anterior superior iliac spine (Fig. 19.20).

4. Shortness and tightness are treated by a series of isometric contractions against resistance with the patient's effort to pull the heel toward the buttock (Fig. 19.21).

Note: An alternative position has the patient hold the posterior aspect of the distal thigh, while the operator extends the knee and resists a knee flexion effort by the patient against the operator's resistance (Fig. 19.22).

5. Strength testing is performed by having the patient prone on the table with the operator resisting patient attempts at knee flexion in a bilateral fashion.

6. Weakness is treated by a series of concentric isotonic contractions through the full range of knee flexion against progressively increasing operator resistance.

7. Retest.

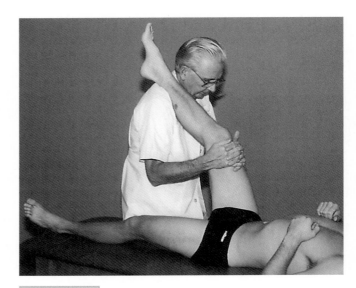

FIGURE 19.21

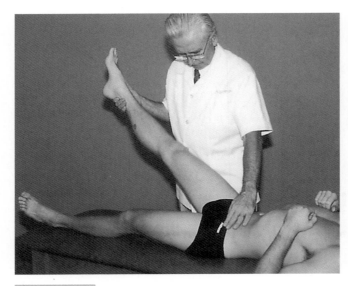

FIGURE 19.20

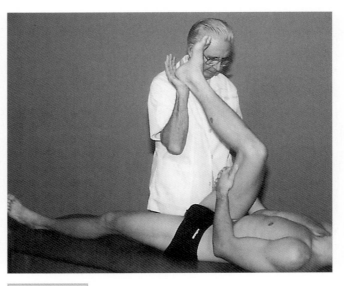

FIGURE 19.22

HIP JOINT

Muscle Energy Technique

Motion Tested: Hip extension

Muscle Tested: Iliopsoas

1. Patient is supine with the pelvis close to the end of the table so that lower extremity below the knee is free of the table.

2. Operator stands at the end of the table facing the patient.

3. Patient's hips and knees are flexed.

4. Patient holds the leg opposite that being tested in a flexed position while the operator passively extends the leg being tested (Fig. 19.23).

5. The normal range is for the back of the thigh to strike the table with the knee fully flexed (Fig. 19.24).

6. Patient performs strength testing by attempting to lift the knee to the ceiling against operator resistance.

7. Comparison is made with the opposite side.

8. Shortness is treated by isometric contraction against operator resistance. Patient is instructed to perform hip flexion. Operator also resists attempts at external rotation of the hip by offering a resistance with the leg against the medial side of the patient's foot and ankle (Fig. 19.25).

9. Weakness is treated by a series of concentric isotonic contractions of hip flexion and external rotation.

10. Retest.

Note: Before testing for length and strength of the iliopsoas, the lumbar spine should be evaluated and treated appropriately. This iliopsoas test puts stress on the lumbar spine, particularly the lumbosacral junction.

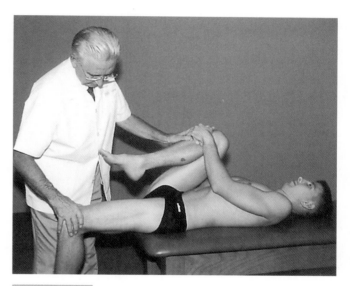

FIGURE 19.24

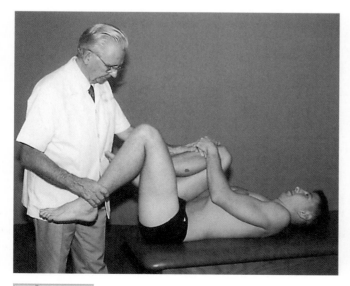

FIGURE 19.23

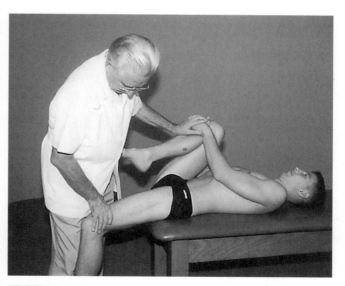

FIGURE 19.25

HIP JOINT

Muscle Energy Technique

Motion Tested: Knee flexion

Muscles Tested: Quadriceps group (rectus femoris, vastus lateralis, vastus intermedius, and vastus medialis)

1. Patient is prone on the table with the operator standing at the foot facing the patient.
2. Operator flexes both knees while holding the patient's ankles (Fig. 19.26).

3. Test is made for range and quality of movement.
4. Operator performs strength testing by asking the patient to extend the knees against resistance with both sides contracting simultaneously.
5. Shortness is treated by a series of isometric contractions against resistance (Fig. 19.27).
6. Weakness is treated by a series of concentric isotonic contraction against progressively increasing operator resistance.
7. Retest.

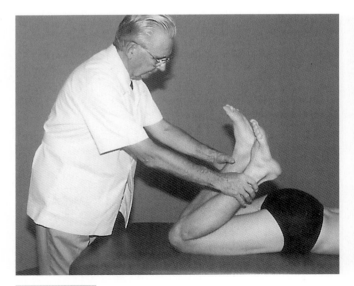

FIGURE 19.26

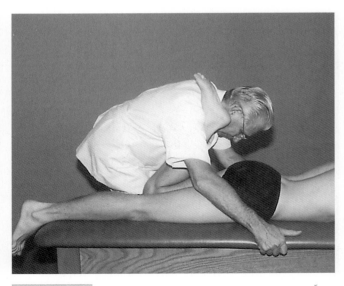

FIGURE 19.27

HIP JOINT

Muscle Energy Technique

Motion Tested: Internal rotation with hips in neutral

Muscles Tested: External rotators (obturator internus, obturator externus, gemellus superior, gemellus inferior, quadratus femoris, and piriformis)

1. Patient is prone on the table with the operator standing at the foot of the table facing the patient.

2. Operator flexes the patient's knees to 90 degrees (Fig. 19.28).

3. Operator tests for range and quality of internal rotation by allowing the feet to drop laterally (Fig. 19.29).

4. Operator performs strength testing by asking the patient to bilaterally pull the feet together against resistance.

5. Shortness is treated by the operator holding the opposite leg with the knee flexed and hip internally rotated, while the patient performs external rotation of the leg in the 90-degree flexed position against operator resistance (Fig. 19.30).

6. Weakness is treated by a series of concentric isotonic contractions through a range of external rotation with the knee at 90 degrees.

7. Retest.

Note: This muscle group is intimately attached to the posterior hip capsule and frequently needs attention with an .altered hip capsular pattern.

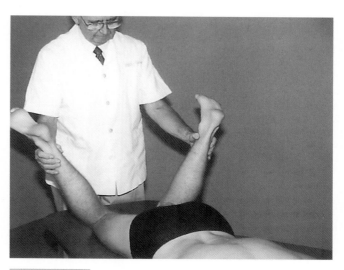

FIGURE 19.29

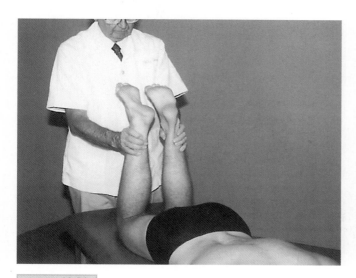

FIGURE 19.28

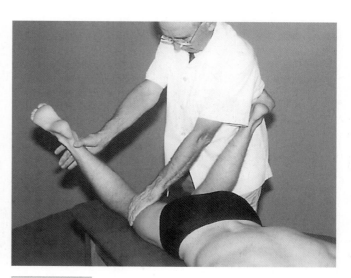

FIGURE 19.30

HIP JOINT

Muscle Energy Technique

Motion Tested: External rotation with the hips at neutral

Muscles Tested: Internal rotators (gluteus medius, gluteus minimus, and tensor fascia lata)

1. Patient is prone on the table with the operator standing at the foot facing the patient.

2. Operator stabilizes the leg opposite the one being tested with slight knee flexion and hip external rotation.

3. The leg being tested is flexed to 90 degrees and externally rotated looking for range and quality of movement (Fig. 19.31).

4. The opposite side is tested in a similar manner (Fig. 19.32).

5. Operator performs strength testing by asking the patient to internally rotate against resistance.

6. Shortness and tightness are treated by a series of isometric contractions of internal rotation against resistance (Fig. 19.33).

7. Weakness is treated by a series of concentric isotonic contractions against increasing operator resistance.

8. Retest.

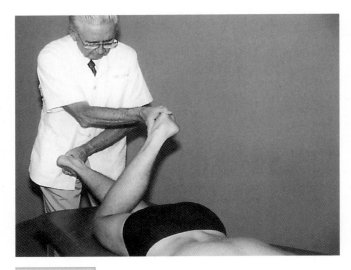

FIGURE 19.32

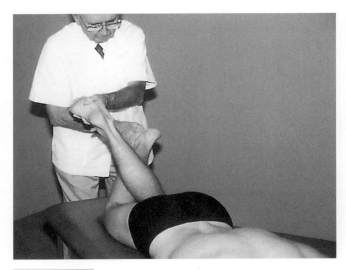

FIGURE 19.31

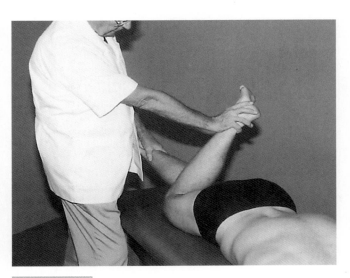

FIGURE 19.33

KNEE JOINT

The primary movement at the knee joint is flexion and extension of the tibia under the femur. The lengths of the medial and lateral femoral condyles are different resulting in an internal–external rotational component to the flexion–extension arc. During extension, the tibia rotates externally, and during flexion, the tibia rotates internally. Dysfunction of the internal–external rotation interferes with normal flexion–extension. The flexion–extension and the internal–external rotation movements depend on a small anteroposterior glide and medial-to-lateral gapping of the opposing joint surfaces. These minor joint play movements are present within the constraints of normal ligamentous stability. The movements are increased when there is ligamentous or cartilage damage within the knee. *The primary somatic dysfunctions of the knee joint are at the medial meniscus and the internal–external rotation of the tibia on the femur.*

KNEE JOINT

Supine

Medial Meniscus Technique

Mobilization without Impulse

1. Patient is supine on the table with the operator standing at the side near the dysfunctional knee.

2. Operator holds the patient's distal leg between the upper arm and chest with both hands surrounding the proximal tibia.

3. Operator's thumbs are placed over the medial joint space with the knee in flexion (Fig. 19.34).

4. Operator's lateral hand exerts a medial compression on the distal femur, while the operator's thumbs maintain posterolateral compressive force on the medial meniscus and the leg is carried into extension (Fig. 19.35).

5. Several repetitions of this procedure may be necessary to release restriction of the medial meniscus.

6. Retest.

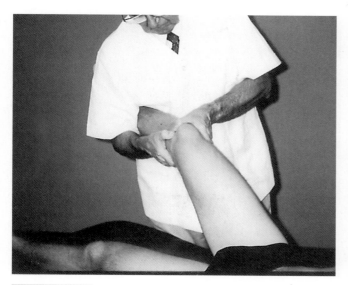

FIGURE 19.34

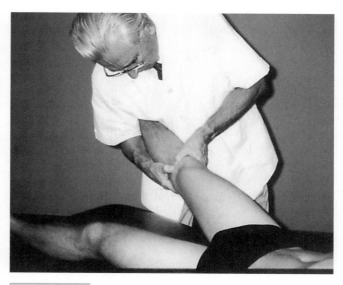

FIGURE 19.35

KNEE JOINT

Supine

Medial and Lateral Meniscus Technique

Mobilization without Impulse Technique

1. Patient is supine on the table with the operator standing at the caudal end facing the patient.

2. Operator supports the patient's dysfunctional leg between the thighs over the edge of the table.

3. Operator's hands grasp the proximal tibia with the thumbs over the anteromedial or anterolateral joint space depending on whether the restriction is of the lateral or medial malleolus (Fig. 19.36).

4. For medial meniscus dysfunction, the operator performs a circumduction movement beginning in flexion, including medial translation with thumb compression over the medial meniscus, while carrying the knee into full extension (Fig. 19.37).

5. For restriction of the lateral meniscus, the operator places the thumbs over the anterolateral aspect of the knee. The circumduction movement begins in flexion and includes lateral translation while carrying the distal leg into extension.

6. Several repetitions may be necessary.

7. Retest.

Note: Restriction of the medial meniscus is much more common than restriction of the lateral meniscus.

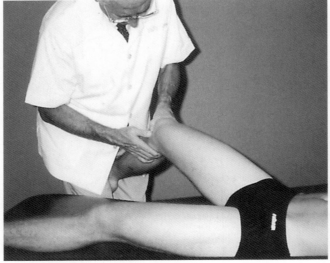

FIGURE 19.36

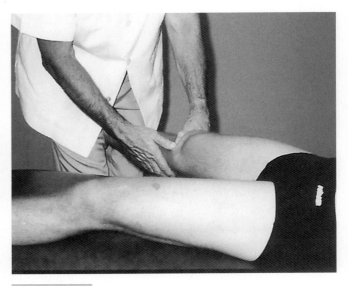

FIGURE 19.37

KNEE JOINT

Supine

Medial and Lateral Meniscal Tracking

Joint Play

1. Patient is supine on the table with the operator standing at the side closest to the dysfunctional knee.

2. Operator controls the dysfunctional leg at 90-degree hip and 90-degree knee flexion positions with the distal hand controlling dorsiflexion of the ankle for close packing, while the proximal hand controls the distal femur with the thumb over the lateral meniscus and the index and middle fingers over the medial meniscus (Fig. 19.38).

3. Operator medially and laterally rotates the tibia through the close-packed ankle joint with progressive extension of the hip and the knee (Fig. 19.39).

4. Several repetitions are necessary. The amount of medial and lateral rotation gradually decreases as the knee extends.

5. Retest.

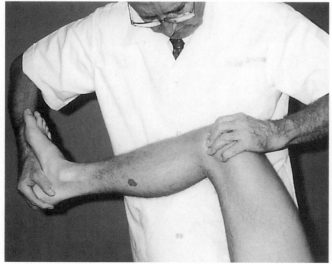

FIGURE 19.38

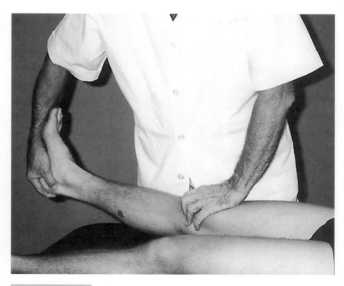

FIGURE 19.39

KNEE JOINT

Supine

Extension Compression Test

1. Patient is supine on the table with the operator standing at the side of the dysfunctional leg.

2. Operator's proximal hand stabilizes the distal femur.

3. Operator's distal hand grasps the patient's heel (Fig. 19.40).

4. Operator carries the distal leg into increased extension at the knee against the stabilizing proximal hand.

5. Comparison is made with the opposite side.

6. Restriction of extension with pain provocation is a positive test and indicates restriction of external rotation and extension of the knee joint or meniscal injury.

KNEE JOINT

Sitting

Diagnosis

Restriction of Internal–External Rotation

1. Patient sits on the edge of the table with the lower legs dangling and the operator sitting in front of the patient.

2. Operator grasps the feet and dorsiflexes the ankle to close-pack position.

3. Operator introduces external rotation (Fig. 19.41) and internal rotation (Fig. 19.42), testing for range, quality of range, and end feel.

4. Operator performs strength testing by asking the patient to internally and externally rotate the tibia against resistance.

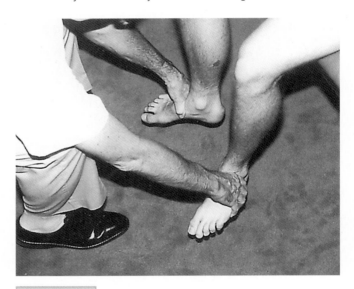

FIGURE 19.41

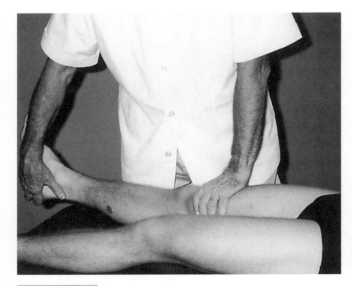

FIGURE 19.40

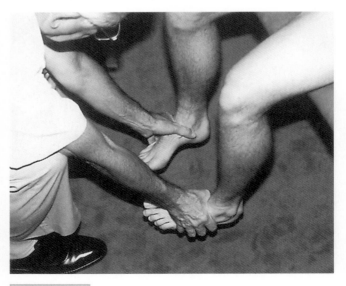

FIGURE 19.42

KNEE JOINT

Sitting

Muscle Energy Technique

Diagnosis

Position: Tibia internally rotated

Motion Restriction: External rotation of tibia

1. Patient sits on the edge of the table with the lower legs dangling and the operator sitting in front of the patient.

2. Operator grasps the heel of the foot in one hand and forefoot in the other.

3. Operator dorsiflexes the foot at the ankle and introduces external rotation to the barrier (Fig. 19.43).

4. Patient internally rotates the forefoot against the operator resistance for 3 to 5 seconds and three to five repetitions.

5. After each patient effort, the operator externally rotates the tibia to the new barrier.

6. Retest.

KNEE JOINT

Sitting

Muscle Energy Technique

Diagnosis

Position: Tibia externally rotated

Motion Restriction: Internal rotation of the tibia

1. Patient sits on the edge of the table with the lower legs dangling and the operator sitting in front of the patient.

2. Operator grasps the heel of the foot in one hand and the forefoot in the other.

3. Operator dorsiflexes the foot at the ankle and introduces internal rotation to barrier (Fig. 19.44).

4. Operator externally rotates the forefoot against operator resistance for 3 to 5 seconds and three to five repetitions.

5. Following each patient effort, the operator internally rotates the tibia to the new barrier.

6. Retest.

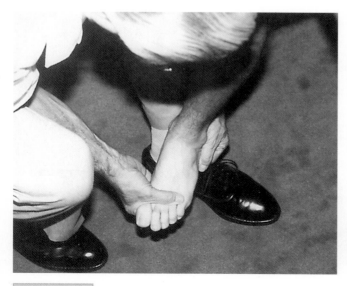

FIGURE 19.43

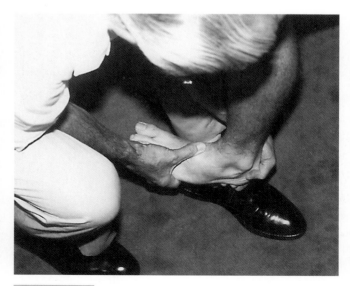

FIGURE 19.44

KNEE JOINT

Prone

Muscle Energy Technique

Diagnosis of Internal–External Rotation

1. Patient is prone on the table with the knees flexed to 90 degrees and the operator standing at the end of the table grasping each foot in each hand.

2. Operator introduces dorsiflexion of the ankle and externally rotates (Fig. 19.45) and internally rotates the tibia (Fig. 19.46), testing for range, quality of range, and end feel.

3. Operator performs strength testing by asking the patient to internally or externally rotate the foot against resistance offered by the operator.

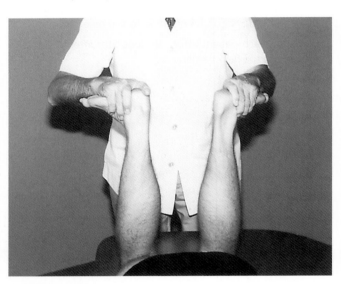

FIGURE 19.45

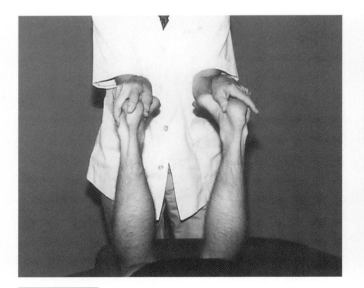

FIGURE 19.46

KNEE JOINT

Prone

Muscle Energy Technique

Diagnosis: Tibia internally rotated

Motion Restriction: External rotation of the tibia

1. Patient is prone on the table with the operator standing on the side of the dysfunctional extremity.

2. Operator flexes the knee to 90 degrees and grasps the heel and the forefoot in each hand.

3. Operator dorsiflexes the ankle and externally rotates the foot to barrier (Fig. 19.47).

4. Patient internally rotates forefoot against operator resistance for 3 to 5 seconds and three to five repetitions.

5. Following each patient effort, the operator externally rotates the foot to the new barrier.

6. Retest.

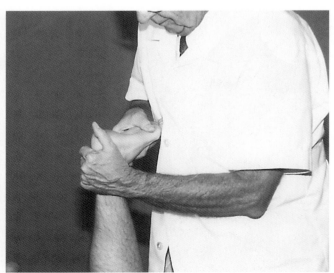

FIGURE 19.47

KNEE JOINT

Prone

Muscle Energy Technique

Diagnosis

Position: Tibia externally rotated

Motion Restriction: Internal rotation of tibia

1. Patient is prone on the table with the operator standing at the side of the dysfunctional extremity.

2. Operator flexes the knee to 90 degrees and grasps the heel and the forefoot of patient.

3. Operator dorsiflexes the ankle and internally rotates the tibia to the barrier (Fig. 19.48).

4. Patient externally rotates the forefoot against operator resistance for 3 to 5 seconds and three to five repetitions.

5. Following each patient effort, the operator internally rotates the foot to the new barrier.

6. Retest.

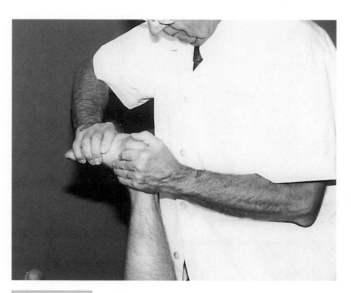

FIGURE 19.48

PROXIMAL TIBIOFIBULAR JOINT

This articulation is intimately related to the knee joint and is equally important in its relation to the ankle. The proximal tibiofibular joint has an anteroposterior glide and is influenced by the action of the biceps femoris muscle inserting at the fibular head. The proximal tibiofibular joint can be restricted either anteriorly or posteriorly. Restoration of the normal anteroposterior glide and its normal relationship to the tibia are the goals of the treatment.

Restoration of normal internal–external rotational movement of the tibia on the femur is accomplished before addressing the proximal tibiofibular joint.

The plane of the joint is approximately 30 degrees from lateral to medial and from anterior to posterior. Testing for the anteroposterior movement of the proximal tibiofibular joint must be within the plane of the joint and can be accomplished with the patient in the supine or sitting position.

PROXIMAL TIBIOFIBULAR JOINT

Testing for Anteroposterior Glide

1. Patient sits on the table with both feet flat for fixation (Fig. 19.49) or the patient sits on the edge of the table with the operator sitting in front holding the medial sides of both feet together (Fig. 19.50).

2. Operator grasps the proximal fibula between the thumb or thenar eminence and *the fingers of each hand being careful not to compress the peroneal nerve against the fibular head.*

3. Operator translates the fibular head anteriorly and posteriorly within the plane of the joint, testing for comparable range on each side, the quality of movement, and end feel.

4. A fibular head that resists anterior translatory movement is positionally a *posterior fibular head*, and a fibular head that resists posterior translatory is positionally an *anterior fibular head*.

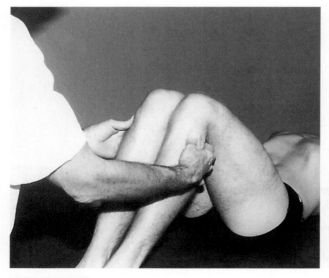

FIGURE 19.49

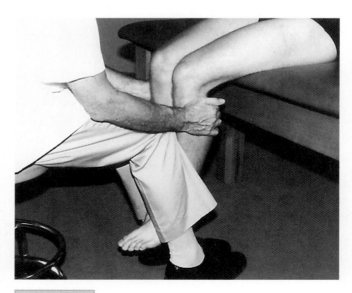

FIGURE 19.50

PROXIMAL TIBIOFIBULAR JOINT

Sitting

Muscle Energy Technique

Diagnosis

Position: Posterior fibular head

Motion Restriction: Anterior glide of the fibular head

1. Patient sits on the edge of the table with the dysfunctional leg dangling and the operator sitting in front with the medial hand grasping the patient's forefoot.

2. Operator inverts and internally rotates the patient's foot while the lateral hand exerts an anterolateral force on the posterior aspect of the fibular head (Fig. 19.51).

3. Patient is instructed to evert and dorsiflex the foot against resistance offered by the operator's medial hand for 3 to 5 seconds and three to five repetitions.

4. Operator engages a new barrier after each patient effort.

5. Retest.

PROXIMAL TIBIOFIBULAR JOINT

Sitting

Muscle Energy Technique

Diagnosis

Position: Anterior fibular head

Motion Restriction: Posterior glide of the fibular head

1. Patient sits on the edge of the table with the dysfunctional leg dangling and the operator sitting in front with the medial hand grasping the patient's forefoot.

2. Operator inverts and externally rotates the patient's foot, while the lateral thumb exerts a posteromedial force against the anterior aspect of the fibular head (Fig. 19.52).

3. Patient everts and plantar flexes the foot against operator resistance for 3 to 5 seconds and three to five repetitions.

4. Operator engages a new barrier after each patient effort.

5. Retest.

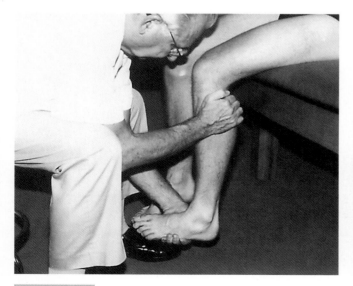

FIGURE 19.51

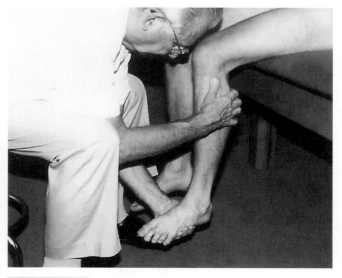

FIGURE 19.52

PROXIMAL TIBIOFIBULAR JOINT

Supine

Mobilization With Impulse Technique

Diagnosis

Position: Posterior fibular head

Motion Restriction: Anterior glide of fibular head

1. Patient is supine on the table with the operator standing at the side of the dysfunction with the caudal hand controlling the patient's foot and ankle.

2. Operator's cephalic hand supports the flexed knee with the metacarpophalangeal joint of the index finger posterior to the fibular head (Fig. 19.53).

3. Operator engages barrier by externally rotating the flexed knee and pinching the metacarpophalangeal joint between the distal femur and the fibular head.

4. Operator performs a mobilization with impulse thrust by exaggerating the knee flexion bringing the fibular head anterior (Fig. 19.54).

5. Retest.

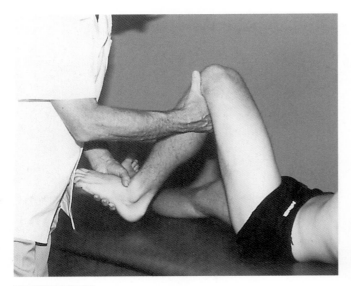

FIGURE 19.53

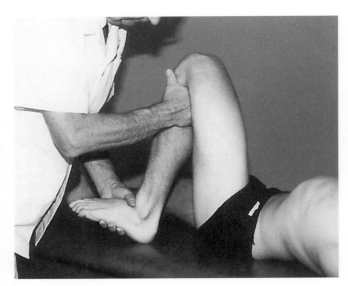

FIGURE 19.54

PROXIMAL TIBIOFIBULAR JOINT

Prone

Mobilization With Impulse Technique

Diagnosis

    Position: Posterior fibular head

    Motion Restriction: Anterior glide of the fibular head

1. Patient is prone on the table with the operator standing at the side of the dysfunction with the distal hand controlling the foot and ankle.

2. Operator's proximal hand is laid over the popliteal space with the metacarpophalangeal joint of the index finger posterior to the fibular head (Fig. 19.55).

3. Operator's knee is flexed pinching the metacarpophalangeal joint between the fibular head and the femur.

4. The barrier is engaged by slight external rotation of the leg and flexion of the knee and the operator performs a mobilization with impulse thrust by exaggerating knee flexion (Fig. 19.56).

5. Retest.

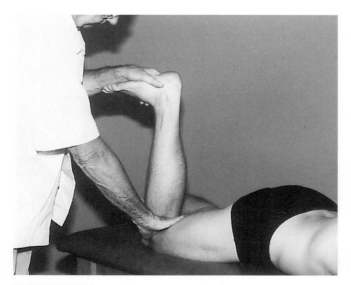

FIGURE 19.55

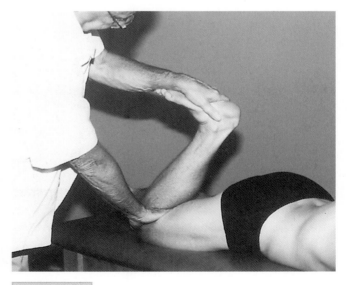

FIGURE 19.56

PROXIMAL TIBIOFIBULAR JOINT

Supine

Mobilization With Impulse Technique

Diagnosis

Position: Anterior fibular head

Motion Restriction: Posterior glide of the fibular head

1. Patient is supine on the table with the operator standing at the side of the dysfunction.

2. Operator's distal hand controls the lower leg in knee extension and internally rotates to approximately 30 degrees.

3. The thenar eminence of the operator's proximal hand is placed over the anterior aspect of the proximal fibula (Fig. 19.57).

4. Operator engages the barrier of the anteroposterior motion of the fibular head by downward compression through the extended arm.

5. When the barrier is engaged, the operator performs a mobilization with impulse thrust by dropping the body weight of the operator through the extended arm onto the anterior aspect of the fibular head.

6. Retest.

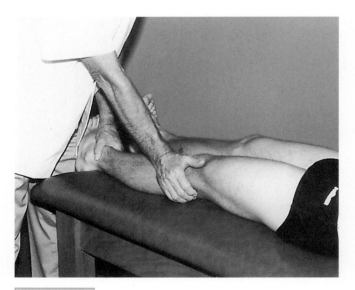

FIGURE 19.57

ANKLE REGION

The ankle region consists of the distal tibiofibular articulation, the articulation of the superior aspect of the talus with the tibiofibular joint mortise, and the talocalcaneal (subtalar) articulation. Although the talocalcaneal joint is frequently classified as being in the foot, it is the key to functional movement of the talus. Talar restriction, from either above or below, significantly restricts ankle motion. The talus is of interest because it has no direct muscular attachments. Its movement is determined by the muscle action on the bones above and below. Dysfunction of the talus at the tibiofibular joint mortise is one of the most common dysfunctions in the lower extremity. Another important anatomic feature of the talus is that its superior surface is wedge-shaped, with the posterior aspect being narrower than the anterior, as it articulates with the tibiofibular joint mortise. The ankle is more stable when dorsiflexed than when plantar flexed. The most common dysfunction at this joint is restricted dorsiflexion.

The distal tibiofibular joint is quite stable and does not have a synovial capsule. It is infrequently dysfunctional. The distal tibiofibular joint is associated with the function of the proximal tibiofibular articulation. Appropriate treatment at the proximal tibiofibular articulation frequently restores function at the distal tibiofibular articulation. Appropriate evaluation and treatment of the proximal and distal tibiofibular articulations should be performed before addressing the talotibiofibular mortise articulation.

ANKLE REGION: DISTAL TIBIOFIBULAR JOINT

Supine

Diagnosis: Distal tibiofibular dysfunction

1. Patient is supine on the table with the operator standing at the foot with the medial hand grasping the posterior and medial aspects of the patient's ankle and heel.

2. Operator's lateral hand grasps the lateral malleolus between the thumb and index finger (Fig. 19.58).

3. Operator's right hand glides the lateral malleolus anteriorly and posteriorly against the fixed foot and ankle.

4. Restriction of anterior movement is a posterior distal tibiofibular joint, and restriction of posterior movement is an anterior distal tibiofibular joint.

5. Comparison is made with the opposite side.

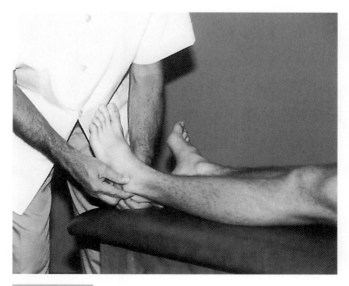

FIGURE 19.58

ANKLE REGION: DISTAL TIBIOFIBULAR JOINT

Supine

Mobilization With Impulse Technique

Diagnosis

Position: Anterior distal tibiofibular joint

Motion Restriction: Posterior movement of the lateral malleolus

1. Patient is supine on the table with the operator standing at the foot.

2. Operator's medial hand grasps the patient's heel and maintains the ankle at 90-degree flexion. The thumb is placed over the anterior aspect of the lateral malleolus (Fig. 19.59).

3. The thenar eminence of the operator's lateral hand is superimposed on the thumb with the fingers curled around the posterior aspect of the ankle (Fig. 19.60).

4. When the barrier is engaged, a mobilization with impulse thrust is performed in a posterior direction against the anterior aspect of the lateral malleolus by a combined effort of the thenar eminence of the lateral hand and the thumb of the medial hand.

5. Retest.

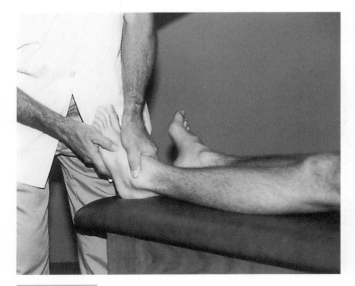

FIGURE 19.59

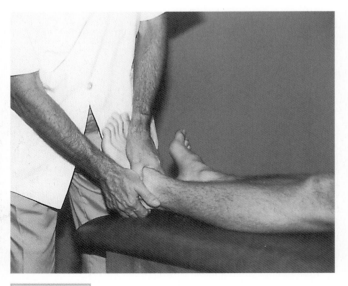

FIGURE 19.60

ANKLE REGION: DISTAL TIBIOFIBULAR JOINT

Prone

Mobilization With Impulse Technique

Diagnosis

Position: Posterior distal tibiofibular joint

Motion Restriction: Anterior movement of the lateral malleolus

1. Patient is prone with the feet over the edge of the table with the operator standing at the foot facing cephalad.

2. Operator's medial hand grasps the foot and ankle maintaining dorsiflexion at the ankle. The thumb is placed over the posterior aspect of the lateral malleolus (Fig. 19.61).

3. Operator's lateral hand places the thenar eminence against the opposing thumb (Fig. 19.62).

4. The barrier is engaged in an anterior direction and a mobilization with impulse thrust is performed by combined activity of the lateral hand's thenar eminence and the medial hand's thumb carrying the lateral malleolus toward the floor.

5. Retest.

ANKLE REGION: TALOTIBIAL JOINT

Diagnosis

1. Patient sits on the table with the legs dangling and the operator sitting in front of the patient.

2. Operator grasps the forefoot and plantar flexes to the barrier evaluating each side for restriction.

3. Each thumb is placed on the anterior aspect of the neck of the talus with the fingers under the forefoot and the operator passively swings the foot toward the table resulting in dorsiflexion of the talotibial joint (Fig. 19.63). Restriction of dorsiflexion is compared from side to side. Frequently, the neck of the talus on the dysfunctional side will be tender.

4. A frequent cause of restricted dorsiflexion of the talotibial joint is shortness and tightness of the gastrocnemius and soleus muscles in the calf.

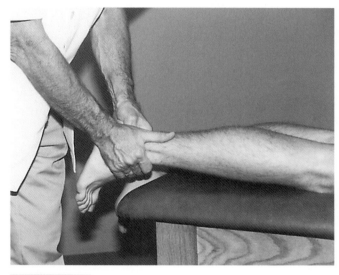

FIGURE 19.62

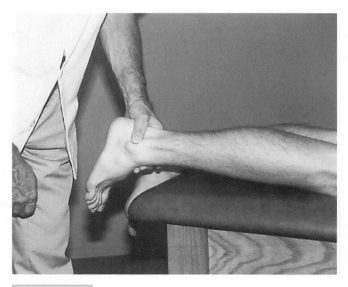

FIGURE 19.61

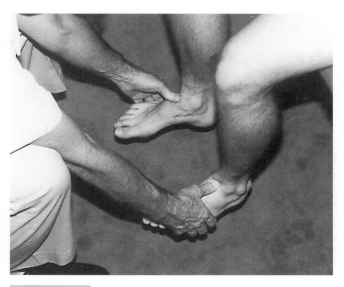

FIGURE 19.63

ANKLE REGION: TALOTIBIAL JOINT

Sitting

Muscle Energy Technique

Diagnosis

Position: Talus plantar flexed

Motion Restriction: Dorsiflexion of the talus

1. Patient sits on the edge of the table with the feet dangling and the operator sitting in front of the dysfunctional talus.

2. Operator places the medial hand under the plantar surface of the forefoot with the web of the lateral hand overlying the neck of the talus (Fig. 19.64).

3. The dorsiflexion barrier is engaged through a combined dorsiflexion movement of the foot and a posterior force on the talar neck.

4. Patient performs plantar flexion muscle effort against equal and opposite resistance for 3 to 5 seconds and three to five repetitions (Fig. 19.65).

5. After each patient effort, additional dorsiflexion is introduced against the resistant barrier.

6. Retest.

Note: It is helpful to have the operator cross the lower legs under the patient's forefoot to assist in resistance of plantar flexion.

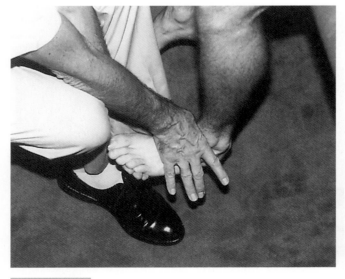

FIGURE 19.64

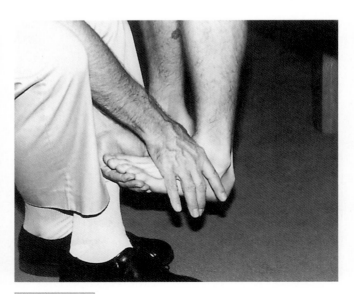

FIGURE 19.65

ANKLE REGION: TALOTIBIAL JOINT

Supine

Mobilization With Impulse Technique

Diagnosis

Position: Talus plantar flexed

Motion Restriction: Dorsiflexion of the talus

1. Patient is supine with the operator standing at the foot of the table.

2. Operator's hands encircle the patient's foot with the middle fingers overlapping the superior aspect of the talar neck and the thumbs on the sole of the foot (Fig. 19.66).

3. Operator engages the barrier by dorsiflexing and long-axis traction.

4. A mobilization with impulse thrust is made by long-axis extension through both hands.

5. Retest.

ANKLE REGION: TALOTIBIAL JOINT

Mobilization with Impulse Technique

Diagnosis

Position: Dorsiflexed or plantar flexed talus

Motion Restriction: Dorsiflexion or plantar flexion of talus

1. Patient is supine on the table with the operator also sitting between the patient's legs, on the table's edge at the dysfunctional side facing caudad.

2. Patient's hip is flexed to 90 degrees and externally rotated. The knee is flexed to 90 degrees with the thigh against the operator's posterior trunk.

3. The webs of the operator's thumb and index fingers are placed on the neck of the talus anteriorly and on the tubercle of the talus posteriorly through the Achilles tendon (Fig. 19.67).

4. The talus is dorsiflexed or plantar flexed against the resistant barrier.

5. When the barrier is engaged, a direct action mobilization with impulse thrust is made in a long-axis distraction direction.

6. Retest.

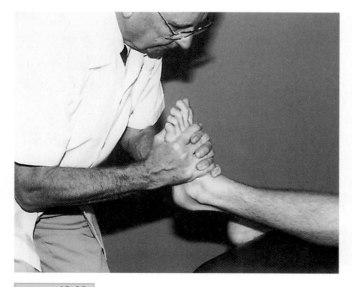

FIGURE 19.66

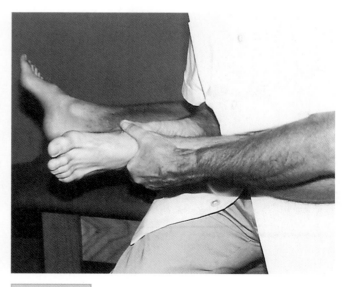

FIGURE 19.67

ANKLE REGION: TALOCALCANEAL (SUBTALAR) JOINT

Testing for Anteromedial-to-Posterolateral Glide

1. Patient is supine on the table with the operator standing at the end facing the dysfunctional ankle.

2. Operator's proximal hand grasps the ankle region with the web of the thumb and index finger over the neck of the talus, the fingers grasping the medial malleolus, and the thumb over the lateral malleolus stabilizing the talus.

3. Operator's distal hand grasps the calcaneus, maintains the foot and ankle at 90 degrees, and translates the calcaneus anteromedially and posterolaterally under the talus sensing for restricted movement (Fig. 19.68).

4. Comparison is made with the opposite side.

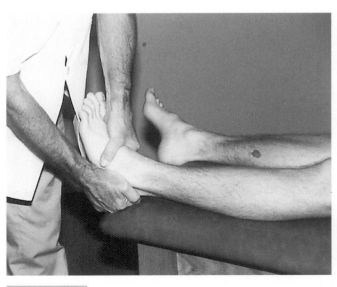

FIGURE 19.68

ANKLE REGION: TALOCALCANEAL (SUBTALAR) JOINT

Supine

Mobilization With Impulse Technique

Diagnosis

Position: Anteromedial or posterolateral talus

Motion Restriction: Posterolateral or anteromedial glide of the talus

1. Patient is supine on the table with the operator sitting between the patient's legs on the table facing caudally.

2. Patient's hip is flexed to 90 degrees and externally rotated with the knee flexed to 90 degrees and the posterior aspect of the thigh being against the operator's trunk.

3. The web between the thumb and index finger of the operator's medial hand contacts the superior aspect of the calcaneus.

4. The web of the thumb and index finger of the operator's lateral hand grasps the anterior and lateral aspect of the calcaneus and incorporates the cuboid. The thumb is on the tarsal navicular.

5. In the presence of an anteromedial talus (calcaneus posterolateral), the calcaneus is medially rotated (inverted to the barrier) (Fig. 19.69).

6. In the presence of a posterolateral talus (calcaneus anteromedial), the calcaneus is laterally rotated (everted) (Fig. 19.70).

7. When the barrier is engaged, a mobilization with impulse thrust is performed through both hands by a long-axis distraction maneuver.

8. Retest.

FOOT

The foot is a complex structure incorporating the tarsals, metatarsals, and phalanges. There are four arches within the foot. The lateral, weight-bearing arch runs from the calcaneus, through the cuboid, to the fourth and fifth metatarsal bones and to the fourth and fifth toes. The key to the lateral weight-bearing arch is the cuboid that rotates medially and laterally around the anterior articulation of the calcaneus. The medial spring arch includes the talus, the navicular, the medial cuneiform, the first metatarsal, and the great toe. The medial and lateral rotations of the navicular around the head of the talus determine the function of the medial spring arch. The transverse arch includes the cuboid laterally and the navicular medially and the accompanying cuneiforms.

The major restrictors of the transverse arch are dysfunction of the cuboid laterally and the navicular medially. The most common dysfunction of the transverse arch is at the cuboid being rotated internally and pronated.

The metatarsal arch is not a true arch but refers to the relation of the heads of the five metatarsals. Restrictions of the metatarsal heads at the metatarsal arch are usually secondary to the dysfunction of the other arches of the foot and are accompanied by restriction of the soft tissues of the foot, primarily the plantar fascia.

Dysfunction at the navicular is either internal or external rotational restriction. Dysfunction usually accompanies that of the cuboid and the most common dysfunction is for the navicular to rotate externally with elevation of its medial tubercle. A less common dysfunction is with the navicular rotating internally with depression of the medial tubercle.

The cuneiforms respond to normal motion or dysfunction of the navicular and the cuboid. The first cuneiform rotates internally and externally on the navicular. The remaining

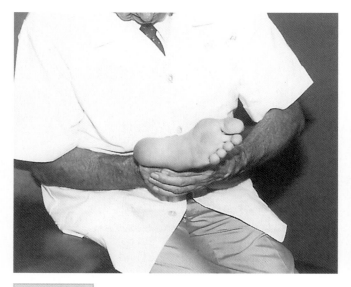

FIGURE 19.69

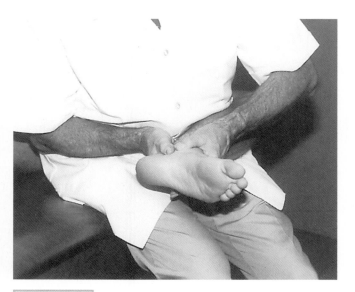

FIGURE 19.70

cuneiforms glide on each other and when dysfunctional, there is usually depression with flattening of the transverse arch.

The first tarsometatarsal joint has movements similar to those of the navicular on the talus and the first cuneiform on the navicular. The remaining tarsometatarsal joints have a dorsal-to-plantar joint play glide motion in response to the transverse tarsal arch. A second joint play movement is medial and lateral rotation.

The metatarsal heads form the pseudometatarsal arch. The second metatarsal appears to be the axis of the forefoot and the first metatarsal is moved on the second, the third on the second, the fourth on the third, and the fifth on the fourth. The joint play movements are dorsal and plantar glide as well as rotation. The most common area of restriction is between the second and third metatarsal heads. When the metatarsal heads are restricted, there is frequent tension and tenderness of the interosseous muscles.

The metatarsophalangeal and interphalangeal joints have primary motions of dorsiflexion and plantar flexion. There are also minor play movements of these joints with medial and lateral tilt and rotation. Restoration of the joint play movements frequently restores pain-free flexion and extension of the metatarsophalangeal and interphalangeal joints.

The primary goals of manual medicine treatment of the foot are to restore functional capacity of the entire mechanism particularly of the cuboid laterally, the navicular medially, the tarsometatarsal joints, the metatarsal heads, and the joints of the phalanges. Appropriate diagnosis and treatment of dysfunctions of the foot frequently restore pain-free movement. Treatment of these dysfunctions strongly influences the remaining lower extremity joints and trunk during the walking cycle.

CALCANEOCUBOID JOINT

Supine

Diagnosis: Cuboid dysfunction

1. Patient is supine on the table with the operator standing at the end.

2. Operator palpates the plantar surface of each cuboid looking for prominence of the tuberosity on the dysfunctional side.

3. Operator palpates the plantar surface of each cuboid for tenderness and tension.

4. Operator motion tests cuboid on each side by having the medial hand grasp and stabilize the calcaneus and the lateral hand grasp the lateral side of the forefoot encircling the cuboid. Internal and external rotations of the forefoot are performed by the lateral hand while simultaneously monitoring for movement at the calcaneocuboid joint (Fig. 19.71).

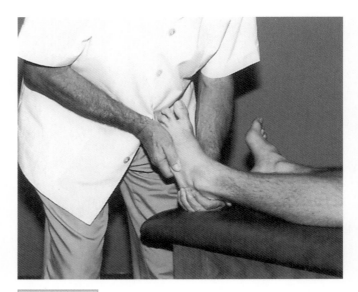

FIGURE 19.71

CALCANEOCUBOID JOINT

Prone

Mobilization With Impulse Technique (J-Stroke Technique)

Diagnosis

Position: Cuboid pronated (internally rotated)

Motion Restriction: Cuboid supination (external rotation)

1. Patient is prone with the dysfunctional leg off the side of the table with the operator standing at the dysfunctional side facing cephalad.

2. Operator's hands grasp and encircle the forefoot.

3. The thumb of the lateral hand is placed over the plantar surface of the cuboid and is reinforced with the thumb of the medial hand (Fig. 19.72).

4. Operator swings the foot in a series of oscillating movements, plantar flexing the forefoot.

5. With engagement of the barrier, the foot is "thrown" toward the floor with acute plantar flexion of the forefoot with the reinforced thumbs carrying the cuboid dorsally and into external rotation (Fig. 19.73).

6. Retest.

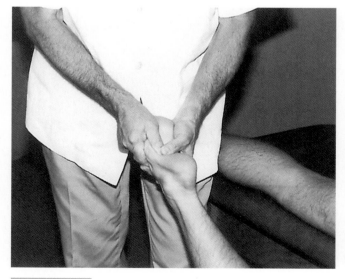

FIGURE 19.72

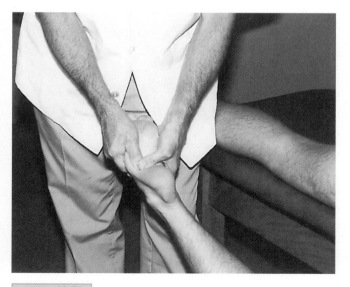

FIGURE 19.73

CALCANEOCUBOID JOINT

Supine

Muscle Energy Technique and Mobilization with Impulse Technique

Diagnosis

Position: Cuboid pronated (internally rotated)

Motion Restriction: Supination (external rotation) of the cuboid

1. Patient is supine on the table with the operator standing at the foot facing the dysfunctional foot.

2. Medial hand grasps the calcaneus and maintains the foot in 90 degrees of ankle flexion.

3. Operator's lateral hand grasps the lateral aspect of the foot with the middle and ring fingers overlying the plantar aspect of the cuboid and the hypothenar eminence over the dorsal aspect of the fourth and fifth metatarsal shafts (Fig. 19.74).

4. Operator engages the resistant barrier by lifting with the middle and ring fingers and depressing the metatarsals with the hypothenar eminence.

5. Patient is instructed to perform dorsiflexion of the little toe against resistance for 3 to 5 seconds with three to five repetitions.

6. Operator engages a new barrier after each effort.

7. With the same localization, the operator performs a mobilization with impulse thrust by an acute lifting maneuver (wrist supination) with the reinforced middle and ring fingers and depression of the fourth and fifth metatarsals (Fig. 19.75).

8. Retest.

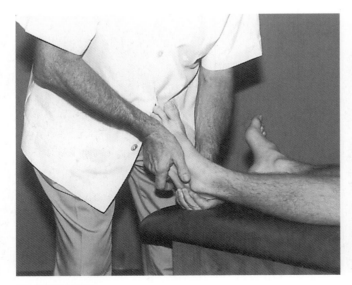

FIGURE 19.74

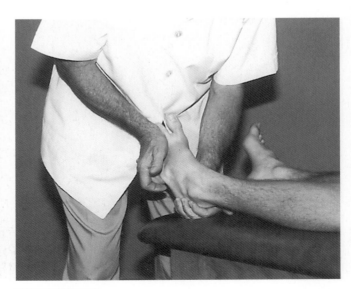

FIGURE 19.75

TALONAVICULAR JOINT

Diagnosis: Internal or External Rotation of the Navicular

1. Patient is supine on the table with the operator standing at the end facing cephalad.

2. Operator palpates the medial tubercle of each navicular for symmetry, tension, and tenderness of the medial and plantar surface.

3. Operator's proximal hand grasps the neck of the talus between the web of the thumb and index finger. The web and index finger of the distal hand surround the navicular. The operator stabilizes the proximal hand and internally and externally rotates with the distal hand in a "ringing" motion testing for the capacity for internal rotation (Fig. 19.76) and external rotation (Fig. 19.77).

4. Comparison is made with the opposite side.

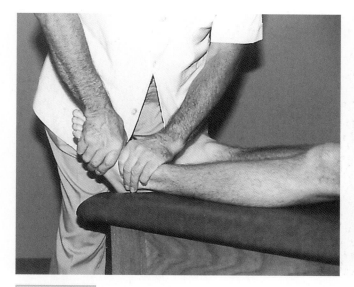

FIGURE 19.76

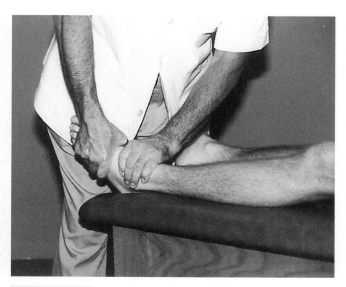

FIGURE 19.77

TALONAVICULAR JOINT

Muscle Energy Technique and Mobilization with Impulse Technique

Diagnosis

Position: Navicular internally rotated or externally rotated

Motion Restriction: Internal or external rotation of the navicular

1. Patient and operator positions are the same as for the diagnostic procedure.

2. With the navicular externally rotated, the operator's distal hand internally rotates the navicular against the resistant barrier (Fig. 19.76). The patient is instructed to invert the foot against resistance for 3 to 5 seconds and repeat three to five times.

3. After each muscle effort, a new barrier is engaged.

4. With the navicular internally rotated, the distal hand externally rotates the navicular to the resistant barrier. The patient is instructed to exert the foot against resistance for 3 to 5 seconds and three to five repetitions (Fig. 19.77).

5. Operator engages a new barrier after each patient effort.

6. A mobilization with impulse thrust activating force can be substituted for the muscle energy activity by mobilizing the distal hand against the proximal.

7. Retest.

CUNEIFORM BONES (INTERTARSAL JOINTS)

Diagnosis: Cuneiform Dysfunction

1. Patient is supine on the table with the operator standing at the foot facing cephalad.

2. Each cuneiform is grasped between the thumb and index finger. While stabilizing one cuneiform, the other is tested for dorsal-to-plantar joint play movement (Fig. 19.78).

3. With the thumbs on the dorsum of the cuneiforms and the fingers of both hands on the plantar surface of the foot, a plantar force is exerted through the thumbs ascertaining the presence or absence of springing movement.

4. Both sides are tested for comparison.

5. Operator can perform a joint play treatment procedure by grasping cuneiform and moving the adjacent one in a dorsal-to-plantar joint play direction.

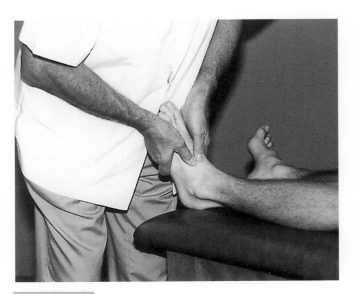

FIGURE 19.78

CUNEIFORM BONES (INTERTARSAL JOINTS)

Muscle Energy Technique

Diagnosis

Position: Depression of cuneiforms

Motion Restriction: Dorsal arching of the cuneiforms

1. Patient is supine on the table with the operator standing at the foot facing cephalad.

2. Operator's proximal hand stabilizes the hind foot with the thumb against the plantar surface of the dysfunctional cuneiform exerting a dorsal force.

3. Operator's distal hand stabilizes the forefoot with the hypothenar eminence over the dorsal aspect of the metatarsal shafts.

4. The barrier is engaged by plantar flexing the forefoot (Fig. 19.79).

5. Patient is instructed to perform a muscle effort of lifting the toes cephalad against equal and opposite resistance for 3 to 5 seconds and three to five repetitions (Fig. 19.80).

6. A new barrier is engaged after each patient effort.

7. Retest.

Note: In the presence of dysfunction of the first cuneiform to the navicular, the muscle energy and mobilization with impulse technique of the navicular on the talus can be modified by the proximal hand grasping the navicular and the distal hand the first cuneiform.

TARSOMETATARSAL JOINTS

Joint Play

Diagnosis: Restoration of dorsal-to-plantar glide

1. Patient is supine with the operator standing at the foot of the table.

2. Operator's thumbs are on the plantar surface of the adjacent metatarsal bases with the fingers on the dorsal side of the proximal metatarsal shafts.

3. Operator holds one metatarsal while the other is moved in a dorsal-to-plantar glide fashion (Fig. 19.81).

4. If restriction is noted, a mobilizing without impulse joint play maneuver is performed enhancing gliding movement between the bases of the metatarsal bones and the tarsometatarsal articulations.

5. Each metatarsal base and shaft is evaluated and treated sequentially.

6. Comparison is made with the opposite side for symmetry.

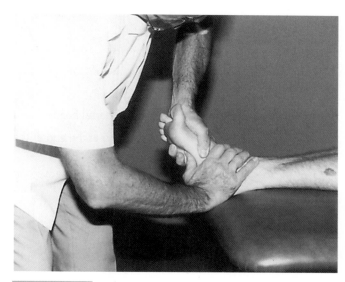

FIGURE 19.80

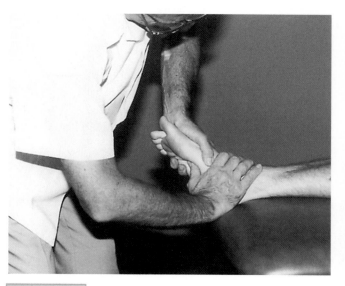

FIGURE 19.79

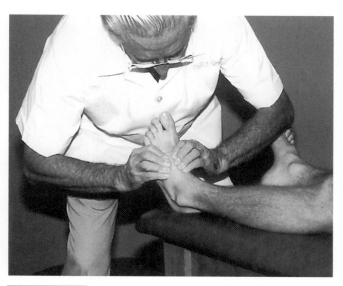

FIGURE 19.81

TARSOMETATARSAL JOINTS

Joint Play

Diagnosis: Evaluation and restoration of medial and lateral rotations

1. Patient is supine with the operator standing at the foot of the table.

2. Operator's proximal hand stabilizes the cuneiform bones through the web of the thumb and index finger.

3. Operator's distal hand dorsiflexes the forefoot and introduces eversion of the forefoot (Fig. 19.82) and inversion of the forefoot (Fig. 19.83).

4. Comparison of eversion and inversion of each foot is made.

5. In the presence of restriction in either direction, a mobilizing with impulse joint play maneuver is performed against the resistant barrier.

6. Retest.

METATARSAL HEADS

Joint Play

Diagnosis: Restriction of joint play at metatarsal heads

1. Patient is supine with the operator standing at the end of the table.

2. Operator's medial hand grasps the shaft of the second metatarsal while the lateral hand grasps the shaft of the third metatarsal (Fig. 19.84).

3. While stabilizing the second metatarsal, the operator's lateral hand dorsi and plantar moves the metatarsal head seeking resistance to motion and provides joint play mobilization if restricted. Comparison is made with the opposite side.

4. Operator's medial hand holds the shaft of the second metatarsal and the lateral hand holds the shaft of the third metatarsal. The lateral hand is rotated medially and laterally testing for rotary capacity of the metatarsal heads. Comparison is made with the opposite side. Joint play rotary mobilization is performed in the presence of restricted motion.

5. Sequentially, the fourth metatarsal is moved on the third, the fifth metatarsal is moved on the fourth, and the first metatarsal is moved on the second in similar fashion.

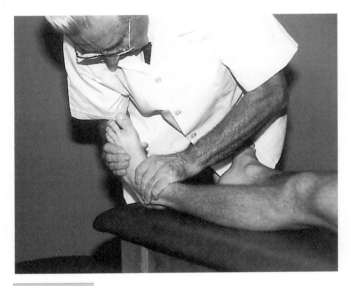

FIGURE 19.83

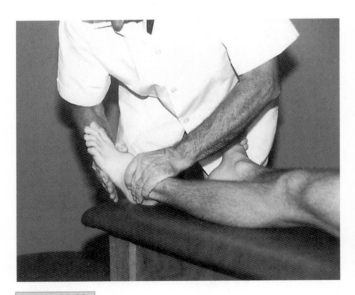

FIGURE 19.82

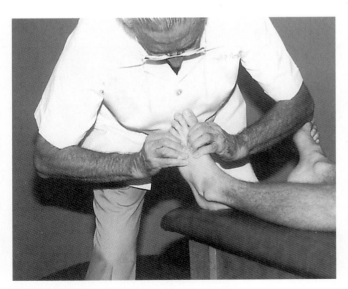

FIGURE 19.84

METATARSOPHALANGEAL JOINTS AND THE INTERPHALANGEAL JOINTS

Motion Testing and Joint Play

Example: First metatarsophalangeal joint

1. Patient is supine with the operator standing at the foot of the table.

2. Operator stabilizes the proximal bone (first metatarsal) with the thumb and fingers.

3. Operator grasps the distal bone (proximal phalanx of the first toe).

4. Flexion–extension, anterior–posterior glide, medial and lateral rotation, and medial and lateral tilt are performed, testing for resistance to movement (Fig. 19.85).

5. Comparison is made with the opposite side.

6. Sequential joint play motions are performed to restore all joint play movements.

7. All other interphalangeal joints can be treated in similar fashion by stabilizing the proximal bone and moving the distal upon it.

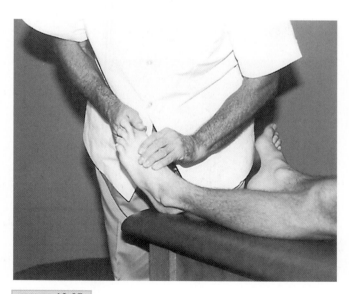

FIGURE 19.85

LOWER LIMB TENSION TESTS

As with the upper extremity, the lower extremity has peripheral nerves encased in the connective tissue, and the nerves need mobility within the covering connective tissue. The reader is encouraged to study the system of neural tension testing and neural and dural mobilization through the work of Butler.[1]

The primary lower extremity tests are really variations of the interpretation of straight leg raising. There are tests using a bias for the femoral nerves as well, but those shown here have been most helpful diagnostically and therapeutically for this author. They are helpful in differentiating pain in the lower extremity coming from neural, muscular, or joint problems. As in many problems of the musculoskeletal system, they are multifactorial. The lower limb tension test maneuvers can be used therapeutically as they are in the upper extremities. It has been observed that the lower limb dural mobilizing maneuvers can profoundly influence the cranial dura when used with traditional cranial technique.

LOWER LIMB TENSION TEST (SCIATIC BIAS)

1. Patient is supine on the table with the operator standing at the side to be tested.

2. Operator grasps the lower leg at the ankle and stabilizes the thigh into knee extension (Fig. 19.86).

3. Operator raises the leg sensing for tension and the provocation of pain (Fig. 19.87). The most common area of pain is in the posterior thigh about two thirds down from the hip joint and it relates to tightness of the hamstring muscles. The pain from the neural system is more to the lateral aspect of the knee.

4. Operator increases the tension by adducting and internally rotating the extended leg (Fig. 19.88).

5. Operator can use dorsiflexion of the foot on the ankle for additional neural and dural tension (Fig. 19.89).

6. When using these maneuvers for dural and neural mobilizations, it is imperative to use an on and off of the tension at the restrictive barrier. Do not use a sustained application of force.

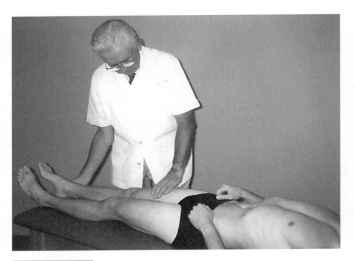

FIGURE 19.86

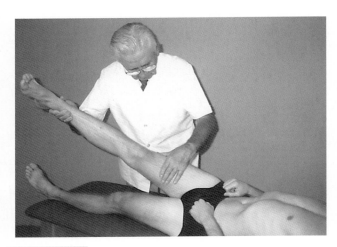

FIGURE 19.88

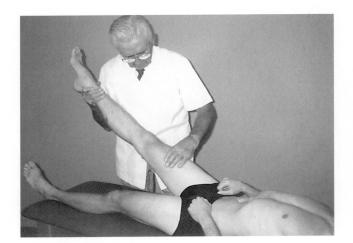

FIGURE 19.87

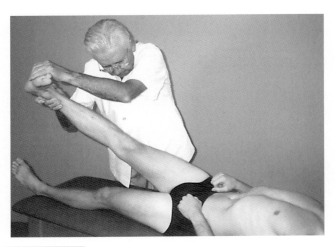

FIGURE 19.89

CONCLUSION

The foot of the lower extremity is the bottom block of the postural structural model. Intrinsic dysfunction within the foot or dysfunction secondary to other dysfunctions within the lower extremity can influence the biomechanical function of the total musculoskeletal system. Lower extremity joint function is essential for symmetric gait. The sole of the foot is a sense organ for sensory motor balance. Evaluation and restoration of function to the foot and lower extremity are essential components of the treatment of patients with musculoskeletal problems.

REFERENCES

1. Butler DS. *Mobilization of the Nervous System*. Melbourne: Churchill Livingstone, 1991.
2. Mennell J McM. *Joint Pain*. Boston: Little, Brown and Company, 1964.
3. Mennell J McM. *Foot Pain*. Boston: Little, Brown and Company, 1964.
4. Mennell J McM. The musculoskeletal system: Differential diagnosis from symptoms and physical signs. Gaithersburg, MD: Aspen Publishers, 1992.

Section

CLINICAL INTEGRATION AND CORRELATION

Chapter
20

COMMON CLINICAL SYNDROMES: EXERCISE PRINCIPLES AND PRESCRIPTIONS FOR THE LOWER QUARTER

Practitioners of musculoskeletal medicine have experience in treating patients with similar clinical presentations. Those who use the structural diagnosis and manipulative treatment aspects of manual medicine will notice that many of these patients present with similar structural diagnostic findings. Appropriate treatment of the areas of somatic dysfunction in some patients results in total symptom resolution, whereas in others, recurrence and persistence occur. Included here are some of the common presentations seen in manual medicine practice, their individual structural patterns, and self treatment approaches.

COMMON COMPENSATORY (UNIVERSAL) PATTERN

Numerous authors have referred to a common "universal" pattern. It is commonly noted that patients are notoriously asymmetric in the functional behavior of their musculoskeletal systems. Symmetric function is ideal but is seldom identified. The universal pattern consists of a cluster of findings including a pronated right foot, an anteriorly rotated right innominate, a posteriorly rotated left innominate, a right inferior pubis, a left superior pubis, a left-on-left forward sacral torsion, a lower thoracic scoliosis convex to the right, a left lumbar scoliosis, an anterior and inferior right shoulder girdle, and a left cervical scoliosis. A number of theories have been postulated to account for this pattern, including the Coriolis force of gravity. It was originally postulated that this pattern was common in the northern hemisphere and that the reverse would be identified in the southern hemisphere, similar to the differences noted in the way that water runs down a drain. This author has been privileged to assess patients in the southern hemisphere in New Zealand and Australia and finds the same universal pattern as found in the northern hemisphere. Obviously, the Coriolis effect is not the cause. Another theory is that it results from right-handedness. Because right-handed people represent a high percentage of the population, this may have some credibility. Our society is dominated by tools and equipment that are made for a right-handed and not a left-handed person, so that even left-handed individuals must live in a right-handed world. Perhaps repetitive movement in this right-handed environment contributes to this universal pattern. This author has often wondered if the fact that most children are delivered in a vertex presentation with the left occiput anterior might be a factor in the development of the functional asymmetry of the musculoskeletal system. The dilemma remains a subject for future research. It is true that this pattern is frequently seen in symptomatic and asymptomatic patients. The question is what is the clinical significance of this common pattern. *Observation shows that if the patient's dysfunctions are out of this pattern, they are more clinically significant. A structural diagnostic finding that does not fit the pattern should alert the diagnostician that the presentation is unusual.* The presence of the common universal pattern can result in practitioners treating patients in a cookbook fashion to restore motion to the segments in this universal pattern. That is poor practice. Patients should be viewed from their individual pattern and how it deviates from that which is more common. Again, dysfunctions out of pattern have been found to be more clinically significant.

MOTOR CONTROL

In addition to the articular restrictions noted in the universal pattern, there are consistent patterns of asymmetric muscle function with some muscles becoming tighter and others becoming inhibited and weak. Motor control of the human function is composed of stabilizing the body in space utilizing postural balance and control in order to move the body through space or function efficiently. Motor control utilizes somatosensory processing at multiple levels, the spinal cord, the brainstem, the cerebellum, the diencephalon, and the cerebral hemispheres, including the cerebral cortex and basal ganglia. This is combined with feed forward and feedback mechanisms from the visual and vestibular systems. The peripheral somatosensory system consists of receptors such as the muscle spindle, golgi tendon organ, joint mechanoreceptors and nociceptors, and cutaneous receptors. It is the peripheral somatosensory system that is most vulnerable to injury.

One's "movement pattern" or "motor program" is the very individualized outcome of his/her motor control processes. It is programmed or hard wired in the sense that the way we move through space is so repetitive that it becomes unconscious. Like learning how to play an instrument, once the senses have developed the pattern of movement required to make the sound it is no longer obvious to the conscious mind. Motor learning is a physiological process that our nervous system utilizes for efficiency of function and recovery of function when injury occurs.

Alterations in the movement pattern occur, primarily due to injuries or disorders in the periphery. According to the work of Vladamir Janda and Karel Lewit, any serious painful disorder at the periphery will cause a central response. The motor program (pattern) will change in order to spare the painful structure, and become permanent even though the painful stimulus is gone. Lewit described this process as a dysfunction in the locomotor system. He and Janda believed that this process could evolve into *muscle imbalance and postural overuse*. The alterations in the motor program (pattern) can occur in the cortical part of the motor system, the muscular or at the joint level. Which ever it may be, this pathology is typically reflex in nature, in a *completely intact nervous system*. Janda defined this pathological process as *functional impairment* and charged that the pathology of the motor system influenced the function of muscles in a typical consistent pattern throughout the neuromusculoskeletal system.[1–5]

1. In the development of tightness and shortness, this involves muscles with predominately *postural function*.
2. In the development of weakness and inhibition, this involves muscles with predominantly *phasic function*.
   a. This development ultimately leads to general imbalance between these two muscle systems with very serious consequences.
3. In the development of inner discoordination of muscles which may produce over activity, overuse or facilitation of some muscle fibers, this leads to tendonopathy or enthesopathy.

Understanding muscles in terms of their global function is not something that is taught in osteopathic school. It is very important, however, in understanding and rationalizing *functional impairment* of muscles and its relationship to our patients as individuals with neuromusculoskeletal dysfunctions. So much so that the classifications of muscle function deserve expansion. The concept of classifying muscles by function gained general acceptability with Margaret Rood's concept of differentiating stabilizer and mobilizer muscles.[6]

- Stabilizer muscles are described as having the characteristics of being monoarticular or segmental, deep, working eccentrically to control movement, and having static holding capacities.
- Mobility muscles are described as biarticular or multisegmental, superficial, working concentrically with the acceleration of movement, and producing power.

Later Bergmark[7] added the concept of local and global muscle systems. In the local system, all muscles have their origin or insertion at the vertebrae for the purpose of controlling the curvature of the spine and providing stiffness for the purpose of maintaining mechanical stability. In the global system, the muscles are more superficial (nonsegmental) and link the thorax and pelvis. These muscles produce large torque and force. Mottram and Comerford[8] added new depth to Rood and Bergmark's models of functional classification of muscles by introducing the local stability, global stability, and global mobility system.

- The local stability muscles have a particular role in maintaining segmental stability. With activity of these muscles there is little length change, so they do not produce range of motion.
- The global stability muscles generate force to control range of movement. They work eccentrically to produce movement with stability.
- The global mobility muscles generate torque to produce large ranges of movement. These muscles work concentrically to produce power and speed and work eccentrically to decelerate high loads.

Functional impairment has been described for each of the various classifications of muscles. Consistently, with injury or joint dysfunction, the local stability and global stability muscles demonstrate inhibition and weakness, whereas the global mobility muscles demonstrate tightness and facilitation.

DYNAMIC JOINT STABILITY

It is amazing how one's movement patterns and his/her articular dysfunction correlate; thus prompting the ever-present question of which came first and which contributes to the persistence of the other. Is it joint or muscle? In all probability, it is a combination of both. This is best exemplified at the vertebral level of the spine with the work of Panjabi.[9] He simplified spinal stability into three subsystems: active, passive, and neural. The *active subsystem* consists of the muscles that control the neutral range of motion of the spine. These muscles are essentially local stabilizers as they are single segment controllers within the neutral range with predominately eccentric contraction. These muscles take their cues "arthrokinematically" from the articular and joint surface mechanoreceptors which signal alteration in the range of segmental motion, length change in muscle, or increased strain on the joint capsule or tendon. The *passive subsystem* consists of bone, the joint capsule, intervertebral disk, and supporting ligaments. The *neural subsystem* consists of the mechanoreceptors within the passive subsystem and the proprioceptors within the active subsystem both of which feedback information to the cord as well as to the active subsystem. Clinical instability of the spine begins with joint dysfunction and ends with spondylosis, degenerative disc changes, and/or stenosis. *Joint dysfunction or somatic dysfunction leads to alteration in feedback control of the vertebral segment due to corrupt neural signaling to the cord, i.e., deafferentation. The active subsystem or stabilizer muscles thus become inhibited and dynamic stability of the joint is lost.*[10] *The segmental neutral range of motion then becomes dependent on the passive subsystem which, with time, hypertrophies or fails.* It is this author's belief that all joints follow the same rules as the spine. All joints have three subsystems which are interdependent for stabilization. All joint subsystems function efficiently within a neutral range of stability.

PRONATION AND SUPINATION

Gary Gray, P.T. is a physiotherapist in Michigan who, along with David Tiberio, Ph.D., P.T. contributed the principle of pronation and supination as having a very sophisticated and important role in musculoskeletal function. Pronation is necessary to eccentrically decelerate forces of gravity, ground reaction, and momentum and load the joint mechanoreceptors and muscle proprioceptors in preparation for concentric unloading or supination. It essentially prepares and allows our body to use the ground in a safe and effective manner for locomotion and propulsion. Pronation is shock absorption while supination is propulsion. Pronation is dominated by deceleration muscle function whereas supination is dominated by acceleration muscle function. Transformation of eccentric muscle function into concentric muscle function requires a great deal of stability and timing. Pronation and supination occur in every joint within the locomotor system and they occur in three planes for each joint, respectively. A good example is to try to jump from a standing position without first pronating or bending at the ankles, knees, or hips. Pronation is the act of loading the joints to allow for supination or acceleration, which is provided by concentric unloading of the stored energy, generated during pronation, against the ground giving height and push. An important aspect of this concept is that pronation, which is dominated by gravity and momentum, is "passive" or "free" whereas supination, which is dominated by concentric muscle function, is "active." Another key aspect is that the timing of motions at the joints is more important than the actual amount of motion.[11]

MUSCLE CO-ACTIVATION

Muscle coactivation involves two groups of muscles contracting synchronously, or cocontracting, to enable a specific motion or action to occur. These two groups of muscles may consist individually of synergists only or may include both agonists and antagonists. The muscles involved may cross one or multiple joints. Coactivating synergist muscles may individually have different fiber types, one type I and the other type II. Antagonist cocontraction serves to increase mechanical stiffness or impedance of the controlled joint, thus fixing its posture or stabilizing its course of movement in the presence of external force perturbations.[12,13]

THE GAIT CYCLE

Many mechanical low back pain syndromes as well as hip and knee problems begin with impairment involving the stability and function of the pelvis, sacrum, and/or lumbar spine during the gait. Efficiency and efficacy of the gait cycle are dependent on many of the concepts defined above. Conceptually, it can be reduced in many ways for easier understanding; however, considering "pronation and supination" as a reference to introduce the gait cycle offers additional access to understanding the muscular etiologies of common neuromusculoskeletal pain syndromes.

Muscular Influences of the Lower Extremity on Pelvic Stability during Gait

Beginning with heel contact with the ground, the joints and ligaments of the foot accommodate and passively transfer the ground reaction forces. This passive transfer of force needs to be harnessed in some fashion to provide efficient and effective locomotion. Immediately following heel contact the dorsiflexed talocrural joint and slightly supinated subtalar joint rapidly plantar flex and pronate, respectively. Secondly, early in the stance phase, the tibia and fibula rotate internally. This activity unlocks the transverse tarsal joint (talonavicular and calcaneocuboid) and activates the tibialis anterior and posterior muscles which act in an eccentric manner to decelerate subtalar eversion and talonavicular abduction as well as to decelerate the medial foot as it pronates, respectively. The tibialis anterior also cocontracts with the tensor

fascia lata and the gluteus medius, stabilizing the pelvis as it passively rotates in the horizontal (transverse) plane over the relatively fixed ipsilateral femur. The peroneus longus eccentrically controls dorsiflexion of the talus; just before the stance phase it cocontracts with the tibialis anterior, acting together as a longitudinal-muscle-tendon-fascia-sling which not only stabilizes the foot but also stabilizes the knee in preparation for it to move over the foot. As the tibia and fibula internally rotate and the fibula begins to descend, the peroneus longus cocontracts with the biceps femoris transferring load into the sacrotuberous ligament to stabilize the ipsilateral sacroiliac joint.[14,15]

Kinematics of the Pelvis during Gait

The right pelvic pronation portion of gait begins at right heel contact and ends at right toe off (0% to 50% of gait). Functionally, during this time the sacrum is turning anteriorly to the right, the pelvis is adducting in the frontal plane (pubic bone and stance femur approximate), the lumbar spine is side bending to the right and rotating to the left, and the pelvis is flexing in the sagittal plane and internally rotating in the transverse plane, toward the stance leg. *Please note that this movement is passive and due to accommodation to the ground reaction forces.*

Kinematically, during this time, the sacrum is moving into right rotation along a right oblique axis, the right innominate is posteriorly rotated and begins to move anterior, the left innominate is anteriorly rotated and begins to rotate posterior, the right pubic rami is moving superior relative to the left, and the lumbar spine has type I motion defined as right side bending and left rotation (Fig. 20.1).

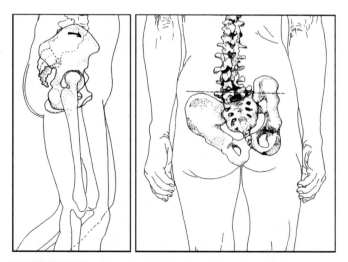

FIGURE 20.1 At right midstance (midleft swing phase), the sacral base on the left begins to move into anterior nutation as it is carried forward by the advancing left ilia. As it begins to rotate to the right it side bends to the left. The oblique hypothetical torsional axis that is produced from this polyaxial movement is right. So, during right midstance gait, the sacrum begins to move into right rotation about a right oblique axis. The lumbar spine will concurrently rotate to the left and side bend to the right.

Muscular Influences of the Pelvis, Hip, and Trunk during Gait

Pronation is passive and occurs in all joints and in all three planes. Because of its passive nature, the muscles involved function in a primarily eccentric fashion to decelerate the joints while simultaneously priming proprioceptors and mechanoreceptors, preparing them for supination or acceleration. *Stabilization of the pelvis is most critical during this stage of gait.* Stabilization of the pelvis in the *frontal plane* is primarily accomplished with the right gluteus medius and minimus. With the assistance of the iliacus, they allow the right (stance leg) tensor fascia lata to eccentrically lengthen, stabilizing the femur as it adducts relative to the pelvis, reducing the valgus torque at the knee. While the abductors and iliacus stabilize the pelvis, the psoas and contralateral quadratus lumborum position the trunk over the center of rotation of the femoral head. In the *transverse plane*, as the pelvis rotates toward the stance leg, the piriformis and other external rotators are eccentrically lengthening, decelerating internal rotation of the right femur relative to the ground. In the *sagittal plane,* the fascial load from the peroneus longus cocontracting with the biceps femoris transfers load into the sacrotuberous ligament to stabilize the ipsilateral sacroiliac joint.[15] Simultaneously, the gluteus maximus is signaled to strongly contract in order to extend the hip and control trunk flexion over the femur. Gluteus maximus also cocontracts with the contralateral latissimus dorsi, via the thoracodorsal fascia, and the lower abdominal musculature in an effort to stabilize the ipsilateral sacroiliac joint as the pelvis moves over the femur.[15] The hip adductors also function in the sagittal plane by cocontracting with the hip extensors and abductors to stabilize the hip.

The role of the trunk in assisting stabilization of the pelvis during the gait cycle cannot be underestimated. The iliopsoas and quadratus lumborum function to provide vertical stability throughout the base of the spine, while the abdominals as well as the transversospinal group of muscles provide intrinsic stabilization to the trunk. The transversospinal muscles are "local stabilizers" as they function to maintain the neutral position of the spine. These muscles cocontract with the transversus abdominus and via the deep layer of the thoracodorsal fascia form a fascial corset around the trunk.

Pelvic and Hip Muscle Dysfunction during Gait

During the first 30% of gait, the pelvis has to rapidly accommodate for passive internal rotation, adduction, and flexion relative to the femur and the trunk. Without decent help from the gluteus muscles and abdominals, the hip has to depend on the external rotators, adductors, iliopsoas, and hamstrings to protect it. Unfortunately this is all too often the case. The gluteus medius muscle produces most of the force at the hip, in fact, it must produce a force twice that of the body weight in order to achieve stability during single-leg stance.[14]

During midstance, as the opposite leg is swinging through, the pelvis becomes even more dependent on the gluteus minimus and medius to stabilize it. Without good assistance from these muscles, the third major abductor, tensor fascia lata, becomes the primary stabilizer, often recruiting the assistance of

quadratus lumborum and the piriformis, whose secondary action is abduction. One would hope at this stage of gait that gluteus maximus is primed and ready to function as the primary hip extensor. If not, again not unusual, the hip has to depend on the biceps femoris to stabilize the sacroiliac joint while the erector spinae extend the trunk against the adductors, especially the posterior fibers of adductor magnus.

As gait proceeds beyond midstance the iliopsoas eccentrically lengthens in order to decelerate ipsilateral hip extension and get primed for hip flexion. Simultaneously, the soleus, gastrocnemius, tibialis posterior, and peroneus musculature are working eccentrically to stabilize the knee and get primed to clear the foot as it swings through with the lower extremity.

Supination of the pelvis during gait consists of external rotation, abduction, and extension. Supination is not free or passive; it must depend on concentric muscle force to provide the acceleration force that is necessary during this last 50% of gait. Hopefully, gluteus maximus has already been working to extend the hip and the iliopsoas, sartororius, tensor fascia lata, rectus femoris, pecineus, and adductor longus are primed and ready to swing the leg forward against a stabilized contralateral pelvis.

Deceleration Overuse Syndromes

As suggested above, pelvic muscle dysfunction during gait may lead to several muscles that having to excessively work in an eccentric manner to decelerate "uncontrolled pronation" burst into concentric action to facilitate joint supination later in the gait cycle. These muscles include the tensor fascia lata, adductors, external rotators (especially piriformis), and hamstrings. Often, under these circumstances, these muscles become short, tight, and can exhibit inner body or insertional tears and/or "trigger points" due to overuse. Clinicians have defined these situations with many terms, i.e., myofascial pain syndromes, tendonopathy, enthesopathy, trigger points, muscle strains, and overuse syndromes. Treatment has typically focused on the problem muscle, with therapies such as stretching, injections, and prolotherapy.

Janda approached the problem as "functional impairment" consistent with facilitation of muscles with predominate "postural" function and inhibition of muscles with predominate "phasic" function. The gluteus muscles in this case are phasic or dynamic in their function. They are also considered "global stabilizers" in that they generate force to control range of movement. These muscles are often inhibited or delayed in contracting, leaving the joint(s) at risk and allowing the postural muscles to become overloaded. Prominent in their function as stabilizers these muscles take their cue from the spinal cord in response to mechanoreceptive information from the sacroiliac joint and the hip capsule. Their delay or inhibition suggests that these muscles have altered afferentation. As such, treatment would begin with manipulation, restoring full function to the joint prior to stretching the facilitated tight muscle. Using appropriate manipulation restores joint mechanoreceptive input into the muscle i.e., it is re-afferentating.[16,17]

Recurrent hamstring pulls are essentially overuse injuries due to functional impairment of the gluteus maximus muscles. The gluteus maximus becomes inhibited with almost any sacroiliac joint dysfunction but in large degree with the posterior torsional dysfunctions. Arthrokinematically, the dysfunctional sacroiliac joint sends corrupt afferent signals to the spinal cord. The information that is sent poorly indicates where the joint is in three-dimensional space and/or inaccurately assumes the relative pressures, speed of motion, and tension within the joint articulation and its associated ligaments. Corrupt efferent information is subsequently communicated back to the respective muscles indicating that the joint is not in a position in space in which it is necessary for it to fire.

Shortly after heel strike as the tibia and fibula internally rotate and the fibula begins to descend, the peroneus longus cocontracts with the biceps femoris, transferring load along the sacrotuberous ligament which assists in stabilizing the ipsilateral sacroiliac joint. As midstance approaches, the gluteus maximus takes over the role of stabilizing the sacroiliac joint, as a component of force closure. If the gluteus maximus is inhibited, the biceps femoris continues to remain contracted in order to offer the stabilizing force across the sacroiliac joint in addition to assisting in preventing the pelvis from flexing excessively over the hip. Without the help of the gluteus maximus, over time, the biceps femoris is assured to become hypertonic, tight, facilitated, and at risk of tears. Stretching the hamstrings does not target the problem but complicates the situation. In this situation, the key is to appropriately restore function to the sacrum and pelvis using manipulative techniques; then maintain the tone of the gluteus maximus muscles, using functional approaches such as squats without weights or lunges.

SENSORY MOTOR BALANCE RETRAINING

The goal of manual medicine is to restore joint function. Maintenance of joint function can be difficult depending on the chronicity of the problem and the adaptations of motor control that have been adopted. Sensory motor balance training is the first and most crucial piece of the home exercise program. It helps restore symmetric muscle firing patterns for control of motor function. Body balance is a complex function and is the result of three primary afferent systems. Our orientation in three-dimensional space results from the visual system, the vestibular system, and the proprioceptive input from the soles of the feet. The body adapts to loss of vision by enhanced proprioception from the extremities and greater dependence on the vestibular mechanism. The visual system compensates for reduced efficiency of proprioceptive input from contact with the ground by the soles of the feet.

Indications for Training

The first indication that a patient may need sensory motor balance training occurs during the screening and scanning examinations, particularly the function of the pelvic girdle. During the one-legged stork test, the patient stands on a single foot. If the patient is so unsteady that it is impossible to perform the test smoothly, an index of suspicion is high that the patient has deficit of proprioceptive sensitivity of the sole of the foot. Initial diagnostic testing includes asking the patient to stand in bare feet, first on one foot and then on the other to see if there is equal balance from right to left. A second level of difficulty of this test is to ask the patient to stand on one leg with arms crossed. This removes the balancing assistance of the upper trunk and

extremities. A third level of difficulty is to ask the patient to stand on one leg with arms crossed and then to close the eyes. The removal of visual perception greatly increases the difficulty. Ideally, the patient should be able to symmetrically stand on one leg with arms crossed and eyes closed for 30 seconds.

Retraining

Sensory motor retraining should be done with bare feet on a carpeted surface. One of the primary goals is to stimulate the proprioceptors of the sole of the foot. One begins by practicing to shorten the foot. The "short foot" is obtained by attempting to grasp the floor with the sole of the foot without excessive curling of the toes. The shortened foot elevates the medial longitudinal arch and enhances the sensitivity of the sole of the foot. All exercises should be done with a shortened foot. A simple home program for sensory motor retraining is shown in Table. 20.1.

TABLE 20.1	*Sensory Motor Examination and Retraining Program*

Do all activities with bare feet

1. Sitting—practice shortening both feet
2. Standing—feet aligned with the hips, neutral pelvis, trunk erect, both knees slightly flexed, and practice shortening both feet

Do the following activities with a neutral pelvis, erect trunk, and shortened feet

1. Standing on one leg
   A. Eyes open, arms down
   B. Eyes open, arms crossed
   C. Eyes closed, arms down
   D. Eyes closed, arms crossed
2. Standing—feet aligned with the hips, practice slight squatting, keep heels on surface, and gradually increase to semisquat (up to 90 degrees)
3. Standing—on one leg—practice squatting
   A. Eyes open, arms down
   B. Eyes open, arms crossed
   C. Eyes closed, arms down
   D. Eyes closed, arms crossed
4. Standing on a rocker board or rebounder
   A. Feet parallel about one foot apart, shift weight from side to side, bringing trunk over each foot
   B. One foot places a short step in front of the other, shift weight from back to front alternate feet
   C. Do both with arms crossed
   D. Do both with eyes closed and arms crossed
5. Standing on one foot on a rocker board or rebounder, repeat with arms crossed and then eyes closed
6. Walk on the floor/balance beam—place one foot directly in front of the other (heel to toe), done first with eyes open and then with eyes closed
7. Walk on the floor/balance beam—place one foot directly behind the other (toe to heel), done first with eyes open and then with eyes closed

The goal of sensory motor balance training is to test the capacity to symmetrically stand on one leg with arms crossed and eyes closed for 30 seconds. The more severe the deficit, the more difficult it will be to achieve the goal. Right-to-left symmetry is the primary objective and the ultimate goal is to achieve the highest level of difficulty with arms crossed, eyes closed, and length of time. The presence of a neurologic deficit of a lower extremity, which frequently follows a lumbar radiculopathy, can make this exercise difficult. Even in the presence of a neurologic deficit, it is advisable to achieve the maximum possible functional capacity to assist in the restoration of more normal muscle firing pattern sequences.

LOWER EXTREMITY
Ankle Sprains

Sensory balance retraining can be difficult for persons with old ankle sprains or injuries. As Dr Greenman commonly states "there is no minor ankle sprain," any degree of inversion ankle sprain can lead to significant joint dysfunction. In addition to destruction of mechanoreceptors in the sprained ligamentous structures

- The talus moves anteriorly and limits appropriate ankle dorsiflexion.
- The subtalar joint inverts and leads to loss of calcaneal eversion.
- The navicula along with the cuboid collapse centrally with loss of the transverse arch.
- Loss of downward motion of the fibula prior to midstance.

The first three dysfunctions also limit the transverse tarsal joint from unlocking and appropriately distributing the ground reaction force transformation during pronation. Each of the above noted joint motions is necessary, as a component of foot pronation, to load the appropriate mechanoreceptors and proprioceptors (neural subsystem) in maintaining joint stability and allowing the fascial and ligamentous force-couples necessary for stabilization of superincumbent joints.

There are several common clinical problems that result from the above joint dysfunctions; in particular, recurrent ankle pain due to poor transformation of ground reaction forces into the lower extremity. For reasons described above, one should not underestimate these joint dysfunctions' influence on medial knee pain, patellofemoral joint pain, iliotibial tract issues, piriformis syndrome, shin splints, chronic hamstring strains, or persistent sacroiliac joint dysfunctions. Appropriate manual medicine treatment for the lower extremity begins at the foot (see Chapter 19) but may continue into the thoracolumbar junction.

The goal of treatment is to restore joint function which

- allows appropriate arthrokinematic feedback into the active subsystem local stabilizers,
- encourages the appropriate and stabilized force-couple into the passive subsystem and global stabilizers,
- allows for appropriate pronation, necessary for loading the passive subsystem mechanoreceptors, storing energy and deceleration of joint motion, and

- allows for appropriate supination, necessary for unloading the passive subsystem, utilizing the stored energy for acceleration during locomotion.

An appropriate expectation for the patient's home exercise program, following manual medicine treatment, begins with restoration of "sensory motor balance" using the above mentioned protocol. Ideally, the patient should be able to symmetrically stand on one leg with arms crossed and eyes closed for 30 seconds.

Supination and Pronation

Overpronation at the foot and ankle leads to deceleration overuse syndromes. If the deceleration problems remain at the foot, the overpronator may present with anterior or posterior tibialis muscle facilitation pain or "shin splints." If the problem is overpronation at the foot combined with an increased valgus strain at the knee, the patient may present with medical knee pain, iliotibial tract syndrome, or even pes anserinus bursitis. If the deceleration problems coexist with poor stability of the pelvis the patient may present with iliotibial tract syndrome or "piriformis syndrome." *Gray makes the point that it is not so much about quantity of motion as it is timing.* For instance, if the patient has, as a normal variant, external tibial torsion, during gait, his/her femur will internally rotate faster than their tibia costing them the stabilization at the knee which is provided by the peroneus longus and tibialis anterior cocontraction during pronation at the foot. Tibial rotation is a critical component of pronation at the foot; if the femur internally rotates, pronation at the hip occurs first before the knee, leaving the knee very vulnerable to inappropriate loading.

Piriformis syndromes are common and are described as recurrent buttock or posterior hip pain, typically unilateral and worse after physical activity. Trigger points can be found anywhere along the muscle and may radiate pain to the sacroiliac region, laterally across the buttock and over the hip region posteriorly or even to the proximal two thirds of the thigh. Timing of pronation of the femur relative to the pelvis determines how fast and furious the piriformis has to fire. Often, increased valgus strain at the knee combined with poor trunk and pelvic control heralds recurrent problems, in particular, if the patient is involved in speed walking or running.

It would be inappropriate not to speak briefly about the "supinator." The example above of the patient with the external tibial torsion is someone that underpronates at the knee. Be it the knee, foot, or hip, the supinator is best approached as underpronator. Just as the overpronator overloads ligaments and muscles, the underpronator overloads the joints. Without an adequate mechanism to dissipate loads, joint surfaces rapidly degenerate.[14]

Treatment of all pronation/supination problems is dependent on the specific diagnosis. Evaluation and treatment would begin at the foot and end at the thoracolumbar junction. Sensory motor balance retraining begins once joint mobility is restored. In some situations, one would consider including a properly cast foot orthosis.

The Hip

Hip osteoarthritis is common and devastating. Understanding how the joint vectors and forces from the ground are utilized by the hip and pelvic musculature is vital in understanding how to treat our patients. During single-leg stance, the gluteus medius, gluteus minimus, and tensor fascia lata contract strongly to stabilize the pelvis, while the psoas and contralateral quadratus lumborum position the trunk over the center of rotation of the femur. The timing and the efficacy of these muscular forces are so very critical in producing an optimal distribution of stress precisely into the acetabular roof. Articular cartilage is very sensitive to an increase or uneven distribution of stress and may be destroyed by a change in orientation of the articular resultant forces.[18]

Functional impairment of the gluteus muscles and facilitation of the tensor fascia lata are a lethal combination for the hip capsule. Recurrent iliotibial tract issues are common, with pain either proximal at the trochanter of the hip or distal at the lateral aspect of the knee. This is a frontal plane overuse issue. What needs to be addressed with these syndromes is any inhibition in firing or coactivation of the gluteus medius muscle. Gluteus medius is a primary stabilizer of the pelvis in the "frontal" plane; it stabilizes adduction and assists in abduction of the pelvis during gait. It is also commonly delayed or inhibited secondary to sacroiliac joint dysfunctions, iliopsoas shortening, and piriformis tightness. These issues need to be addressed first, before stretching the iliotibial band and tensor fascia lata. A home exercise program geared toward stretching the iliopsoas and piriformis (see below) and strengthening the gluteus muscles is highly recommended after disinhibiting the muscle using appropriate manipulation (Figs. 20.2a–c and 20.3).

GLUTEUS MEDIUS MUSCLE

Retraining

1. Patient lies in the lateral recumbent position with the knees flexed to 45 to 60 degrees and the upper hand overlying the gluteus medius muscle (Fig. 20.2a).

2. Maintaining the feet together, patient lifts the top knee toward the ceiling, holds for 5 to 7 seconds, slowly lowers the leg, and repeats five to seven times (Fig. 20.2b).

3. This muscle may fatigue rapidly with this exercise, and the patient must be cautious about the number of repetitions.

4. The knee should not be elevated too far because this will increase the contraction of the piriformis muscle as the external rotator (Fig. 20.2c).

5. Repeat on the opposite side for balance.

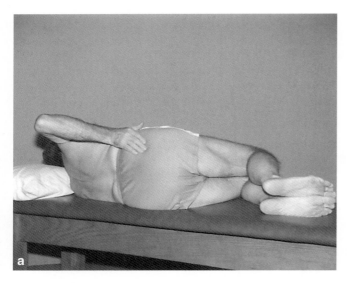

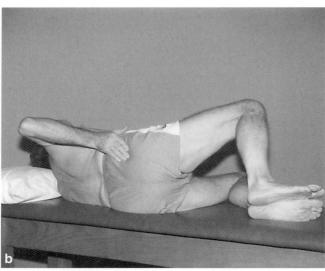

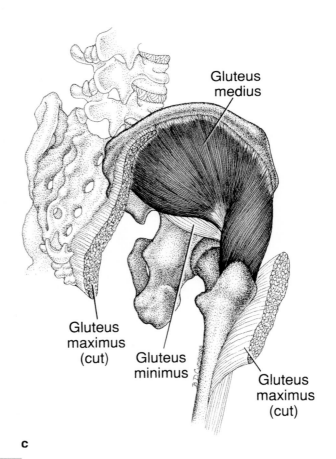

Gluteus medius

Gluteus maximus (cut)

Gluteus minimus

Gluteus maximus (cut)

FIGURE 20.2

GLUTEUS MEDIUS MUSCLE (FIG. 20.3)

Retraining

1. Patient is in the lateral recumbent position against the wall with the shoulders and pelvis perpendicular to the table or floor and the upper leg extended.

2. Patient's upper arm is placed on and pushes into the table or floor while dorsiflexing the upper foot.

3. Patient slowly raises the upper leg to the hip level, keeping the heel in contact with the wall, holds for 5 to 7 seconds, and lowers the leg slowly. This is repeated five to seven times.

4. Externally rotating the leg reduces the influence of the tensor fascia lata muscle, and elongating the leg reduces the influence of the quadratus lumborum muscle and isolates action more to the gluteus medius.

5. Repeat on the opposite side for symmetric balance.

6. As progress is made, the exercise may be done with the knees at 90 degrees. Added difficulty is to raise both legs toward the ceiling.

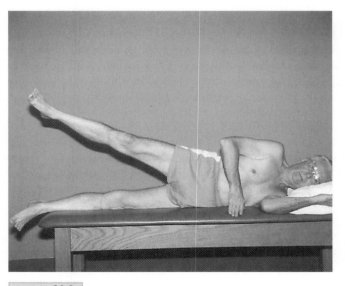

FIGURE 20.3

Nonneutral lumbar mechanics can also cause havoc on the hip capsule, limiting the trunk's ability to move over the center of gravity of the femur during single-leg stance. Nonneutral lumbar mechanics must be addressed in any patient with hip joint complaints. In particular, in young patients with what appears to be a hip labral tear, look for FRS dysfunctions, with rotation towards the side of hip pain, in the upper lumbar or thoracolumbar junction.

LOW BACK PAIN SYNDROMES
The "Dirty Half Dozen" in the Failed Lower Back Syndrome

Disability from lower back pain continues to be a major societal problem. The cost of care to the patient with industrial back pain continues to escalate and frustrates the health care delivery system, the insurance industry (both public and private), and employers. For the patient, it can be catastrophic with the loss of income, reduced activities of daily living, loss of self-esteem, and dependency. The prevention of the failed lower back syndrome and the rehabilitation of its sufferers are indeed challenges.

Structural diagnostic and manual medicine practices have demonstrated a cluster of findings in patients presenting with the failed lower back pain syndrome. This cluster has been designated the "dirty half dozen." The dirty half dozen consists of dysfunction within the lumbar spine, pelvis, and lower extremities. They are

1. Nonneutral dysfunction within the lumbar spine, primarily flexed, rotated, and side bent (FRS) dysfunctions in the segments of the lower lumbar and thoracolumbar spine,
2. Dysfunction at the symphysis pubis,
3. Restriction of anterior nutational movement of the sacral base, either a posterior (backward) torsion or a posteriorly nutated (extended) sacrum,
4. Innominate (hip) shear dysfunction,
5. Short-leg, pelvic-tilt syndrome, and
6. Muscle imbalance of the trunk and lower extremities.

Dr. Greenman studied 183 patients (79 men and 104 women) with an average age of 40.8 years who were disabled for an average of 30.7 months.[19] All patients had disability with 53% working less than full-time and disabled for some activities of daily living, 42% were not working and had disability of most of the activities of daily living, and 5% were totally disabled and needed assistance for activities of daily living. Eighteen percent had previous surgical treatment suggesting that most cases of failed lower back syndrome are a failure of previous nonoperative care. The 18% surgical failure rate is close to the national average of 15%. In these patients, the primary presentation was of back pain with some radiation to the buttock and thigh and in 38% some radiation below the knee. None of the patients presented with leg pain alone. The primary presentation was back, buttock, and thigh pain. The yield from standard neurologic and orthopedic testing was low. Ten percent had some reflex change at the patellar or Achilles levels. Less than 5% showed evidence of significant muscle weakness. Seven percent showed some

sensory loss. The classic straight-leg raising with positive dural response was only identified in 2%. None had the classic crossed, straight-leg raising sign pathognomonic of discogenic radiculopathy. Assessment of the dirty half dozen found 84% to have FRS or extended, rotated, and side bent (ERS) dysfunctions in the lumbar spine clustered at the L4 and L5 levels. Seventy-five percent had unleveling of the symphysis pubis. A total of 48.6% had restriction of anterior nutation of the posterior sacral base. Sixty percent of the failed surgical patients had a posterior sacral base. This high incidence leads one to consider that this functional pathology may be associated with the structural pathology or that the original symptoms were not due to the structural but the functional pathology. In the past, laminectomy was done with the patient in a flattened lumbar lordosis, but today the preservation of a functional lumbar lordosis is the goal of a spinal surgeon. Twenty-four percent showed the presence of hip bone shear with a female to male ratio of 2:1. The short-leg, pelvic-tilt syndrome was found in 63%. This is consistent with a number of previous studies showing two of three people with back and lower extremity disability having inequality of leg length as compared to 8% to 20% of the asymptomatic population. Muscle imbalance was found in almost all of the patients.

Only five patients (2.7%) failed to demonstrate any of the dirty half dozen. Fifty-five percent of the population showed three or more of the dirty half dozen. Despite an average of 2.5 years of disability, 75% of this population returned to full employment and active activities of daily living following a treatment plan directed toward the findings.

Pelvic Dysfunctions
Pubic Symphysis Dysfunctions

During the gait cycle, the pubic rami move superior and inferior in response to the ground and the superincumbent weight. Motion of the pubic rami helps to distribute these forces equally from the femur into the pelvis and across the sacroiliac joints. Dysfunction of the pubic symphysis distorts the pelvic brim and places increased load into the sacroiliac joints (this is why this dysfunction will distort the findings of the seated flexion test). Very commonly dysfunctional in low back pain, this joint exhibits a common pattern, inferior right and superior left. Recurrent pubic symphysis dysfunctions occur commonly due to neuromuscular imbalance between the short tight adductors and weak lower abdominals. The hip adductors function in the sagittal plane by forming a force-couple with the hip extensors and abductors to stabilize the hip; thus, recurrent pubic symphysis dysfunctions due to tight right adductors may be a sign of delayed or poor gluteus maximus tone.

The patient can use exercise to maintain correction of joint dysfunction or to self-treat in the presence of recurrence. This assists patients in taking control of their musculoskeletal systems. In the pelvis, the symphysis pubis can be self-mobilized with isometric activation of the hip adductor musculature (Fig. 20.4). Appropriate balancing of the abdominal musculature above and the hip adductor musculature below the symphysis pubis should follow self-treatment and become a component of one's home program (Fig. 20.5).

SYMPHYSIS PUBIS (FIG. 20.4)

Self-correction Position: Supine

1. Patient is supine with the feet together.

2. Patient abducts knees and places a noncompressible object between them.

3. Patient performs a symmetric 5- to 7-second isometric activity of both legs, trying to bring the knees together.

4. Repeat five to seven times.

HIP ADDUCTOR MUSCLES (FIG. 20.5a,b)

Self-stretch Position: Sitting

1. Patient sits with the buttocks as close to the wall as possible with the lumbar spine in neutral. A pillow or towel may be placed under the ischial tuberosities to provide an anterior pelvic tilt. The patient may begin by sitting on a low step.

2. Patient puts the soles of the feet together, pulling the feet toward the body, and actively externally rotates and abducts both legs.

3. Patient places both hands behind hips to assist in lifting and anteriorly rotating the pelvis and assuming the 6 o'clock position.

4. The stretch is held for 10 to 15 seconds and repeated three to four times with increasing external rotation and abduction with each effort.

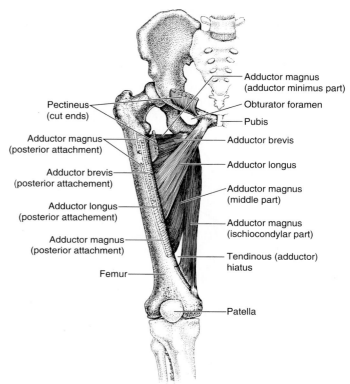

a

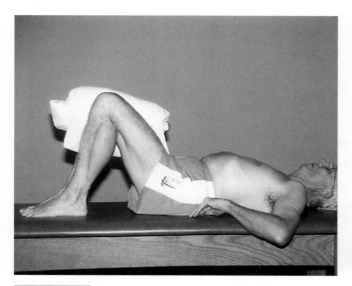

FIGURE 20.4

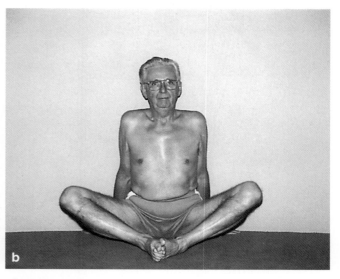

FIGURE 20.5

Anterior or Posterior Innominate Rotations

Anterior or posterior innominate rotations in and of themselves are not painful and are not part of the "dirty half dozen." They do, however, indicate one of the two common problems: short-leg, pelvic-tilt syndrome and/or neuromuscular imbalance. Recurrent anterior innominate dysfunctions can be an adaptation to a short ipsilateral lower extremity. The acetabulum of the femur sits anteriorly to the center of rotation of the innominate; anterior rotation of the ilia thus functionally lengthens the lower extremity. Tightness of the rectus femoris relative to weak lower abdominals will also anteriorly rotate the innominate. Appropriate balancing of the abdominal musculature above and the quadriceps below (Fig. 20.6), the dysfunctional innominate should follow self-treatment and become a component of one's home program. Appropriate treatment of the unequal leg length may also be prudent, in particular, if other cardinal signs of adaptation to the leg length discrepancy are noted, such as anterior sacral base on and lumbar convexity toward the short side.

RECTUS FEMORIS MUSCLE (FIG. 20.6a,b)

Self-stretch Position: Standing

1. Patient stands with the foot of the leg to be stretched on a table or chair with the knee flexed.

2. Patient contracts abdominal and gluteal muscles in the 12 o'clock position. If stretch is felt in the anterior thigh, patient is asked maintain it for 10 to 15 seconds and repeat three times.

3. As length increases, additional stretch is obtained by flexing the opposite knee. Stretch is felt in the anterior thigh.

4. This is repeated on the opposite side for symmetric muscle balance.

5. A dual outcome results with stretching of one side, while strengthening on the side of active knee flexion.

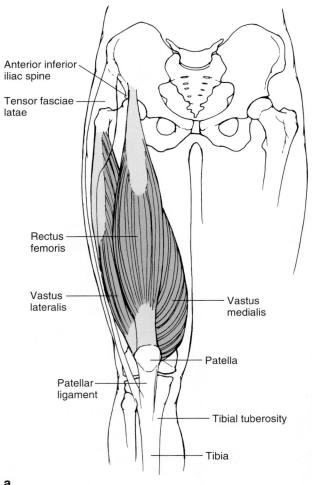

Anterior inferior iliac spine

Tensor fasciae latae

Rectus femoris

Vastus lateralis

Vastus medialis

Patella

Patellar ligament

Tibial tuberosity

Tibia

a

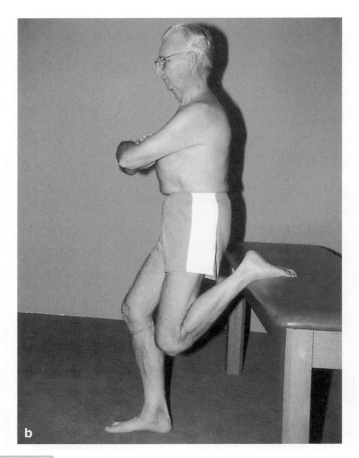

b

FIGURE 20.6

Sacral Dysfunctions

Recurrent sacroiliac joint dysfunctions can be a huge frustration for the patient as well as the clinician. When faced with this situation, it is critical to document the dysfunctional pattern(s) so that an appropriate home exercise program can be instituted. The goal of appropriate manual medicine treatment in the pelvis is to restore the motion of the sacrum during the gait cycle (see Chapter 17); which includes restoration of anterior motion around oscillating oblique axes (R/R and L/L).

CLINICAL PEARL

From this author's personal perspective, the sacral mechanics cannot be properly understood in light of a pubic symphysis dysfunction or certainly an innominate shear dysfunction. Once appropriate manual medicine treatment of the pelvis is complete, it is imperative that the clinician repeat the functional evaluation from the beginning (standing flexion, stork test, and seated flexion test), prior to appreciating the sacral landmarks.

Posterior Sacral Torsions

Loss of nutation of the sacrum is the primary cause of pain and dysfunction for two reasons: loss of form and loss of force closure of the sacrum. According to Vleeming, "Form closure refers to a stable situation with closely fitting joint surfaces, in which no extra forces are needed to maintain the state of the system." Force closure refers to "compression generated by muscles and ligaments that can be accommodated to the specific loading situation."[20]

The sacrum is wider superiorly than it is inferiorly and wider anteriorly than posteriorly. This "keystone-shape" configuration is necessary for the sacrum to wedge itself anteriorly between the ilia (see Chapter 5). The sacroiliac joints are relatively flat and like most flat articular surfaces they lack the ability to resist shear forces. Given the location of the sacrum, the lack of resistance to shear forces can be a problem. The shape of the sacrum and its ability to anteriorly nutate between the ilia protect it from shear; but the sacrum requires sophisticated continuous muscular and ligamentous tensile forces to protect it from vulnerability and yet allow function.

Force closure of the sacrum begins in the lower extremity just after heel strike, with the force-couple of the peroneus longus and biceps femoris into the sacrotuberous ligament and across the ipsilateral sacroiliac joint. At midstance, the biceps femoris' downward pull is replaced by the force-couple between the gluteus maximus ipsilaterally and the latissimus dorsi contralaterally, through the lumbodorsal fascia. This stabilizing force closure of the sacrum is a longitudinal muscle–tendon–fascial sling which is temporally precise. In other words, if there is a delay in the firing of any of the coactivated muscles, the stability factor of the whole system decreases. This is precisely what happens with sacroiliac joint dysfunctions, in particular, posterior torsions of the sacrum. Counternutation of the sacrum places the sacroiliac joint(s) into a very vulnerable position, primarily because nutation, which is the characteristic feature of form closure, is lost. Counternutation

also leads to deafferentation and inhibition of the gluteus maximus muscle arthrokinematically, which subsequently diminishes the force closure capability of the sacrum.

Other factors that inhibit or delay the firing of gluteus maximus also interfere with force closure across the joint and may contribute to recurrent sacroiliac dysfunctions and chronic low back syndromes. These include loss of subtalar eversion following an ankle sprain,[21] and restriction of the hip capsule both posteriorly or anteriorly due to tightness of the piriformis and iliopsoas, respectively.

The most common inciting posture for the posterior torsion is bending forward at the waist while twisting. Bending and twisting to the right takes the lumbar spine into forward flexion, right side bending, and right rotation. Concurrently, it takes the sacrum into its vulnerable counternutation and left rotation. The only axis in which this rotation can occur is right, which means the left sacral base moves posteriorly. If the fifth lumbar remains in a dysfunctional FRS right position (consistent with the bending and twisting posture) with the sacrum preferring left rotation along a right axis, the L5–S1 intervertebral disk will be exposed to a great deal of torque and the patient may present with discogenic low back pain. If in this case the patient has preexisting nonneutral FRS dysfunctions at segments consistent with psoas innervation, the thoracolumbar junction, they may likely present with an acute iliopsoas syndrome.

Diagnosis and treatment of the sacrum should always follow treatment of any innominate shear, symphysis pubis, or lumbar spine dysfunctions. Once treated, disinhibition of the gluteus maximus can be observed by requesting the patient actively hip extend while in the prone position (Fig. 20.7). Diagnosis and treatment of ankle and hip capsule dysfunction should proceed if gluteus maximus inhibition persists. Maintenance of nutation of the sacrum begins by insisting that the patient avoids excessive

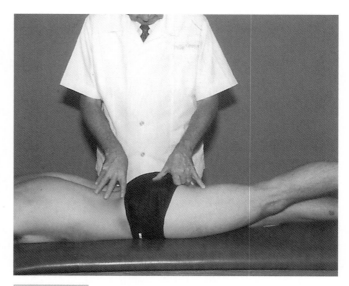

FIGURE 20.7 Hip extension observing gluteus maximus contraction. The patient is instructed to keep the leg straight and lift the knee two inches off the table.

forward bending and bending–twisting postures. Patients with recurrent low back pain will frequently attempt to self-stretch by bending forward or bring their knee to their chest to stretch into the pain, both of which only add to the problem. Self-stretching of the iliopsoas muscles (Figs. 20.8 and 20.9) and retraining the gluteus medius muscles will help to keep the sacrum stable (Fig. 20.2).

ATTACHMENTS OF THE RIGHT PSOAS MAJOR, PSOAS MINOR, AND ILIACUS MUSCLES (FIG. 20.8a)

The psoas major crosses many articulations including T12, the lumbar spine and the lumbosacral, sacroiliac, and hip joints. It does not attach to L5. The psoas minor does the same, except that it does not cross the hip joint. The iliacus, on the other hand, crosses only the hip joint.

PSOAS MUSCLE (FIG. 20.8b)

Self-stretch Position: Kneeling

1. Patient kneels and internally rotates the femur on the side to be stretched with the opposite hip and knee flexed to 90 degrees.

2. Patient places a hand on the buttock, voluntarily contracts the gluteus maximus, flattens the stomach, and maintains a 12 o'clock posterior pelvic tilt.

3. Patient maintains the trunk in an upright position, uses the opposite leg to pull the body forward, leading with the involved hip and maintaining contraction of the gluteal muscles throughout the stretch that is felt in the front of the hip and thigh.

4. Patient performs a series of contract–relax stretches for 1 to 2 minutes or a sustained 30-second stretch and repeats two or three times. The opposite side should be stretched in the same manner to achieve symmetric balance.

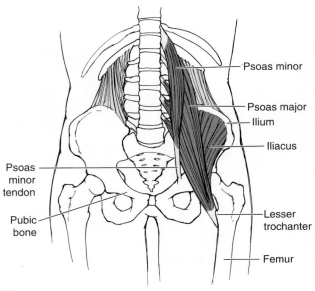

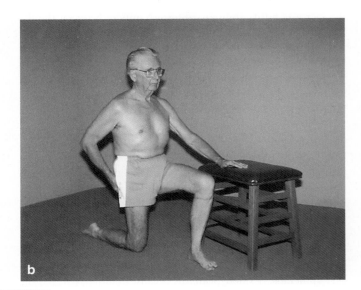

FIGURE 20.8

GLUTEUS MAXIMUS MUSCLE (FIG. 20.9a–c)

1. Patient lies on the back with knees flexed and feet flat.

2. Patient stabilizes the trunk by voluntary contraction of the transversus abdominus muscle, squeezes the buttocks together, and lifts the buttocks from the table (Fig. 20.9b). The pelvis should remain level and the lumbar spine in neutral.

3. Patient holds the position for 5 to 7 seconds, slowly returns to the table, and repeats five to seven times.

4. When able to perform easily, patient progresses to straighten one leg while in the bridged position (Fig. 20.9c) and repeats the 5- to 7-second hold for five to seven repetitions on each side. It is important that the pelvis remains level during the one-legged bridge.

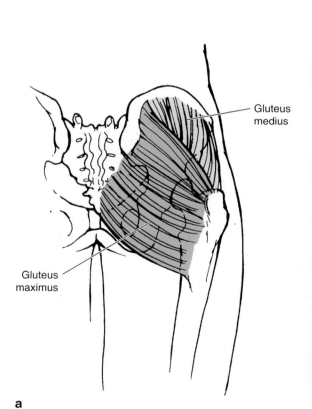

Gluteus medius

Gluteus maximus

a

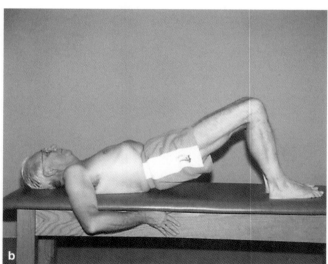

b

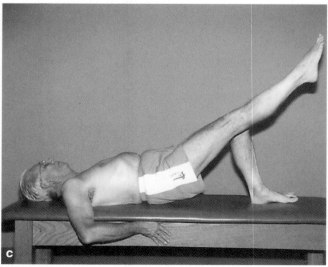

c

FIGURE 20.9

Anterior Sacral Torsions

Anterior torsions of the sacrum can be recurrent and typically define one of two common situations: the short-leg, pelvic-tilt syndrome or a chronically tight piriformis on the side of the anterior sacral base. During the gait cycle the sacrum in someone with an anatomically short, right, lower extremity will remain in the left-on-left position longer than the right-on-right, due to the relatively increased time spent in left gait stance. Anterior torsions in and of themselves will not lead to failed back syndrome and are thus not part of the "dirty half dozen." If suspected based on anatomical landmark levels and combined with a recurrent anterior innominate on and lumbar convexity toward the side of the short lower extremity, it would be prudent to correct the leg length discrepancy.

A unilateral chronically tight piriformis is not unusual in runners or those who speed walk for exercise. The syndrome has been previously described and, typically due to the muscles, needs to decelerate the hip during overpronation or uncontrolled pronation. The piriformis attaches proximally on the anterior surface of the sacrum and functions as a hip external rotator and abductor. When facilitated, it has the tendency over time to bring the sacral base forward and can contribute to recurrent anterior sacral torsions. In addition to treating the sacral dysfunction and stretching the hip external rotators, treatment consists of limiting the overpronation or uncontrolled pronation (see above) (Fig. 20.10).

PIRIFORMIS MUSCLE BELOW 90 DEGREES (FIG. 20.10a,b)

Self-stretch Position: Supine

1. Patient is supine with the leg on the involved side flexed at the hip and knee and with the foot lateral to the opposite knee.

2. Patient grasps the distal thigh and maintains adduction and internal rotation of the leg while stabilizing the pelvis with the other hand on the anterosuperior iliac spine. If the arm is too short, a belt or towel can be placed around the distal thigh to offer resistance.

3. Patient pushes the knee laterally against resistance and without rotating the pelvis.

4. Patient performs a series of contract–relax muscle efforts for 5 to 7 seconds with five to seven repetitions.

PIRIFORMIS MUSCLE ABOVE 90 DEGREES (FIG. 20.10c)

Self-stretch Position: Supine

1. Patient lies on the back and grasps with both hands the ankle and knee on the involved side.

2. The knee is pulled toward the opposite shoulder until a stretch is felt in the buttock.

3. Patient performs a sustained 30-second stretch repeated twice or a series of 5- to 7-second contract–relax muscle efforts repeated five to seven times.

4. The opposite side is stretched to balance.

PIRIFORMIS MUSCLE (FIG. 20.10d)

Self-stretch Position: Prone

1. Patient begins on the hands and knees and places the foot of the involved side in front of the opposite knee, with the foot pointing toward the ceiling and the knee lateral to the trunk. The involved leg is flexed, externally rotated, and abducted.

2. The opposite leg is stretched distally while keeping the pelvis level until stretch is felt in the buttock.

3. A sustained 30-second stretch is repeated twice.

4. The position is reversed to stretch the opposite side to balance.

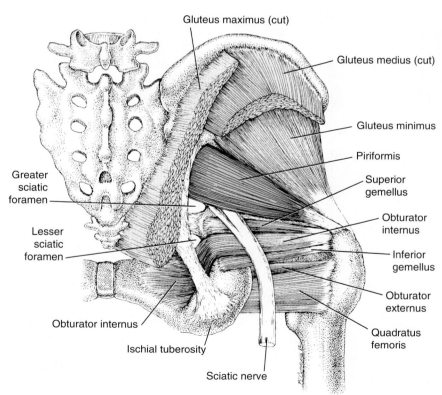

a

FIGURE 20.10

EXTERNAL ROTATORS OF THE HIP (FIG. 20.10e)

Self-stretch Position: Supine

The external rotators of the hip beside the piriformis are assessed and treated in relation to the posterior hip capsule (see Figs. 19.7 and 19.8). The manual stretch for this group of external hip rotator muscles is found in Chapter 19 (Figs. 19.29 and 19.30).

1. Patient is supine on the table with the uninvolved leg crossed over the involved leg and serving as a stabilizer.

2. Patient rotates the pelvis away from the involved hip sufficient to get the buttocks off the table.

3. With the uninvolved leg preventing movement of the involved leg, the patient attempts to pull the buttock of the involved side back to the table by a 5- to 7-second contraction repeated five to seven times.

4. The pelvis is rotated away from the involved hip by the other leg between each contraction.

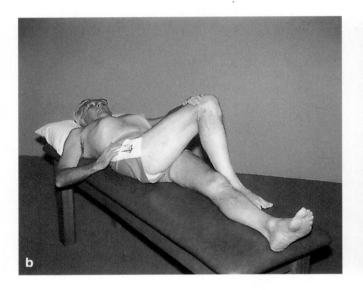

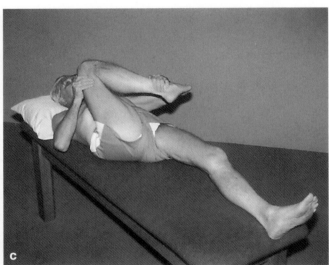

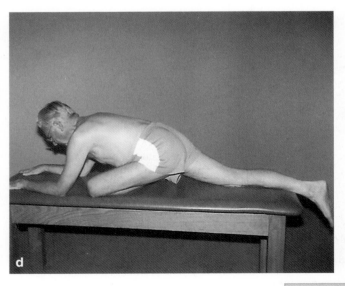

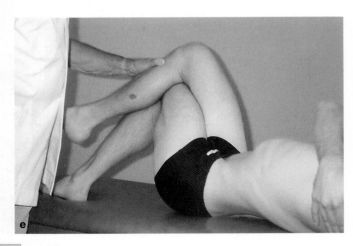

FIGURE 20.10   Cont'd

Unilateral Sacral Dysfunctions

Patients with recurrent unilateral sacral dysfunctions present with chronic recurrent disabling back pain with minimal radiation to the lower extremity below the buttocks. They find it difficult to stand for any period because the back pain progressively increases while standing without being mobile, hence the term "cocktail party syndrome." It is of major significance in patients who must stand in a confined area for long periods such as workers on assembly lines or cashiers at checkout counters. The pain is lessened by walking activities or by sitting. People who suffer from this problem are frequently one-legged standers who do not bear weight symmetrically on their lower extremities resulting in chronic postural imbalance.

The structural diagnostic findings in this population usually consist of the problem on the left side with the left pubis being superior, the left sacrum being anteriorly nutated (flexed), the left innominate posterior, and an L5 with ERS dysfunction to the left. From a muscle imbalance perspective, they frequently present with tight erector spinae muscles, weak pelvic stabilizers and weak abdominals. Patients presenting out of pattern, i.e., a right sacral nutation (flexion) or left sacral counternutation (extension) are more likely present in patients following pelvic fractures or major pelvic trauma.

Treatment of these patients is difficult and frequently frustrating. Recurrent exacerbations are common. Self-treatment should begin with derotating the innominate and self-mobilizing the sacrum (Figs. 20.11 and 20.12). They may require appropriate manual medicine treatment for the dysfunctions described and a lifelong exercise program to maintain pelvic, trunk, and abdominal muscle control. The patient must learn not to be a one-legged stander and to maintain balanced standing posture. Modifications of the work activity may be necessary to provide the patient with the opportunity to move on a frequent basis and to minimize standing in the nonmobile posture.

ANTERIOR INNOMINATE ROTATION (FIG. 20.11a)

Self-correction Position: Supine

1. Patient is supine on the table with involved hip and knee flexed.

2. Keeping the opposite knee straight, the patient grasps both hands below the involved knee and attempts hip extension by a 5-to 7-second muscle contraction.

3. After each relaxation, the patient increases hip flexion and repeats 5 to 7 times.

POSTERIOR INNOMINATE (FIG. 20.11b)

Self-correction Position: Supine

1. Patient is supine with the involved leg off the edge of the table or bed.

2. Patient flexes the opposite hip and knee bringing the knee to the chest.

3. At full exhalation, patient contracts the gluteal muscles to further extend the leg and holds for 5 to 7 seconds.

4. Five to seven repetitions are made with increasing amounts of hip extension.

POSTERIOR NUTATED (EXTENDED) SACRUM OR ANTERIOR NUTATED (FLEXED) SACRUM (FIG. 20.12)

Self-correction Position: Prone

1. Patient is prone with the involved leg slightly abducted and externally rotated on the table and the opposite foot placed on the floor.

2. Patient performs a push-up and maintains a sagging abdomen while forcefully exhaling.

3. Five to seven respiratory cycles are made with an attempt to increase the push-up with each effort.

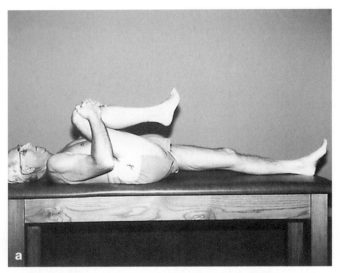

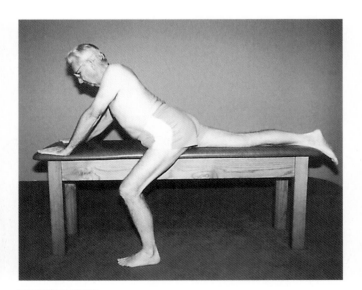

FIGURE 20.11

FIGURE 20.12

Lumbar Spine Dysfunctions

Lumbar segmental joint dysfunctions, in particular those that limit extension, lead to nonneutral behavior of the lumbar spine during gait. More importantly, lumbar segmental dysfunction inhibits the transversospinal muscle function that is critical for segmental stabilization during function of any sort. The coactivation of the multifidi with transversus abdominus lifts each lumbar segment against the vertical load provided by the iliopsoas and the quadratus lumborum muscles. This synergistic system also includes the thoracoabdominal and pelvic diaphragms which together allow for optimized intra-abdominal pressures, vital for overall trunk stability in addition to optimized venous and lymphatic flow from below upwards into central circulation.

Unopposed vertical loading from the iliopsoas and quadratus lumborum, together with loss of segmental control, leads to inappropriate segmental compression and torque. With time the lumbar intervertebral disks can lose height and fluid content. Loss of vertebral height leads to increased segmental movement which, without segmental control, will eventually lead to annular tears and facet hypertrophy heralding clinical instability, spondylosis, and spinal stenosis.

Segmental treatment of the lumbar spine should follow with iliopsoas stretches and quadratus lumborum stretches (Figs. 20.8b and 20.13). The "Pelvic Clock" is a diagnostic exercise for trunk and pelvic control and can also be useful in the diagnosis and self-management of lumbar spine dysfunctions (Fig. 20.14). The patient is taught how to assess the lumbar spine by touching each number of the clock sequentially, both clockwise and counterclockwise. The inability to symmetrically touch each number of the clock identifies the presence of dysfunction. Inability to touch 1 and 2 o'clock identifies an extended, rotated, and side bent left (ERS_{left}) dysfunction, 4 and 5 o'clock, an FRS_{left} dysfunction, 7 and 8 o'clock, an FRS_{right} dysfunction, and 10 and 11 o'clock, an ERS_{right} dysfunction. If the patient cannot move from 3 to 9 o'clock and from 9 to 3 o'clock easily and has some discomfort in trying, there is usually a sacroiliac dysfunction present. The inability to go to 3 'clock identifies restricted left rotation of the sacrum. Inability to go to 9 o'clock relates to restricted right rotation of the sacrum. These restrictions are most commonly due to a posterior sacral base on one side, either a posteriorly nutated sacrum or a backward torsion. Useful self-mobilizing procedures are of two types. One is release by position wherein the patient assumes a body position exactly opposite the number of the clock denoting restriction; for example, if unable to touch 5 o'clock, the patient moves as far toward 11 o'clock as possible and holds that position for 60 to 90 seconds, using a counterstrain principle. Then the patient slowly returns to neutral and again attempts 5 o'clock. The second procedure for the same dysfunction calls for moving all the way to 11 o'clock, then to 5 o'clock as far as possible, then back again to 11 o'clock, and repeat as mobilizing without impulse self-mobilization. With each repetition, an attempt to go further into 5 o'clock is made until symmetry is achieved. Other self-correction procedures for lumbar spine dysfunctions of the FRS type are modifications of Mackenzie's procedure to reduce the lateral shift and then incorporate extension. Procedures that have been found useful include standing and side gliding into the wall (Fig. 20.15) and while facing the wall (Fig. 20.16). This procedure allows fine-tuning of the amount of lateral shift and extension. Prone press-ups (Fig. 20.17) and backward bending while standing (Fig. 20.18) are then used to enhance trunk extension. Lumbar spine rotational strengthening and control can be performed with trunk rotational reeducation (Fig. 20.19).

Self-correction for ERS dysfunctions first needs to restore flexion. Single and bilateral knees to the chest in the supine position can achieve flexion but puts the sacrum at risk for posterior nutation. Another very effective exercise is a prayer stretch in the hands and knees position (Fig. 20.20). To restore flexion, rotation, and side bending together, the diagonal hip sink in the hands and knees position has been effective (Fig. 20.21). This exercise is also useful for stretching the quadratus lumborum and strengthening the gluteus medius and minimus muscles. Forward bending in step standing (Fig. 20.22) is also effective in self-correcting ERS lumbar dysfunction.

QUADRATUS LUMBORUM MUSCLE (FIG. 20.13a,b)

Self-stretch Position: Lateral Recumbent

1. Patient lies in the lateral recumbent position with the involved side uppermost.

2. Patient flexes the bottom leg to 90 degrees, with the involved leg extended and adducted off the side of the table or bed.

3. Patient's arm on the involved side reaches overhead, adding to the stretch by the weight of the involved leg.

4. The stretch is held for 10 to 15 seconds and repeated three times or a sustained stretch for 30 seconds.

5. The opposite side is stretched to balance.

QUADRATUS LUMBORUM MUSCLE (FIG. 20.13c)

Self-stretch Position: Standing

1. Patient stands with the arm of the involved side stretched overhead.

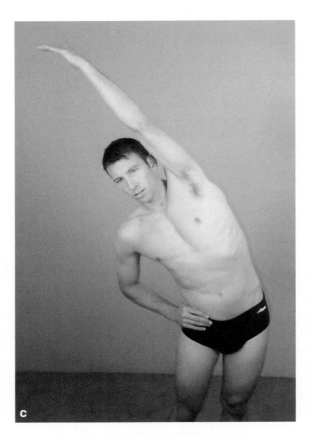

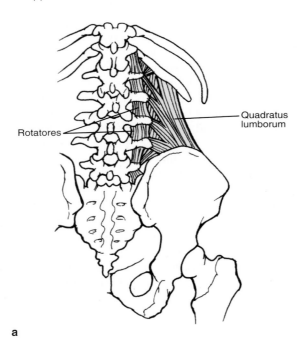

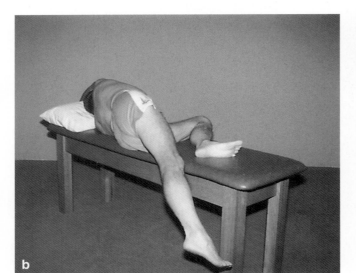

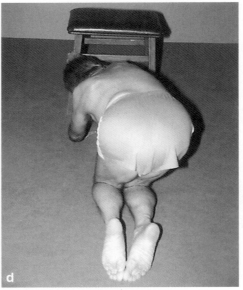

FIGURE 20.13

2. Patient laterally translates the pelvis toward the involved side as the trunk is side bent away from the involved side.

3. The position is sustained for 15 to 30 seconds and repeated two to three times.

4. The opposite side is stretched to symmetry.

QUADRATUS LUMBORUM AND LATISSIMUS DORSI MUSCLES (FIG. 20.13d)

Self-stretch Position: Kneeling

1. Patient on hands and knees reaches forward with the hand of the involved side and grasps a chair or stool with the hand internally rotated.

2. Patient shifts the pelvis laterally toward the involved side and then sits back, elongating the involved side with each repetition and increasing the diagonal drop of the pelvis.

3. The stretch is held for 10 to 15 seconds and repeated three to four times.

4. Externally rotating the hand adds an increase in the stretch of the latissimus dorsi.

5. The opposite side is stretched to balance.

PELVIC CLOCK (FIG. 20.14)

The pelvic clock is a diagnostic exercise for trunk and pelvic control. It can also be useful in the diagnosis and self management of lumbar spine dysfunction.

HIP SHIFT (FIG. 20.15)

Self-correction Position: Standing

1. Patient stands about 2 ft (60 cm) away from the wall with one shoulder, upper arm, and elbow against the wall.

2. Patient translates the pelvis toward the wall but avoids side bending of the spine.

3. Patient's other hand assists by pushing the pelvis to the wall.

4. Position is held for 5 to 7 seconds and repeated five to seven times.

5. This exercise deals with the side-bending component of a flexed, rotated, and side-bent lumbar dysfunction.

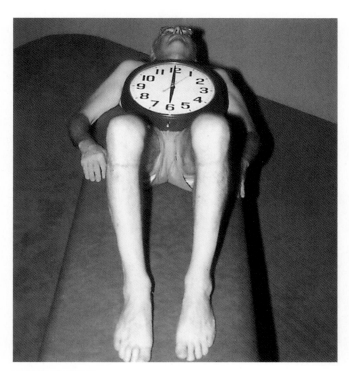

FIGURE 20.14

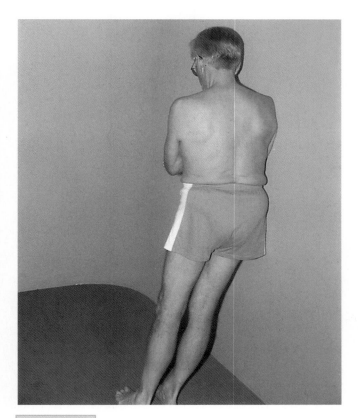

FIGURE 20.15

LUMBAR SPINE FLEXED, ROTATED, AND SIDE-BENT DYSFUNCTION (FIG. 20.16)

Self-correction Position: Standing

1. Patient stands facing the wall with feet acetabular distance apart and hands on the wall at shoulder height.

2. Patient shifts hips laterally from side to side toward restriction four to five times with increasing movement into the restrictive barrier (Fig. 20.16a).

3. Patient introduces extension by sagging the trunk forward while maintaining the arms straight (Fig. 20.16b).

4. The side shifting and extension components are gradually increased with five to seven repetitions.

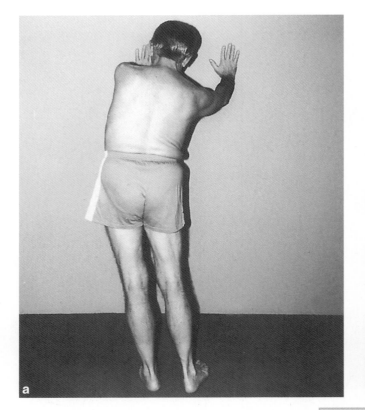
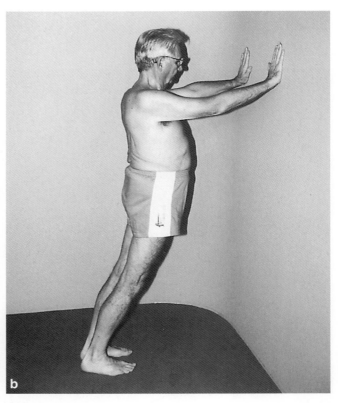

FIGURE 20.16

LUMBAR SPINE EXTENSION RESTRICTION (FIG. 20.17)

Self-correction Position: Prone

1. Patient is prone with hands on the table or floor.

2. Patient straightens the elbows and extends the trunk from above downward.

3. Spinal muscles are relaxed, and the stretch should be felt in the front of the chest and abdomen.

4. Position is held for 5 to 7 seconds and repeated five to seven times.

LUMBAR SPINE EXTENSION RESTRICTION (FIG. 20.18)

Self-correction Position: Standing

1. Patient stands with hands on posterolateral buttock and feet acetabular distance apart and slightly externally rotated.

2. Patient extends trunk from the head and neck downward and the hips shift anteriorly.

3. Patient repeats five to seven times with an increase in the trunk extension each time.

4. This exercise can be added to the hip shift (Fig. 20.15) to correct the extension component of a flexed, rotated, and side-bent lumbar dysfunction.

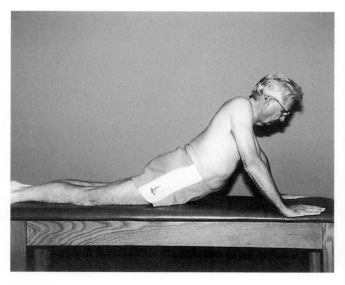

FIGURE 20.17

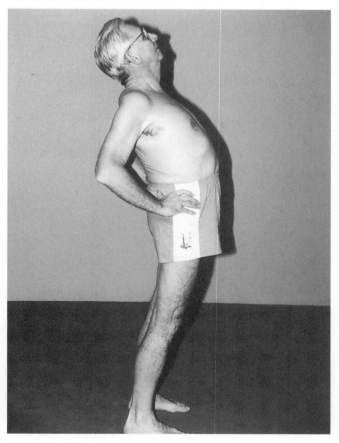

FIGURE 20.18

TRUNK ROTATION (FIG 20.19)

Reeducation Position: Supine

1. Patient lies with knees and hips flexed and feet together and flat on the table or floor. Arms are extended with palms down.

2. Patient's knees are slowly dropped to one side and held for a 5- to 7-second stretch (a).

3 Knees are slowly brought back to neutral by touching each spine segment from above downward to the table or floor. Hip and thigh muscles are passive; the motion comes from the trunk muscles (b).

4. The other side is exercised in a similar manner. Repeat five to seven times.

5. This exercise is good for the rotational component of lumbar nonneurtral dysfunctions.

LUMBAR SPINE "PRAYER STRETCH" (FIG. 20.20)

Self-correction Position: Prone

1. Patient begins in the hands and knees position with feet and knees hip-width apart.

2. Patient sinks back, attempting to touch buttocks to the heels.

3. Patient drops head and neck into flexion, allowing the spine to flex and the chest to drop to the floor.

4. The hands remain in contact with the floor.

5. Stretch is held for 10 to 15 seconds and is repeated three to four times.

6. This stretch deals with the flexion component of lumbar non-neutral dysfunctions.

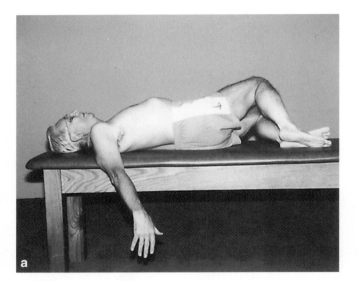

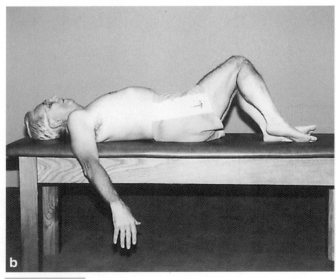

FIGURE 20.19

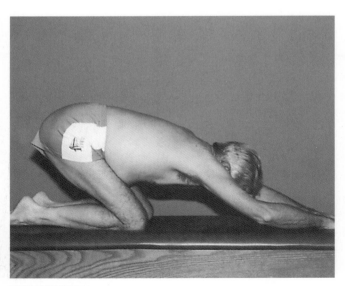

FIGURE 20.20

LUMBAR SPINE EXTENDED, ROTATED, AND SIDE-BENT DYSFUNCTIONS (FIG. 20.21)

Self-correction Position: "Diagonal Hip Sink"

1. Patient begins in hands and knees position.

2. Patient sits back diagonally, (toward the dysfunctional facet) introducing flexion, side bending, and rotation.

3. Position is held for 5 to 7 seconds and repeated five to seven times.

4. With each repetition, an increased amount of "hip sink" is done, increasing the mobility of the dysfunctional facet.

5. This exercise also strengthens the gluteal muscles. The operator may offer resistance alternately to the buttocks and opposite shoulder as the gluteal muscles are made to work eccentrically and concentrically.

6. This exercise is useful for self-correction of the anteriorly nutated sacrum, which is combined with an extended, rotated, and side-bent dysfunction at L5. Deep inhalation respiratory activating force is combined with the stretch position.

LUMBAR SPINE EXTENDED, ROTATED, AND SIDE-BENT DYSFUNCTION (FIG. 20.22)

Self-correction Position: Standing (Example: ERS$_{right}$)

1. Patient stands and places one foot on a chair or stool with the other leg straight.

2. Patient places both hands on the sides of the knee and bends forward, drawing the chest toward the knee as the hands slide down the leg to the ankle.

3. Position is held for 5 to 7 seconds and repeated five to seven times with increased trunk flexion with each effort.

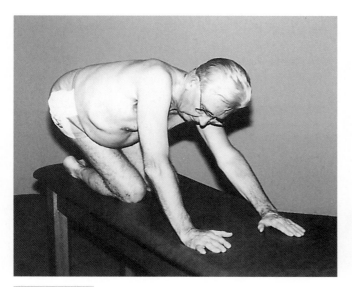

FIGURE 20.21

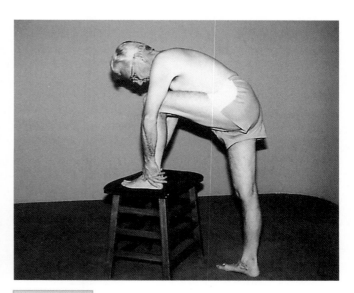

FIGURE 20.22

ABDOMINAL MUSCLES

The abdominal muscles as a group are notoriously weak and inhibited. They are essential for the maintenance of core stability, particularly the transversus abdominus. Recent research has found that the transversus abdominus muscle is the first to contract when movement occurs in the upper or lower extremity.[22,23] In patients with lower back pain, the activation of the transversus abdominus is delayed. There are a large number of exercises for strengthening the abdominal muscles, but few exercise all components of the them. One way to begin is to lay supine, place a hand under the lumbar lordosis, and contract the transversus abdominus by pulling the navel posteriorly without losing the lumbar lordosis. Another is to be on the hands and knees with a neutral lumbar lordosis and lift the navel without changing the lumbar curve. These exercises are done voluntarily but need to be programmed to occur subconsciously. More advanced abdominal strengthening exercises can be utilized once the patient has the capability to find and hold his/her transversus abdominus, without firing the superior obliques (depressing the rib angles) and continue to breathe comfortably (Figs. 20.23–20.24).

ABDOMINAL MUSCLES (FIGS. 20.23 AND 20.24)

Retraining with Curl-up

1. Patient lies supine with hips and knees flexed.

2. Patient extends arms in front and slowly curls up beginning in the cervical spine and up to the upper back while reaching toward the knees.

3. Position is held for 5 to 7 seconds and then the spine is slowly lowered segmentally to the starting position.

4. Placing the hands behind the neck increases the difficulty.

Note: This mainly exercises the rectus abdominus with concentric and eccentric contraction.

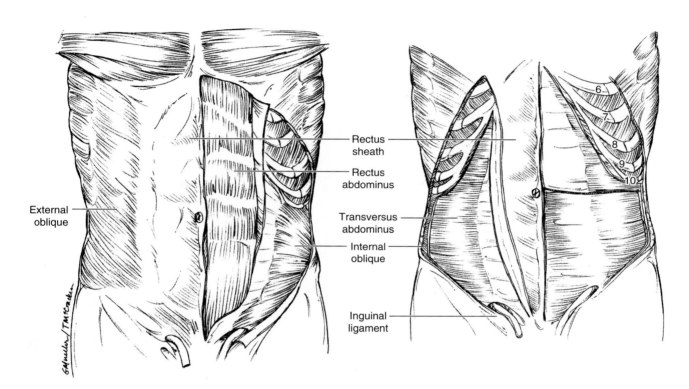

FIGURE 20.23

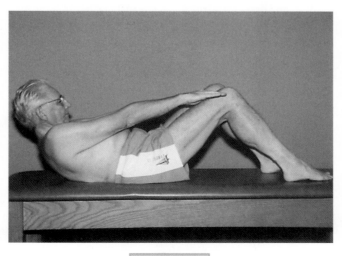

FIGURE 20.24

ABDOMINAL MUSCLES (FIG. 20.25)

Retraining

Heel Slides and Norwegian

1. Patient lies with the knees and hip bent and feet on the table or floor.

2. Patient contracts the transversus abdominus and slowly slides one leg down on the table or floor without losing the neutral lumbar lordosis and returns to the starting position. Each leg is alternately extended with 6 to 10 repetitions (Fig. 20.25a).

3. An alternative is to assume the 12 o'clock position for the lumbar spine and pelvis and slide the heel as far as possible without allowing the lumbar spine to extend and repeat on each side for 6 to 10 repetitions. The leg does not extend as far as it did in the first in this variation.

4. The Norwegian exercise begins in the same starting position, both hips and knees are flexed, and one leg at a time alternately touches the table or floor (Fig. 20.25b).

5. The patient increases the difficulty by touching the heel with gradually more extension of the hips and knees (Fig. 20.25c).

6. The lumbar lordosis must be maintained throughout these exercises by the contraction of the transversus abdominus muscle. Keeping a hand under the lumbar spine monitors the lordosis.

7. The goal is to perform the Norwegian leg extension for 2 minutes while counting aloud to prevent holding the breath.

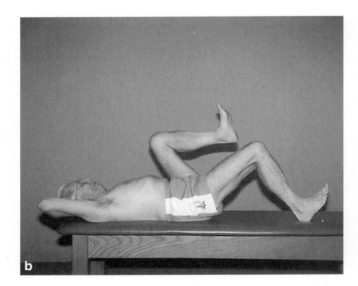

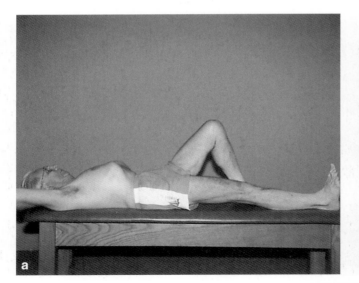

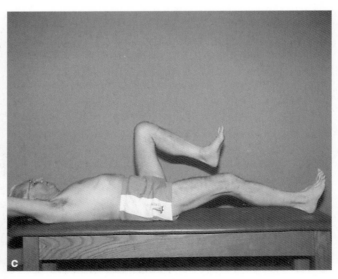

FIGURE 20.25

ABDOMINAL MUSCLES (FIG. 20.26)

Retraining with Sit Backs

1. Patient sits with hips and knees bent, the heels digging into the table or floor, and the toes plantar flexed.
2. Patient maintains the lumbar spine in neutral mechanics and extends the arms over the knees.
3. The patient sits back from this position as far as possible without lifting the heels and while maintaining the neutral lumbar spine. This is held for 5 to 7 seconds and then returned to the starting position. This is repeated five to seven times (step 1).

4. Patient places hands across the chest or behind the neck to increase the difficulty of performing the same and sits back for five to seven repetitions with a 5- to 7-second hold (step 2).
5. When proficient at step 2, patient progresses but rotates the shoulders while maintaining the neutral lumbar spine and performing the sit back with the right elbow pointed to the left knee, then returning to the starting position, rotating with the left elbow pointing to the right knee and repeating. Again, five to seven repetitions of a 5- to 7-second hold are made on each side.

Note: This is the favorite abdominal exercise of Dr. Greenman because it automatically activates the transversus abdominus subconsciously, exercises both obliques and the rectus abdominus in the lengthened position, and maintains a neutral lumbar spine.

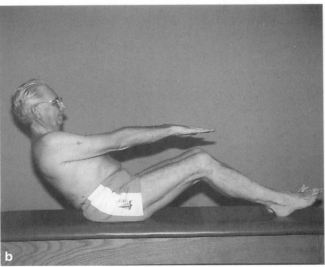
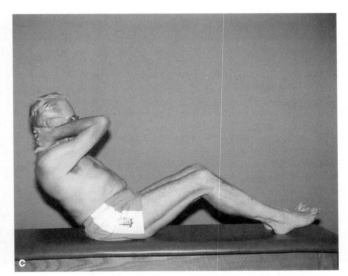
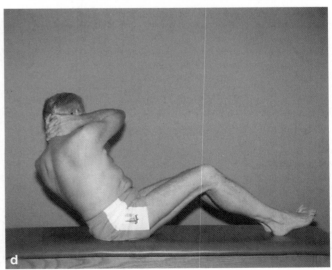
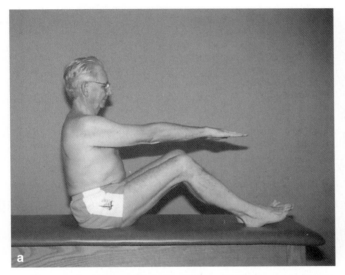

FIGURE 20.26

CONCLUSION

Exercise is a powerful tool in the management of patients with chronic musculoskeletal disorders and enhances the effectiveness of manual medicine interventions. The principles enumerated here focusing on centrally mediated and controlled motor balance, followed by stretching, and subsequently with strengthening (retraining), have been most effective. A properly designed and executed exercise program gives patients control of their level of musculoskeletal health and is very cost-effective.

REFERENCES

1. Janda V. Muscle and motor control in cervicogenic disorders: Assessment and management. In: Grant R, ed. *Physical Therapy of the Cervical and Thoracic Spine, Clinics in Physical Therapy*. New York: Churchill Livingstone, 1994:195–216.
2. Janda V. Muscle weakness and inhibition (pseudoparesis) in back pain syndromes. In: Grieve GP, ed. *Modern Manual Therapy of the Vertebral Column*. Edinburgh, UK: Churchill Livingstone, 1986:197–201.
3. Janda V. Muscles as a pathogenic factor in back pain. In: *The Treatment of Patients. Proceedings of the 4th Conference on International Federation of Orthopedic Manipulative Therapists*, Christchurch, New Zealand, 1980:1–23.
4. Janda V. Muscles: Central nervous motor regulation and back problems. In: Korr I, ed. *The Neurobiologic Mechanisms in Manipulative Therapy*. New York: Plenum Publishing, 1977:27–41.
5. Lewit K. *Manipulative Therapy in Rehabilitation of the Motor System*. 2nd Ed. Oxford: Butterworth, 1991.
6. Goff B. The application of recent advances in neurophysiology to Miss M. Rood's concept of neuromuscular facilitation. *Physiotherapy* 1972;58(12):409–415.
7. Bergmark A. Stability of the lumbar spine. A study in mechanical engineering. *Acta Orthop Scand Suppl*. 1989;230:1–54.
8. Mottram S, Comerford, M. Stability, dysfunction and low back pain. *J Orthop Med* 1998;20(2):13–18.
9. Panjabi MM. The stabilizing system of the spine. Part I. Function, dysfunction, adaptation, and enhancement. *J Spinal Disord* 1992;5(4):383–389.
10. Hides JA, Stokes MJ, Saide M, et al. Evidence of lumbar multifidus muscle wasting ipsilateral to symptoms in patients with acute/subacute low back pain. *Spine* 1994;19(2):165–172.
11. Gray G, *Understanding Pronation & Supination*. Wynn Marketing, Inc., November 2000.
12. Inman VT, Saunders FRCS, Abbott LC. Observations on the function of the shoulder joint. *J Bone Joint Surg* 1944;26A:1–30.
13. Kuo KH, Clamann HP. Coactivation of synergistic muscles of different fiber types in fast and slow contractions. *Am J Phys Med* 1981;60(5):219–238.
14. Neumann DA. *Kinesiology of the Musculoskeltal System: Foundations for Physical Rehabilitation*. St Louis: Mosby, 2002.
15. Vleeming A, Mooney V, Dorman T, et al. *Movement Stability and Low Back Pain: The Essential Role of the Pelvis*. New York: Churchill Livingstone, 1997.
16. Bullock-Saxton JE, Janda V, Bullock MI. Reflex activation of gluteal muscles in walking. *Spine* 1993;18:704.
17. Herzog W, Sheele D, Conway PJ. Electromyographic response of back and limb muscles associated with spinal manipulative therapy. *Spine* 1999;24(2):146–152.
18. Sims K. The development of hip osteoarthritis: Implications for conservative management. *Man Ther* 1999;4(3):127–135.
19. Greenman PE. Syndromes of the lumbar spine, pelvis, and sacrum. *Phys Med Rehabil Clin N Am* 1996;7(4):773–785.
20. Vleeming A, Stoeckaert R, Volkers ACW, et al. Relation between form and function in the sacroiliac joint. Part I: Clinical anatomic aspects & Part II: Biomechanical aspects. *Spine* 1990;15(2):130–136.
21. Bullock-Saxton JE, Janda V, Bullock MI. The influence of ankle sprain injury on muscle activation during hip extension. *Int J Sports Med* 1994;15:330–334.
22. Hodges PW, Richardson CA. Inefficient muscular stabilization of the lumbar spine associated with low back pain: A motor control evaluation of transversus abdominis. *Spine* 1996;21:2640–2650.
23. Hodges PW, Richardson CA. Altered trunk muscle recruitment in people with low back pain with upper limb movement at different speeds. *Arch Phys Med Rehabil* 1999;80:1005–1012.

ADJUNCTIVE DIAGNOSTIC PROCEDURES

The manual medicine practitioner primarily uses the structural diagnostic process to determine the presence or absence of somatic dysfunction, and its clinical significance, before instituting a manual medicine treatment. Adjunctive diagnostic procedures are frequently of assistance in determining the presence or absence of organic pathology of the musculoskeletal system in addition to the dysfunction. It is helpful to know whether the symptom presentation is due to organic pathology, dysfunction, or a combination of both. In most instances, it is a combination of both and the practitioner needs to address all components of the patient's presentation. Manual medicine must be practiced within the context of total patient care.

IMAGING PROCEDURES

The appropriate use and inappropriate abuse of imaging procedures remain controversial within the health care system. Imaging procedures can be expensive and can carry some risk, demonstrate both false-positive and false-negative results, and provide information that may be of little assistance in patient care. An admonition for all musculoskeletal medicine practitioners is to treat patients and not images. The following sections are not designed to be comprehensive but to share with the reader the opinions of this author on the assistance imaging procedures can have in manual medicine practice.[1]

Plain Films

Plain films of the lumbar spine and pelvis are not necessary before performing a manual medicine intervention. If the history and the physical examination lead the practitioner to a high index of suspicion of organic bone or joint disease, plain films are indicated, because they are relatively inexpensive, reveal osseous and joint anatomy, and can be of assistance in ruling out major traumatic, neoplastic, and inflammatory diseases. Plain films should be included as a minimum anteroposterior (AP) (Fig. 21.1) and lateral projections (Fig. 21.2). Right oblique (Fig. 21.3) and left oblique (Fig. 21.4) studies, while not routinely performed, provide good visualization of the zygapophysial joints and of the pars interarticularis. These views visualize the "Scottie dog" appearance of the posterior elements of the lumbar spine. The Scottie dog's eye is the pedicle, the associated transverse process is the nose, the superior facet joint is the ear, the inferior facet joint is the front leg, and the neck is the pars interarticularis. A defect through the pars interarticularis is identified as "spondylolysis" and the separation of the defect is termed "spondylolisthesis." Another commonly used view is a spot lateral projection of the lumbar sacral junction, particularly to look at the L5-S1 disc space. Preference is given to a 30-degree cephalic angled study (sunshine view) (Fig. 21.5), because it

provides excellent visualization of the lumbosacral disc space and both the sacroiliac joints and is of great assistance in the detailed assessment of transitional lumbosacral vertebrae. Note the bat wing transverse process with a pseudoarthrosis to the sacrum and to the ilium in Figure 21.5. This structural variation is one of the few predictors of future pathology and disability within the lumbar spine. The disc above the transitional vertebra is statistically at risk for herniation and the development of discogenic radiculopathy.[2,3]

Plain Film Postural Study. If the practitioner has suspicion of a short-leg, pelvic-tilt syndrome on the basis of the clinical finding of unleveling of the iliac crest and greater trochanter in the standing position, plain film postural study is useful in confirming the diagnosis and in determining the amount of the leg inequality and unleveling of the sacral base.[4,5] The postural study includes an AP projection of the lumbar spine and pelvis with the patient standing (Fig. 21.6) and in the lateral projection (Fig. 21.2). Great care by the technician is necessary to obtain quality images for postural analysis. The important technical factors are as follows:

1. An upright Bucky level with floor or footrest of the table
2. 14 × 17 in. film loaded level in the cassette
3. Cassette loaded level in Bucky
4. Patient standing erect with equal weight distribution on each feet 15 cm (6 in.) apart at the medial malleolus
5. One meter (40 in.) target-to-film distance
6. Vertical film centered at iliac crest
7. Central ray projected at center of film

The AP and erect films are measured in the following fashion:

1. AP projection
   A. A horizontal line is drawn across the top of each femoral head.
   B. A horizontal line is drawn across the sacral base. Three variations are provided in the order of their reliability.[6]
      (i) Across the most posterior aspect of the posterior margin of S1 body;
      (ii) Inferior aspect of sacral notch (transverse process S1); and
      (iii) Medial corner of S1 facet at the junction with the sacral body.
   C. Two vertical lines are drawn from the bottom of the film through the highest point of the femoral head to the line drawn across the sacral base.
   D. The difference in the distance from the femoral head to the bottom of the film is the leg length deficit.
   E. The difference in distance from the sacral base line to the bottom of the film on each side is the amount of sacral base unleveling.

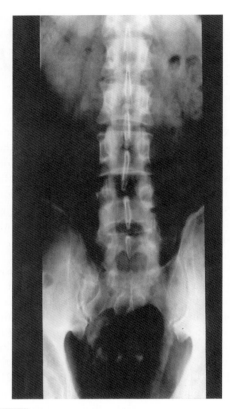

FIGURE 21.1 AP lumbar spine (supine).

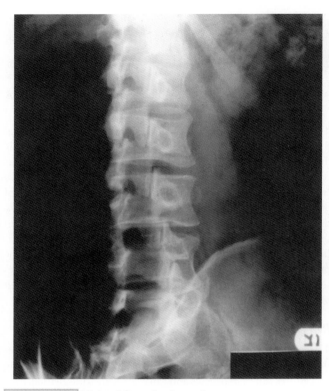

FIGURE 21.3 Right oblique lumbar spine.

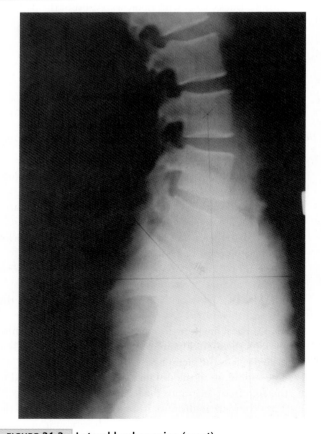

FIGURE 21.2 Lateral lumbar spine (erect).

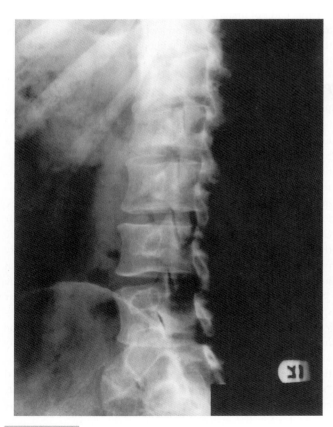

FIGURE 21.4 Left oblique lumbar spine.

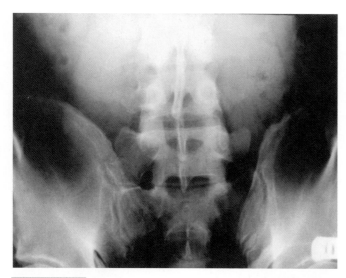

FIGURE 21.5 Sunshine view of the sacroiliac and lumbosacral joints.

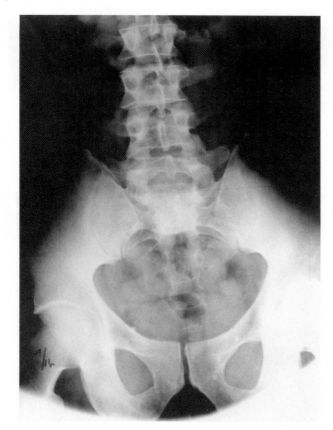

FIGURE 21.6 AP lumbar spine, erect, for postural analysis.

2. Lateral projection
   A. A line is drawn across the superior aspect of the body of S1 to meet a horizontal line drawn parallel to the bottom of the film at the level of the anterior aspect of S1. The resultant acute angle is called the "sacral base angle." In the erect position, the normal sacral base angle is 40 degrees plus or minus 2 degrees.
   B. The midportion of the third lumbar body is identified and a vertical line is dropped from the midthird lumbar body. Normally, this line should strike on the superior aspect of S1.

3. Lumbar scoliosis
   A. Assessment is made of the lumbar scoliosis in the AP projection. The normal adaptive process should show a lumbar convexity toward the side of the sacral base unleveling.[7]

Experience has shown that interrater and intrarater reliability using this methodology is 1 mm of difference. Unless the history and the physical examination require the plain film study before the initiation of treatment, it is advisable to treat the lumbar spine and pelvis to maximum biomechanical balance before performing a postural radiographic study.[8] Occasionally, dysfunction of the lumbar spine and pelvis, particularly dysfunction associated with major muscle imbalance, makes the study technically difficult and the measurements less than reliable. The study is best performed with the patient at maximum biomechanical function of the lumbar spine, pelvis, and lower extremities.[9]

Dynamic Studies

Plain films are frequently supplemented by dynamic studies in the erect position performing AP right-side bending (Fig. 21.7), left-side bending (Fig. 21.8), backward-bending (Fig. 21.9), and forward-bending lateral projections (Fig. 21.10). Assessment is made of the dynamic changes in the AP and lateral projections and compared with the neutral AP and lateral views. In the side-bending dynamic films, assessment is made of the presence or absence of neutral or nonneutral lumbar vertebral coupling. Figure 21.7 demonstrates side bending to the right with a rotation of the vertebrae into the concavity consistent with nonneutral vertebral mechanics in the lumbar spine. Figure 21.8 shows side bending to the left with a rotation of the lumbar vertebrae to the right, consistent with neutral vertebral motion in the lumbar spine. By overlying one film on another, it is frequently possible to identify which segment within the lumbar spine is resisting side bending to the right or to the left. In the forward-bending and backward-bending lateral projections, analysis is made of the intersegmental mobility. Again, by overlying one film on the other, in reference to the neutral lateral projection, it is possible to identify the vertebral segment that resists forward or backward bending. Coupling the neutral or nonneutral behavior of the lumbar spine in side bending with the intersegmental restriction of flexion or extension can assist in the evaluation of nonneutral vertebral dysfunction within the lumbar spine. The role of dynamic studies remains controversial because of difficulty in the biomechanical research of the methodology. Despite this concern, clinical experience has shown them to be of assistance in the collaboration of the structural diagnostic finding.

Special Imaging Studies

There are a number of special imaging studies that have use in musculoskeletal problems particularly in lower back and lower

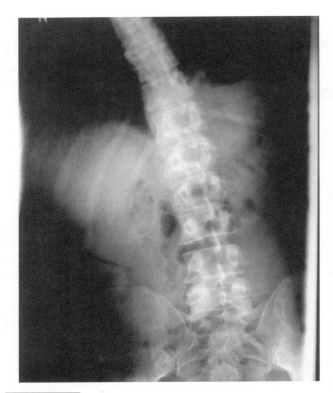

FIGURE 21.7 AP erect, right-side bending dynamic film.

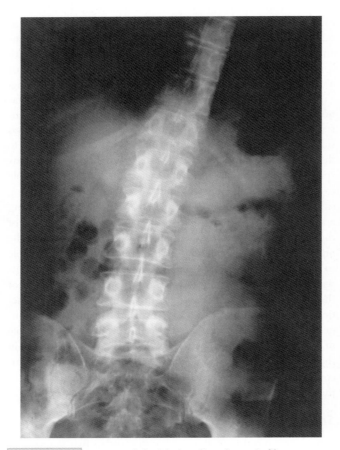

FIGURE 21.8 AP erect, left-side bending dynamic film.

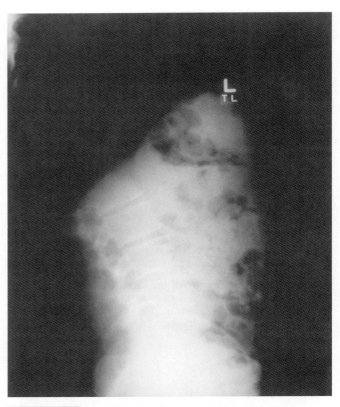

FIGURE 21.9 Lateral backward-bending dynamic film.

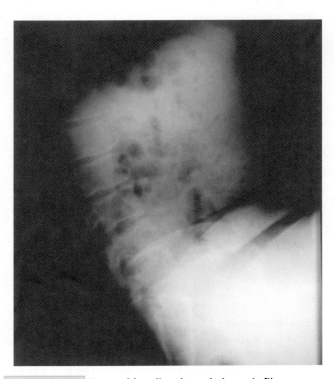

FIGURE 21.10 Forward-bending, lateral, dynamic film.

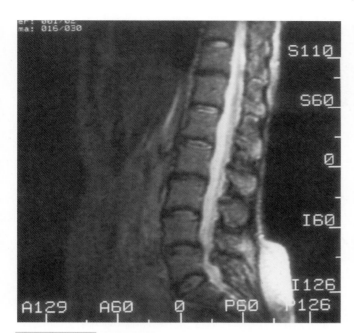

FIGURE 21.11 MRI, lumbar spine, sagittal view.

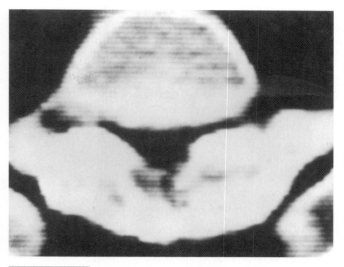

FIGURE 21.12 CT scan, lumbar spine, bone window.

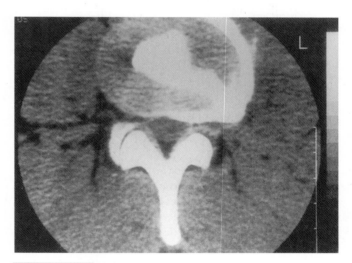

FIGURE 21.13 Lumbar spine, discogram CT.

extremity pain syndromes. Before ordering a special imaging study, the practitioner should show care in selecting a procedure that will provide the information desired. Different imaging studies provide different information. Special imaging studies should be done to confirm the impressions gained from the clinical examination.

Magnetic Resonance Imaging. Special images such as magnetic resonance imaging (MRI) should not be used as a screening tool to look for pathology in a patient presenting with back pain. MRI has many advantages in the diagnostic process and provides the best information about the soft tissues of the musculoskeletal system. It has become the imaging method of choice for diagnosis of disc herniation, cord lesions, brain lesions, and many of the less common developmental variants like syringomyelia and tethered cord (Fig. 21.11). MRI can provide images that demonstrate the nucleus of the disc similar to those revealed in a discogram and outline the spinal canal and its contents similar to those of a myelogram. The procedure involves no ionizing radiation, is noninvasive, and has few contraindications, namely metal implants and pacemakers. MRI gantries are becoming larger so that the patient is less likely to become claustrophobic in the machine. One drawback to MRI studies is the difficulty in obtaining dynamic studies because of the dimensions of the gantry and the fact that the patient is in an unloaded position. With special technical effort, it is possible to obtain some dynamic flexion and extension studies of the cervical spine. Dynamic studies of the lumbar spine are much more difficult. Upright MRI technology has recently been developed and is currently being used in research studies of spinal mechanics in the loaded position. In the future, this technology may become available for clinical use and is exciting to contemplate.[10]

Computed Tomography. Computed tomography (CT) studies have a longer history than MRI. CT is the imaging method of

choice when looking for morphology of the osseous system. It is also useful in identifying disc disease, including herniation with extrusion of nuclear material into the central and lateral vertebral canals as well as lateral and interior herniations (Fig. 21.12). This technology is particularly useful in the assessment of central and lateral recess stenosis as seen in Fig. 21.12. CT can be combined with discography and myelography to provide additional diagnostic information (Fig. 21.13). Plain CT is noninvasive but does require the patient to be exposed to ionizing radiation. Metallic implants are not a contraindication, but the images are frequently distorted by artifact. A discogram CT and myelogram CT require an accompanying invasive procedure.

Myelography. Myelography is one of the older special imaging methods in the diagnosis of spinal pathology. Historically, it has been used for localization of disc pathology, neural compression, blockage of cerebral spinal fluid, and intraspinal pathology such as cord tumor. It is an invasive procedure and some of the dye material used in the past was toxic and led to complications.

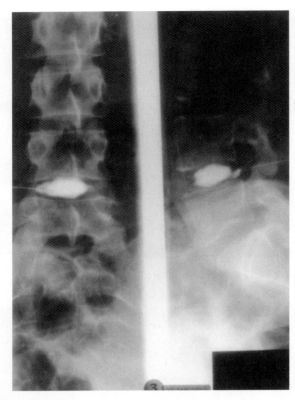

FIGURE 21.14   Disc AP and lateral projections.

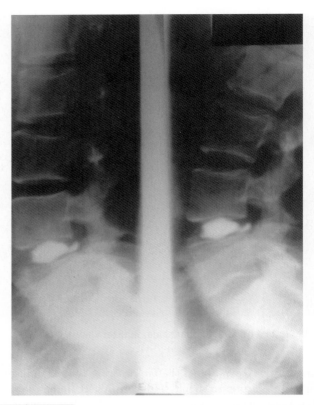

FIGURE 21.15   L4-L5 lumbar discogram, erect, forward bending and backward bending.

There is a statistically significant increase in arachnoiditis with pantopaque myelography. Currently, water-soluble contrast materials are much less toxic, but they are contraindicated in a few individuals who are iodine-sensitive. False negatives in myelography are common for disc disease at the L5-S1 level. Myelography occasionally becomes a procedure of choice, particularly in association with CT imaging, in certain diagnostic challenges.

Discography. Discography continues to have its advocates and detractors. It is an invasive procedure with considerable technical difficulty. Radiopaque material is injected into the nucleus of the disc and images are made for assessment of intradiscal pathology (Fig. 21.14). Discography also provides the opportunity to assess whether a disc is a pain generator. An injection into a normal disc is usually not painful. Injection into a diseased disc is frequently painful, and if it replicates the patient's pain complaint, gives some corroboration of the disc as the site of pain generation. In the presence of disc herniation, there is commonly exacerbation of the associated radiculopathy. Like myelography, the procedure is invasive and requires the introduction of a foreign substance that carries some allergic risk. Another value of discography is the ability to perform the study with the patient loaded and unloaded. In the erect loaded position, flexion and extension can be performed to further assist in the diagnostic process (Fig. 21.15). Note in Fig. 21.15 that there was additional extrusion of the opaque nuclear material in a posterior direction during trunk backward bending. Like discography,

myelography can be performed in the standing loaded position, and the patient can be subjected to dynamic stress of forward bending, backward bending, and right- to left-side bending.

Diagnostic Blocks and Injections

On occasion, additional special studies can be of assistance in determining the location of the pain generator and the significance of altered anatomy. These procedures include zygapophysial and sacroiliac joint injections, selected nerve blocks, and the previously discussed discography. These procedures require fluoroscopic control, the use of contrast material, and the instillation of anesthetic agents to determine if the structure is painful and responds to a local block (Figs. 21.16 and 21.17). Figures 21.16 and 21.17 show the role of a zygapophysial injection in determining if the spondylolisthesis at this level was symptomatic. Note that the needle is placed in the L4-L5 joint, but with instillation of contrast material there, the image shows delineation of the pars' defect and the zygapophysial joint at L5-S1. The procedure was pain free for the patient and the conclusion is that this defect is not pain producing. The sacroiliac joint can be challenged and visualized by arthrography (Figs. 21.18–21.20). Under fluoroscopic control, the inferior margin of the synovial portion of the sacroiliac joint can be entered and contrast material injected. Like zygapophysial joint injection, if the joint is contributing to pain generation, the injection is painful to the patient. Instillation of local anesthetic with relief of concordant pain identifies this structure as a pain generator. Figures 21.18 through 21.20 show an

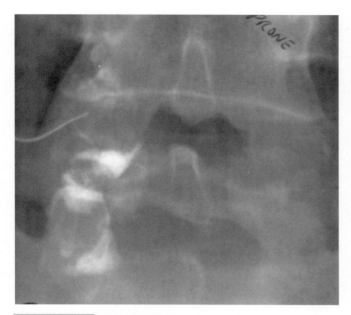

FIGURE 21.16 L4-L5 joint block, AP projection.

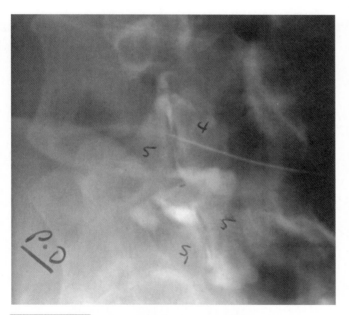

FIGURE 21.17 L4-L5 zygapophysial joint block, oblique projection.

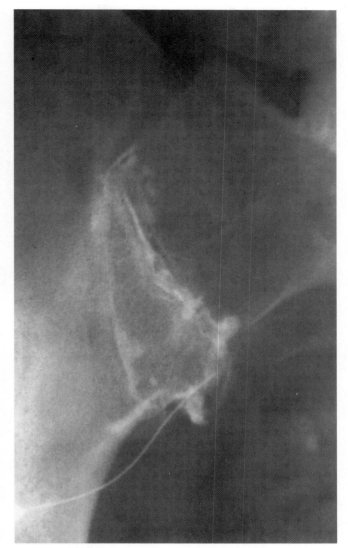

FIGURE 21.18 Left sacroiliac arthrogram, AP view.

example of anterior capsular diverticula in the presence of a joint that was positive to the challenge of injection. After instillation of local anesthetic, the patient experienced complete removal of the concordant pain. This confirmed the left sacroiliac joint as a pain generator contributing to the patient's presentation. Figure 21.21 is a special CT view of the sacroiliac joints in the case represented in Figures 21.18 through 21.20. Note the asymmetric relationship of the anterior aspects of the sacrum to the posterior aspects of the ilium as shown by the horizontal lines. This finding was imaging confirmation of the palpatory assessment of sacral torsion in this patient. Occasionally, information can be obtained about the

functional capacity of the anatomy that is so well displayed by such imaging techniques. Selective nerve blocks require fluoroscopic guidance and again seek to identify whether a specific nerve root and its sheath are contributing to pain generation. This technology has greater value in the diagnosis of acute discogenic radiculopathy than it does in the dysfunctional pathology dealt with by manual medicine.

Special Magnetic Resonance Imaging Studies

MRI is an excellent technology for distinguishing differences in soft tissues. For the past 2 years, a special protocol for MRI imaging of the upper cervical spine has been used to identify selective fatty replacement of rectus capitis posterior minor and rectus capitis posterior major muscles. This fatty replacement is seen in 87% of patients presenting with posttraumatic cervical cranial pain syndromes and is not found in 100% in a normative

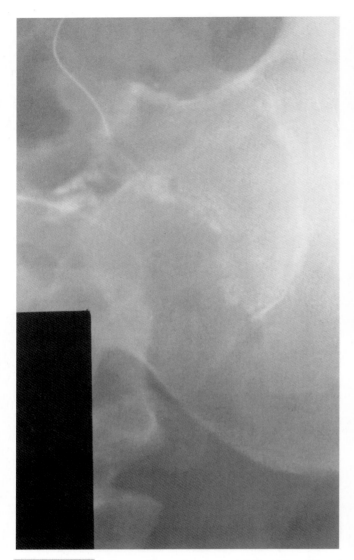

FIGURE 21.19   Left sacroiliac arthrogram, right anterior oblique.

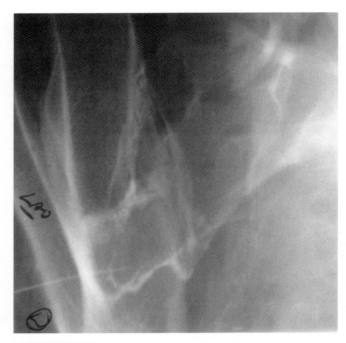

FIGURE 21.20   Left sacroiliac arthrogram, left anterior oblique.

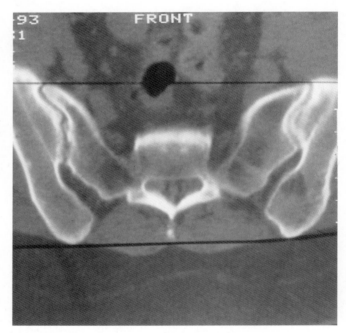

FIGURE 21.21   CT scan of sacroiliac joints.

population (Figs. 21.22 and 21.23).[11–13] Figure 21.22 shows good definition of both the rectus capitis posterior major and minor, with muscle densities identified with arrows, in an asymptomatic patient with no history of trauma. Figure 21.23 shows fatty replacement of rectus capitis posterior major and minor muscles (arrows) in a patient 2 years after a motor vehicle injury with flexion–extension of the cervical spine and resultant pain in the upper cervical region with radiation of head pain anteriorly from the cranial base. The cause of the fatty replacement is under study and its overall significance is yet to be determined. Intuitively, one would assume that if a muscle has been replaced by fat and has lost its contractile properties, this might contribute to persistent symptoms and the lack of response to manual medicine using muscle energy activating force.

Electrodiagnostic Studies

The use of electromyography and nerve conduction studies can be of assistance in the differential diagnosis of cervicobrachial

and lower extremity pain syndromes to rule in or rule out the presence of significant radiculopathy from discogenic disease or other causes. Nerve conduction studies are of particular value in documenting the presence of the carpal tunnel or tarsal tunnel syndromes. There are many sophisticated neurophysiologic tests available but they are seldom needed in the practice of manual medicine. Electromyography in the presence of acute radiculopathy is not diagnostic for the initial 3-week period: A negative

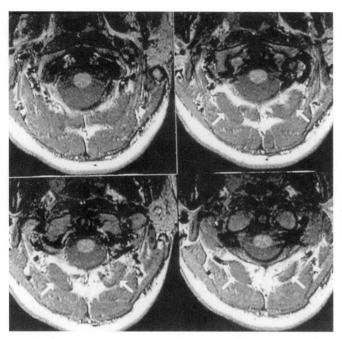

FIGURE 21.22 Cervical spine MRI in nontrauma, nonsymptomatic patient.

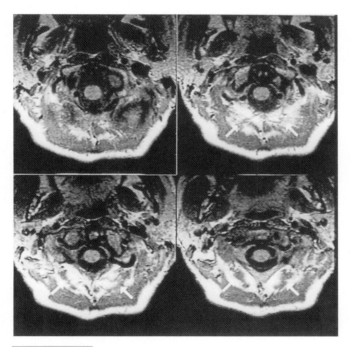

FIGURE 21.23 Cervical spine MRI in posttraumatic symptomatic patient.

author uses confirmatory EMG studies before subjecting patients to surgical intervention for disc disease.

Electromyography of the rectus capitis posterior muscles identified by MRI (Fig. 21.23) has shown that they have denervation changes. The fatty replacement is not disuse atrophy; it is true neurologic change.[13] The posterior primary division of C1 innervates the superior and inferior oblique muscles and the rectus capitis posterior major and posterior minor muscles. This leads one to wonder why fatty replacement of the obliques has never been seen and is rarely seen in the rectus capitis posterior major muscle. The rectus capitis posterior minor innervation is from the terminal branch of C1 and travels through the belly of the rectus capitis posterior major. Perhaps the answer is that during the flexion–extension injury, the terminal branch is avulsed and the rectus capitis posterior minor is dennervated. It is interesting to note that during these EMG studies, the muscle is most active during anterior translation of the head and not during extension. The apparent role of the rectus capitis posterior minor muscle is to reduce forward translation of the occiput during flexion movement.

Fine-wire and surface EMG are of diagnostic assistance in the determination of normal or abnormal muscle firing pattern sequences. Janda has described normal muscle firing sequences for hip extension,[14] hip abduction, and shoulder abduction. Fine-wire and surface EMG studies have been used in the research that has defined the major role of the transversus abdominis muscle in core stability.[15] These aberrations can be documented by fine-wire and surface EMG study and the technology can be of assistance in documenting the response to treatment interventions.

Laboratory Testing

A practitioner has a vast array of laboratory diagnostic tests available. In musculoskeletal medicine, there are a few that can be of assistance, particularly in ruling out rheumatologic conditions and in identifying general systemic illness. It has been said that the sedimentation rate takes the temperature of the musculoskeletal system. It is a valuable screening test requiring additional laboratory testing if positive. Basic rheumatologic tests are found within the arthritic profile, and the findings may direct the clinician toward more extensive antinuclear antibody and DNA studies. Vitamin D deficiency can present as musculoskeletal pain. The populations with the greatest risk include the homebound elderly, people with pigmented skin, people with cultural and social avoidance of the sun, people who live in wintertime in climates above and below latitudes of 35 degrees, and people with gastrointestinal malabsorption.[16] Assessment of thyroid function is frequently of assistance in patients with chronic pain. Borderline hypothyroidism is frequently seen in patients with primary and secondary fibromyalgias. Not all patients who present with musculoskeletal pain syndromes are experiencing biomechanical dysfunction. The alert practitioner uses all the tools available, including laboratory testing, to assess the total patient.

Psychological Evaluation

Psychological assessment of patients with musculoskeletal pain syndromes, particularly those with chronic pain, is frequently of

study in an early presentation does not rule out the presence of radiculopathy. A positive electromyogram (EMG) with acute changes can help confirm the diagnosis of discogenic radiculopathy in a patient who presents with classic clinical findings when the positive findings are consistent with the diagnosis. This

assistance in patient management. Psychosocial factors play a large role in back pain disability. There are a number of standardized tests such as the Minnesota Multiphasic Personality Inventory test that have had extensive use in assessing the psychological and psychiatric status of a patient. A one-on-one psychological evaluation by a trained clinical psychologist conversant with musculoskeletal pain syndromes can be of great assistance. Psychological evaluation, particularly the neuropsychological examination, is of considerable value in identifying the presence and severity of traumatic brain injury. Traumatic brain injury is frequently seen in patients with chronic pain syndromes and is probably underdiagnosed. A probing history will frequently identify trauma resulting in transient unconsciousness and disorientation.

Occupational Therapy Assessment

A cognitive, perceptual, motor evaluation by a skilled occupational therapist is another test useful in the diagnosis of traumatic brain injury. Assessment of the work site, particularly in those patients presenting with repetitive strain injuries, can be very useful in total patient management. Work-site modification is frequently beneficial in the rehabilitation of disabled patients as well as in the prevention of injuries in the future.

Nutritional Evaluation

The services of a skilled nutritionist can be of assistance in the rehabilitation process. Many patients with musculoskeletal pain syndromes have poor nutrition with heavy use of caffeine, alcohol, and high-inflammatory or fast foods. A poor diet contributes to an unhealthy musculoskeletal system and interferes with the normal neurologic control of the motor system function. Obesity continues to be a societal problem particularly in patients with chronic musculoskeletal problems that reduce the patients' activity level. Smoking contributes to poor response to both nonoperative and operative care of spinal problems. Reduction in smoking, alcohol, and drugs, plus a well-balanced diet resulting in an appropriate weight, can be of major significance in the recovery of patients with musculoskeletal problems.

CONCLUSION

The manual medicine practitioner should be aware of the role of adjunctive diagnostic procedures in patient assessment.

Knowledge of the attributes and shortcomings of many of the aforementioned diagnostic procedures is necessary for their appropriate use. The practitioner should become acquainted with the expertise of other disciplines that can be included in the patient management process. Such knowledge will lead to the appropriate use and not the inappropriate abuse of medical technology.

REFERENCES

1. Greenman PE. Clinical use of the roentgen examination in the low back syndrome. *J Am Osteopath Assoc* 1974;73(7):554–563.
2. Bron JL, van Royen BJ, Wuisman PI. The clinical significance of lumbosacral transitional anomalies. *Acta Orthop Belg* 2007;73(6):687–695.
3. Luoma K, Vehmas T, Raininko R, et al. Lumbosacral transitional vertebra: Relation to disc degeneration and low back pain. *Spine* 2004;29(2):200–205.
4. Greenman PE. Lift therapy: Use and abuse. *J Am Osteopath Assoc* 1979;79(4):238–250.
5. Friberg O. Clinical symptoms and biomechanics of lumbar spine and hip joint in leg length inequality. *Spine* 1983;8(6):643–651.
6. Irwin RE. Reduction of lumbar scoliosis by use of a heel lift to level the sacral base. *J Am Osteopath Assoc* 1991;91:34–44.
7. McCaw ST, Bates BT. Biomechanical implications of mild leg length inequality. *Br J Sports Med* 1991;25(1):10–13.
8. Brady RJ, Dean JB, Skinner TM, et al. Limb length inequality: Clinical implications for assessment and intervention. *J Orthop Sports Phys Ther* 2003;33(5):221–234.
9. Hoffman KS, Hoffman LL. Effects of adding sacral base leveling to osteopathic manipulative treatment of back pain: A pilot study. *J Am Osteopath Assoc* 1994;94(3):217–220, 223–226.
10. Alyas F, Connell D, Saifuddin A. Upright positional MRI of the lumbar spine. *Clin Radiol* 2008;63(9):1035–1048.
11. Hallgren RC, Greenman PE, Rechtien JJ. Atrophy of suboccipital muscles in patients with chronic pain: A pilot study. *J Am Osteopath Assoc* 1994;94(12):1032–1038.
12. Hack GD, Koritzer RT, Robinson WL, et al. Anatomic relation between the rectus capitis posterior minor muscle and the dura mater. *Spine* 1995;20(23):2484–2486.
13. Andary MT, Hallgren RC, Greenman PE, et al. Neurogenic atrophy of suboccipital muscles after a cervical injury: A case study. *Am J Phys Med Rehabil* 1998;77(6):545–549.
14. Janda V. Muscle spasm – a proposed procedure for differential diagnosis. *J Man Med* 1991;6(4):136–139.
15. Hodges PW, Richardson CA. Feedforward contraction of transversus abdominisis not influenced by the direction of arm movement. *Exp Brain Res* 1997;114:362–370.
16. Heath KM, Elovic EP. Vitamin D deficiency: Implications in the rehabilitation setting. *Am J Phys Med Rehabil* 2006;85(11):916–923.

ADJUNCTIVE THERAPEUTIC PROCEDURES

Manual medicine is a powerful tool in the management of many health problems, particularly those involving the musculoskeletal system. In some cases, manual medicine is the primary therapeutic intervention. Other therapies may be used with manual medicine. When using manual medicine techniques, it is essential that it be done within the context of total patient care and the practitioner must determine that the manual medicine interventions are appropriate for the patient's physical condition.

The following are comments on a variety of other therapeutic interventions that this author has found to be most useful.

MEDICATION

In using an oral or injectable medication, the practitioner should be knowledgeable about the actions, reactions, and iatrogenic effects of any substance used. The medication protocol should be as simple as possible. A general observation is that the more potent the medication is for its effectiveness, the more common are its side effects and reactions.

Medication for pain control is of great importance in the management of musculoskeletal conditions. The longer the nociceptive process is ongoing, the more likely it is that sensitization of pain pathways and deprogramming of motor control will occur.[1,2] The management of pain associated with acute tissue injury is quite different from the management of pain that has been present for months or years. Acute pain is characterized by its specific localization, lancinating quality, and associated tissue damage in a specific structure of the musculoskeletal system. Chronic musculoskeletal pain is quite different. It is characterized by being less well localized, more diffuse, and frequently a burning quality.

Analgesics and Narcotics

Analgesics and narcotics are most useful for the acute painful condition. In acute pain, it is advisable to see that the dose is adequate in strength and availability to control the painful perception. The persistence of nociceptive pathway stimulation has a negative effect on the patient's nervous system and can lead to chronicity. The dose should be adjusted to avoid peaks and valleys of pain relief and increased pain perception.

It is unknown when acute pain changes to chronic pain. Some view chronicity as being related to time, with the changeover being from 3 to 6 months. Some believe that pain pathway stimulation for 30 days is sufficient to change central pain processing pathways. In chronic pain, the patient continues to perceive pain despite the lack of ongoing tissue damage. This is commonly frustrating for both the attending physician and the patient because of the absence of an identifiable cause of persistent pain. However, to the patient, the pain is real and it needs

appropriate attention just as the more commonly recognized acute pain associated with acute tissue damage. Chronic pain in the absence of identifiable tissue damage is managed quite differently from the chronic pain of patients with associated diseases such as malignancy, inflammatory joint disease, and associated rheumatologic conditions. In these conditions, the appropriate mix of medications to assist the patient in the control of pain is clearly indicated. In the patient with chronic pain without ongoing tissue damage or disease process, medications are mainly contraindicated. Analgesics and narcotics seem to contribute to, rather than ameliorate, the chronic pain system. These patients need to be weaned off potent medications as rapidly as possible. During their rehabilitative process, particularly with increasing activity during an exercise program, there may be exacerbation of the tissue reaction, which results in short bursts of acute pain. Appropriate acute pain medication at this time is clearly beneficial, but needs to be discontinued as rapidly as possible. Acetaminophen in adequate doses seems to work well in these instances. The treatment of the patient with chronic pain syndrome requires an integrated team approach with only one physician being responsible for the medication prescriptions.

Antiinflammatory Agents

Another group of medications of great adjunctive use in the management of musculoskeletal conditions is the antiinflammatory agents. The nonsteroidal antiinflammatory drugs (NSAIDs) are quite popular and are available over the counter. The classes of NSAIDs differ primarily in the balance of analgesic and antiinflammatory effects and the length of action. Almost all are irritating to the gastrointestinal tract and caution must be used in prescribing these agents for patients with peptic ulcer disease, gastritis, and irritable bowel syndrome. Aspirin is the oldest and least expensive of this group; if tolerated by the patient, it is as good as any. In general, it is most effective to use short-acting NSAIDs in adequate antiinflammatory doses and then wean the patient off the medication as rapidly as possible. This author has found that 2,400 to 3,200 mg of ibuprofen in daily divided doses for 7 to 10 days is very useful for the patient with acute pain as well as for the acute exacerbation in the patient with chronic pain undergoing active manual medicine intervention and early exercise programming. Caution should be used for the longer acting NSAIDs because patients metabolize these drugs differently and toxic levels can be achieved with little warning. Injectable ketorolac tromethamine (Toradal) is frequently of value in achieving control of acute pain, particularly that associated with acute tissue injury and the acute flare following an active manual medicine intervention. In the long-term management of

521

patients using NSAIDs, careful monitoring of gastrointestinal, hepatic, renal, and hematologic functions is prudent.

The newest of this group are the Cox-2 inhibitors (Celebrex and Vioxx are examples), which have longer action and are somewhat less irritating to the gastrointestinal tract when compared with NSAIDs, but recently there have been more reports of gastrointestinal problems, myocardial infarction, and stroke with their long-term use. Although Vioxx has been taken off the market, Celebrex is worth considering in patients with arthritis, both osteoarthritis and rheumatoid disease.

Corticosteroids

Corticosteroids have a place in the management of musculoskeletal conditions, particularly during the acute phase. Oral and injection formulations are available and corticosteroids have particular value in the management of acute radiculopathy. Spinal and caudal epidural steroids have long been used in the management of acute radiculopathies and both have their advocates and their critics. The problem with caudal instillation is the difficulty in achieving levels high enough to affect radiculopathies above S1. Spinal epidurals can be more precise in the localization of steroid effect. Both of these invasive procedures should be done under fluoroscopic control to ensure correct needle placement and appropriate instillation of therapeutic material.

Oral Steroids

Oral steroid use in the presence of radiculopathy has been effective for many years. A regime beginning with 60 to 80 mg of prednisone in divided doses, decreasing daily by 10-mg increments, is effective and inexpensive. Again, caution must be expressed about the patient's tolerance to steroids, particularly from the perspective of the gastrointestinal tract. Cardiovascular and psychic alterations from long-term steroid use are always a risk, as is the danger of aseptic necrosis in the shoulder and hip joints. A guiding principle can be that steroids are useful in short-term application for acute conditions; they are much less useful in chronic conditions. Patients requiring long-term steroid use for the management of systemic disease should be monitored closely for deleterious side effects.

Antidepressants

Another class of drugs found to be useful in musculoskeletal conditions is those that deal with depression associated with chronic pain and in the restoration of the sleep cycle. The tricyclics benefit these patients.[3,4] There are a number of tricyclic antidepressants, but this author has found amitriptyline (Elavil) to be useful if the patient can tolerate the drug. Doses from 10 to 150 mg may be necessary to restore a normal sleep cycle. There is some evidence that tricyclics have a positive effect on chronic pain pathways. Duloxetine (Cymbalta, Yentreve) is a serotonin–norepinephrine reuptake inhibitor used for major depressive disorder, generalized anxiety disorder, and pain related to diabetic neuropathy and fibromyalgia.[5] Although the exact mechanisms of the antidepressant and central pain inhibitory action of duloxetine in humans are unknown, they are believed to be related to its potentiation of serotonergic and noradrenergic activity in the CNS.

Muscle Relaxants

The muscle relaxants are very popular in the treatment of acute and chronic musculoskeletal conditions; however, this author has found their use to be quite disappointing. Many of them are central-acting depressants rather than local muscle relaxants. Oral and injectable diazepam (Valium) is somewhat useful in dealing with acute muscle spasm, and if a muscle relaxant is deemed necessary, it is probably the drug of choice.

Medication use requires that the patient understands the prescribed drug's beneficial effects, side effects, length of action, and allergy potential. Simpler medication programs are better. The prescribing physician must know what over-the-counter medications the patient is taking and the drugs prescribed by other physicians for other health problems. Iatrogenic drug interactions contribute greatly to health care cost and should always be on the physicians' mind when picking up a pen and prescription pad.

Injections

Different injection techniques have been useful in musculoskeletal conditions. These techniques have indications and contraindications and require that the practitioner be skilled in their use. Various injection techniques have both diagnostic and therapeutic indications. The use of epidural steroids in radiculopathy has been referred to in the Corticosteroids section. Concurrent selective nerve blocks are of assistance in identifying the nerve root involved with pain generation. These procedures require adequate training and sufficient volume to maintain the skill for the procedure. They all require fluoroscopic control.

Acupuncture

One of the oldest injection procedures is classic acupuncture. There are a number of different schools of acupuncture that can all be classified as peripheral stimulating treatment. In selected cases, acupuncture has been very useful in assisting in pain control, particularly in patients experiencing postsurgical or dental pain. However, not all patients respond to acupuncture; appropriate selection of the patient, as well as the practitioner, is essential for success.

Trigger Points

Simons and Travell have long advocated the treatment of the primary and secondary trigger points. Some practitioners have found spray and stretch techniques useful. This author has found the injection technique of classic Travell triggers more effective than spray and stretch. A clear relationship between the presence of somatic dysfunction and myofascial trigger points has been observed. Adequate treatment of the somatic dysfunction frequently relieves the trigger points. In other instances, the trigger points persist despite adequate treatment of the somatic dysfunction. Appropriate treatment of the trigger points would then seem indicated.[6] The reverse has also been found true. Primary treatment of trigger points has reduced observable somatic dysfunction in related parts of the musculoskeletal system, but it is not 100% effective. This author prefers to treat them in an integrated fashion and uses dry-needling or lidocaine hydrochloride (Xylocaine) injection to trigger points if they are present after adequate treatment of somatic dysfunction, or if they considered a primary contributor to the patient's presentation. It is interesting to note that trigger points are more common in phasic muscles. The two tonic muscles that seem to have the most persistent trigger points are the quadratus lumborum and the levator scapulae. This author's experience has been that these are the two muscles that may need treatment by injection for resolution. Follow-up treatment of trigger point therapy requires adequate and appropriate exercise, regardless of whether spray and stretch or injection technique is used.

Sacroiliac Injections

The use of injections in the sacroiliac syndrome is useful from the diagnostic and the therapeutic perspectives.[7,8] Injection into the capsular portion of the joint requires fluoroscopic guidance and is best done from the inferior aspect of the joint. Both pain generation and arthrographic appearance can be used in diagnosing the painful sacroiliac joint. Occasionally, injection of the capsular portion of the joint demonstrates extravasation of contrast material in an anterior direction outlining the L5 and S1 nerve roots. This mechanism may account for the lower extremity pain seen in the sacroiliac syndrome. From a therapeutic perspective, injection into the posterior ligamentous portion of the sacroiliac joint can be useful. If local analgesic infiltration of the posterior sacroiliac joint results in reduction or relief of the patient's pain, the sacroiliac joint is likely the pain generator. Steroid injection into the posterior sacroiliac ligaments for the antiinflammatory effect coupled with appropriate manual medicine and exercise programs have been useful in the management of the sacroiliac syndrome. Infiltration of the posterior sacroiliac ligamentous structures can be done without fluoroscopic control if one is familiar with the anatomy and skilled in the procedure. Instillation of steroids into the posterior sacroiliac ligaments is usually done no more than twice.

A similar, but less commonly used, procedure is the infiltration of local anesthetic and steroid into the posterior aspect of the zygapophysial joint in the lower lumbar spine.[9] This is not the classic facet injection that requires fluoroscopic control to ensure that you are in the posterior facet. Without fluoroscopy, it is possible to walk a spinal needle along a bone to the base of the transverse process, and by moving slightly above and below, one can instill local anesthetic and steroid into the posterior aspect of the capsule of the joint. This can be useful in short-term management of an acute zygapophysial joint pain syndrome. Again, adequate training and practice are essential to successful performance of this procedure. Complications are exceedingly rare, but must always be considered.

Prolotherapy

A number of musculoskeletal medicine practitioners advocate the injection of proliferent solutions into ligaments. Gedney[10] popularized this procedure in the osteopathic profession and Hackett[11] in the allopathic medical profession. The principal concept is to inject material that stimulates proliferation of collagen in ligament to strengthen the ligament, particularly its attachment to bone, and to reduce ligamentous-related pain. Historically, a number of solutions have been advocated. The most popular solution currently is that advocated by Ongley et al.[12] and consists of hypertonic glucose, glycerin, and phenol, diluted with water and then combined with lidocaine hydrochloride (Xylocaine) for injection. The reader is referred to the text *Injection Technique in Orthopaedic Medicine* by Dorman and Ravin for definitive information on this system.[13] Prolotherapy, as it is currently called, has undergone basic and clinical research study and appears to have value in selected cases. As with all injection techniques, there is a learning curve and adequate instruction and practice are essential. This author has found prolotherapy useful in selected patients with recurrent sacroiliac syndrome, particularly those with hypermobility associated with hip bone (innominate) shear dysfunction and chronic recurrent anteriorly nutated sacroiliac dysfunction with a significant inferior translatory component. Fluoroscopic control is not necessary but is advisable if available. Recently, some researchers have injected proliferent material into the intervertebral disk for the treatment of annular tear. This requires high-level skill and fluoroscopic control.

Recent experience in a small number of cases of fatty replacement of the rectus capitis posterior minor muscle using proliferent injection into the occipital attachments of the muscle and the zygapophysial joints at C1-C2 has been effective in the relief of the classic occipital headache radiating toward the orbit in these patients.

Prolotherapy is quite uncomfortable for the patient and pre-injection medication is frequently useful. Like many technologies, prolotherapy can be overused in the hands of an enthusiastic practitioner. For the right patient with the right diagnostic criteria, it is clearly a technology that can be useful.

ORTHOTIC DEVICES

There are numerous orthotic devices available to the manual medicine practitioner. The following are those that have been found most useful by this author.

Lumbar Corsets

There are numerous lumbar corsets and supporting belts. A contoured belt individualized to the patient by heating of the material can be useful in acute conditions. It stabilizes the patient's trunk during the acute phase, but should be replaced as rapidly as possible by an exercise program of trunk stabilization and control. Dependency on supporting corsets can easily occur. Patients should be cautioned that the corsets are for temporary use only and appropriate exercise is the long-term goal of the treatment plan.

Sacroiliac Cinch Belt

The orthotic device found most useful is the Hackett sacroiliac cinch belt manufactured by Brooks Appliance Company (Marshall, MI). These varying-sized belts without padding over the sacrum provide dynamic tension around the pelvis and assist

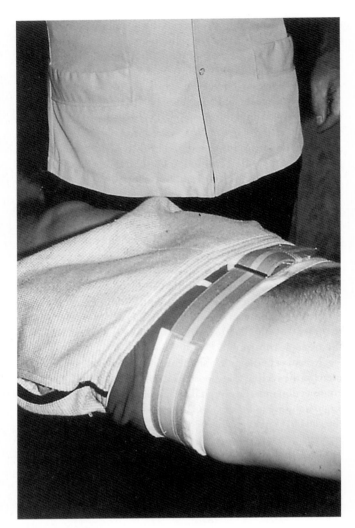

FIGURE 22.1 Sacroiliac cinch belt.

in stability during the rehabilitative process (Fig. 22.1). All patients with hip bone shear dysfunction use them while weight bearing for a minimum of 6 weeks. If the hip bone shear does not recur within a 6-week period, the belt is discontinued except during strenuous exercise and long motor vehicle trips. Occasionally, the same device is used for patients with chronic recurrent lower back pain syndrome associated with an anteriorly nutated sacrum, a posteriorly rotated hip bone, and a superiorly displaced pubic bone. This device allows free mobility of the pelvis during the walking cycle. Other devices that restrict the sacrum by a compressive pad have limited value in this author's experience.

Heel Lift

The most commonly used orthotic device is a heel lift for the long-term management of the short-leg, pelvic-tilt syndrome. The amount of shortness of a lower extremity and the amount of pelvic tilt that are clinically significant differ greatly from author to author. This author has found that sacral base unleveling of 6 mm or more is clinically significant in patients with lower back and lower extremity pain syndromes, particularly those recurrent

in nature. The methodology for the diagnosis of the short-leg, pelvic-tilt syndrome has been described in Chapter 21. There are times when one does not wish to expose the patient to additional radiologic procedures. Clinical assessment of short leg and pelvic tilt can be quite accurate if plain films are available showing the shape and symmetry of the two hip bones and the sacrum. The practitioner can use a series of shims, which are placed under the supposed short lower extremity, to restore functional balance to the pelvis and lumbar spine. The 1/8-, 1/4-, 3/8-, and 1/2-in. shims are easily obtainable from a lumber dealer. When the adequate manual medicine intervention has restored mobility to the lumbar spine and pelvis, the patient is evaluated in the erect position sequentially using shims to achieve a level of greater trochanter height, level iliac crest, and symmetric trunk side bending behavior of the lumbar spine (Fig. 22.2). When the amount of lift needed has been identified, either by radiologic study or clinical assessment as described above, temporary lifts can be placed inside the heel of the shoe to be followed by permanent additions to the heel and sole to balance lumbopelvic mechanics. In most cases, any shoemaker can add the appropriate amount of lift to the heel and sole. In some instances, a specialized prescription to an orthotist or pedorthist is necessary. Ideally, both heel and sole lifts should be used so that the device does not alter foot and ankle mechanics. Empiric reports indicate that most people can tolerate 3/8-in. heel lift without additional sole lifting, but this must be individualized for each patient.

The following is a suggested prescription sequence for the use of lift therapy. If the desired lift is 3/8 in. or less, a single addition of a heel lift to the side with short leg and pelvic tilt is sufficient. Despite past recommendations that lifts be increased in 1/8-in. increments, most patients tolerate 3/8 in. in a single application. If the sacral base angle is more than 42 degrees or the clinical assessment shows an increased lower lumbar lordosis, it is advisable that the heel on the long leg be reduced by the appropriate amount, rather than adding to the short leg. One does not want to increase the anterior tilt of the pelvis more than necessary. If the lift needed is more than 3/8 in., but less than 3/4 in., it should be applied in two stages. First, add half the amount needed to the heel of the short leg, followed in 3 to 6 weeks by reducing the other half from the heel of the long leg. If the amount of lift needed is more than 3/4 in., it should be staged in a maximum of 3/8-in. increments, ultimately resulting in heel and sole lifts of the required amount. It is rare that a patient cannot tolerate lift therapy if the condition is appropriately diagnosed and treated. Caution must be used in the presence of significant degenerative joint disease, particularly of the hip, and in the presence of pelvic girdle osseous asymmetry when using a lift to the long leg to level the sacral base declination. In the latter case, this places additional stress on the hip joint and the lateral stabilizers of the hip, particularly the gluteus medius and minimus muscles. The lumbar spine usually adapts to the short-leg, pelvic-tilt syndrome by scoliosis convex to the side of the sacral base declination and short lower extremity. Appropriate lift therapy reduces the severity of the adaptive scoliosis and assists in restoring neutral lumbar mechanics that are more normal. Complications of lift therapy are rare but occasionally occur.

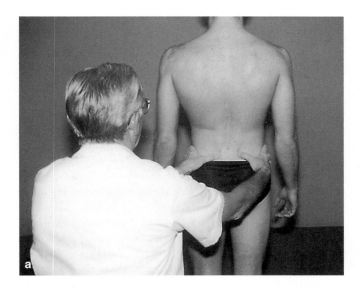

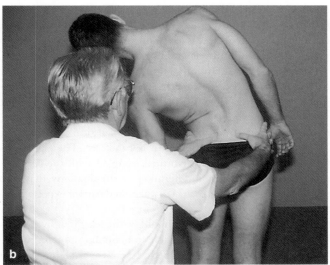

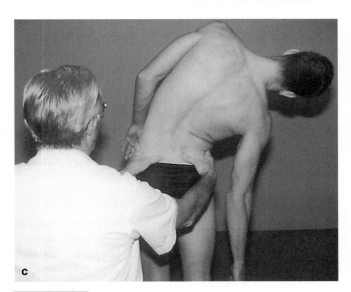

FIGURE 22.2 a: Iliac crest height. b: Trunk side bending left. c: Trunk side bending right.

These are usually related to the foot and ankle. Lifting a heel changes talotibial mechanics and potentially increases instability of the joint. Appropriate sole lifting in addition to the heel can prevent this. The second complication involves the plantar fascia and results in heel pain caused by stress on the plantar side of the calcaneus. This is alleviated by appropriate heel and sole lift or using the lift with a foot orthotic device. It usually takes 6 to 8 weeks for a patient to adjust to lift therapy. Appropriate stretching exercises should be prescribed to assist the patient in achieving myofascial balance. The patient must be cautioned that lift therapy use is continuous and must be incorporated into all footwear. The amount of lift does not change unless there is subsequent fracture or rapidly progressive degenerative joint disease in a lower extremity.

Foot Orthotics

Foot orthotic devices can be used to assist the patient in restoring musculoskeletal balance. A podiatrist can individually customize appropriate orthotic devices for foot mechanics. *Orthotic devices should never be prescribed until the joints and fasciae of the foot and ankle have been treated maximally by appropriate manual medicine.* Great care must be exercised when using lift therapy with an orthotic device. Incorporation of the appropriate amount of lift to the orthotic device is frequently sufficient. Occasionally it is necessary to change the outside of the shoe to correct the requirement of the short-leg, pelvic-tilt syndrome and to use appropriate orthotic correction inside of the shoe for foot mechanics.

MODALITIES

Several treatment modalities are extensively used in the health care delivery system despite the paucity of research evidence for their effectiveness. The opinions expressed here are based on the author's clinical experience.

Ice

Ice packs are frequently used for acute soft-tissue injuries. The classic athletic medicine principle of RICE (Rest, Ice, Compression, and Elevation) is appropriate for many conditions. Ice packs are used after treatment to reduce the inflammatory response after stimulating chronic dysfunctional musculoskeletal tissues. Frequent short-term applications are most effective. Caution must be used to not chill the skin.

Heat

External heat has wide acceptance by most patients and, while comforting, is frequently abused. A frequent history for a patient with an acute lower back injury is to continuously apply a heating pad overnight while asleep and find it impossible to get out of bed the next day. Short-term application of heat does enhance circulation to the body part and can be effective in mobilizing the inflammatory process. However, too much heat applied for too long a period can overly congest a part and contribute to the inflammatory process. Hot packs, particularly moist heat, are very useful prior to extensive manual stretching. For home use, the patient is advised to apply heat, either moist or dry, for no longer than 15 minutes and no more frequently than every 2 hours, with a maximum of six applications per day.

Ultrasound

Ultrasound is used to provide deep "heat" to tissue by its "stimulation." It is used mainly in the shoulder region in preparation for more extensive stretching and rehabilitation exercises.

Traction

The application of external traction, by static devices or machines, is used extensively in musculoskeletal medicine. Research evidence of the effectiveness of traction in the literature is sparse, but the empiric use of traction in certain conditions has been deemed valuable. Pelvic traction at 90 degrees of hip flexion and 90 degrees of knee flexion in acute lumbar discogenic disease can be helpful. In this instance, the patient's body weight provides the appropriate amount of traction and distraction of the lower lumbar spine in a flexed position.

Residential Inversion Table type lumbar traction devices are widely available online. Their effectiveness has not been clinically proven[14]; however, many patients with discogenic disease find the low cost and ease of use worth the benefits in pain relief they obtain.

Traction is more frequently used in the cervical spine, particularly in home programs.

Head-halter cervical traction is an effective adjunctive intervention. The patient needs adequate instruction in positioning the head halter to avoid compression on the jaw and irritation to the temporomandibular joint. The recommended weight is 5 to 8 lb (2.25 to 3.6 kg) and should be maintained up to 20 minutes twice daily. Small increments of flexion–extension and rotation right–left exercises while unloaded seem to assist in the management of acute and chronic conditions of the cervical spine.

TENS (Transcutaneous Electric Nerve Stimulation)

TENS units are quite popular with health professionals and the laity. This author has been personally disappointed in their effectiveness. Electrical stimulation therapy has also been helpful to some practitioners. For this author (like the TENS unit), the results have been disappointing.

Surgery

Spinal surgery has two major objectives. The first is to decompress neural structures compromised by trauma or degenerative disease. The second is to stabilize hypermobile and unstable vertebral segments. There is a vast array of options available for both decompression and stabilization. A successful surgical outcome depends on identifying the right procedure for the right patient at the right vertebral level at the right time and its being performed by the right surgeon. The goal of any surgical intervention is to assist in the restoration of maximal functional capacity of the musculoskeletal system in postural balance. Before any surgical intervention is performed, the patient should have adequate and appropriate diagnostic studies and nonoperative care. The diagnostic

studies should reveal a surgical pathology that contributes to or causes the patient's pain complaint. Appropriate nonoperative care should be aggressive and comprehensive and not consist of bed rest, modalities, and analgesics.

Most discogenic radiculopathies will respond to aggressive nonoperative care such as appropriate manual medicine, antiinflammatory agents, analgesics, short-term rest, and exercise. If the patient does not respond to nonoperative care and shows evidence of progressive neurologic deficit, surgical consultation and intervention should be obtained as soon as possible. The neurologic deficits of maximum concern are the cauda equina syndrome and progressive muscle weakness or increasing dural tension signs despite appropriate nonoperative care. The diagnostic workup should identify a surgical pathology consistent with the patient's presentation and should be confirmed by electrodiagnostic studies.

For successful surgical outcome, the patient should receive both prehabilitation and rehabilitation. Adequate nonoperative care before surgery should prepare the patient's musculoskeletal system for the surgical intervention. Postsurgical rehabilitation occurs as soon as possible. Even in the presence of a stabilization procedure, early isometric stabilization exercise can be done before ambulation. Restoration of mobility, muscle control, and balance is the goal of postoperative rehabilitation. A successful surgical outcome is based on the preparation of the patient for the anticipated outcome. Many patients expect total pain relief and restoration of a normal back following a surgical intervention. They should be cautioned that it is not the case. The pathology for which the surgery is performed, coupled with the surgical procedure itself, results in alteration of the anatomy that can never be restored to "normal." Unwarranted patient expectations should be avoided.

The surgical intervention should be the least invasive possible. Every attempt should be made to maintain the integrity of the anatomy. Postsurgical magnetic resonance imaging studies show fatty replacement infiltration of the deep fourth-layer muscles of the spinal complex. Following fatty replacement, muscles no longer provide the proprioceptive information essential for muscle control and a good functional outcome. It is for this reason that the postoperative patient performs an intensive exercise program.

Exercise

Of all of the adjunctive therapeutic procedures, the one of most value to this author has been exercise. Exercise is fundamental to maintaining the therapeutic effectiveness of manual medicine intervention.

SUMMARY

Manual medicine practitioners should avail themselves of any adjunctive therapeutic procedure that assists in patient management. The broader the physician's armamentarium, the more likely its success. Each patient must be individually evaluated and the devised treatment plans unique to that individual. Adjunctive therapeutic procedures, like manual medicine, should not be prescribed in a cookbook fashion.

REFERENCES

1. Mense S, Simons DG. Central pain and centrally modified Pain. In: *Muscle Pain: Understanding Its Nature, Diagnosis, and Treatment*. Philadelphia, PA: Lippincott Williams & Wilkins, 2001.
2. Winkelstein BA. Mechanisms of central sensitization, neuroimmunology & injury biomechanics in persistent pain: Implications for musculoskeletal disorders. *J Electromyogr Kinesiol* 2004;14(1):87–93.
3. Sindrup SH, Otto M, Finnerup NB, et al. Antidepressants in the treatment of neuropathic pain. *Basic Clin Pharmacol Toxicol* 2005;96(6):399–409.
4. McCleane G. Antidepressants as analgesics. *CNS Drugs* 2008;22(2):139–156.
5. Arnold LM, Lu Y, Crofford LJ, et al. A double-blind, multicenter trial comparing duloxetine with placebo in the treatment of fibromyalgia patients with or without major depressive disorder. *Arthritis Rheum* 2004;50(9):2974–2984.
6. Simons DG. New views of myofascial trigger points: Etiology and diagnosis. *Arch Phys Med Rehabil* 2007;88(12):1658–1661.
7. Fritz J, Henes JC, Thomas C, et al. Diagnostic and interventional MRI of the sacroiliac joints using a 1.5-T open-bore magnet: A one-stop-shopping approach. *AJR Am J Roentgenol* 2008;191(6):1717–1724.
8. Hansen HC, McKenzie-Brown AM, Cohen SP, et al. Sacroiliac joint interventions: A systematic review. *Pain Physician* 2007;10(1):165–184.
9. Sehgal N, Dunbar EE, Shah RV, et al. Systematic review of diagnostic utility of facet (zygapophysial) joint injections in chronic spinal pain: An update. *Pain Physician* 2007;10(1):213–228.
10. Gedney EH. Hypermobile joint. *Osteop Prof* 1937;4:30–31.
11. Hackett GS. *Joint Ligament Relaxation Treated by Fibro-osseus Proliferation*. 2nd Ed. Springfield: Charles C. Thomas, 1957.
12. Ongley MJ, Klein RG, Dorman TA, et al. A new approach to the treatment of chronic back pain. *Lancet* 1987:143–146.
13. Dorman TA, Ravin TH. *Diagnosis and Injection Techniques in Orthopedic Medicine*. Philadelphia, PA: Lippincott Williams & Wilkins, 1991.
14. Clarke J, van Tulder M, Blomberg S, et al. Traction for low back pain with or without sciatica: An updated systematic review within the framework of the Cochrane collaboration. *Spine* 2006;31(14):1591–1599.

Page numbers followed by "f" denote figures; those followed by "t" denote tables.

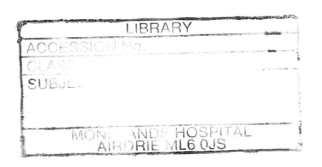